Essentials of Pediatric Radiology

A Multimodality Approach

Essentials of Pediatric Radiology

A Multimodality Approach

Heike E. Daldrup-Link
Associate Professor of Radiology and Pediatrics, Department of Radiology and Biomedical Imaging,
University of California San Francisco Medical Center, San Francisco, USA

Charles A. Gooding
Professor Emeritus of Radiology and Pediatrics, Department of Radiology and Biomedical Imaging,
University of California San Francisco Medical Center, San Francisco, USA

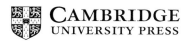

CAMBRIDGE
UNIVERSITY PRESS

CAMBRIDGE UNIVERSITY PRESS
Cambridge, New York, Melbourne, Madrid, Cape Town, Singapore,
São Paulo, Delhi, Dubai, Tokyo

Cambridge University Press
The Edinburgh Building, Cambridge CB2 8RU, UK

Published in the United States of America by
Cambridge University Press, New York

www.cambridge.org
Information on this title: www.cambridge.org/9780521515214

© Cambridge University Press 2010

First published 2010

Printed in the United Kingdom at the University Press, Cambridge

A catalog record for this publication is available from the British Library

Library of Congress Cataloging-in-Publication Data
Essentials of pediatric radiology : a multimodality approach / edited
by Heike E. Daldrup-Link, Charles A. Gooding.
        p. ; cm.
    Includes bibliographical references and index.
    ISBN 978-0-521-51521-4 (Hardback)
1. Pediatric radiology.   I. Daldrup-Link, Heike E.   II. Gooding,
Charles A.   III. Title.
    [DNLM: 1. Diagnostic Imaging–methods.   2. Child.
3. Infant.   WN 240 E78 2010]
    RJ51.R3E87 2010
    618.92'00757–dc22
                                                              2010022609

ISBN 978-0-521-51521-4 Hardback

Additional resources for this publication at
www.essentials-of-pediatric-radiology.com

Contents

v

Contributors

Paul Babyn, MD
Radiologist in Chief,
Hospital for Sick Children,
Toronto, Ontario, Canada

Kevin M. Baskin, MD
Assistant Professor of Radiology,
University of Pittsburgh School of Medicine Chief,
Vascular and Interventional Radiology,
Children's Hospital of Pittsburgh of UPMC,
Pittsburgh, PA, USA

Soonmee Cha, MD
Associate Professor of Radiology,
Department of Radiology and Biomedical Imaging,
Neuroradiology Section, University of California,
San Francisco, CA, USA

Govind Chavhan, MD, DNB
Clinical Fellow,
The Hospital for Sick Children,
Toronto, Ontario, Canada

Soni C. Chawla, MD
Assistant Professor of Radiology,
Department of Radiological Sciences,
Olive View–UCLA Medical Center,
University of California Los Angeles,
Los Angeles, CA, USA

John J. Crowley, MD
University of Pittsburgh School of Medicine Section
Head Neuroradiology,
Children's Hospital of Pittsburgh of UPMC,
Pittsburgh, PA, USA

Heike E. Daldrup-Link, MD, PhD
Associate Professor of Radiology and Pediatrics,
Pediatric Radiology Section,
Department of Radiology and Biomedical Imaging,
University of California San Francisco Medical Center,
San Francisco, CA, USA

Charles R. Fitz, MD
Professor of Radiology,
University of Pittsburgh School of Medicine Section
Head Neuroradiology, Children's Hospital of
Pittsburgh of UPMC, Pittsburgh, PA, USA

Donald P. Frush, MD
Professor of Radiology and Pediatrics and Chief,
Division of Pediatric Radiology, Duke University
Medical Center, Durham, NC, USA

Robert Goldsby, MD
Associate Professor of Clinical Pediatrics,
Division of Pediatric Hematology/Oncology,
University of California San Francisco,
San Francisco, CA, USA

**Charles A. Gooding, MD, FACR, FRCR
(London, Honorary)**
Professor Emeritus of Radiology and Pediatrics,
Department of Radiology and Biomedical Imaging,
University of California San Francisco Medical Center,
San Francisco, CA, USA

Thomas E. Herman, MD, FACR
Associate Professor of Radiology,
Washington University School of Medicine,
Mallinckrodt Institute of Radiology, and Associate
Radiologist, St. Louis Children's Hospital,
St. Louis, MO, USA

Jane Kim, MD
Assistant Professor of Radiology,
San Francisco General Hospital,
Neuroradiology Section, University of California,
San Francisco, CA, USA

Keith A. Kronemer, MD
Assistant Professor of Radiology,
Washington University School of Medicine,
Mallinckrodt Institute of Radiology, and Radiologist,
St. Louis Children's Hospital,
St. Louis, MO, USA

Alison Meadows, MD, PhD
Assistant Professor of Clinical Radiology and Pediatrics,
Department of Radiology and Department of Cardiology,
University of California San Francisco,
San Francisco, CA, USA

Beverley Newman, MD
Associate Professor of Radiology,
Department of Radiology,
Stanford University School of Medicine,
Associate Chief of Pediatric Radiology,
Lucile Packard Children's Hospital,
Stanford, CA, USA

Catherine M. Owens, BSc MBBS MRCP FRCR
Director Cardiothoracic CT and Consultant Radiologist,
Great Ormond Street Hospital for Children,
London, UK

Kate M. Park, BA BM BCh MRCP FRCR
Radiology Fellow,
Department of Imaging,
Great Ormond Street Hospital for Children,
London, UK

Karl Schneider, MD
Professor of Radiology and Pediatrics and
Radiologist-in-Chief,
Department of Pediatric Radiology,
Children's Hospital of the University of Munich,
Munich, Germany

David Stringer, MD
Head of Department,
Diagnostic and Interventional Imaging,
KK Women's and Children's Hospital,
Singapore

Harvey Teo, MD
Department of Diagnostic and Interventional Imaging,
KK Women's and Children's Hospital,
Singapore

Laura Varich, MD
Department of Pediatric Radiology,
Lucile Packard Children's Hospital,
Stanford University School of Medicine,
Stanford, CA, USA

Max Wintermark, MD
Associate Professor of Radiology and Director,
Neuroradiology Division,
University of Virginia,
Department of Radiology,
Charlottesville, VA, USA

Sandra Wootton-Gorges, MD
Director of Pediatric Imaging and Professor of
Clinical Radiology,
University of California,
Davis Medical Center and UC Davis Children's Hospital,
Sacramento, CA, USA

Preface

Do a little bit more than average and from that point on your progress multiplies itself out of all proportion to the effort put in.

Paul J. Meyer

Two types of radiology textbooks exist: One type is the easily readable, ultra-short book which covers the most basic essentials and permits the reader to "survive" in the field. The second type is the comprehensive compendium which represents a valuable resource for in-depth information on certain topics, but is too extensive to be read from cover to cover. Our book, "Essentials of Pediatric Radiology" attempts to blend these two types by providing a detailed overview of selected topics which are commonly encountered in the daily practice of pediatric radiology. Our book is concise enough to be read completely, yet it provides more detailed information compared to other brief textbooks in the field, thereby allowing the reader to acquire more in-depth knowledge.

The topics presented have been chosen based upon practical considerations and include commonly encountered topics in pediatric radiology (such as neonatal chest disorders and trauma imaging), challenging topics (such as bone dysplasias and transplant imaging) and practical "hot topics" (such as correct positioning of medical devices and radiation protection). Recognizing recent advances in imaging technologies, all presented topics cover the full gamut of up-to-date radiological diagnostic techniques, including conventional radiography, ultrasound, Doppler ultrasound, current CT (computed tomography) and MRI (magnetic resonance imaging) techniques, and PET-CT (positron emission tomography-CT). Chapters are arranged according to pathology rather than organ system.

This provides the reader with clinically oriented information when employing "whole-body" techniques or analyzing scans which involve multiple anatomical sites. Each chapter is richly illustrated with high-quality images, as well as graphs, tables and decision flowcharts, in order to feature as many cases as possible and to train the reader to consider differential diagnoses.

Realizing that no single author can be an expert in every topic, this book has been written by a team of distinguished pediatric radiologists from renowned universities and children's hospitals. This book is intended to provide pediatric radiology fellows, advanced radiology residents, general radiologists, pediatricians and pediatric surgeons with state-of-the-art information regarding the most common, the most important and the most challenging topics in pediatric radiology. In order to allow trainees to test their diagnostic proficiency for Board examinations or CAQ examinations, the book is complemented by online presentations of cases as "unknowns."

It is our sincere desire to provide our readers with a tool to develop a thorough understanding of practical pediatric imaging, so that they may improve their diagnostic proficiency and excel in their profession. This book is dedicated to the children in hospitals worldwide who, hopefully, will receive more accurate diagnoses and enhanced treatment because well trained physicians have taken the time and effort to educate themselves beyond minimum requirements.

Heike E. Daldrup-Link
Charles A. Gooding

Free-access website at www.essentials-of-pediatric-radiology.com
This book is complemented by a free access website of sample cases, containing questions and answers that enable readers to test their diagnostic proficiency.

Chapter 1

The normal child: growth and development of the infant and child; frequent and important normal variants

Karl Schneider

General remarks on the development of the human body

The body proportions and the size of the organs vary greatly in different age groups from birth to adolescence. In early life, 0–1 years of age, the head is very large, the neck extremely short and the trunk is long with a relatively short chest in relation to the abdomen (Figure 1.1). On the other hand, the arms and legs are relatively short in the first years. During the growth spurt, which starts at about eight years, the long bones of the extremities lengthen considerably, the neck becomes longer and the head smaller. The technician and the radiologist have to consider these extreme differences of body proportions for patients of different age groups. For example, if the radiographer does not collimate the exposure field for a chest radiograph closely in small premature babies, a cumulative high eye lens dose can result as a deterministic radiation effect. Of course, correct coning is also important at the lower field edge of a chest X-ray, because a great number of abdominal organs are exposed to radiation. Figure 1.2 shows the increase of optimally coned field size in radiographs of the chest and abdomen. A similar problem exists in multidetector CT of the chest in young children. This effect is called over ranging and must be kept as low as possible in small patients.

Concurrently with the changes of the body proportions there is a shift of the red bone marrow from the head and the long bones in infants to the axial skeleton (spine, pelvic bones, ribs and sternum) in older children. This process is nearly completed at about 15 years of age (Figure 1.3). Of note, Cristy *et al.* described bone marrow conversion, but did not mention the extramedullary hematopoiesis within the liver, spleen and the kidneys in the first three months. The distribution of red and yellow bone marrow is readily apparent on magnetic resonance (MR) images. The most significant changes occur in the long bones. In newborns the long bones of the arms and the legs are entirely filled with red marrow. After infancy the yellow marrow begins to extend from the center of the bone to the metaphyseal ends. The conversion of fatty marrow occurs earlier in the epiphyses and diaphyses

than in the metaphyses. The partly converted normal marrow in children aged 10 years or older appears isointense or hyperintense to skeletal muscle on plain T1-weighted MR images, while focal neoplasms appear hypointense. In adults, only small areas of hematopoietic bone marrow persist in the vertebrae as well as proximal metaphyses of the femur and humerus.

Skull

Ossification of the skull (calvaria and skull base) starts prenatally at the 12th week. The ossification at the skull base is of the enchondral type, in the cranial vault of the desmal type. The synchrondroses at the base of the skull are widely open at birth. This growing cartilage of the synchrondroses at the skull base is relatively soft and can accidentally be passed by tubes and catheters. The cranial vault grows along the sutures depending on the intracranial pressure. The infant's head has six physiological gaps, so-called fontanels, which diminish in size gradually during the first 12 months. The great (anterior) fontanel between the frontal and parietal bones is the largest. It closes normally between 8 and 24 months. The posterior fontanel is very small and lies between the parietal bones and occipital bone. In most term neonates it is closed. The lateral fontanels are anterior and posterior to the squamous bones. All fontanels allow access to perform ultrasound of the brain and to perform Doppler examinations of intracranial vessels.

In infants there is great variation in the head shape: one example is a long skull with a large anterior–posterior (ap) diameter; and the opposite, a short head with large bitemporal diameter. The neurocranium in the first two years is considerably larger than the viscerocranium. In term infants the ratio is 4 to 1 and will reduce to a value of 2.5 at five years. The cranial sutures begin to close at the age of about seven years. Complete closure is noted in adulthood, between 30 and 40 years.

Wormian bones represent normal variants in skull growth, and are apparent as small bones located in and between normal sutures, frequently in the Lambda and Mendoza sutures. If abundant, Wormian bones may indicate an

Essentials of Pediatric Radiology, ed. Heike E. Daldrup-Link and Charles A. Gooding. Published by Cambridge University Press.
© Cambridge University Press 2010.

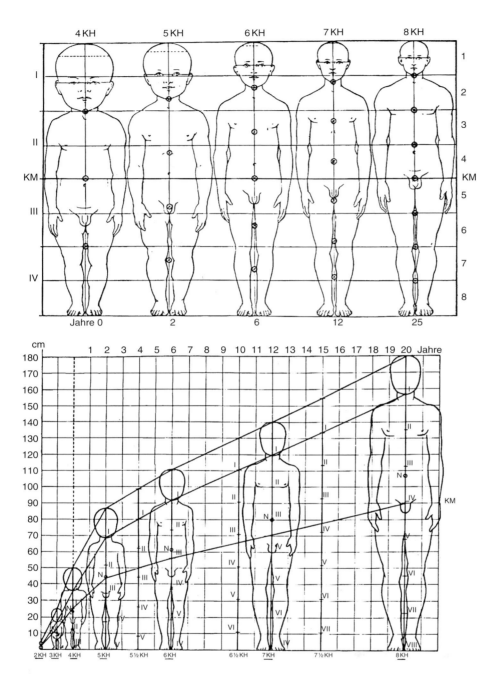

Figure 1.1 Body proportions during growth from newborn to adult. Illustration modified from *Handbuch der Anatomie des Kindes*, Bergmann Verlag München, 1938. KM (*Körper Mitte*) = body center; KH (*Kopfhöhe*) = length of the head. Body length can be calculated from KH; it is equivalent to 4 KH for a newborn and 8 KH for an adult.

osteogenesis imperfecta or cleidocranial dysplasia. A large extra bone located between the occipital and the parietal bones has been named "Inca bone." Sometimes, it is difficult to discern the sutures in skull radiographs, especially if the sutures are partially fused. In such cases, CT can be very helpful (Figure 1.4). Premature closure of the sutures occurs shortly after birth, or even prenatally, and is associated with typical abnormalities of the head shape, e.g. trigonocephaly or scaphocephaly. Convolutional markings (impressiones digitatae) may be seen in later childhood, mainly in school children. These striking findings in skull films are *not related* to an increased intracranial pressure, but are presumably caused by

the pulsation effects of cortical arteries. Convolutional markings must be differentiated from the lacunar skull in patients with myelomeningocele and Arnold-Chiari II malformation, which is always present at birth. Other modeling effects on the tabula interna can be caused by Pacchioni granulations, parietal sinus and diploe veins. They are all harmless and need no further diagnostic work-up. Occasionally, a prominent protuberantia occipitalis externa must be distinguished from an occipital horn.

The development of facial bones and the orbits is greatly influenced by the development of the paranasal sinuses and the dentogenesis. The ethmoid cells and the antrum of the mastoid bone are already developed in newborns. Other parts of the paranasal sinuses develop at the same time from very tiny cavities to large mucosa-lined structures, starting with the maxillary sinuses at the age of about two years and the sphenoidal sinus at four to five years. The frontal sinus starts its development at the age of eight years, and the mastoid cells pneumatize fully with puberty. There are two main deviations of the normal process of pneumatization of the facial bones and the skull base: hypo- and hyperpneumatization (Figure 1.5). The teeth in the maxilla and mandible are visible at birth. Dentition normally starts at the age of six months; the first permanent molar tooth erupts at seven years of age.

Brain

Many anatomical details of the developing brain can be imaged with US and MR. MR provides more-detailed

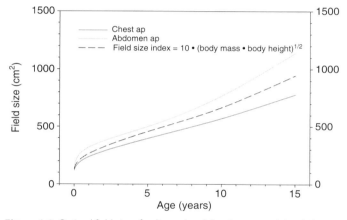

Figure 1.2 Optimal field size of radiographs of the chest ap and the abdomen ap from the newborn to 15 years of age. The dashed line represents calculations from body weight and height using the Lindskoug model (Lindskoug, 1992).

information because the contrast resolution is better than with US. Diffusion-weighted imaging and tractography are very sensitive for the detection of brain edema and can differentiate it further. Finally, the arteries and veins can be depicted with magnetic resonance angiography. On the contrary, pulsed-wave (PW) US can not only demonstrate very fine cerebral vessels (Figure 1.6), but also provide hemodynamic information of cerebral blood flow.

The development of the brain can be easily followed in premature babies with high frequency sonography looking at the appearances of specific gyri and sulci. Also, the size and shape of the lateral ventricles and extracerebral spaces filled with cerebrospinal fluid (CSF) are evaluated. There are four sonographic criteria to follow normal brain development (Figure 1.7):

1. The brain surface before the 26th week is totally smooth with no sulci and widely open insular regions of the temporal lobes.
2. The first gyrus which can be seen at the 28th week is the gyrus cinguli.
3. The operculation of the temporal lobes is nearly completed in the 34th week.
4. At the 40th week, the brain has developed further with many sulci and the gyri at the surface. The brain completely fills the intracranial space at that time.

In addition, deeper cerebral structures, e.g. the basal ganglia, can be imaged with US. Especially, the caudate nucleus is very well suited for evaluation of the deep brain parts. Before the 32nd week, the head of the caudate nucleus is very echogenic, more than the adjacent internal capsule and the thalami. After the 34th week, the echogenicity of the head of the caudate nucleus has totally reversed. In very small premature babies, the external CSF spaces are wide; to a lesser extent also the ventricular system.

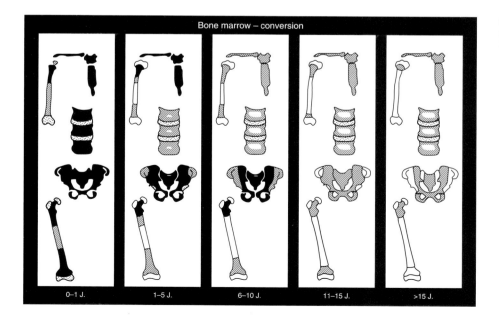

Bone marrow – conversion

0–1 J.   1–5 J.   6–10 J.   11–15 J.   >15 J.

Figure 1.3 Age- and anatomic-site-dependent conversion from hematopoietic (black) to fatty (white) bone marrow (Kricun, 1985).

(A)

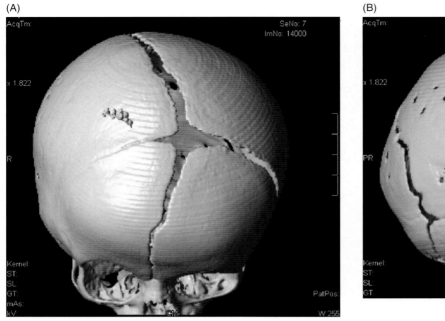

(B)

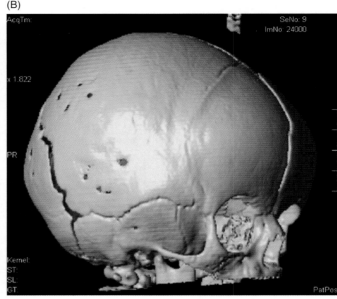

Figure 1.4 Unilateral synostosis of the right coronal suture clearly seen on (A) 3D-CT (bird's-eye perspective); (B) (right lateral aspect).

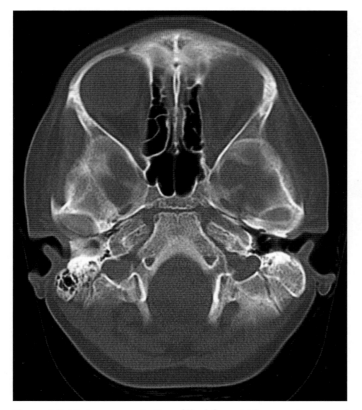

Figure 1.5 Missing pneumatization of the left mastoid process in a normal child.

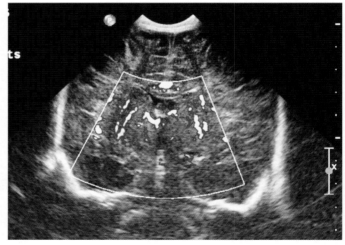

Figure 1.6 Prominent arteriae lenticulostriatae in a newborn brain visualized with power Doppler.

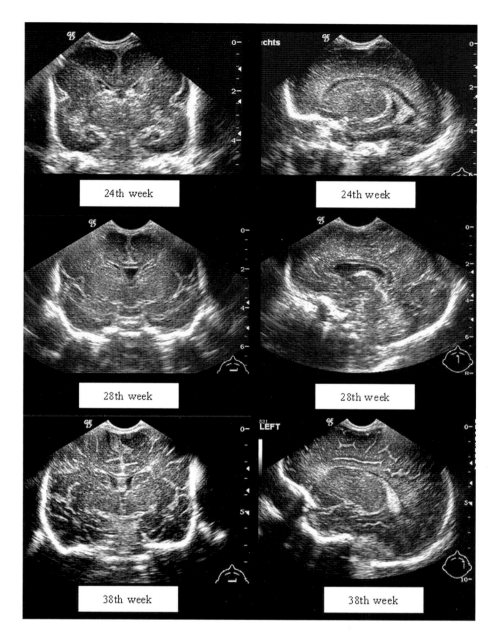

24th week   24th week
28th week   28th week
38th week   38th week

Figure 1.7 Brain development in premature babies illustrated in mid-coronal and parasagittal sections from extremely premature to mature babies.

There are many publications dealing with measurements of the size of the ventricular system, parenchymal thickness and the width of the extracerebral CSF space. A very simple measurement and a comparable value for all cross-sectional-imaging methods is the transverse diameter of the third ventricle. In all pediatric age groups the upper normal value for the third ventricle is 4.5 mm in horizontal and/or coronal sections.

A normal variant is the persistence of the cavum septi pellucidi. In premature babies the cavum vergae and the cavum septi pellucidi gradually regress. Most term babies have a septum with disappearance of the cavum. Other normal variants are: ventricular bands; tiny plexus cysts; round, or otherwise funny looking choroidal plexus. Beyond eight years, small

intracranial calcifications can be detected in the falx, choroidal plexus, and the pineal gland on skull X-rays or on CT exams.

In addition to US, the myelination of the brain can be evaluated by a thorough analysis of MR images. At birth, the myelination is sparse and can be seen in the pons, pedunculi cerebelli, vermis, and the posterior crus of the internal capsule and very subtly in the gyrus praecentralis. A graph with a timetable shows the myelination in Figure 1.8. The myelination has progressed to the corpus callosum and the centrum semiovale in the eight-month-old infant. In addition, the myelin will then extend to the splenium, frontal and occipital lobes. This is the final progress of the myelination and is also called "arborization." MR is the optimal method to follow the development of sulci and gyri.

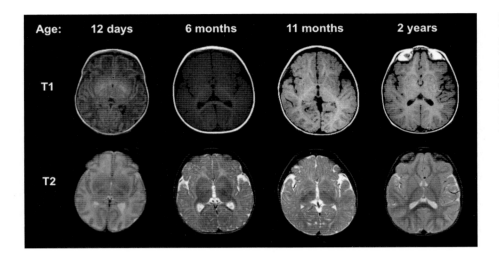

Figure 1.8 Normal appearance of the brain on T1- and T2-weighted MR images for children of different ages. The MR signal of white and gray matter shows an inversion from birth to 2 years of age. Myelination of the white matter during the first 6 to 8 months of life is best apparent on T1-weighted images, and myelination between 6 and 24 months of life is best evaluated on T2-weighted images. The myelination progresses with increasing age from caudal to cephalad and from dorsal to ventral.

PW-Doppler US can provide flow curves from specific blood vessels (cerebral arteries, cerebral veins, dural sinus). These curves represent a spectral distribution of different velocities sampled in the investigated vessel. Two measurements of velocity curves are of practical importance: peak systolic velocity (S), and end-diastolic velocity (D) of the Vmax curve. Using these two values, the resistive index can be calculated as $(S - D)/S$. Deeg *et al.* reported normal values of blood flow velocities and resistive indices of the main cerebral arteries for different age groups. The resistive indices are considerably higher in the first six months than in older children. In neonatal intensive care medicine, the Doppler examination of the anterior cerebral artery is a quick and simple method to detect hemodynamic effects on the cerebral circulation, e.g. caused by large left-to-right shunts such as a wide-open patent ductus arteriosus (PDA).

Table 1.1 Comparison of scan length of chest CT in pediatric patients of different age and size. Measurements of 275 spiral CT examinations

Age group	Mean values ± 2 SD of scan length for chest CT (cm)		
	Galanski et al., 2005/2006[a]	Theocharopoulos et al., 2007	Munich, 2007[b]
Newborn	10.1	8	11.0 ± 1.7
1 year	12.3	11	15.4 ± 4.4
5 years	16.4	15	17.9 ± 2.2
10 years	20.4	20	22.7 ± 3.2
15 years	26.0	24.3	28.0 ± 2.2
Adult	31.0	27	30.0 ± 2.0

Notes:
[a] Galanski et al., 2007.
[b] Unpublished data.

Airways and chest

The diameters and the lengths of the chest change remarkably during development from the newborn to the child and adolescent. The shape of the newborn chest is at first a relatively short cylinder with a similar ap and lateral diameter. Beginning with the second year of life, the chest enlarges in the longitudinal direction (apicobasal) due to growth of the lungs (Table 1.1); later also in the transverse plane, and more in the horizontal than in the sagittal direction. In teenagers, the chest transverse diameter will have increased by a factor of two compared to the ap diameter (Figure 1.9).

The air-filled trachea is composed of two parts: a flexible cervical, and a nearly fixed thoracic part. Depending on the height of the diaphragm/respiratory phase, the intrathoracic part of the trachea slightly deviates to the right side. This effect is more evident in expiration (Figure 1.10). The reason is that, on the left side, two great arterial vessels (aortic arch and left pulmonary artery (PA)) cross the left main stem bronchus.

This deviation is called tracheal scoliosis (old-fashioned, but more appropriate, is the term "bayonet shape"). It is a simple sign of the presence of a normal left-sided aortic arch. The normal trachea does not collapse completely. In patients with tracheomalacia, the trachea collapses completely on expiration. This can be due to a deficiency in the cartilaginous rings (primary tracheomalacia) or extrinsic compression (secondary tracheomalacia).

Infants normally have a large thymus which often increases further in size up to the age of two years. As the thymus can partially overlie the right and left heart border and can obscure the heart on chest X-rays, the term cardio-thymic shadow can be used. The shape of the thymus can vary greatly. If the thymus imitates a sail, this is called the sail or spinnaker sign. The thymus often has a cervical portion which is located behind the manubrium sterni and can move from the retrosternal position into the suprasternal fossa. The diagnosis of

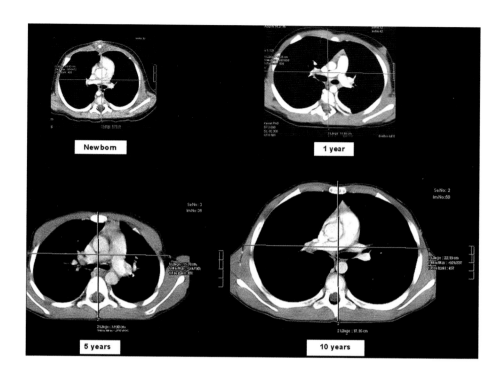

Figure 1.9 Axial CT sections through the level of the tracheal bifurcation are shown using the same magnification for patients of different ages.

(A)

(B)

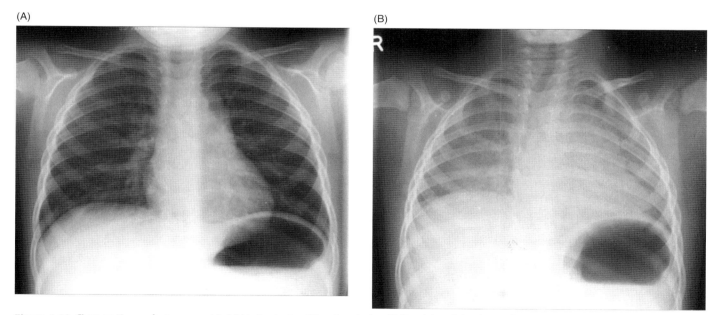

Figure 1.10 Chest pa X-rays of a two-year-old child in inspiration (A) and expiration (B). Variability of the shape of the trachea, heart and thymus size is clearly demonstrated.

thymus tissue is possible with US or MR. The normal cervical extension of a normal thymus must be differentiated from an ectopic cervical thymus, which appears as a cervical mass, which is discontinuous with the orthotopic thymus in the mediastinum and can be mistaken for a tumor or enlarged lymph node. The size of the thymus greatly depends on the respiratory phase, i.e. from the inflation of the lungs. In expiration the thymus is wide; in inspiration much smaller (Figure 1.10). After severe stress and in patients with severe and/or chronic diseases, the normal thymus decreases dramatically within a few days. Following chemotherapy, the thymus can show a "rebound" phenomenon with markedly increased size. Homogeneous texture, lack of mass effect on adjacent mediastinal vessels and flexible movement with inspiration and expiration on US can help to differentiate normal thymus from mediastinal masses.

The size of the heart can be measured using the cardiac index method. In newborns, the cardio-thoracic index is larger (up to 0.7) than in later childhood (0.5). There are some transitional effects related to incomplete expansion of the chest, less inflation of the lungs, open fetal shunts and high blood volume. In older infants, the use of the cardio-thoracic index requires a correct ap (anterior–posterior) or pa (posterior–anterior) projection of the chest radiograph, which very often is not achievable in young patients less than five years of age. Thus, a diagnosis of a cardiomegaly may be difficult in young children. In an unclear clinical situation we recommend an echocardiography.

In the first days after birth the mediastinum may be enlarged. In premature babies with an open ductus arteriosus, a prominent "ductus bump" may be seen at the aortic arch. The permanent closure of the ductus does not occur before the 12th week after birth. In older children, the area of the closed ductus appears in the aortopulmonic window as a ligament, which may be calcified and should not be mistaken for a calcified lymph node.

The lateral pleural recesses in young children are much deeper than in older children or young adolescents. In infants, the diaphragm can descend considerably in inspiration with completely flat contours on lateral chest films. The anterior recesses are not developed at this age. This explains why diaphragmatic borders are not well visible on inspiratory ap chest X-rays of young infants. Concurrently with the increase in length of the chest cage, these pleural recesses deepen considerably. These changes finally lead to the formation of the diaphragmatic dome.

The trachea and the bronchi (main, lobar and segmental bronchi) have relatively large diameters compared to the small peripheral bronchi. These anatomical findings are more marked in smaller children. This is the explanation of why in neonates a very prominent air bronchogram is visible even with normal lungs. Even more pronounced is the difference between the central and peripheral pulmonary arteries in the first three months. The reason for this finding is the high resistance of the small pulmonary arteries. These arterioles still have thick muscle walls persisting for a few months after birth, i.e. physiological transitory pulmonary hypertension. Therefore, following a transitional "wet-lung" syndrome, the lungs of young babies may show very few and small lung vessels. In addition, the interstitial lung tissue in early age is more prominent, which leads to an increased lung density compared to older children. Premature babies and, to a lesser proportion, term neonates can have hazy opacifications of the lungs on chest X-rays. In some cases there is an increase in pulmonary water as a transient phenomenon of immature lungs. But this finding may also be related to the predominantly lying position in the first months and the insufficient expansion of the chest by the respiratory muscles. Therefore, it is not surprising that the density of the lung parenchyma of infants and children of less than five years is higher in CT compared to older children and adolescents. The development of the human lung with all alveoli and capillaries continues throughout early childhood until approximately the age of eight years.

The degree of inflation of the lungs and the size of pulmonary vessels in young children is mainly influenced by external factors. Extreme crying or high fever without bronchopulmonary infection can simulate or even cause marked lung hyperemia and simulate a left-to-right shunt. In some cases, deep inspiratory effort can look like severe air-trapping and simulate bronchiolitis or asthma. If the inspiration is shallow, the normal prominent interstitium in infants can be mistaken for an interstitial lung disease. In small patients, especially in the first year, rotation of the chest can simulate an overinflation of a lung or even a pneumothorax. In neonates, skinfolds can be misdiagnosed as a pneumothorax. Critical analysis of the radiographs will lead to the right diagnosis in most cases.

Anomalies of the thoracic skeleton are relatively frequent. We often see fork ribs, which can simulate a rib tumor, but are harmless. Synchrondroses between the first and second rib are also occasionally seen. Abnormally shaped/shortened claviculae or scapulae are pathological findings and associated with certain syndromes, such as the VACTERL syndrome or certain skeletal dysplasias, such as very rare acamptomelic camptomelic dysplasias or cleidocranial dysplasias etc. Anomalies of the vertebra, e.g. butterfly vertebra, hemivertebra and more complex malformations are important markers for a hidden pathology, e.g. neurenteric cyst, esophageal duplication and Alagille syndrome.

Neck

Uncomplicated separation of the airway and feeding path in the middle of the pharynx requires a normal morphology of the epiglottis, larynx and esophagus. In addition, a normal swallowing process must coordinate the closure of the larynx, opening of the upper esophageal sphincter and the timely constriction of the lower pharyngeal muscles. Some newborns have transient coordination problems which may lead to aspirations of feedings (Figure 1.11); other newborns may have isolated or additional pharyngo-nasal reflux because of velopalatine insufficiency. These coordination problems often disappear within a few days. Lateral neck radiographs may show prominent prevertebral soft tissues, which show a decreasing thickness with increasing age. As a "rule of thumb," in infants between two and five years of age, the retrotracheal soft tissues should have approximately the thickness of the C5 vertebral body, and the retropharyngeal soft tissues should have approximately the thickness of $0.5 \times C5$. Between the ages of two to eight years the adenoids can be very large, obstructing the nasopharynx. If tracheal stenosis is suspected, evaluation of the airways with CT has replaced tracheal radiographs with a high kV technique. N. T. Griscom has published normal values of tracheal cross-sectional areas measured with CT.

Gastrointestinal tract

A "barium swallow" (we prefer low-osmolar iodinated contrast media) will delineate three physiological narrowings of the esophagus. The first narrowing is the normal upper esophageal

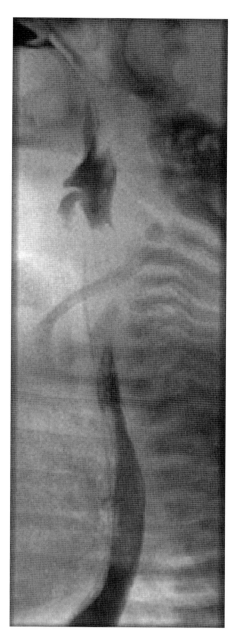

Figure 1.11 Intermittent minimal aspiration during swallowing in a normal newborn. Single frame from a digital video loop.

in a slight gliding of the cardia. However this finding should not be interpreted as hiatus hernia, because it can disappear with further growth. The peristalsis of the esophagus is not fully developed in the first six months. Although the fast longitudinal contraction of the proximal third of the esophagus is well developed in the newborn, there are various abnormalities of the other parts often visible in healthy infants:

1. The entire esophagus may be intermittently wide and atonic.
2. Strong circumferential contractions may be intermittently visible in the mid-portion.
3. Jo-Jo peristalsis of the entire esophagus may be seen.
4. A hypertonic cardia may cause delayed passage in the distal esophagus.

All of these functional abnormalities gradually disappear by the end of the first year. Gastric emptying is a complex process of concurrent actions and can be influenced by extrinsic and intrinsic factors. The position of the stomach is related to the position of the atria of the heart. The normal anatomy is concordant between the left-sided heart (left atrium), left-sided stomach and left bilobed lung. In situs inversus, there is a mirror-image situation. In heterotaxia syndromes, the situation is disconcordant; e.g. the heart can be left sided, but the stomach is on the right side with many associated abnormalities which are beyond the scope of this chapter.

The duodenum and the small bowel rotate several times with subsequent fixation of the bowel at the posterior abdominal wall. The normal duodenojejunal junction is located to the left of the spine and at the level of the pyloric canal (Figure 1.12). This important landmark is connected with the hiatus oesophagei via the Treitz' ligament. The small bowel mesentery runs from the duodenojejunal junction in the left upper abdominal quadrant, in an oblique and caudal direction to the right iliac fossa (RIF), where it ends at the right-sided colon with the free cecum and appendix. Consequently, the jejunum is located in the left upper abdomen, and the ileum in the right lower part of the abdomen. The main bowel artery is the superior mesenteric artery which is normally to the left of the superior mesenteric vein. In most patients with malrotation, this anatomical situation is reversed. However, exceptions occur. The evaluation of the normal position of the duodenojejunal junction via an upper GI study is considered a more reliable indicator for exclusion of a malrotation than evaluation of the position of the cecum via an enema. The neonatal colon has a small lumen and typically no haustra. The position of the cecum in the young infant is higher than in adults and in most cases in the mid-position between the right colonic flexure (Figure 1.13) and its future final position in the right lower quadrant. The lengths of the sigmoid colon and of both colonic flexures are very variable. The rectum is often dilated compared to other parts of the large bowel. Haustra of the large bowel are observed at three to six months after birth.

The baby swallows air even in the birth canal, i.e. before the first cry and first breath. Air in the stomach rapidly passes the pylorus and the small bowel. Intraluminal air has reached

sphincter. In infants the contraction of lower constrictor pharyngeal muscle can simulate a true esophageal stenosis. However, this is only a transient functional disturbance in young children, which disappears spontaneously with increasing age. The second narrowing is the crossing of the aortic arch and the adjacent left main stem bronchus with the mid-portion of the esophagus. The third narrowing of the esophagus is the lower esophageal sphincter, i.e. cardia. These narrowings are important in foreign-body ingestion. The pressure zone in the lower esophageal sphincter is not fully developed in infants up to the age of six to eight months. This can result in gastroesophageal reflux. Similarly, the fixation of the esophagus in the hiatus of the diaphragm is not very tight, which can result

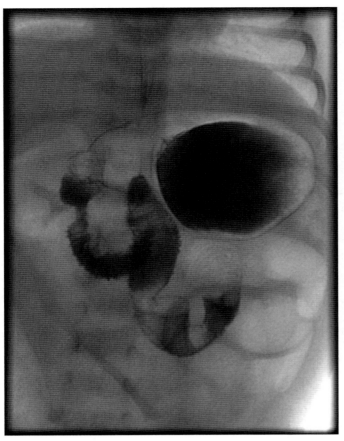

Figure 1.12 Normal stomach and duodenum in an infant.

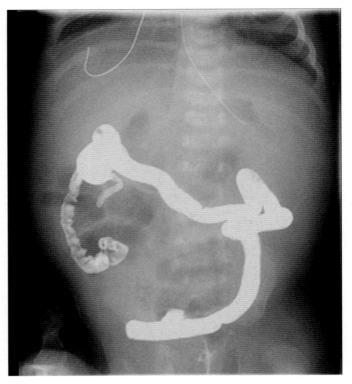

Figure 1.13 Normal colon in a newborn.

the colon after 4–8 hours, and the rectum after 12–24 hours. Concurrently with the progress of bowel air, the newborn will pass the meconium. In premature babies the air and meconium passage is often delayed.

In infants, air is noted in all bowel loops, including the rectum. In older children, the stomach and small bowel are filled with various amounts of swallowed air, while there is little gas and stool in the large bowel. Some otherwise normal children swallow air all the time and may have a large air-filled stomach and a lot of air in the whole bowel. This is called aerophagia. This is a self-limited and transitory phenomenon and must be differentiated from meteorism and bowel obstruction of any cause.

Kidney and ureters

The main diagnostic procedures are sonography and renal scintigraphy with ^{99m}Tc MAG3 (technetium 99m mercaptylacetyltriglycine). The normal proximal and juxtavesical segments of the ureter can be sonographically visualized in the well-hydrated child with a full bladder. However, even markedly dilated ureters can be missed with ultrasound when a lot of bowel air/gas is present. In some patients, ^{99m}Tc DMSA (technetium 99m-labeled dimercaptosuccinic acid) is indicated, e.g. to evaluate the functional renal cortex, e.g. in

pyelonephritis. MR is helpful in evaluation of obstructive uropathies, and crucial for the comprehensive diagnosis of complex genitourinary malformations. Doppler sonography and MR angiography are useful for the evaluation of renal vessel abnormalities. Forty percent of normal patients with normal kidneys have more than one renal artery. Low dose CT is the method of choice in suspected urolithiasis.

The kidneys develop from seven ventral and seven dorsal renculi. A renculus is the smallest anatomical element which is composed of a cortical cap, a medullar pyramid, a calyx and surrounding blood vessels. The newborn kidney has a typical lobulated surface caused by the incomplete fusion of the renculi. During renal growth, the fusion of the renculi progresses continuously. The smoothing of the surface of the upper and lower poles of the kidney starts between year one and two of age. The fusion is incomplete at two sites, ventro-medially at the upper pole of the right kidney, and dorsally in the mid-portion of both kidneys. This finding has been described by F. Hoffer as the interrenicular junction (Figure 1.14).

In many infants during the first year, the renal cortex is narrow and hyperechoic compared to the liver parenchyma on US (Table 1.2). The triangular medullar pyramids at this age are large, compared to the overlying cortex, and extremely hypoechoic. Starting at the age of six months, the echogenicity of the renal cortex decreases gradually. Beyond infancy the cortex is hypoechoic compared to the liver. The renal sinus becomes enlarged by the deposition of fat, which begins at about six to eight years and progresses during puberty, reaching

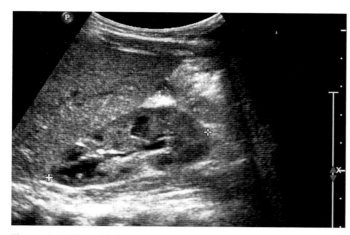

Figure 1.14 Normal kidney in a young child with interrenicular junction, an echogenic focus between two renculi of the kidney, which should not be mistaken for a scar.

Table 1.2 Echogenicity of the parenchyma of various abdominal and retroperitoneal organs. Reference for the echogenicity is the right diaphragmatic crus, and the psoas muscle which is always very hypoechoic

Age	Liver	Renal cortex	Pancreas	Spleen
0–1 years	High	Very high	Very high	High
1–5 years	Intermediate	Low	Intermediate	High
5–10 years	Intermediate	Low	Low	High
10–15 years	Intermediate	Low	Intermediate	High
>15 years	Intermediate	Low	High	High

the appearance of an adult kidney. Renal growth is completed between 12 and 16 years. Similar morphological changes can be observed with MR. Following intravenous injection of gadolinium contrast media, an initial nephrographic phase with a bright cortex is noted, followed by a transitional phase with enhancement of the medullar pyramids and a delayed pyelographic phase with the enhancement of the renal collecting system. Frequent normal variants are:

1. interrenicular junction defects;
2. pyelectasia;
3. parenchymal inclusion or "bridge" between the renal calixes, simulating duplicated collecting systems.

If the ureters are of major interest, special T2-weighted "3D MR urography" sequences, e.g. RARE (rapid acquisition with relaxation enhancement) or similar sequences, are used. The normal ureters have a straight course along the psoas muscles with a slight dilatation of their middle parts. The proximal and distal parts are often contracted.

The renal function measured as glomerular filtration rate (GFR) is very low at birth, about $10\,\mathrm{ml\,min^{-1}m^{-2}}$. But it increases rapidly within four to six weeks to about $30\,\mathrm{ml\,min^{-1}m^{-2}}$. During childhood the GFR increases with the growth of the

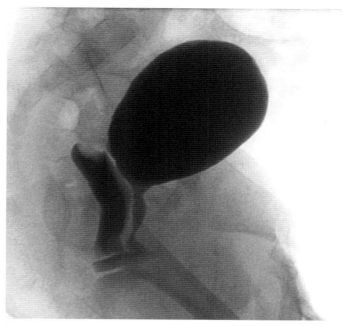

Figure 1.15 Normal female urethra. Spotfilm in a true lateral projection during maximal voiding shows vaginal influx.

kidneys and reaches adult values with puberty. The MAG3 scintigraphy is used mainly for the determination of the individual renal function and the evaluation of the severity of obstruction.

Urinary bladder and urethra

Sonography and voiding cystourethrography (VCUG) are the basic investigations of uroradiology. Very rarely retrograde urethrography and antegrade ureteropyelography are performed as well. US is the ideal method to investigate the full urinary bladder regarding bladder wall thickness as well as extra- and intravesical pathology, such as ureteroceles, diverticula, stones etc. US can also be used to evaluate the bladder after voiding regarding residual urine volume in the bladder. Furthermore, the juxtavesical ureters with their peristalsis, the intramural segments and the ureter jets can be easily assessed. In male infants we can see, occasionally, the dilated posterior urethra suggesting urethral obstruction.

The gold standard to show anatomical details and the function of the bladder and the urethra is the VCUG. Fluoroscopic spot views (e.g. with the "last image hold" mode) or short fluoroscopic videos of the bladder base and urethra should be obtained in a true lateral or slightly oblique projection during maximal voiding (Figure 1.15). Normal findings are a small utriculus at the posterior urethra in boys, and a vaginal influx during voiding in girls. A slightly irregular posterior bladder wall during contrast filling is a normal finding on VCUGs and should not be mistaken for cystitis, bladder diverticula or a neurogenic bladder. Incomplete bladder emptying during a VCUG is a normal finding caused by the investigation procedure itself. Bladder "ears" are also a normal variant and occur predominantly in infants. Another frequent finding is asynchronous conversion of the bladder base anterior and posterior part during voiding, a wide bladder neck and spinning top urethra. Of note, some uroradiologists believe that the "spinning top urethra" may be a pathological finding. Finally, slight asymmetric indentations of the male urethra are pure functional abnormalities.

Uterus and ovaries/testes

The uterus undergoes at least three phases of development. In newborn girls the uterus is strikingly large. This enlargement is limited to the cervix uteri with hyperplasia of the glands, and presumably caused by hormonal stimulation. This enlargement of the uterus persists for three to four months. Then the cervix decreases in size and the ratio of cervix to the corpus is about 1 : 1, with no substantial growth during the next six to eight years. At the age of about six to eight years, the uterus starts to grow under hormonal influence, with the corpus uteri becoming larger than the cervix. The length of the corpus uteri increases to 4 cm until the age of 10 years. After puberty the size has quadrupled. MR may show more details of the growing uterus, especially different muscle layers, which are not visible with US. Duplication anomalies of the uterus and the vagina are due to incomplete fusion of the müllerian ducts, and show a large spectrum of variation. These malformations are difficult to detect in young girls and even in older patients with transabdominal ultrasound; MR is the diagnostic method of choice to evaluate these complex abnormalities.

Similarly to the growth of the uterus, the ovaries do not significantly change in size and appearance on US and MR between 0 and 6 years of age. The main growth of the ovaries occurs after the age of 10 years. Sometimes, an unusual position of the ovary is suspected with sonography. Again, MR is more sensitive than US to detect abnormal positions of the ovaries. During the whole development, the normal ovaries show multiple small follicular cysts with remarkably low echogenicity on US in young children, and higher echogenicity after 10 years of age. Occasionally, large ovarian cysts can be detected in symptom-free patients. Such cysts are occasionally seen even prenatally. In most cases these cysts have no hormonal effects and regress within a few months; very rarely they can cause an ovarian torsion.

The descended testes can be visualized with US. US and MR can detect undescended testes. Sonographically, the echogenicity of the testicular tissue and epididymis is slightly different. Occasionally, small Morgangi cysts can be seen in the head of the epididymis. The prostate is very small and may not be clearly delineated before puberty, but it is clearly visible on US and MR post-puberty. MR is the best approach to image the seminal vesicles with cross-sectional techniques in young individuals.

Liver and biliary system

The liver is the largest organ in all age groups and is particularly big at birth. The right lobe can extend into the right iliac fossa; the left lobe can displace the stomach caudally and posteriorly. Within the first year, the growth of the liver is less than the growth of the whole body. The growth of the left liver lobe lags behind the right lobe. Therefore, the left liver lobe is often very small in adolescents.

Sonography and MR have become very important imaging methods for evaluation of the liver in pediatric patients, especially if all available US modalities (B-mode, color Doppler, PW-Doppler) and multiple MR sequences are used. A complete US and MR examination of the liver should show:

1. the parenchyma of the whole liver;
2. liver edges (sharp or round);
3. the intrahepatic blood vessels (hepatic artery, portal vein, hepatic veins) from the liver hilus to the periphery;
4. intrahepatic course of the inferior vena cava;
5. the biliary system (gallbladder, intra- and extrahepatic ducts);
6. the tributaries of the portal vein system with their flow characteristics;
7. the spleen.

In young patients of less than eight years, US examinations with high frequency transducers allow the depiction of very fine anatomical details of the intrahepatic structures. The liver parenchyma in infants is homogeneous and slightly echogenic. This pattern changes with age, with a slight decrease of echogenicity and more coarse parenchymal echoes (Table 1.2).

The portal vein system in neonates is characterized by the recessus umbilicalis of Rex, i.e. the entry of the umbilical vein into the left-sided portal vein. A dilatation of the left portal vein remains visible throughout life and can vary in size from patient to patient. At birth, the main portal vein is often small. In the following months, with higher bowel perfusion the vascular bed of the whole portal venous system enlarges. The ductus venosus Arantii is a natural intrahepatic shunt between the recessus umbilicalis and the inferior vena cava (IVC). This pathway is used for insertion of an umbilical vein catheter. However, this fetal shunt closes shortly after birth with permanent closure at about two months. The portal venous system, especially the peripheral intrahepatic branches, seems very prominent in some young children between three and eight years (Figure 1.16). This is either a normal variant or may be related to enteroviral infections. Other frequent variants are the number of hepatic veins, often more than three, and a deep entry of a supernumerary branch of the right hepatic vein directly into the vena cava. Another variant is a small liver bump, which is associated with a small eventration of a part of the right leaflet of the diaphragm. This must be differentiated from a true eventration of the diaphragm.

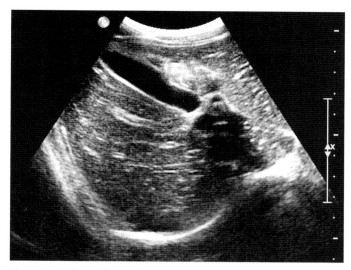

Figure 1.16 Normal liver with prominent peripheral portal vein branches.

The biliary system, i.e. the gallbladder and the intra-/ extrahepatic bile ducts, is very tiny in young patients. It can be investigated with high-frequency linear US and concomitant use of color Doppler. In some cases, MRCP (magnetic resonance cholangiopancreaticography) is needed for a better overview of the anatomical relationships, especially in congenital anomalies.

Spleen

The normal spleen lies in the left upper abdomen with or without contact to the diaphragm. The tissue echogenicity on US is, in all age groups, higher than the echogenicity of the normal liver, and no vessels are visible in the parenchyma (Table 1.2). The position of the hilum of the spleen is very variable, depending on the course of the tail of the pancreas. In most cases the pancreas is slightly ascending towards the left diaphragm. However, in some cases the pancreas courses horizontally and in others caudally. The spleen has a variety of forms: the organ can have one or many clefts; round shape, banana or boomerang form. Therefore, sonographic measurements should be interpreted with caution. Relatively frequently, one or two splenules can be seen at the hilum. Cross-sectional scanning with contrast-enhanced CT or MR in the early arterial phase may show sometimes peculiar enhancement patterns, named zebra-spleen or rosette-spleen.

Pancreas

The pancreas is located in the retroperitoneum in front of the large abdominal vessels (aorta (Ao), inferior vena cava (IVC), superior mesenteric artery, confluens). The normal pancreas is very long. It extends from the right side (with its head next to the descending part of the duodenum) to the splenic hilum in the left upper abdomen. In newborns the pancreas is small and very echogenic on US, with no

lobular structure (Table 1.2). In small children, over one year, the size of the pancreas increases rapidly and the lobular structure appears. Especially the pancreatic body and tail can become relatively large in children. Normal variants are anomalies of the shape, e.g. croissant type, dumbbell type and anvil type with local thickening and narrowing of the glandular tissue. The size of the pancreas increases during growth, more in the corpus and tail and less in the head. The echogenicity of the pancreas changes three times during childhood, in contrast to other abdominal organs (Table 1.2). The hypoechoic pancreas of slim schoolchildren is a striking US finding. With the exception of neonates and young infants, the lobular structure of the pancreas is a typical finding and independent of the basic echogenicity. These sonographic findings have no counterpart in MR. MRCP is the best procedure to depict the pancreatic duct stenosis or if dilatation is suspected.

Endocrine glands

The pituitary gland is best imaged with MR. In infancy, it has a relatively higher signal than in older children. The pituitary gland is composed of the large adenohypophysis, the pituitary stalk and the neurohypophysis, which is located behind, and in the majority of cases fused with the larger anteriorly positioned adenohypophysis. The size of the pituitary gland is greatest in puberty, especially in females.

The thyroid gland is located in front of the larynx and the proximal trachea, immediately under the skin and easily accessible to high-resolution US. The normal thyroid gland is highly echogenic with a fine structure and is heavily vascularized. The common carotid arteries are in close contact with the lateral borders of both lobes. Normal variants are: hypoplasia of one lobe, long isthmus representing a pyramidal lobe, and sometimes a small isthmus. Hemiagenesis of one lobe with or without an isthmus is a rare anomaly. If no thyroid gland is found in the normal position, the gland may be ectopic and is most frequently found at the base of the tongue or the upper neck, above the hyoid bone. Scintigraphy and MR are indicated in such cases. The thyroid slowly enlarges before puberty, with many reports on normal size and/or the volume. Nevertheless, it is difficult to provide normal values for the volume of the thyroid gland due to large interindividual variations. Differing growth curves in various publications can be explained by the heterogeneity of the populations screened and highly variable iodine intake of normal individuals. All reports show a steep increase of thyroid size beyond 10 years of age. The parathyroid glands are only 2–5 mm in size and oval shaped. Two of the four parathyroid glands are frequently located at the lower poles of the thyroid. The site of the parathyroids can vary extremely from the skull base to the diaphragm.

The adrenal glands are remarkably large in newborns with a typical triangular shape. Because of their large size in neonates, they partially overlie the upper poles of the kidneys.

In this age group, we can differentiate three layers in the adrenal glands. The size of the adrenals decreases after the neonatal period. The shape of an adrenal gland is dependent on the shape of the adjacent kidney. In renal agenesis the ipsilateral adrenal has a pencil-like shape. Very rarely, the adrenals are fused in the midline, forming a horseshoe adrenal.

Peripheral skeleton and the pelvis

In term neonates, no ossification is seen in the epiphyses of long or short bones of the upper and lower extremities. The X-ray of the hand of a term newborn shows no ossification of carpal bones. The X-ray of the foot shows an ossified talus, calcaneus and cuboid. The neonatal knee is an exception. Even in premature babies of the 32nd week of gestational age, there are small epiphyseal ossifications in the distal femur epiphysis, and, from the 34th week on, also in the proximal tibial epiphysis. The bone age in the first two years can be determined by evaluating the size of the epiphyseal ossification on ap and lateral radiographs of the knee. In older children, radiographs of the left hand are taken and compared with standards in the *Radiographic Atlas of Skeletal Development of the Hand and the Wrist* of Greulich and Pyle.

The appearance of the epi- and apophyseal ossifications of all bones is listed in reference tables with percentile lists and curves, separately for females and males. These lists also show the chronology of the ossification of various bones, but, also, the wide variation between different individuals and ethnic groups. In addition, there is a difference between females and males, with significantly earlier ossification of bones in females of all age groups. The ossification of the human skeleton is completed with the closure of upper pelvic rim apophyses, which occurs at approximately 21 years in females and at 25–28 years in males.

The growth of the long bones occurs in a longitudinal direction at the physis and in a circular direction along the periosteum. In infants, a periosteal bone formation of long bones, e.g. humeri, is frequently seen. This normal finding involves all long bones in a symmetric fashion and must not be mistaken for a disease, e.g. osteomyelitis, battered child or Caffey's disease. The growth potential of the physes of the long bones differs greatly. The physes with the greatest growth potential are the distal physes of the femora.

Special knowledge of the time of appearance, the site and the size of epiphyseal or apophyseal ossification centers is crucial for the correct diagnosis of abnormalities. This is especially important for the elbow (Figure 1.17), because fractures of the distal humerus, the proximal radius and the proximal ulna are often very complex and may involve displacement of ossification centers. In complex cases, CT or MR may be indicated. An example for a frequent false positive diagnosis with a suspected fracture is the normal apophysis of the fifth metatarsal simulating a fracture. Sometimes, the ossification of the humeral or femoral epiphyses may appear abnormal. A common normal variant is Meyer's dysplasia. As the hip is the joint which has to bear the whole body weight, the early diagnosis of developmental abnormalities of the neonatal/infantile hip joint is of great importance.

The sonographic evaluation of the hips is possible within the first 12 weeks, because the cartilaginous femoral head is translucent during this time. Later, the femoral ossification centers appear and prevent hip US beyond the age of five months. Graf recommends performing the US examination of the hip in a coronal section through the center of the acetabulum (Figure 1.18). Four ultrasonographic criteria for a correct section plane are defined:

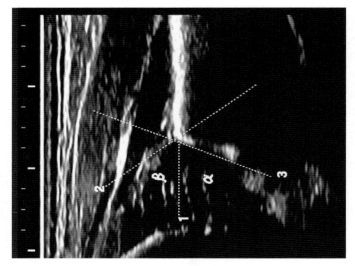

Figure 1.18 Coronal hip ultrasound. Normal hip type I, according to the Graf classification. The extension of the iliac crest (1) dissects the head of the femur. The alpha angle between the iliac crest and a line drawn from the inferior point of the iliac bone tangential to the bony acetabulum (3) reflects the depth of the bony acetabular roof, and should be greater than 60° in a mature infant of more than six to eight weeks. The beta angle is the angle between the iliac crest and a line drawn from its inferior point to the acetabular labrum (2), and is used for subclassifications of hip dysplasias. The beta angle should be less than 50° in a normal infant.

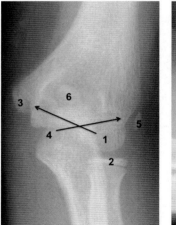 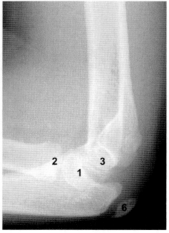

Figure 1.17 Elbow ossification centers (1 capitulum; 2 radial head; 3 internal condyle; 4 trochlea; 5 external condyle; 6 olecranon; numbered according to the sequence of their appearance. Memo: CRITOE).

1. visibility of the lowest point of the iliac bone bordering the Y-cartilage;
2. visibility of the edge of the acetabular roof;
3. visibility of the labrum acetabulare;
4. visibility of the ossified metaphysis of the proximal femur.

Graf defined four different types of developing hips: type I to type IV. Type I is a normal well-developed hip; type II is still normal, but the development is delayed. Type II involves several subtypes which cannot be fully discussed here. Type III was named a dysplastic hip joint with some degree of subluxation, and type IV is a complete dislocation of the femoral head into the fossa glute009. In contrast to Graf's one standard section technique, Harcke recommended a dynamic sonographic technique. X-rays of the pelvis are diagnostically useful with the appearance of the femoral head ossification, i.e. at about six months. MR could be used as well, especially in patients who are treated for hip dysplasia.

Normal variants of the pelvis and the hip joints are relatively frequent. The ossification of the inferior ramus of the pubic bone may be delayed up to three months. Patients with bladder extrophy have a diastasis of the pubic bone and no pubic symphysis. The synchrondrosis ischiopubica may be enlarged and may simulate a bone tumor. The acetabular roof often is irregular with small additional ossification centers. At the inferior anterior spine of the pelvis, an extra ossification center may be present simulating an avulsion. The same false positive diagnosis is often made for the apophyseal ossification rim of the os ischium. Finally, even the normal major or minor trochanter may be misinterpreted as a femoral fracture.

Spine, spinal canal and myelon

The ossification of the spine begins very early prenatally, at about the ninth week of gestation in three portions of the vertebrae: both neural arches and in the vertebral body. Two or even more ossification centers can appear in the vertebral bodies, and these ossification centers have often not yet fused in full-term newborns. As many vertebrae in early infancy are not sufficiently ossified, spine radiographs have a limited diagnostic value. Especially, the neurocentric synchrondroses appear very wide because they are totally cartilaginous. Similarly, the ribs

are also only partially ossified. The paraspinal medial portions of the ribs are also of cartilage. MR is therefore a very good alternative imaging modality to answer special questions in infancy, e.g. battered child syndrome, infection etc.

On the other hand, the delayed ossification of the spinal processes is the precondition to perform a spinal US (Figure 1.19). Using this technique, the myelon, nerve roots, epidural space with vessels and the longitudinal ligaments and partially the intervertebral discs can be visualized. Using the real-time qualities of US, the motion characteristics of the cauda equina can be studied with M-mode US. Beyond the first trimester, MR is the method of choice to depict the vertebral bodies, the paraspinal soft tissue structures, the spinal canal and the spinal cord.

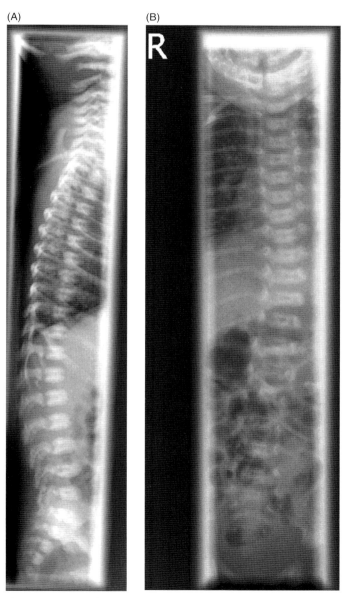

Figure 1.20 Normal ap (A) and lateral (B) spine in a newborn.

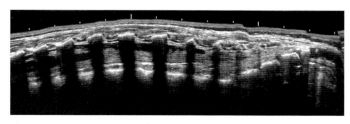

Figure 1.19 Panoramic view of the spinal cord: sagittal longitudinal section in a neonate.

The development and the growth of the spine and the spinal cord go hand in hand. The spinal nerves leave and reach the spinal cord in the spinal canal via the intervertebral foramina. Because the spinal nerves C4 to T2 form the brachial plexus, the lower cervical spinal cord is slightly thicker than the thoracic myelon. This leads to wider transverse and sagittal diameters of the cervical part of the spinal canal. On the other hand, the thoracic part of the spinal canal is relatively small. The lumbar spine has a wider spinal canal, because the end of the myelon is thickened and forms the conus medullaris which gives rise to the cauda equina. In the last fetal months, the conus medullaris ascends from L3/L4 to L1/L2 because of the faster growth of the spine compared with the spinal cord.

The size and shape of the single vertebra in different segments of the spine change in the first year, when the main favorite posture is upright (sitting, standing, walking). In newborns and young infants, the so-called bone-in-bone appearance can be observed (Figure 1.20). In later childhood, the vertebral bodies first show small carvings at the upper and lower edges. Later, ring apophyses appear. During the growth of the spine the intervertebral discs decrease considerably in height. Calcification of the discs can be observed before 10 years of age. This predominantly occurs in the cervical and thoracic spine.

Parts of the spine are depicted on chest and abdominal X-rays. Very often, the pathology of the spine is detected in these radiographs, but not clearly seen. A coned view of the thoracic spine will then be needed to make the final diagnosis, for example a butterfly vertebra of the lower thoracic spine, may be associated with Alagille syndrome. Radiographs of the whole spine in infants are rarely indicated. But they may be needed in patients with unclassified skeletal dysplasia, suspected battered child syndrome and metabolic disease.

The spine in the newborn is straight. The physiological bending in the sagittal plane will not develop before the age of six months: lordosis of the cervical spine, slight kyphosis of the thoracic spine and lordosis of the lumbar spine. However, the slight kyphosis of the sacrum is of developmental origin and not acquired by functional effects as the cervical lordosis. The enormous mobility of the cervical spine causes the phenomenon of pseudoluxation of the upper cervical spine at the levels C2/3 and C3/4 in neutral position or slight kyphosis. A minimal lateral deviation (scoliosis) of the mid-thoracic spine in adolescence is very frequent, and should not be considered to be pathological. Idiopathic scoliosis must be differentiated from painful postural scoliosis which can occur with infection of the spine, paraspinal tissue, or an intra-abdominal abscess, and very rarely with a tumor.

Further reading

Allison JW, Faddis LA, Kinder DL et al. (2000) Intracranial resistive index (RI) values in normal term infants during the first day of life. Pediatr Radiol 30, 618–20.

Argyropoulou M, Perignon F, Brunelle F et al. (1991) Height of normal pituitary gland as a function of age evaluated by magnetic resonance imaging in children. Pediatr Radiol 21, 247–9.

Barghouth G, Prior JO, Lepori D et al. (2002) Paranasal sinuses in children: size evaluation of maxillary, sphenoid, and frontal sinuses by percentile curves. Eur Radiol 12, 1451–9.

Barkovich AJ Pediatric Neuroimaging, 4th edn. (Philadelphia: Lippincott Williams and Wilkins, 2005).

Bar-Ziv J, Barki Y, Itzchak Y et al. (1984) Posterior mediastinal accessory thymus. Pediatr Radiol 14, 165–7.

Berdon WE, Baker DH, James LS (1965) The ductus bump. A transient physiologic mass in the chest roentgenograms in newborn infants. AJR Am J Roentgenol 95, 91–8.

Blane CE, Bockstein F, DiPietro M et al. (1985) Sonographic standards of normal infant kidney length. AJR Am J Roentgenol 145, 1289–92.

Brodeur AE, Silberstein MJ, Graviss ER Radiology of the Pediatric Elbow (Boston: Hall, 1981).

Budorick NE, Pretouius DH, Grafe MR et al. (1991) Ossification of the fetal spine, Radiology 181, 561–5.

Byrd SE, Darling CF, Wilczynski MA (1993) White matter of the brain. Neuroimaging Clin N Am 3, 247–66.

Chiara A, Chirico G, De Vecchi E, Rondini G (1989) Ultrasonic evaluation of kidney length in term and preterm infants. Eur J Pediat 149, 94–5.

Cohen HL, Shapiro MA, Mandel FS, Shapiro ML (1993) Normal ovaries in neonates and infants: sonographic study of 77 patients 1 day to 24 months old. AJR Am J Roentgenol 160, 583–6.

Cohen MM Jr, McLean RE (eds.) Craniosynostosis (New York: Oxford University Press, 2000).

Cristy M (1981) Active bone marrow distribution as a function of age in humans. Phys Med Biol 26, 389–400.

Deane MGM, Burton EM, Harlow SA et al. (2001) Swallowing dysfunction in infants less than 1 year of age. Pediatr Radiol 31, 423–42.

Deeg KH, Rupprecht T (1989) Pulsed Doppler sonographic measurement of normal values for the flow velocities in the intracranial arteries of healthy newborn. Pediatr Radiol 19, 71–8.

Dinkel E, Ertl M, Dittrich M et al. (1985) Kidney size in childhood sonographical growth charts for kidney length and volume. Pediatr Radiol 15, 38–43.

Dittrich M, Milde S, Dinkel E et al. (1983) Sonographic biometry of liver and spleen size in childhood. Pediatr Radiol 13, 206.

Edwards DK, Higgins CB, Gilpin EA (1981) The cardiothoracic ratio in newborn infants. AJR Am J Roentgenol 136, 907–13.

Engelbrecht V, Scherer A, Rassek M et al. (2002) Diffusion-weighted MR imaging in the brain in children: findings in the normal brain and in the brain with white matter disease. Radiology 222, 410–18.

Enriquez G, Correa F, Lucaya J et al. (2003) Potential pitfalls in cranial sonography. Pediatr Radiol 33, 110–17.

Enriquez G, Correa F, Aso C et al. (2006) Mastoid fontanel approach for sonographic imaging of the neonatal brain. Pediatr Radiol 36, 532–40.

Fischer JK (1978) Technical notes: skin fold vs. pneumothorax. AJR Am J Roentgenol 130, 791–2.

Fraser-Hill MA, Atri M, Bret PM *et al.* (1990) Intrahepatic portal venous system: variation demonstrated with duplex and color Doppler US. *Radiology* 177, 523–6.

Friedman DM, Schacht RG (1991) Doppler waveforms in the renal arteries of normal children. *J Clin Ultrasound* 19, 387–92.

Galanski M, Nagel H-D, Stamm G (2007) (in German) Pädiatrische CT Expositionspraxis in Deutschland. *ROFO* 179, 1110–11. www.drg-apt.de.

Gallego C, Miralles M, Marin C *et al.* (2004) Congenital hepatic shunts. *Radiographics* 24, 755–72.

Girodias JB, Azouz EM, Maarton D (1991) Intervertebral disk space calcification. A report of 51 children with a review of the literature. *Pediatr Radiol* 21, 541–6.

Gollogly S, Smith JT, White SK *et al.* (2004) The volume of lung parenchyma as a function of age: a review of 1050 normal CT scans of the chest with three-dimensional volumetric reconstruction of the pulmonary system. *Spine* 29, 2061.

Gooding CA Cranial sutures and fontanelles. In *Radiology of the Skull and Brain,* vol. 1 *The Skull,* ed. TH Newton, DJ Potts (St. Louis: Mosby, 1971) pp. 216–40.

Gooding CA, Neuhauser EBD (1965) Growth and development of the vertebral bodies in the presence and absence of normal stress. *AJR Am J Roentgenol* 93, 388–93.

Graf R (1984) Classification of hip joint dysplasia by means of sonography. *Arch Orthop Trauma Surg* 102, 248–55.

Graf R, Tschauner C, Klapsch W (1993) Process in prevention of late developmental dislocation of the hip by sonographic newborn hip "screening": results of a comparative follow-up study. *J Pediatr Orthop* 2, 115–21.

Grattan-Smith JD, Jones RA (2006) MR urography in children. *Pediatr Radiol* 36, 1119–32.

Gressens P, Hüppi PS Normal and abnormal brain development. In *Fanaroff and Martin's Neonatal-Perinatal Medicine: Diseases of the Fetus and Infant*, 8th edn., ed. RJ Martin, AA Fanaroff, MC Walsh (Philadelphia: Mosby, 2006) pp. 883–908.

Greulich WW, Pyle SI *Radiographic Atlas of Skeletal Development of the Hand and the Wrist*, 2nd edn. (Stanford: Stanford University Press, 1959).

Griscom NT (1982) Computed tomographic determination of tracheal dimensions in children and adolescents. *Radiology* 145, 361.

Haber HP, Mayer EI (1994) Ultrasound evaluation of uterine and ovarian size from birth to puberty. *Pediatr Radiol* 24, 11–13.

Han BK, Babcock DS (1985) Sonographic measurements and appearance of normal kidneys in children. *AJR Am J Roentgenol* 145, 611.

Harcke HT (1995) The role of ultrasound in diagnosis and management of developmental dysplasia of the hip. *Pediatr Radiol* 25, 225–7.

Harcke HT, Grissom LE (1990) Performing dynamic sonography of the infant hip. *AJR Am J Roentgenol* 155, 837–44.

Hernanz-Schulman M, Ambrosino MM, Freeman PC *et al.* (1995) Common bile duct in children: sonographic dimensions. *Radiology* 195, 193–5.

Hoffer FA, Hanabergh AM, Teele RL (1985) The interreniculare junction: a mimic of renal scarring on normal pediatric sonograms. *AJR Am J Roentgenol* 145, 1075–8.

Jequier S, Rousseau O (1987) Sonographic measurements of the normal bladder wall in children. *AJR Am J Roentgenol* 149, 563–6.

Katz ME, Siegel MJ, Shackelford GD *et al.* (1987) The position and mobility of the duodenum in children. *AJR Am J Roentgenol* 148, 947–51.

Keats TE, Anderson MW *Atlas of Normal Roentgen Variants that may Simulate Disease*, 7th edn. (St. Louis: Mosby, 2001).

Kendall KA, McKenzie S, Leonard RJ *et al.* (2000) Timing of events in normal swallowing: a videofluoroscopic study. *Dysphagia* 15, 74–83.

van der Knapp MS, van Wezel-Meijler G, Barth PG *et al.* (1996) Normal gyration and sulcation in preterm and term neonates: appearance on MR images. *Radiology* 200, 389–96.

Kramer SS (1989) Radiologic examination of the swallowing impaired child. *Dysphagia* 3, 117–25.

Kricun ME (1985) Red-yellow marrow conversion: its effect on the location of some solitary bone lesions. *Skeletal Radiol* 14, 10–19.

Lachman RS *Taybi and Lachman's Radiology of Syndromes, Metabolic Disorders, and Skeletal Dysplasias*, 5th edn. (Philadelphia: Mosby, 2007).

LeQuesne GW, Reilly BJ (1975) Functional immaturity of the large bowel in the newborn infant. *Radiol Clin North Am* 13, 331–42.

Libicher M, Troger J (1992) US measurement of the subarachnoid space in infants: normal values. *Radiology* 184, 749–51.

Lindskoug BA (1992) Reference man in diagnostic radiology dosimetry. *Radiat Prot Dosim* 43, 111–14.

Martin RJ, Fanaroff AA, Walsh MC (eds.) *Fanaroff and Martin's Neonatal-Perinatal Medicine: Diseases of the Fetus and Infant*, 8th edn. (Philadelphia: Mosby, 2006).

McAlister WH, Askin FB (1983) The effect of some contrast agents in the lung: an experimental study in the rat and dog. *AJR Am J Roentgenol* 140, 245–51.

Metrewelli C, So NM, Chu WC, Lam WW (2004) Magnetic resonance cholangiography in children. *Br J Radiol* 77, 1059–64.

Okada Y, Aoki S, Barkovich A *et al.* (1989) Cranial bone marrow in children: assessment of normal development with MR imaging. *Radiology* 171, 161–4.

Ontel FK, Ivanovic M, Ablin DS *et al.* (1996) Bone age in children of diverse ethnicity. *AJR Am J Roentgenol* 167, 1395–8.

Oppenheimer DA, Carroll BA, Yousem S (1983) Sonography of the normal neonatal adrenal gland. *Radiology*, 157–60.

Osenfeld DL, Schoenfeld SM, Underberg-Davis S (1997) Coarctation of the lateral ventricles: an alternative explanation for subependymal pseudocysts. *Pediatr Radiol* 27, 895–7.

Pettersson H, Ringertz H *Measurements in Pediatric Radiology*, 1st edn. (London: Springer, 1991).

Pyle SI, Hoerr NL *A Radiographic Standard of Reference of the Growing Knee* (Springfield: Charles C. Thomas, 1969).

Ricci C, Cova M, Kang Y *et al.* (1990) Normal age-related patterns of cellular and fatty bone marrow distribution in the axial skeleton: MR imaging study. *Radiology* 177, 83–8.

Richter E, Lierse W *Imaging Anatomy of the Newborn* (Baltimore: Urban and Schwarzenberg, 1991).

Robbins WJ, Brody S, Hogan AG *Growth* (New Haven: Yale University Press, 1928).

Robinson M, Chumlea WC (1982) Standards for limb bone length ratios in children. *Radiology* 143, 433–6.

Rosen L, Bowden DH, Uchida I (1957) Structural changes in pulmonary arteries in first year of life. *AMA Arch Pathol* **63**, 316–17.

Rosenberg HK, Markowitz RI, Kolbert H *et al.* (1994) Normal splenic size in infants and children: sonographic measurement. *AJR Am J Roentgenol* **157**, 119.

Sacton HM, Borzyskowski M, Mundy AR *et al.* (1988) Spinning top urethra: not a normal variant. *Radiology* **168**, 147–50.

Scammon RE, Norris EH (1918) On the time of the post-natal obliteration of the fetal blood-passage (foramen ovale, ductus arteriosus, ductus venosus). *Anat Rec* **15**, 165–80.

Schlesinger AE, White DK, Mallory GB *et al.* (1995) Estimation of total lung capacity from chest radiography and chest CT in children: comparison with body plethysmography. *AJR Am J Roentgenol* **165**, 151.

Schumacher R, Knoll B, Schwarz M, Ermert JA (1992) M-mode sonography of the caudal spinal cord in patients with meningomyelocele: work in progress. *Radiology* **184**, 263–5.

Shopfner CE (1966) Periosteal bone growth in normal infants: a preliminary report. *AJR Am J Roentgenol* **97**, 154–63.

Shopfner CE, Hutch JA (1967) The normal urethrogram. *Radiol Clin North Am* **6**, 165–89.

Siegel MJ, Martin KW, Worthington JL (1987) Normal and abnormal pancreas in children: US studies. *Radiology* **165**, 15.

Skandalakis JE, Gray SW (eds.) *Embryology for Surgeons*, 2nd edn. (Baltimore: Williams and Wilkins, 1994) pp. 414–50.

Slovis TL (ed.) *Caffey's Pediatric Diagnostic Imaging* (Philadelphia: Mosby, 2008).

Staudt M, Schropp C, Staudt F *et al.* (1993) Myelination of the brain in MRI: a staging system. *Pediatr Radiol* **23**, 169–76.

Swischuk LE (1977) Anterior displacement of C2 in children: physiologic or pathologic?

A helpful differentiating line. *Radiology* **122**, 759–63.

Swischuk LE Alimentary tract, esophagus. In *Imaging of the Newborn, Infant, and Young Child*, ed. LE Swischuk (Philadelphia: Lippincott Williams and Wilkins, 2004) pp. 342–9.

Swischuk LE Alimentary tract, esophagus. In *Imaging of the Newborn, Infant, and Young Child*, ed. LE Swischuk (Philadelphia: Lippincott Williams and Wilkins, 2004) pp. 539–41.

Swischuk LE, Swischuk PN, John SD (1993) Wedging of C-3 in infants and children: usually a normal finding and not a fracture. *Radiology* **188**, 523–6.

Taccone A, Oddone M, Dell'Acqua AD *et al.* (1995) MRI "road-map" of normal age-related bone marrow. II. Thorax, pelvis and extremities. *Pediatr Radiol* **25**, 596–606.

Taccone A, Oddone M, Occhi M *et al.* (1995) MRI "road-map" of normal age-related bone marrow. I. Cranial bone and spine. *Pediatr Radiol* **25**, 588–95.

Teitel DF, Iwamoto HS, Rudolph AM (1987) Effects of birth-related events on central blood flow patterns. *Pediatr Res* **22**, 557–66.

Theocharopoulos N, Damilakis J, Perisinakis K, Gourtsoyiannis N (2007) Energy imparted-based estimates of the effect of z overscanning on adult and pediatric patient effective doses from multi-slice computed tomography. *Med Phys* **34**, 1139–52.

Tola V, Kuhns L, Kauffman R (1993) Correlation of gastric emptying at one and two hours following formula feeding. *Pediatr Radiol* **23**, 26–8.

Ueda D (1987) Sonographic measurement of the pancreas in children. *J Clin Ultrasound* **17**, 417.

Unsinn KM, Geley T, Freund MC, Gassner I (2000) US of the spinal cord in newborn: spectrum of normal findings, variants,

congenital anomalies, and the acquired diseases. *Radiographics* **20**, 923–38.

Vock P, Malanowski D, Tscheappeler H *et al.* (1987) Computed tomographic lung density in children. *Invest Radiol* **22**, 627.

Waitches G, Zawin J, Poznanski A (1994) Sequence and rate of bone marrow conversion in the femora of children as seen on MR imaging: are accepted standards accurate? *AJR Am J Roentgenol* **162**, 1399–1406.

Walsh E, Cramer B, Pushpanthan C (1990) Pancreatic echogenicity in premature and newborn infants. *Pediatr Radiol* **20**, 323.

Wittenborg MH, Gyepes MT, Crocker D (1976) Tracheal dynamics in infants with respiratory distress, stridor and collapsing trachea. *Radiology* **88**, 653–62.

Wolf S, Schneble F, Troger J (1992) The conus medullaris: time of ascendence to normal level. *Pediatr Radiol* **22**, 590–2.

Wolf G, Wolfgang A, Kuhn F (1993) Development of the paranasal sinuses in children: implications for paranasal sinus surgery. *Ann Otol Rhinol Laryngol* **102**, 705–11.

Wolpert SM, Osborn M, Anderson M *et al.* (1988) Bright pituitary gland: a normal MR appearance in infancy. *AJNR Am J Neuroradiol* **9**, 1–3.

Zerin JM, DiPietro MA (1992) Superior mesenteric vascular anatomy at US in patient with surgically proved malrotation of the midgut. *Radiology* **183**, 693–4.

Zimmermann MB, Hess SY, Molinari L *et al.* (2004) New reference values for thyroid volume by ultrasound in iodine-sufficient schoolchildren: a World Health Organization/Nutrition for Health and Development Iodine Deficiency Study Group Report. *Am J Clin Nutr* **79**, 231–7.

2

Neonatal imaging

Beverley Newman and Laura Varich

2A SPECTRUM AND SUBDIVISION OF CAUSES OF NEWBORN RESPIRATORY DISTRESS

Newborn respiratory distress can be caused by a large number of different entities, including intrapulmonary and intrathoracic as well as extrathoracic lesions (Table 2.1). This chapter will focus predominantly on the intrapulmonary entities.

The intrapulmonary causes of neonatal respiratory distress are readily subdivided based on their tendency to affect premature versus full-term infants or both, as well as the likelihood that they will produce symmetric or asymmetric radiographic changes (Table 2.2). The asymmetric lesions are often associated with mediastinal shift and are more likely to require surgical rather than medical management. Under- or over-aeration of the lung as well as specific pulmonary patterns of abnormality are additional useful differentiating features for the medical conditions (Table 2.3).

Systematic evaluation of newborn chest radiographs

Systematic evaluation of newborn chest radiographs includes assessment of the placement of tubes and catheters (Figures 2.1–2.3) as well as the overall chest configuration and aeration, appearance of the heart and vessels, pleura, musculoskeletal and abdominal structures and presence of mediastinal shift (Figures 2.4, 2.5) before reviewing the details of the pattern and symmetry of pulmonary abnormality. The radiographic appearance should be correlated with clinical history and findings.

Surfactant deficiency disease

Surfactant deficiency disease (SDD; also variously called hyaline membrane disease or respiratory distress syndrome) occurs in premature newborn infants of less than 36 weeks gestation because of absence or immaturity of pulmonary

Table 2.1 Causes of neonatal respiratory distress

1. Intrapulmonary abnormality — Medical / Surgical

2. Intrathoracic extrapulmonary
   Cardiac – congenital or acquired
   Vascular enlargement, rings/slings
   Airway abnormality
   Tracheoesophageal fistula
   Mediastinal mass
   Congenital diaphragmatic hernia

3. Extrathoracic
   Upper airway obstruction
   Musculoskeletal abnormality
   Abdominal pathology
   Central nervous system lesions
   Metabolic/hematological disorders

Table 2.2 Intrapulmonary abnormalities in newborn infants

	Preterm	Term	Both
Symmetric	Surfactant deficiency disease	Transient tachypnea of the newborn	Lymphangiectasia
			Bilateral lung hypoplasia
Asymmetric	Pulmonary hemorrhage	Fetal aspiration	Pneumonia
			Atelectasis
			Airleak
			Unilateral agenesis/hypoplasia
			Hydrothorax
			Bronchopulmonary malformation
			Tumor

Essentials of Pediatric Radiology, ed. Heike E. Daldrup-Link and Charles A. Gooding. Published by Cambridge University Press.
© Cambridge University Press 2010.

surfactant resulting in diffuse alveolar collapse. The lungs are therefore characterized radiographically by underinflation with diffuse ground-glass opacity ranging from mild fine granularity to complete lung whiteout (Figure 2.6). Because of early treatment including continuous positive airway pressure (CPAP) and/or intubation with intratracheal surfactant administration, underaeration may be less apparent and radiographic findings mitigated, with a coarser granular appearance (Figure 2.7). The combination of prenatal steroid and postnatal surfactant has been the most effective way of preventing or mitigating SDD and its complications in premature infants.

Reopacification of the lungs in an infant with treated SDD raises the differential diagnosis of recurrent or incompletely treated SDD, pulmonary edema or pulmonary hemorrhage (Figure 2.7). The two latter entities are often associated with a patent ductus arteriosus.

Bronchopulmonary dysplasia

Chronic lung disease in the form of bronchopulmonary dysplasia (BPD) is the most serious consequence of SDD (Figures 2.7, 2.8). BPD can also follow other neonatal diseases that require prolonged intubation, pressure ventilation and

Table 2.3 Pattern of lung abnormality – medical conditions

	Underaeration	Overaeration	Granular	Streaky/patchy
SDD	X		X	X (Post-surfactant)
TTN		X		X
Aspiration		X		X
Pneumonia	X	X	X	X

SDD = surfactant deficiency disease.
TTN = transient tachypnea of the newborn.

oxygen administration, including neonatal pneumonia, meconium aspiration and cardiac disease. Persistent pulmonary opacity, interstitial and/or cystic changes are suggestive of evolving chronic lung disease as early as 10 to 14 days of age, but the specific diagnosis is made based on a continued need for supplemental oxygen along with radiographic changes beyond 28 days of life.

Transient tachypnea of the newborn

Transient tachypnea of the newborn (TTN), meconium aspiration and persistent pulmonary hypertension tend to occur more commonly in full-term or post-term infants. TTN is associated with a delay in the normally rapid process of removal of fetal lung fluid and replacement by air. TTN is seen most often in the context of decreased thoracic squeeze (cesarean section delivery) or decreased respiratory effort at birth. TTN is characterized radiographically by mild hyperinflation, increased interstitial markings and sometimes small pleural fluid with rapid clinical and radiographic improvement, usually normalizing within 48 hours (Figure 2.9). Focal fluid retention also occurs in areas of lung that have an abnormal or obstructed bronchial supply, such as congenital lobar hyperinflation, bronchial atresia and congenital pulmonary airway malformation (CPAM) (Figure 2.10).

Persistent pulmonary hypertension, perinatal asphyxia and meconium aspiration

Persistent pulmonary hypertension (PPHN) occurs most commonly in the setting of perinatal asphyxia. Persistent hypoxemia and acidosis result in pulmonary vasoconstriction with decreased pulmonary blood flow and right-to-left atrial and ductal shunting: so-called persistence of the fetal circulation pattern. Hypoxemia and pulmonary vasoconstriction can become a vicious and unrelenting life-threatening cycle. The chest radiograph may be completely normal or show

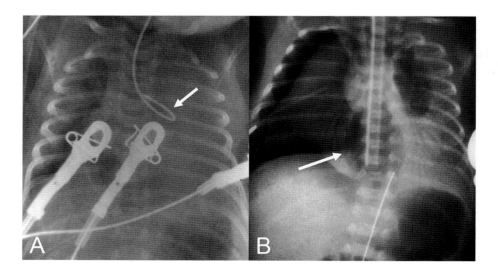

Figure 2.1 Frontal chest radiographs on two different neonates. (A) Feeding tube coiled in the left mainstem bronchus (arrow) with opacification of the left lung. (B) Carinal perforation by endotracheal tube (ETT) with airleak producing a posterior pneumomediastinum (arrow) and tension right pneumothorax with cardiomediastinal shift to the left.

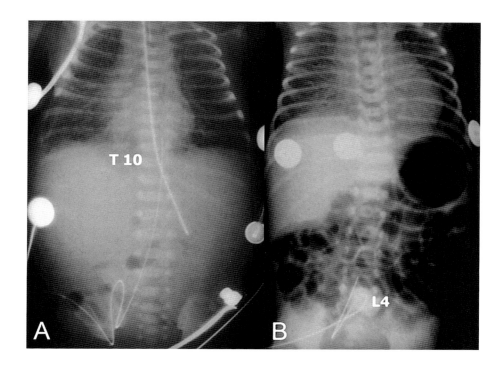

Figure 2.2 Umbilical arterial (UA) line course and placement. (A) High line (tip T10) is the more common location. Optimal position is T6 to 10, away from major vessel branch orifices. (B) Low line (tip L4) is a less common placement. Optimal position is L3 to 5. The major concern is inadvertent removal of the low line and catastrophic hemorrhage. Note the typical course of a UA line from the umbilical artery in the umbilicus initially extending inferiorly in the external iliac artery and then superiorly in the internal iliac artery to the aorta.

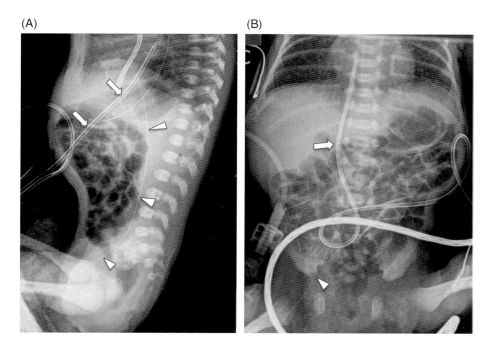

Figure 2.3 Umbilical venous (UV) and femoral venous lines. (A) Lateral and (B) frontal abdominal views demonstrate the anterior course of the umbilical venous catheter (arrows) from the umbilicus directly superiorly in the umbilical vein. Although the course appears relatively straight through the liver, the catheter courses from the umbilical vein to the left portal vein, then to the hepatic venous confluence and IVC/right atrium via the ductus venosus. While the femoral venous (arrowheads) and umbilical venous catheters are partially superimposed on the frontal view, the lateral view shows the posterior course of the femoral catheter (femoral vein to iliac vein to IVC; arrowheads).

mild oligemia in the setting of PPHN. Radiographic abnormalities more commonly reflect accompanying or underlying conditions including perinatal asphyxia (Figure 2.11), meconium aspiration, pneumonia and pulmonary hypoplasia (such as in congenital diaphragmatic hernia). With meconium aspiration, radiographic findings are those of partial or complete airway obstruction and possibly superimposed infection. They include hyperinflation, airleak, patchy consolidation and atelectasis (Figure 2.12). In the presence of a congenital diaphragmatic hernia, the chest radiograph may show intrathoracic bowel or viscera with contralateral mediastinal shift and atelectasis (Figure 2.13). High frequency ventilation along with inhaled nitric oxide as a vasodilator and, if necessary, extracorporeal membrane oxygenation (ECMO) (Figure 2.13) are used to treat pulmonary hypertension.

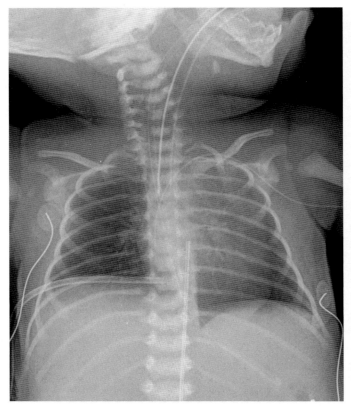

Figure 2.4 Note very thin ribs in this ventilator-dependent newborn with amyotonia congenita and probable pulmonary hypoplasia.

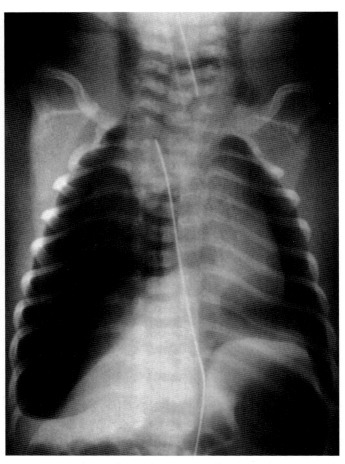

Figure 2.5 Newborn infant with Potter's syndrome (renal agenesis) with bilateral pulmonary hypoplasia, bell-shaped chest and marked airleak including pneumothoraces, pneumomediastinum and subcutaneous air dissecting in the neck.

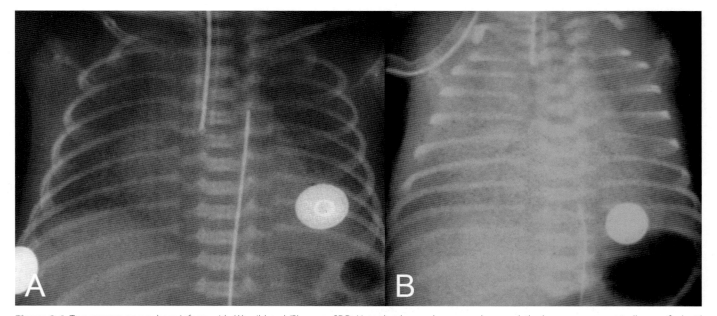

Figure 2.6 Two premature newborn infants with (A) mild and (B) severe SDD. Note that lung volumes are decreased; the lungs are symmetrically opacified with mild to severe diffuse ground-glass opacity.

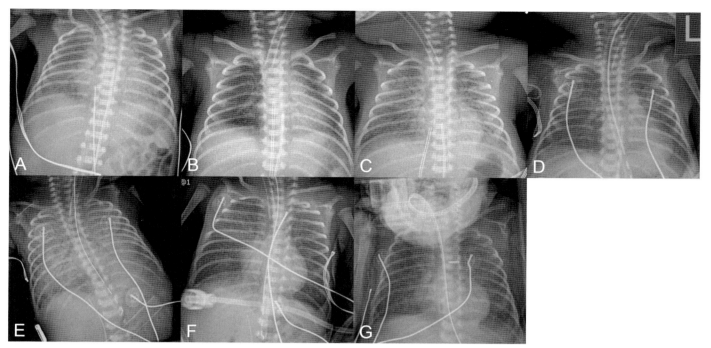

Figure 2.7 (A) A 1-day-old, 27-week-gestation infant, already intubated, with decreased lung volumes and moderate diffuse hazy ground-glass opacity typical of SDD. Note good position of UV line just within the right atrium and UA line at T6. (B) Day 1: diffuse, although somewhat coarsened, clearing pattern of lung abnormality post-surfactant. (C) Day 4: recurrent SDD with reopacification of the lungs and development of diffuse PIE (streaky linear lucencies) concurrent with increased ventilator settings. (D) Day 10: mild residual hazy opacity of resolving SDD. (E) Day 13: new dense diffuse alveolar opacification obscuring the heart and accompanying suctioning of blood from the ETT suggesting pulmonary hemorrhage. (F) Day 16: clearing pulmonary hemorrhage with asymmetric alveolar-to-interstitial pattern most marked in the right upper lobe. (G) One month: moderate chronic lung changes (BPD) with diffuse increased interstitial markings. Note: clip on occluded PDA.

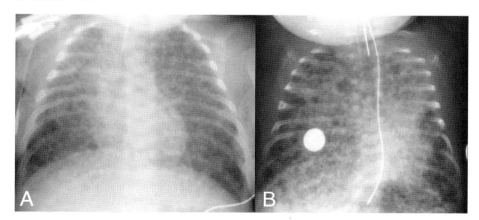

Figure 2.8 Two previously premature infants still intubated at one month of age, with (A) moderate and (B) severe chronic lung changes of broncho-pulmonary dysplasia. Characterized by irregular patchy mottled and streaky linear, sometimes cystic, opacities.

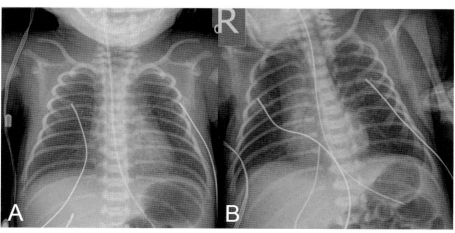

Figure 2.9 Transient tachypnea of the newborn (TTN). Near-term newborn infant with respiratory distress. Mild hyperinflation and perihilar increased markings (A). There was both clinical and radio-graphic (B) resolution by 48 hours of life.

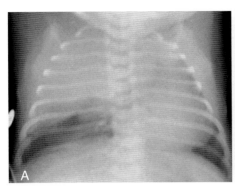
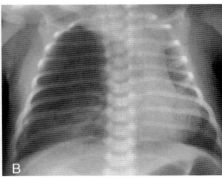

Figure 2.10 Congenital lobar hyperinflation. (A) Chest radiograph at two hours of age with opacified right lung and cardiomediastinal shift to the left. (B) By 48 hours of age, the fluid retained in the abnormal right upper lobe has been replaced by hyperinflated lung compressing the right middle and lower lobe and herniating across the midline.

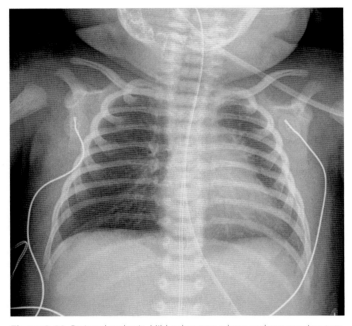

Figure 2.11 Perinatal asphyxia. Mild pulmonary edema and anasarca in a two-day-old with severe perinatal asphyxia. Mild cardiac and moderate renal dysfunction, along with intracranial edema, are likely contributors to the pulmonary edema.

Neonatal pneumonia

Although transplacental infectious pneumonia can occur (TB, syphilis, *Listeria*), *Streptococcus* group B is the most common cause of perinatal pneumonia, usually acquired via ascending infection associated with prolonged rupture of membranes or aspiration during passage through the birth canal. The appearance can be very variable, ranging from streaky interstitial or scattered patchy to diffuse granular changes mimicking almost every other type of neonatal lung disease (Figure 2.14). Superimposed infection is not uncommon in association with other lesions such as aspiration and SDD. The presence of a pleural effusion is a helpful feature in neonatal infection. Recurrent bacterial and/or viral respiratory infections are common in chronically hospitalized, ventilated infants and may contribute to the development of BPD.

Atelectasis and airleak

Atelectasis and airleak occur commonly in the sick newborn infant either as part of ventilation and airway compromise in conditions such as SDD, aspiration and pneumonia, or related to mucous plugging and iatrogenic tube malpositions (Figure 2.15).

Airleak, often starting as pulmonary interstitial emphysema (PIE), is common in ventilated neonates (Figures 2.7, 2.16). The presence of PIE may be the harbinger of air dissecting elsewhere, including pneumomediastinum (Figures 2.1, 2.5, 2.16), pneumothorax (Figures 2.1, 2.5, 2.13, 2.17), pneumopericardium (Figure 2.18), pneumoperitoneum and subcutaneous

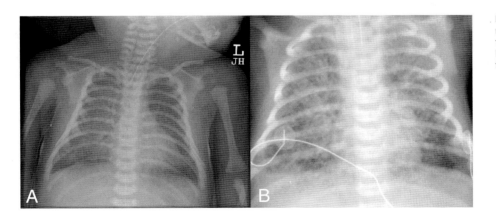

Figure 2.12 Meconium aspiration in two neonates. (A) Asymmetric, patchy airspace consolidations, right > left. (B) Coarse patchy bilateral opacities. Note moderate overinflation and asymmetry of lung findings.

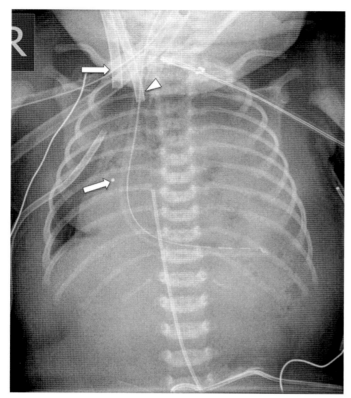

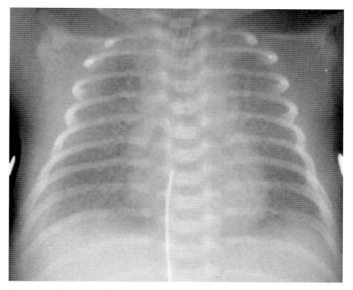

Figure 2.14 1-day old newborn with group B streptococcal pneumonia. The lungs demonstrate diffuse granular opacities mimicking SSD. The right pleural effusion is indicative of pneumonia and would be unusual for SSD.

Figure 2.13 Left congenital diaphragmatic hernia on ECMO. Note endotracheal tube, nasogastric tube and umbilical arterial line displaced to the right. Right chest tube with small right pneumothorax. Bowel loops and solid density (liver) are herniated into the left chest with cardiomediastinal shift to right. Note appropriately placed ECMO catheters: jugular venous catheter tip in right atrium (arrow); this line has a nonopaque section proximal to the tip (marked by a radiographic dot – arrow); the ECMO arterial line is in the right carotid artery with the tip close to the aortic arch (arrowhead). There is marked body wall edema due to third-spacing of fluid.

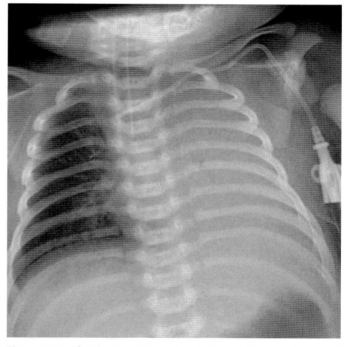

Figure 2.15 Left atelectasis with ipsilateral mediastinal shift secondary to right main bronchus entubation.

air (Figure 2.5). PIE is seen as linear or cystic lucencies initially clustered perihilar and then extending peripherally in a perivascular distribution (Figures 2.7, 2.16, 2.18). Pneumomediastinum is recognized radiographically as medial air adjacent to the heart, frequently displacing the thymus from the heart (Figures 2.16, 2.19), and may extend partially around the heart and along the medial diaphragm. Posterior mediastinal air collections are more commonly associated with esophageal or tracheal perforation, often iatrogenic (Figure 2.1).

A small pneumothorax may be very difficult to recognize because the abnormal lung does not readily collapse and air tends to collect anteromedially in a supine infant (Figure 2.17). Unilateral hyperlucency with unusually sharp mediastinal and diaphragmatic borders should raise suspicion for a pneumothorax, which can be confirmed with a lateral decubitus view. A large pneumothorax with mediastinal shift and/or diaphragmatic eversion is readily recognized (Figures 2.1, 2.5). Beware of mistaking a superimposed skinfold for a pneumothorax (Figure 2.20).

Pneumopericardium is recognized radiographically by the presence of air completely surrounding the heart (Figure 2.18).

Pulmonary agenesis and hypoplasia

Pulmonary agenesis (Figure 2.21) and hypoplasia are uncommon and may be difficult to recognize. Pulmonary hypoplasia is most often unilateral and right sided, frequently associated with underlying vascular anomalies including absent ipsilateral pulmonary artery or veins and scimitar syndrome (Figure 2.22)

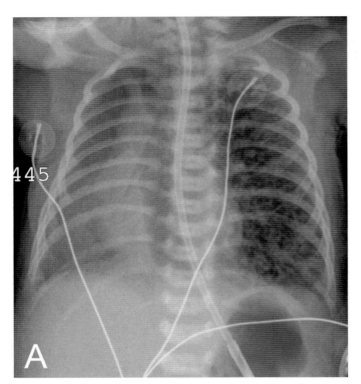

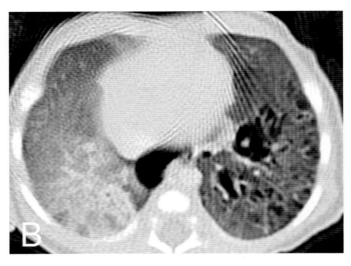

Figure 2.16 Pulmonary Interstitial Emphysema (A) Neonate with persistent coarse linear and rounded lucencies in the left lung on chest radiograph with contralateral shift. (B) CT confirms that the lucencies are due to persistent interstitial air that tracks around and adjacent to the vessels.

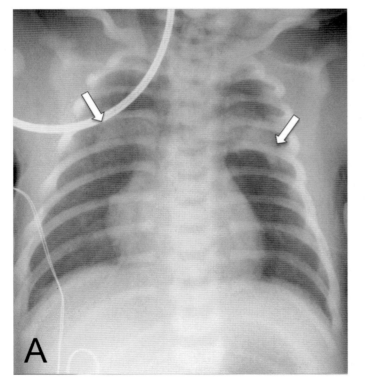

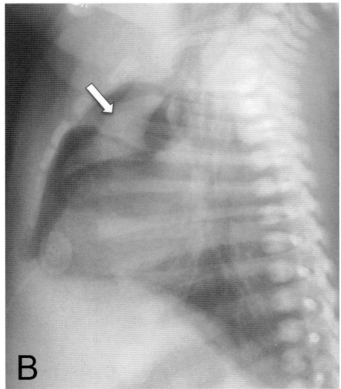

Figure 2.17 Newborn with mild respiratory distress. Note characteristic appearance of pneumomediastinum elevating the thymus (arrows) away from the mediastinum on both frontal (A) and lateral (B) views (courtesy of L. Varich).

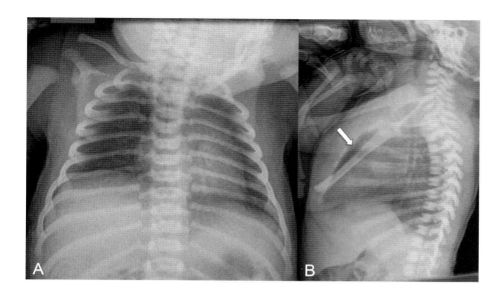

Figure 2.18 Newborn with respiratory distress and pneumothorax. (A) Frontal radiograph – there is subtle hyperlucent right lung especially medially, as well as an unusually sharp right hemidiaphragm. (B) The lateral view confirms free pleural air anteriorly (arrow).

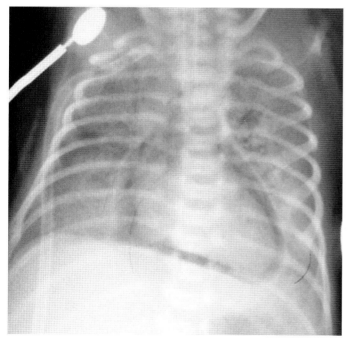

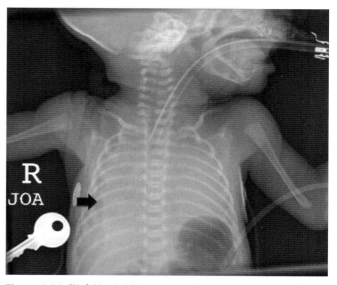

Figure 2.20 Skinfold mimicking pneumothorax in a premature infant with severe hyaline membrane disease. Skin folded under the infant (arrow) simulating the edge of a pneumothorax. If uncertain, obtain a cross-table lateral or a decubitus view for confirmation with the side in question up.

Figure 2.19 Ventilated newborn infant with airleak including perihilar interstitial emphysema and pneumopericardium. Note the air completely surrounding the heart (courtesy of L. Varich).

or in utero intra- or extrathoracic compression including congenital diaphragmatic hernia, most often left sided (Figure 2.13), large bronchopulmonary malformation or pleural effusion (usually chylothorax) (Figure 2.23). Bilateral pulmonary hypoplasia is likewise associated with in utero chest restriction including oligohydramnios (most often with severe renal dysfunction or agenesis) (Figure 2.5), abnormal chest wall (e.g. asphyxiating thoracic dystrophy), decreased pulmonary blood flow and

decreased respiratory motion in utero (e.g. amyotonia congenita) (Figure 2.4). On occasion pulmonary hypoplasia is idiopathic or associated with primary lung maldevelopment as in alveolar capillary dysplasia. PPHN is a common and often life-threatening component of pulmonary hypoplasia.

Bronchopulmonary malformations and other pulmonary masses

Pulmonary masses are uncommon in infants. By far the most common lesions are the bronchopulmonary malformations including CPAM, congenital lobar overinflation (CLO)/

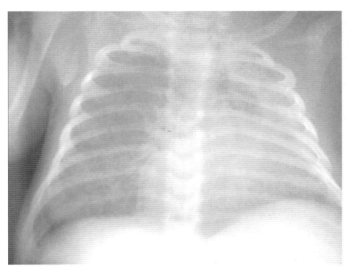

Figure 2.21 Left lung agenesis. Note marked left-sided mediastinal shift with herniation of the right lung across the midline and an underdeveloped left chest wall. Compare with mediastinal shift in atelectasis (Figure 2.15).

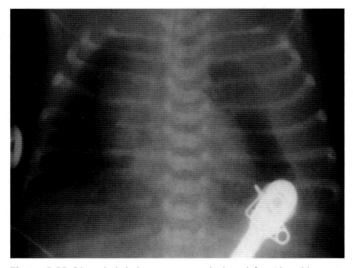

Figure 2.23 Bilateral chylothorax more marked on left, with mild contralateral shift.

bronchial atresia (Figures 2.10, 2.24), pulmonary sequestration and bronchogenic cyst. These entities are likely the spectrum of an obstruction malformation complex with in utero airway obstruction, most often bronchial atresia, at varying stages of lung development, with subsequent dysplastic and cystic lung changes. While they differ somewhat in their typical appearance, there is considerable imaging and pathological overlap with many hybrid lesions containing features of more than one entity, especially the small cyst form of CPAM and pulmonary sequestration. Many of these are now discovered and followed in utero with ultrasound or MR imaging (Figure 2.24). They frequently peak in size in the second trimester and get progressively smaller to the point where they

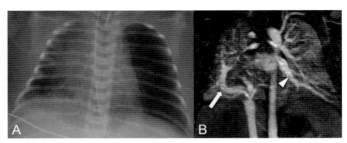

Figure 2.22 One-week-old infant with persistent respiratory distress. (A) Chest radiograph with small-volume, partially opacified right lung, persistent on all radiographs since birth. (B) Scimitar syndrome shown on coronal MIP (maximal intensity projection) MRA with a small right lung and scimitar-shaped right pulmonary vein draining anomalously to the IVC (arrow). Note the normal left pulmonary venous drainage to the left atrium (arrowhead). (Reproduced with permission from Springer Science and Business Media: *Pediatric Radiology*, Congenital bronchopulmonary foregut malformations: concepts and controversies, volume 8, 2006, p. 773, Figure 2.10.)

may be extremely subtle on postnatal radiographs and only visible on CT (Figure 2.24). They have a variable radiographic appearance, usually of a small or large cystic or solid-appearing mass. CT imaging is often performed to provide detailed anatomy; important features to evaluate are size, location, presence and size of cysts, bronchial atresia/mucoid impaction, connection to airway, systemic arterial supply, and other anomalies including multiple lesions, GI connection, cardiac, laryngotracheal, vascular and bone abnormalities. Many of these lesions are removed surgically, although there is an increasing tendency to treat them conservatively if they are asymptomatic, especially the lesions that have typical imaging features of CLO, bronchial atresia or sequestration. The bronchopulmonary malformation lesions may be a source of recurrent postnatal infection and there is concern about the possibility of malignant pleuropulmonary blastoma occurring in preexisting CPAM lesions. This connection has been reported in the literature in a very small number of cases; whether the lesions were originally benign or not is controversial.

Esophageal duplication and neurenteric cysts and the spectrum of congenital tracheoesophageal fistula (TEF) are also often included in the spectrum of bronchopulmonary malformations, and typically appear radiographically as a mediastinal mass or cyst or dilated air-filled esophageal pouch with or without distal fistula in the case of TEF (Figure 2.25).

Pulmonary neoplasms are extremely rare in neonates. There have been some reports of pulmonary or chest wall myofibroblastic tumors or fibrosarcoma, mesothelioma and pleuropulmonary blastoma, the last usually a predominantly cystic mass in infants, radiographically almost indistinguishable in appearance from large cyst CPAM. Accompanying pneumothorax and solid nodules can be helpful in distinguishing features (Figure 2.26).

Mediastinal masses can produce respiratory symptoms by compressing the airway. These include bronchopulmonary cysts as well as cystic hygroma/lymphangioma and teratoma.

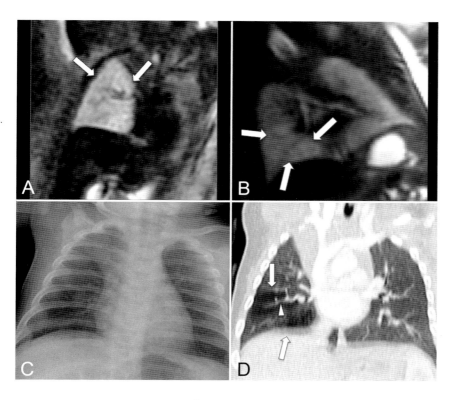

Figure 2.24 (A) Prenatal MR (coronal T2) at 22 weeks gestation demonstrates a large, high-signal right lung mass with (B) considerable reduction in size by 32 weeks (arrows). (C) Chest radiograph at birth demonstrates a subtle lucent area in the right lower lobe. (D) Coronal reconstruction from a CT demonstrates two areas of hyperlucent lung in the right lower lobe, corresponding well to the abnormality on MR (arrows). The larger hyperlucency contains linear branching mucoid impaction (arrowhead). Findings suggest multifocal segmental bronchial atresia.

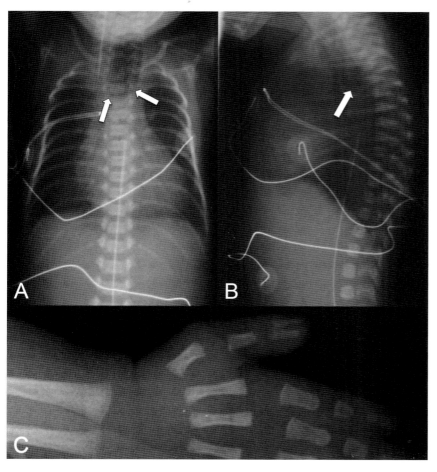

Figure 2.25 Newborn infant with respiratory distress and inability to pass a nasogastric tube. (A), (B) Frontal and lateral radiographs demonstrate the dilated air-filled pouch of esophageal atresia (arrows). Absence of air in the stomach indicates that there is no distal tracheoesophageal fistula. Tracheoesophageal fistula spectrum is frequently associated with other anomalies, termed the VACTERL association (vertebral, imperforate anus, cardiac, tracheoesophageal fistula, renal and limb anomalies). (C) Abnormal thumb with duplication of the distal phalanx. The infant also had a ventricular septal defect on cardiac echo.

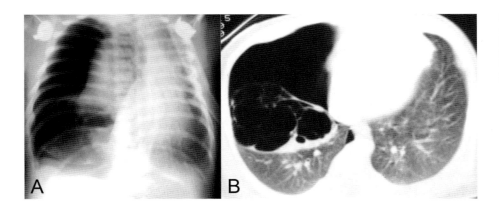

Figure 2.26 Two-week-old infant, previously well, with acute respiratory distress. The chest radiograph (A) demonstrates a large right pneumothorax with a lower lobe cystic lesion, confirmed at CT (B). The lesion was resected and on pathology proved to be a cystic pleuropulmonary blastoma.

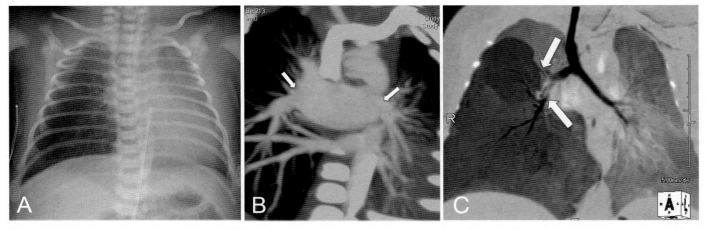

Figure 2.27 Newborn with respiratory distress. (A) Chest X-ray: there is abnormal pulmonary aeration with markedly overaerated right lung and contralateral mediastinal shift. There is soft tissue fullness in the right hilum. (B) CT angiogram at two days of age: a coronal MIP reconstruction demonstrates aneurysmally dilated central pulmonary arteries (arrows) compressing the airways; predominantly right upper lobe and bronchus intermedius as seen in the coronal MINIP (minimum intensity projection) reconstruction (C) (arrows). This CT appearance is characteristic of tetralogy of Fallot with absence of the pulmonary valve leaflets.

Vascular lesions, especially vascular rings and slings and aneurysmally enlarged vascular structures, may cause airway compressive symptoms (Figure 2.27) and abnormal pulmonary aeration with air-trapping or atelectasis.

Summary

There are many causes of respiratory problems in the newborn; only a few of them are represented here. Careful and thorough evaluation of newborn chest radiographs includes assessment of: tubes and lines; chest configuration and aeration; mediastinal shift; pattern and symmetry of pulmonary abnormality; cardiac silhouette and pulmonary vascularity; mediastinal, pleural, musculoskeletal and abdominal structures. The radiographic appearance should be correlated with clinical history and changes over time.

Further reading

Bulas D, Slovis TL Prenatal and neonatal imaging. In *Caffey's Pediatric Diagnostic Imaging*, ed. TL Slovis (Philadelphia: Mosby, 2008) pp. 73–138.

Cleveland RH (1995) A radiologic update on medical diseases of the newborn chest. *Pediatr Radiol* **25**, 631–7.

Kunisaki SM, Fauza DO, Nemes LP *et al.* (2006) Bronchial atresia: the hidden pathology within a spectrum of prenatally diagnosed lung masses. *J Pediatr Surg* **41**, 61–5.

Langston C (2003) New concepts in the pathology of congenital lung malformations. *Semin Pediatr Surg* **12**, 17–37.

Newman B (1999) Imaging of medical disease of the newborn lung. *Radiol Clin North Am* **37**, 1049–65.

Newman B (2006) Congenital bronchopulmonary foregut malformations: concepts and controversies. *Pediatr Radiol* **36**, 773–91.

Pumberger W, Hormann M, Deutinger J *et al.* (2003) Longitudinal observation of antenatally detected congenital lung malformations (CLM): natural history, clinical outcome and long-term follow-up. *Eur J Cardiothorac Surg* **24**, 703–11.

Swischuk LE Respiratory system. In *Imaging of the Newborn, Infant, and Young Child*, 4th edn., ed. LE Swischuk (Baltimore, MD: Williams and Wilkins, 1997) pp. 25–108.

2B NEONATAL ABDOMEN

Normal newborn gastrointestinal tract

The gastrointestinal tract begins its development and function in early fetal life. Ingestion of amniotic fluid along with intestinal mucosal secretions and sloughed cells contributes to the formation of meconium that is passed into the fetal colon.

The normal newborn gastrointestinal tract demonstrates a pattern quite distinct from that of the normal adult. Following an infant's first breath, air begins descending through the gastrointestinal tract (Figure 2.28). Air is seen to pass from the stomach through the small intestine and finally into the colon within approximately 24 hours of initial inspiration. The normal newborn pattern is that of "multiple polygons" or a "chicken-wire" appearance in which multiple, thin-walled loops of gas-filled bowel are present throughout the abdomen (Figure 2.29).

Abdominal distension, vomiting and failure to pass meconium represent the first signs of neonatal bowel obstruction or

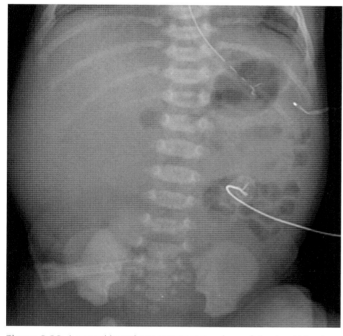

Figure 2.28 A normal bowel gas pattern at two hours following birth, demonstrating passage of air into the stomach and proximal small intestine. A paucity of gas in the right hemi-abdomen is due to lack of gas filling of the distal small bowel and should not be confused with a right-sided abdominal mass.

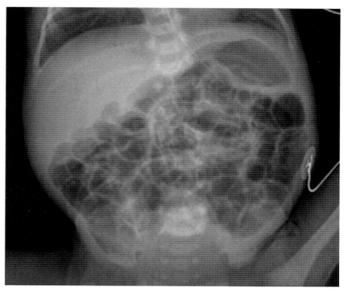

Figure 2.29 A normal bowel gas pattern at 24 hours. Gas is seen filling multiple intestinal loops throughout the abdomen, with the appearance of "multiple polygons." It is difficult to differentiate small from large intestine on radiographs in the newborn period.

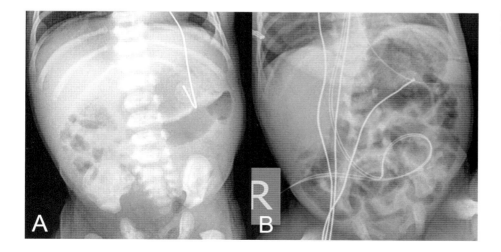

Figure 2.30 (A), (B) Early changes in necrotizing enterocolitis include separation and unfolding of bowel loops.

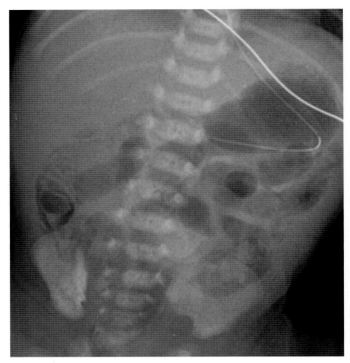

Figure 2.31 Linear pneumatosis is seen in the right lower quadrant of a patient with necrotizing enterocolitis.

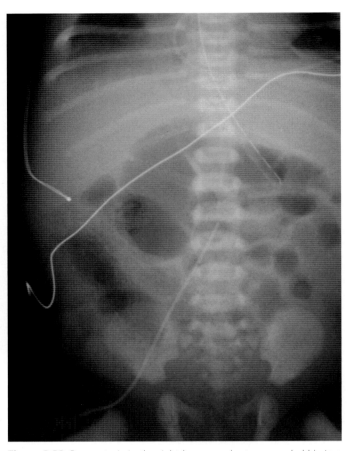

Figure 2.32 Pneumatosis in the right lower quadrant appears bubbly in a patient with necrotizing enterocolitis.

dysfunction. Etiological considerations vary depending on the gestational age of the baby. Evaluation of symptoms referable to the bowel in neonates includes plain radiography, with subsequent ultrasonography and fluoroscopy as required.

Necrotizing enterocolitis

In the premature infant, abdominal distension, gastric retention and vomiting can represent signs of necrotizing enterocolitis (NEC). The NEC pathological process is not thoroughly understood but is believed to result from a combination of bowel infection and ischemia. The earliest anatomical change is inflammation of the mucosa and submucosa that can progress to full-thickness bowel wall involvement. Bowel thickening, therefore, is the earliest radiographic sign of NEC and is demonstrated by unfolding and separation of the bowel loops (Figure 2.30). With further NEC progression, bacteria from within the bowel lumen can invade into the bowel wall. These bacteria produce gas, giving the radiographic appearance of intramural gas (pneumatosis intestinalis), presenting in either a linear (Figure 2.31) or bubbly (Figure 2.32) pattern. Ultrasound can be beneficial in identifying bowel wall thickening and pneumatosis intestinalis, seen as echogenic foci within the bowel wall (Figure 2.33). Gas within the bowel wall can occasionally travel via the superior and inferior mesenteric veins into the portal venous system. Gas within the portal venous system is usually transient and can be visualized on

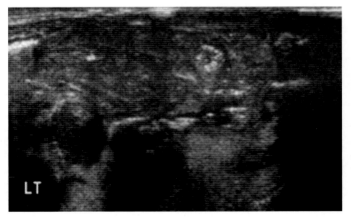

Figure 2.33 Pneumatosis appears as punctate echogenic foci circumferentially involving the bowel wall on ultrasound in a patient with necrotizing enterocolitis.

radiographs as lucent, linear branching structures within the periphery of the liver (Figure 2.34). Portal venous gas can also be identified by ultrasound as branching, echogenic structures within the portal triads of the liver (Figure 2.35). Continued involvement of the bowel by infection and ischemia can result in full-thickness bowel wall necrosis. Ultrasound can detect bowel wall thinning and lack of perfusion, suggestive of non-viable bowel that is at risk for perforation. In its most severe form, NEC can result in complete loss of bowel wall integrity, and perforation, with identifiable free air.

In cases of early NEC, prior to loss of bowel viability and perforation, medical management includes cessation of enteric feeding, total parenteral nutrition (TPN) administration, and antibiotics. In the presence of bowel perforation, emergent surgical management is required, with complete resection of all perforated and nonviable bowel. However, bowel-sparing treatment of perforation, utilizing early percutaneous drainage and avoidance of emergent bowel resection, is now being utilized.

The most common delayed complication of NEC is stricture formation. Strictures are most often identified at the splenic flexure of the colon but can occur throughout the large or small intestine.

Pneumoperitoneum

Pneumoperitoneum in the newborn is most frequently a result of bowel perforation secondary to spontaneous gastric perforation in infants with neonatal stress, iatrogenic rectal perforation, or necrotizing enterocolitis. Because the newborn is radiographed in the supine position, free air manifests as central lucency located within the upper abdomen, and is often seen overlying the liver. When there is a large amount of free air, a continuous diaphragm sign (intraperitoneal air extending across the undersurface of the diaphragm), Rigler's sign (both sides of the bowel wall defined by intraluminal and extraluminal gas), or the football sign (a large central lucency outlining the falciform ligament) may be identified (Figure 2.36). Lateral decubitus and

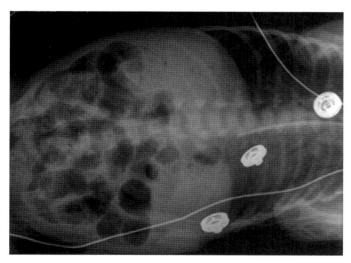

Figure 2.34 Left lateral decubitus examination demonstrates evidence of portal venous gas with linear lucencies seen in the liver of a patient with necrotizing enterocolitis. Also seen is pneumatosis within a bowel loop in the right and mid lower abdomen, compatible with NEC.

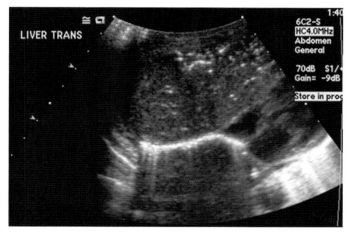

Figure 2.35 Portal venous gas on ultrasound appears linear, branching and echogenic, and conforms to the location of the portal triads in a patient with necrotizing enterocolitis.

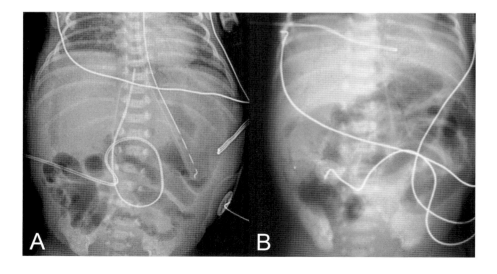

Figure 2.36 Two patients with necrotizing enterocolitis, bowel perforation and free abdominal air. (A) Perforation is evidenced by the football sign (lucency over the upper abdomen and outlining of the falciform ligament by air). (B) Perforation, apparent by an ill-defined lucency projecting on the liver. This patient also demonstrates pneumatosis in the right lower quadrant, and portal venous gas.

cross-table lateral examinations are more sensitive for identifying free air, and are often performed adjunctively to the supine view in this clinical setting.

Neonatal bowel obstruction

Newborn infants who present with symptoms of bowel obstruction should initially be evaluated by plain radiographs. The major initial key radiographic determination will be whether a high or low obstruction is present, and this differentiation will guide further imaging. In patients with a high obstruction, little additional radiological evaluation (if a midgut volvulus is suspected) or no further imaging (if midgut volvulus is not suspected) is required, and surgical intervention provides the diagnosis. Patients with suspected low intestinal obstruction require additional imaging utilizing a contrast enema, which itself may be therapeutic.

High obstruction

Patients with high gastrointestinal obstruction (defined as obstruction occurring proximal to the mid-jejunum) often present with vomiting, and their radiographs will demonstrate few (usually three or fewer) dilated loops of small bowel. The differential diagnosis of high neonatal bowel obstruction

includes midgut volvulus (MGV), duodenal atresia, duodenal stenosis, duodenal web, annular pancreas, and proximal jejunal atresia.

Patients with a classic "double-bubble" sign at birth and no evidence of distal gas are considered to have duodenal atresia, and no further radiological evaluation is required. If there are findings of duodenal obstruction with distal gas identified, the differential diagnosis includes MGV, duodenal stenosis, duodenal web, and annular pancreas. In this situation, where MGV is a possible etiology, an upper gastrointestinal (GI) series should be urgently obtained. Barium or nonionic isotonic water-soluble contrast medium can be administered orally. Hyperosmolar agents should never be used for evaluation of the upper gastrointestinal tract in infants because aspiration of these agents can result in massive pulmonary edema.

Cases of duodenal atresia represent the failure of bowel recanalization in the fetus. This obstruction is therefore complete and long-standing. The radiograph will demonstrate the classic double-bubble appearance, with a gas-filled, dilated stomach and duodenum (Figure 2.37). In duodenal atresia, the obstruction occurs in the second portion of the duodenum, in the region of the ampulla of Vater, and no gas will be visualized distal to the level of obstruction.

Duodenal atresia is the most severe entity in a spectrum of diseases that includes duodenal stenosis, duodenal web, and annular pancreas. These related entities usually cause incomplete obstruction and, therefore, demonstrate evidence of distal bowel gas and less duodenal distension on radiographs (Figure 2.38). Duodenal atresia and stenosis are associated with Down syndrome and the VACTERL sequence.

Midgut volvulus (MGV) is a life-threatening emergency in which the mesenteric root of the bowel is abnormally fixed,

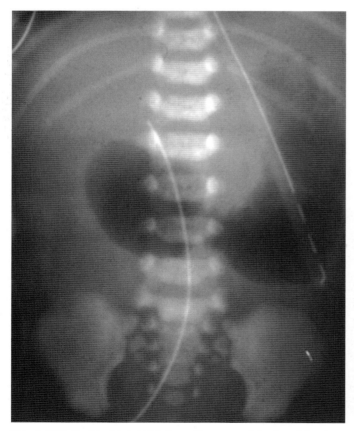

Figure 2.37 The "double-bubble" sign, with gaseous distension of the stomach and proximal duodenum in a patient with duodenal atresia.

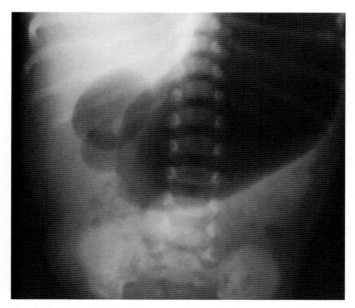

Figure 2.38 A double-bubble-type configuration is present in this patient with duodenal stenosis, but air is identified within distal bowel loops.

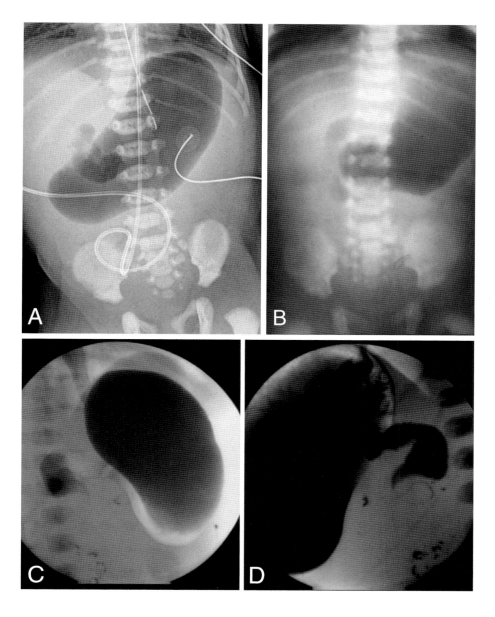

Figure 2.39 (A), (B) Two cases of midgut volvulus, with distension of the stomach and less distension of the duodenum than seen in cases of congenital duodenal obstruction. Small foci of distal air are seen in each case. (C), (D) Typical signs of MGV on an upper GI fluoroscopy with "beak sign" of the proximal duodenum (C) and "whirlpool sign" of the twisted bowel (D).

thereby making the entire mesenteric root prone to rotate around the mesenteric vasculature, resulting in bowel ischemia (see Chapter 5). As MGV produces acute obstruction at the mid-duodenum, it can be confused radiographically with congenital duodenal obstruction if MGV occurs in the neonatal period. Both entities can demonstrate a gas-distended stomach and duodenum. Differentiating features of MGV include a patient who is clinically very ill, a less dilated duodenum (as it has not been obstructed chronically), and the presence of distal gas (Figure 2.39).

Low obstruction

Abdominal distension and failure to pass meconium signal a lower intestinal tract obstruction (involving the distal jejunum, ileum or colon). Radiographs will demonstrate multiple loops of dilated bowel within the abdomen (Figure 2.40). The differential diagnosis of neonatal low bowel obstruction includes meconium ileus, ileal atresia, Hirschsprung disease and meconium plug syndrome.

Contrast enema studies are routinely performed for evaluation of low bowel obstruction. The preferred agent is an isotonic to mildly hypertonic water-soluble contrast agent that also has the therapeutic potential to relieve the obstructing meconium in patients with meconium ileus and meconium plug syndrome.

Meconium ileus is strongly associated with cystic fibrosis. In these infants, thick, inspissated secretions within the bowel lumen produce tenacious meconium that obstructs the distal ileum. Proximal to the obstruction, the small intestine is dilated and filled with meconium. The colon distal to the obstruction is unused and of extremely small caliber; this is

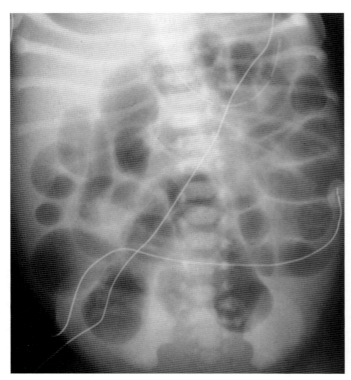

Figure 2.40 Multiple dilated loops of bowel are consistent with low (distal) bowel obstruction. A contrast enema should be performed.

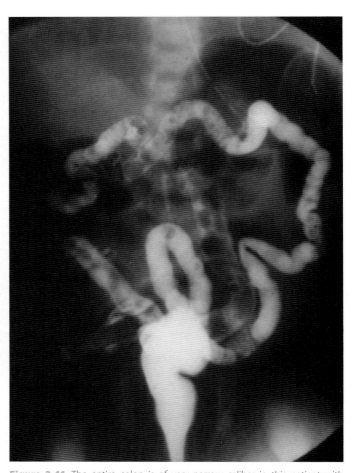

Figure 2.41 The entire colon is of very narrow caliber in this patient with microcolon.

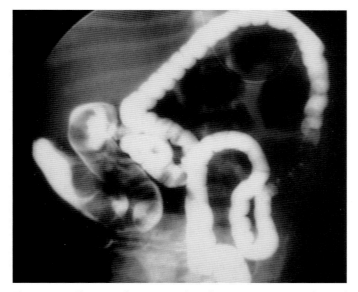

Figure 2.42 This case of meconium ileus demonstrates a microcolon and reflux of contrast into the dilated, obstructed and meconium-filled distal ileum.

called a "microcolon" (Figure 2.41). Microcolon is defined as involvement of the entire colon, with a luminal diameter on contrast enema of less than 1 cm. A microcolon signals a significant obstruction at the distal ileum, allowing little or no passage of meconium into the colon. A microcolon is therefore seen in cases of meconium ileus and ileal atresia. Meconium ileus may be "complicated" or "uncomplicated." In complicated cases, the obstructed and dilated segment may twist, resulting in volvulus. A volvulus can obstruct the blood supply, causing atresia, stenosis and perforation of the involved bowel segment. Abdominal radiographs in meconium ileus patients can demonstrate the classic bubbly appearance in the right lower quadrant, a result of the mixing of ingested air and meconium. On enema examination, a microcolon will be noted. Attempts should be made to reflux contrast into the obstructed small bowel loops. If contrast is passed in retrograde fashion into the dilated, obstructed and meconium-filled loops, the study may be both diagnostic and therapeutic (Figure 2.42). Often, multiple water-soluble contrast enema examinations are performed before relief of the obstruction is accomplished. In cases where contrast cannot be refluxed into the dilated segment, ileal atresia remains a diagnostic consideration. If relief of obstruction is not achieved, complicated meconium ileus should be suspected, and surgical exploration is warranted.

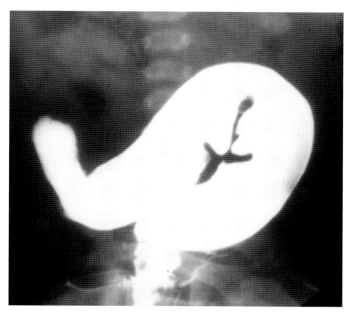

Figure 2.43 In this patient with Hirschsprung disease, the transition zone is apparent at the rectosigmoid junction, identified as a change in luminal caliber. The proximal, normally innervated colon is dilated. The distal noninnervated segment is of small caliber. The rectosigmoid index is abnormal.

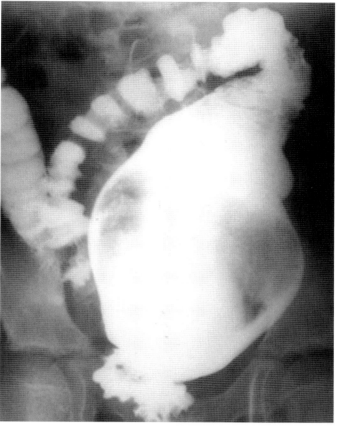

Figure 2.44 Hirschsprung disease diagnosed in a nine-year-old patient. The transition zone is well defined and seen within the distal sigmoid colon.

Jejunal and ileal atresia are conditions caused by in utero vascular insult leading to necrosis and resorption of the affected segment of bowel. The bowel loops proximal to the obstruction will appear dilated at birth. In cases of distal jejunal or ileal atresia, the colon will appear underused (microcolon); however, the bowel caliber will depend on the level of the obstruction. In proximal small bowel atresias, some secretions from the distal intestine pass into the colon, causing the colon to attain a more normal caliber. Conversely, distal ileal obstructions produce a very narrow caliber microcolon. In these cases, contrast enema will demonstrate a microcolon, but because there is discontinuity of the bowel, contrast will not be refluxed into the dilated segment proximal to the obstruction.

Hirschsprung disease is a common cause of neonatal bowel obstruction and is caused by arrest in the normal proximal-to-distal migration of the neural cell ganglia that populate the bowel wall. Because the distal ganglia are laid down last, the anus will always be involved in Hirschsprung disease. There may be proximal extension in a continuous fashion to involve a variable length of colon and even small intestine (termed "total colonic aganglionosis"). Lack of innervation results in an absence of normal peristalsis within the involved segment, leading to a functional obstruction. This condition presents clinically with a classic triad of symptoms in the neonatal period: delayed passage of meconium, vomiting and abdominal distension. If undiagnosed at birth, patients will suffer severe constipation and may present with severe and life-threatening enterocolitis and toxic megacolon later in life. Radiographs obtained shortly after birth will demonstrate

findings of distal bowel obstruction. In cases of Hirschsprung disease, the aganglionic segment is relatively normal in caliber. The more proximal, normally innervated bowel (proximal to the functional obstruction) will appear dilated. It is this change in caliber that is termed the "transition zone" and signals the change from normal to aganglionic bowel. Contrast enema is performed with the patient initially placed in the lateral position, with the goal of identifying a transition zone and evaluating the caliber of the rectum and sigmoid colon (Figure 2.43). Contrast is administered in a slow and controlled fashion to prevent overfilling of the colon and possible obscuration of the transition zone. The transition zone becomes more prominent with advancing patient age (Figure 2.44) and may be very difficult to identify in the newborn. In the newborn period, a more common finding is an abnormal "rectosigmoid index." This index is defined as the ratio of rectal-to-sigmoid caliber, and should always be greater than one in normal infants. In a child with Hirschsprung disease, the rectum will be narrower than the sigmoid colon, resulting in a rectosigmoid index of less than one (Figure 2.45). The definitive diagnosis is made by rectal wall biopsy and evaluation of intramural ganglia. Treatment consists of surgical resection of the abnormally innervated

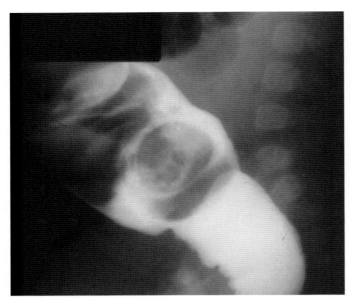

Figure 2.45 In this patient with Hirschsprung disease, the rectum is smaller than the sigmoid colon, resulting in an abnormal rectosigmoid index.

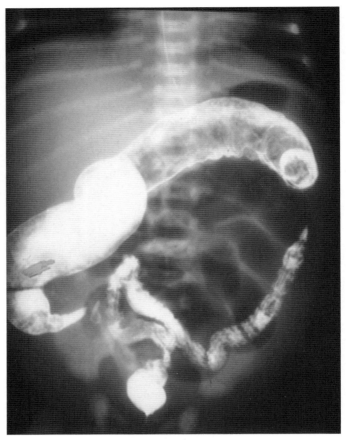

Figure 2.46 There is a change in caliber of the colon at the splenic flexure in this meconium plug syndrome patient. Filling defects within the colon are meconium plugs.

segment and a "pull-through" procedure to maintain bowel continuity.

Meconium plug syndrome is a disorder of "immaturity" of the colon that results in a functional obstruction at the splenic flexure. This condition is associated with maternal diabetes, prematurity and maternal drug intake (including magnesium sulfate for eclampsia). Contrast enema examination will demonstrate a change in caliber of the colon at the splenic flexure. The distal colon will appear narrow and can have meconium plugs within it. Colon proximal to the splenic flexure will be dilated and distended with meconium (Figure 2.46). This condition may be confused with Hirschsprung disease in which the transition zone is present at the splenic flexure; however, meconium plug syndrome differs in that the rectum appears distensible and patient symptoms should resolve in hours to days following enema examination.

Meconium peritonitis and pseudocyst

Conditions of the bowel that cause perforation in utero can result in the development of intraperitoneal calcifications. The meconium spilled into the peritoneal cavity following in utero bowel perforation incites an inflammatory reaction that leads to calcification. The calcification can be seen at birth along the serosal surfaces of the abdomen and can extend through the patent processus vaginalis into the scrotum, causing calcified scrotal masses. If the perforated and necrotic segment of bowel is walled-off by the inflammatory process, a focal calcified mass (meconium pseudocyst) can develop (Figure 2.47).

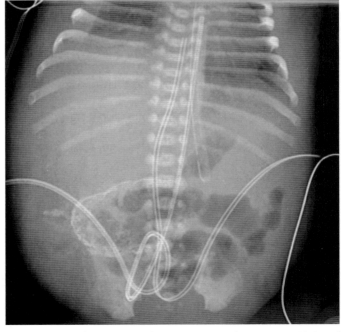

Figure 2.47 In this patient with meconium pseudocyst, an ovoid rim of calcification is visible within the right lower quadrant.

Further reading

Epelman M, Daneman A, Navarro OM *et al.* (2007) Necrotizing enterocolitis: review of state-of-the-art imaging findings with pathologic correlation. *Radiographics* **27**, 285–305.

Kirks DR *Practical Pediatric Imaging*, 3rd edn. (Philadelphia: Lippincott-Raven, 1998).

Lewis NA, Levitt MA, Zallen GS *et al.* (2003) Diagnosing Hirschsprung's disease: increasing the odds of a positive rectal biopsy result. *J Pediatr Surg* **38**, 412–6.

Martucciello G (2008) Hirschsprung's disease, one of the most difficult diagnoses in pediatric surgery: a review of the problems from clinical practice to the bench. *Eur J Pediatr Surg* **18**, 140–9.

Moss RL, Dimmitt RA, Barnhart DC *et al.* (2006) Laparotomy versus peritoneal drainage for necrotizing enterocolitis and perforation. *N Engl J Med* **354**, 2225–34.

Slovis TL *Caffey's Pediatric Diagnostic Imaging*, 11th edn. (St. Louis: Mosby, 2007).

Chapter 3

Congenital cardiac malformations

Alison Meadows

Introduction

Relatively recent advances in pediatric cardiovascular surgery, catheter-based interventional therapies, intensive care and medical management have dramatically changed the landscape of the field of congenital heart disease (CHD). The complexity of the anatomy and physiology of patients surviving with CHD is increasing exponentially, and the majority will survive to adulthood. These changes are placing new demands on imaging to diagnose and plan medical management. There are a number of imaging modalities available to the clinician and radiologist when it comes to these evaluations. The primary modalities, and the ones highlighted in this chapter, include the chest X-ray (CXR), echocardiography, cardiac catheterization with X-ray angiography, cardiac magnetic resonance imaging (MRI) and cardiac CT angiography (CTA).

The following chapter is divided into (1) left-to-right shunt lesions: atrial septal defects (ASDs), ventricular septal defects (VSDs), patent ductus arteriosus (PDA), common atrioventricular canal defects (CAVCs) and partial anomalous pulmonary venous return (PAPVR); (2) obstructive lesions: coarctation of the aorta (CoA); (3) cyanotic lesions: tetralogy of Fallot (TOF), truncus arteriosus (TA), D-transposition of the great arteries (D-TGA), total anomalous pulmonary venous return (TAPVR) and the univentricular heart, and finally, (4) great vessel anomalies: aortic rings and pulmonary artery slings. For each defect, the anatomy, physiology, natural history and approach to repair are briefly discussed before presenting diagnostic imaging examples.

Left-to-right shunt lesions

Atrial septal defects

Isolated secundum atrial septal defect (ASD) occurs in 5–10% of all CHD, and about 30–50% of children with CHD have an ASD. ASDs occur twice as frequently in females. There are four types of atrial septal defect; these include secundum ASDs, sinus venosus defects, primum ASDs and coronary sinus defects (Figure 3.1).

Secundum ASDs are the most common, accounting for 50–70% of all ASDs. Secundum ASDs are the result of a defect in the septum primum; the tissue that covers the fossa ovalis (Figures 3.2, 3.3).

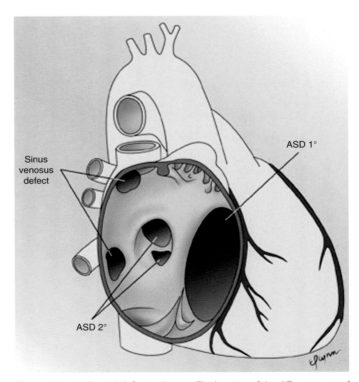

Figure 3.1 Atrial septal defect – diagram. The location of the different types of atrial septal defect (ASD) are demonstrated. Secundum ASDs (ASD 2°) are the result of fenestrations in, or deficiency of, septum primum. Primum ASDs (ASD 1°) represent deficiencies in the endocardial cushion portion of the atrial septum. Sinus venosus ASDs occur at the junction of the superior vena cava with the right atrium, or less frequently, at the junction of the inferior vena cava with the right atrium. *From the Multimedia Library of Congenital Heart Disease, Children's Hospital, Boston, MA, editor Robert Geggel, MD,* www.childrenshospital.org/mml/cvp *with permission.*

Essentials of Pediatric Radiology, ed. Heike E. Daldrup-Link and Charles A. Gooding. Published by Cambridge University Press.
© Cambridge University Press 2010.

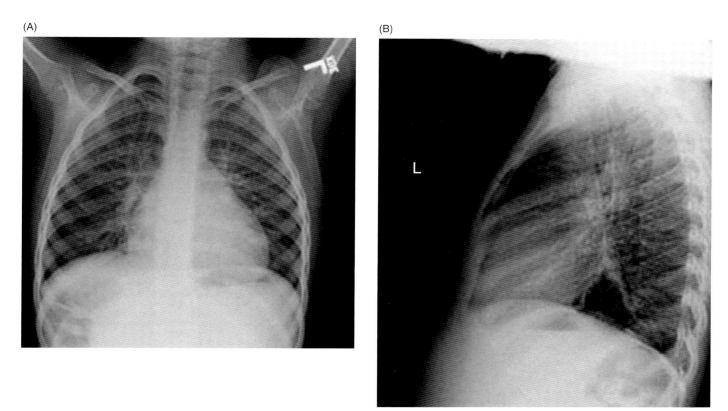

Figure 3.2 Atrial septal defect – chest X-ray. (A) Anteroposterior CXR in a young child with a large ASD reveals mild cardiomegaly and increased pulmonary vascular markings. (B) Lateral CXR reveals enlargement of the right ventricle with opacification of the retrosternal space.

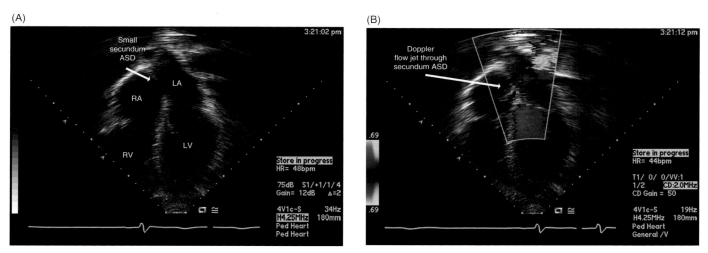

Figure 3.3 Secundum atrial septal defect – echocardiogram. Apical four-chamber view of the atrial septum (A) with and (B) without Doppler in a patient with a small secundum ASD. The right ventricle is normal in chamber size. Echocardiogram is still the gold standard for diagnosing this defect.

Isolated primum ASDs account for 15% of all ASDs. They are the result of an endocardial cushion defect. These defects are usually quite large as both the atrial and ventricular septae are deficient (Figure 3.4). A primum ASD differs from a complete atrioventricular canal defect in that the atrioventricular valve tissue is displaced downward to attach to the crest of the septum, thus minimizing intraventricular shunt. There is, however, still deficiency of both the atrial and ventricular septae. Primum ASDs are commonly associated with a cleft mitral valve.

Sinus venosus defects account for approximately 10% of all ASDs; most commonly they are of the superior vena cava (SVC) type located at the entry of the superior vena cava into the right atrium. Occasionally they occur at the entrance of the inferior vena cava to the right atrium. This defect is almost always associated with anomalous drainage of the right upper

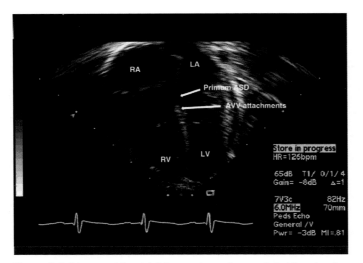

Figure 3.4 Primum atrial septal defect – echocardiogram. Apical four-chamber view in this patient with a primum atrial septal defect. There is deficiency of both the atrial and ventricular septum (endocardial cushion defect); however, there is no intraventricular shunt because the atrioventricular valve (AVV) leaflets are displaced downward and attached to the crest of the ventricular septum. As a result, the atrioventricular valves are attached in the same plane, characteristic of this defect.

and sometimes right middle pulmonary veins into the superior vena cava (Figure 3.5).

A coronary sinus defect is quite rare. It occurs when there is unroofing of the coronary sinus leading to direct communication between the coronary sinus and the left atrium. The os of the coronary sinus then allows free communication between the atria. The physiology is similar to other atrial septal defects.

Physiology of ASDs

The physiology of ASDs is that of a left-to-right shunt. What determines the degree of shunting is the size of the defect and the relative compliance of the right and left ventricles.

Imaging diagnosis

Chest X-rays do not show any abnormality in the case of relatively small ASDs. Relatively large ASDs may be associated with an increased heart size, especially involving the right ventricle (Figure 3.2). The pulmonary vascularity may be increased and the aortic knob is typically small. Transthoracic *echocardiography* directly diagnoses an atrial septal defect, and color flow imaging

(A)

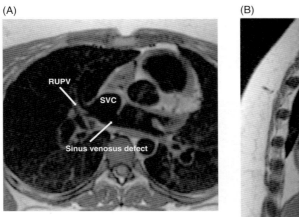

(B)

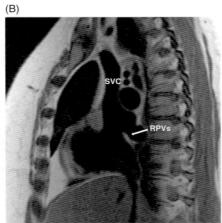

Figure 3.5 Sinus venosus defect – MRI. (A) Axial black blood imaging of a superior sinus venosus defect. The right upper pulmonary vein (RUPV) is shown to drain into the superior vena cava (SVC) at the location of the intra-arterial communication. (B) Sagittal oblique black blood imaging of the same defect. The confluence of the right pulmonary veins (RPVs) and the superior vena cava (SVC) at the intra-atrial communication is demonstrated.

(A)

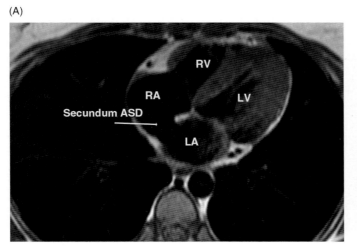

(B)

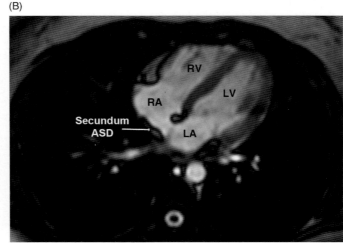

Figure 3.6 Secundum atrial septal defect – MRI. (A) Axial black blood imaging of a secundum septal defect. (B) Axial bright blood cine image of the same secundum septal defect. There is mild right ventricular enlargement.

(A)

(B)

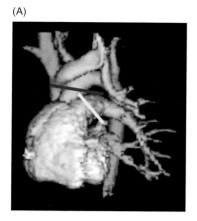

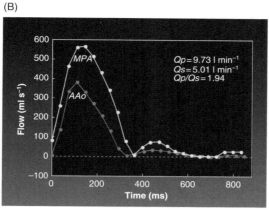

Figure 3.7 Atrial septal defect – MRI. MR phase-contrast (velocity-encoding) techniques can be used to measure flow across a vessel or valve of interest. In atrial septal defects, the decision to close the defect is determined by the presence of right ventricular enlargement and a pulmonary-to-systemic flow ratio ($Q_p : Q_s$) of greater than 1.5 : 1. (A) Planes of flow image acquisition perpendicular to the direction of flow in the main pulmonary artery (MPA; yellow) and ascending aorta (AAo; pink). (B) Graph of the net flows demonstrating a pulmonary-to-systemic flow ratio of greater than 1.9 : 1. Q_p = pulmonary blood flow; Q_s = systemic blood flow (or cardiac output).

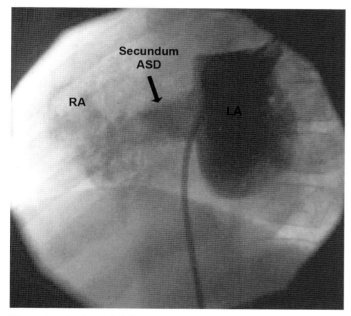

Figure 3.8 Atrial septal defect – angiography. Depicted is a still image of an angiogram with a catheter across the atrial septum and positioned in the left atrium. Contrast crosses the atrial septum into the right atrium.

may visualize a jet of blood from the left atrium (LA) to the right atrium (RA) (Figures 3.3, 3.4). MR or CT also directly visualize the septal defect and may show associated anomalous drainage of right pulmonary veins into the superior vena cava (Figures 3.5, 3.6). MR phase-contrast (velocity-encoding) techniques can be used to measure flow across a vessel or valve of interest (Figure 3.7). Angiography may be used to confirm the diagnosis and to determine the extent and direction of shunt hemo-dynamics (Figure 3.8).

Natural history of ASDs

Many secundum ASDs diagnosed in infants will close spontaneously. In fact, 100% of secundum ASDs < 3 mm, and 80%

of secundum ASDs between 3 and 8 mm will close spontaneously. ASDs > 8 mm rarely close on their own. Primum ASDs, sinus venosus defects and coronary sinus defects do not close spontaneously. Hemodynamically significant ASDs (left-to-right shunt greater than 1.5 : 1) can lead to right ventricular failure and atrial arrhythmias if left unrepaired. Rarely, patients with large ASDs will develop pulmonary arterial hypertension (PAH) and ultimately reversal of shunt (Eisenmenger physiology).

Repair of ASDs

Many secundum ASDs can be closed percutaneously with septal occluder devices. The exceptions are when there are deficient rims or the defect is too large. All other hemodynamically significant ASDs require surgical closure.

Ventricular septal defects

Ventricular septal defects (VSDs) are the most common form of CHD accounting for 15–20% of all CHD, not including VSDs associated with more complex CHD. There are a number of different types of VSD, including membranous VSDs, muscular VSDs, inlet (atrioventricular canal-type) VSDs and outlet (infundibular) VSDs (Figure 3.9).

Membranous VSDs are the most common form of VSD, accounting for approximately 70% of all VSDs. The membranous septum is a small portion of the septum just below the aortic valve. Defects in the membranous septum frequently extend beyond the membranous septum into the inlet septum, muscular septum or outlet septum, and thus are frequently referred to as "perimembranous" VSDs.

Outlet VSDs are rarer and account for only 5–7% of all VSDs (although they are more common in the Far Eastern countries). They occur in the infundibulum just beneath the aortic and pulmonary valves and thus are frequently termed supracristal, conal, or subarterial VSDs. The right coronary cusp of the aortic valve often prolapses into this defect, warranting closure even if the shunt is small.

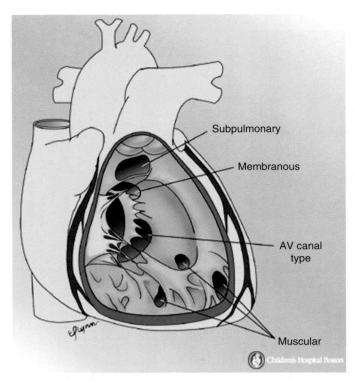

Figure 3.9 Ventricular septal defect – diagram. The location of the different types of ventricular septal defect (VSD) is demonstrated. Subpulmonary VSDs are caused by deficiency of the conal septum. Membranous VSDs are defects in the membranous septum and are located behind the septal leaflet of the tricuspid valve. Atrioventricular (AV) canal-type defects are caused by deficiency of the endocardial cushion portion of the ventricular septum. Muscular VSDs can occur in any portion of the muscular septum. The diagram does not depict malalignment defects (see Tetralogy of Fallot section). *From the Multimedia Library of Congenital Heart Disease, Children's Hospital, Boston, MA, editor Robert Geggel, MD, www.childrenshospital.org/mml/cvp with permission.*

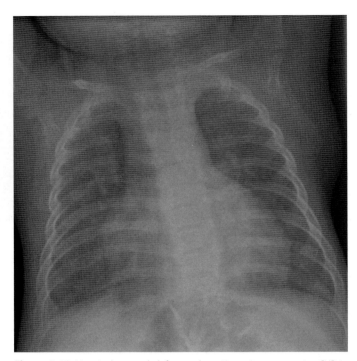

Figure 3.10 Ventricular septal defect – chest X-ray. Anteroposterior CXR in a young child with a large VSD reveals cardiomegaly and pulmonary edema.

Inlet VSDs account for 5–8% of all VSDs. They occur posterior and inferior to the membranous septum just below the septal leaflet of the tricuspid valve.

Muscular VSDs account for 5–20% of all VSDs. Muscular VSDs are further separated into central, marginal and apical defects. Apical muscular VSDs are difficult to visualize and repair. Marginal muscular VSDs are usually multiple and tortuous. Muscular VSDs are frequently multiple.

Physiology of VSDs

The physiology of VSDs is that of a left-to-right shunt. The amount of shunt is determined by the size of the lesion and the ratio of systemic-to-pulmonary vascular resistance. Shunting occurs during ventricular systole. As a result, the left side of the heart is volume loaded, resulting in left atrial and left ventricular dilatation.

Imaging diagnosis

Chest X-rays are typically normal if the VSD is small. If the VSD is large, chest X-rays may show cardiomegaly, increased pulmonary vascularity and a pulmonary edema (Figure 3.10). The left atrium is often enlarged, which leads to an increased splaying of the carina with an angle of more than 90° between the main stem bronchi. The aortic knob is typically small. Echocardiography may provide more specific information concerning the type of defect as well as the extent and direction of shunt hemodynamics (Figures 3.11–3.13). Cine MR imaging can be used to identify and quantify flow jets associated with shunt lesions (Figure 3.14). Chronic, unrepaired VSD may result in right ventricular hypertrophy and Eisenmenger syndrome (Figure 3.15). Angiography is the gold standard for establishing the diagnosis (Figure 3.16).

Natural history of VSDs

VSDs can range from small, resulting in hemodynamically insignificant shunt, to large, resulting in congestive heart failure in infancy and pulmonary arterial hypertension if left unrepaired. Spontaneous closure occurs in 30–40% of patients with muscular and membranous VSDs during the first year of life. This obviously occurs more commonly in small defects. Inlet and outlet defects do not close spontaneously. Closure is indicated if there is a large right-to-left shunt leading to refractory congestive heart failure and/or failure to thrive in infancy or if the Qp : Qs ratio is greater than 2 : 1.

Repair of VSDs

Some VSDs can be closed percutaneously with septal occluder devices. These are limited to muscular VSDs and patch margin VSDs, and limited to a few centers that specialize in this procedure. The majority of VSDs, if deemed hemodynamically significant, require surgical closure. The surgical approach depends on the type and size of the defect.

(A)

(B)

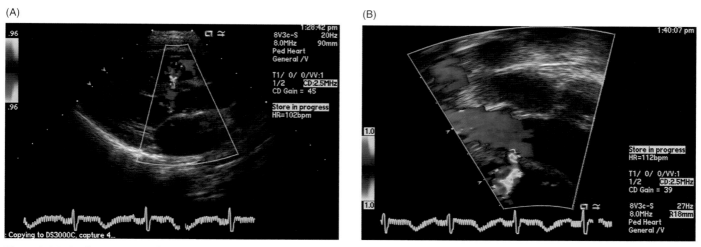

Figure 3.11 Membranous ventricular septal defect – echocardiogram. (A) Parasternal long axis and (B) apical four-chamber echocardiographic images in a patient with a membranous ventricular septal defect. Both images are colored with Doppler, demonstrating left-to-right flow during ventricular systole.

(A)

(B)

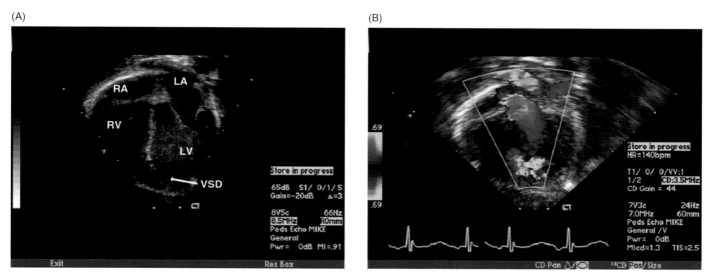

Figure 3.12 Muscular ventricular septal defect – echocardiogram. (A) Still frame in an apical four-chamber view of a muscular ventricular septal defect. (B) Same image with color Doppler applied to evaluate flow across the defect.

(A)

(B)

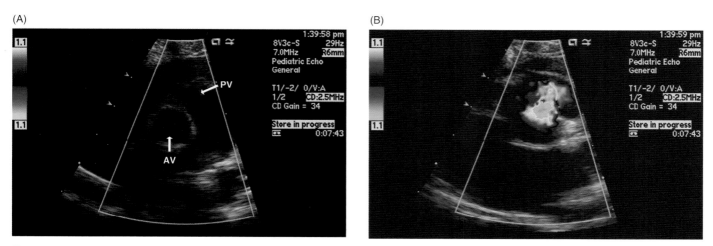

Figure 3.13 Subarterial (supracristal) ventricular septal defect – echocardiogram. (A) Parasternal short-axis view demonstrating the relationship between the aortic (AV) and pulmonary (PV) valves. (B) Doppler applied in the same plane demonstrates the ventricular septal defect in the infundibulum so that it is committed to both great vessels.

(A)

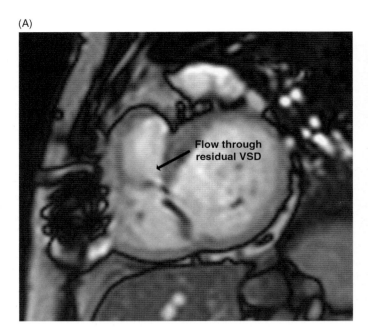

(B)

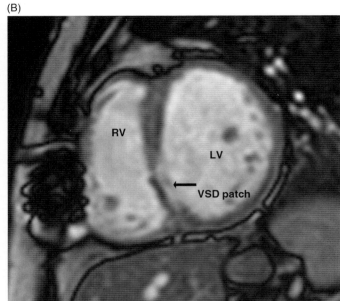

Figure 3.14 Patch margin ventricular septal defect – MRI. Cine MR imaging can be used to identify flow jets associated with shunt lesions, as demonstrated in this set of images. This patient underwent repair of a common atrioventricular canal defect as a youth, and now has a residual patch margin ventricular septal defect. The images represent a single plane in the short-axis plane across the right and left ventricle at two time points (systole and diastole). The patch is visualized as hypointense to the rest of the myocardium. (A) A flow jet is seen during systole. (B) A dilated left ventricle is seen at end diastole. By MR flow assessment, the pulmonary-to-systemic flow ratio was greater than 1.5 to 1, and closure was recommended.

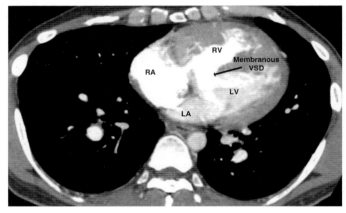

Figure 3.15 Membranous ventricular septal defect – CT scan. Axial contrast-enhanced CT image of a large unrepaired membranous VSD in an older man with Eisenmenger syndrome. There is right ventricular hypertrophy, as would be expected for a right ventricle experiencing chronic pressure overload.

Patent ductus arteriosus

Excluding premature infants, isolated patent ductus arteriosus (PDA) occurs in 5–10% of all CHD. The pathology is persistent patency of the ductus arteriosus; a normal vascular structure in the fetal heart, usually connecting the proximal left pulmonary artery to the descending aorta, that allows diversion of blood from the pulmonary vascular bed to the descending aorta.

Physiology of PDAs

The physiology of PDAs is that of left-to-right shunt. They produce left atrial and left ventricular volume overload and potentially pulmonary arterial pressure overload (Figures 3.17 and 3.18).

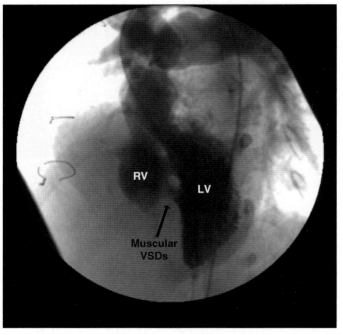

Figure 3.16 Multiple muscular ventricular septal defects – angiography. A lateral angiogram with contrast injection into the left ventricle reveals two jets of contrast flowing across two muscular VSDs.

Imaging diagnosis

Chest X-rays may be normal or show a cardiomegaly, increased pulmonary vascularity and a pulmonary edema. The left atrium is often enlarged, the aortic knob may be prominent and an enlarged ductus arteriosus may form a "ductus bump," a soft tissue shadow at the level of the aortic knob. Echocardiography may show a jet of ductal flow going into the proximal left pulmonary artery (Figure 3.19). Cine MR imaging may demonstrate the anatomy in more detail and provide additional functional information regarding shunt hemodynamics (Figure 3.20). CT scans, obtained for other reasons, may sometimes reveal calcifications in the area of the (usually closed) ductus, or incidental findings of a small open ductus (Figure 3.21). Angiography may confirm the diagnosis of an open ductus and may be used to place ductus closure devices in older patients via interventional procedures (Figure 3.22).

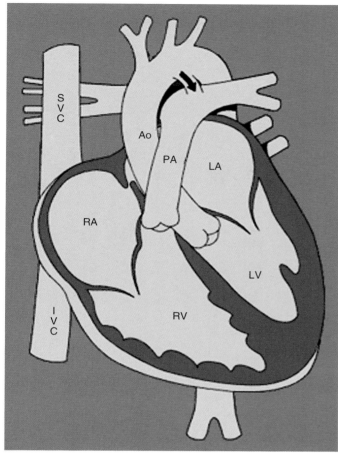

Figure 3.17 Patent ductus arteriosus – diagram. The patent ductus arteriosus (PDA) connects the aorta (Ao) and pulmonary artery (PA) and is associated with a left-to-right shunt (arrow). IVC = inferior vena cava; SVC = superior vena cava. *From the Multimedia Library of Congenital Heart Disease, Children's Hospital, Boston, MA, editor Robert Geggel, MD, www.childrenshospital.org/mml/cvp with permission.*

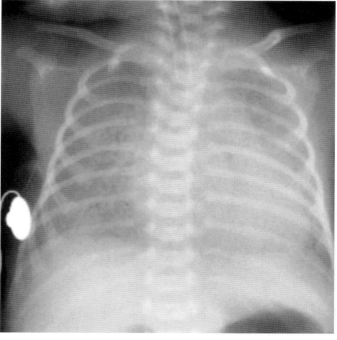

Figure 3.18 Patent ductus arteriosus – CXR. Anteroposterior CXR in a newborn with a patent ductus arteriosus. There is cardiomegaly (enlargement of the left atrium and left ventricle) as well as increased pulmonary vascular markings.

(A)

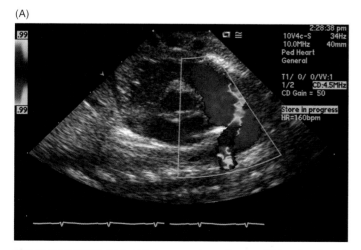

(B)

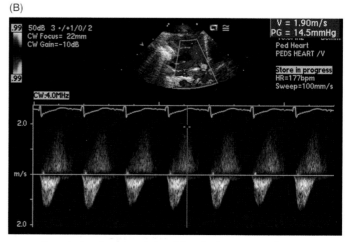

Figure 3.19 Patent ductus arteriosus – echocardiogram. (A) Imaging from the suprasternal notch showing a jet of ductal flow (red) going into the proximal left pulmonary artery (blue). (B) Pressure gradient measured by Doppler is only 14 mmHg, suggesting this is an unrestrictive patent ductus arteriosus.

(A)

(B)

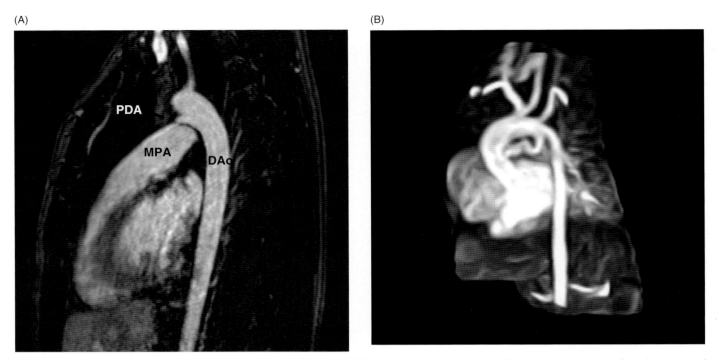

Figure 3.20 Patent ductus arteriosus – MRI. (A) Cine imaging in the sagittal oblique plane demonstrating a small patent ductus arteriosus from the isthmus of the descending aorta (DAo) to the left pulmonary artery in a young teen. (B) Gadolinium-enhanced 3D MIP MRA image of a tortuous patent ductus arteriosus in a newborn. MPA = main pulmonary artery.

(A)

(B)

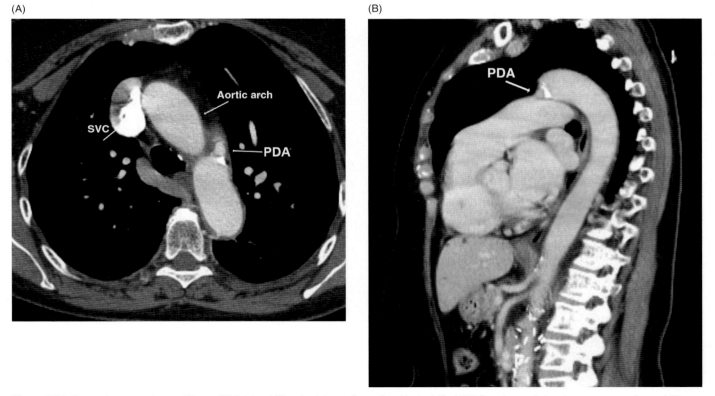

Figure 3.21 Patent ductus arteriosus – CT scan. (A) Axial and (B) sagittal views of a small residual calcified PDA found serendipitously on contrast-enhanced CT scan. SVC = superior vena cava.

Natural history of PDAs

In full-term infants, PDAs typically do not close spontaneously. When small and restrictive, PDAs are asymptomatic. Rarely, bacterial endocarditis can occur. Large and unrestrictive PDAs result in torrential pulmonary blood flow and systemic pulmonary arterial pressures and, ultimately, left heart dilatation and congestive heart failure, early, with the development of pulmonary arterial hypertension and Eisenmenger physiology later. There is debate about indications for closure in small PDAs for the prevention of endocarditis. Large PDAs should be closed to prevent the aforementioned complications.

Repair of PDAs

In premature infants, PDA closure may be achieved via indomethacin (indometacin) treatment. If indomethacin treatment

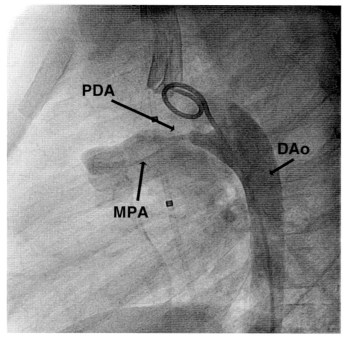

Figure 3.22 Patent ductus arteriosus – angiography. Angiogram with injection via a catheter in the descending aorta (DAo) demonstrates opacification of a small ductus arteriosus and main pulmonary artery (MPA).

does not result in closure, PDAs are usually closed via an external clip, placed via endoscopic procedures. In older patients, transcatheter approaches are usually preferred for the closure of PDAs, although surgery is still available for large PDAs not amenable to percutaneous closure.

Complete common atrioventricular canal defects

Complete common atrioventricular canal defects (CAVC) or complete endocardial cushion defects occur in 2% of all CHD. Approximately 30% of all children born with CAVC have Down syndrome, and CAVC defects account for 40% of all defects associated with Down syndrome (Figure 3.23).

The pathology associated with this type of defect includes defects in the tissue derived from the endocardial cushions, including the inferior portion of the atrial septum, inlet portion of the ventricular septum, and atrioventricular valves. A partial endocardial cushion defect, or primum ASD, occurs when there is deficient atrial and ventricular septal tissue, but the atrioventricular valves are displaced downward to attach to the crest of the ventricular septum such that there is no interventricular shunt (see description in ASD section). A complete endocardial cushion defect consists of a common atrioventricular valve with both interatrial and interventricular communication with varying degrees of valve leaflet attachments to the ventricular septum.

In the majority of cases, the atrioventricular valves are equally committed to the two ventricles (balanced CAVC). CAVC defects associated with Down syndrome are almost always balanced. More rarely, the atrioventricular valves are committed to one or the other ventricle while the other is hypoplastic. Associated lesions such as tetralogy of Fallot and PDA occur in 10% of all cases.

Physiology of CAVC

The physiology associated with a CAVC is that of a left-to-right shunt with both right- and left-sided volume overload. The degree of chamber enlargement is complex and determined by multiple factors including the size of the defect, the amount of atrial level shunting and ventricular level shunting, the compliance of the ventricles, and the ratio of systemic to pulmonary vascular resistance.

(A)

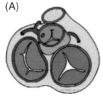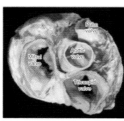

(B)

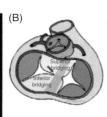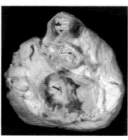

(C)

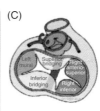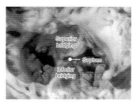

Figure 3.23 Common atrioventricular canal defect – diagram. Depicted in this diagram are (A) the normal atrioventricular valves, and the atrioventricular valves in partial (B) and complete (C) endocardial cushion defects (viewed from above). *From the Multimedia Library of Congenital Heart Disease, Children's Hospital, Boston, MA, editor Robert Geggel, MD, www.childrenshospital.org/mml/cvp with permission.*

Imaging diagnosis

Chest X-rays may reveal cardiomegaly of all four chambers as well as increased pulmonary vascular markings and a pulmonary edema (Figure 3.24). Echocardiography demonstrates the atrial and ventricular septal defects as well as the common atrioventricular valve (Figure 3.25). Cine MR imaging may reveal crowding of the left ventricular outflow tract, commonly referred to as the "gooseneck deformity", which is the result of an anterior displacement of the aorta and main pulmonary artery (Figure 3.26). Angiography may provide further detail regarding shunt hemodynamics (Figure 3.27).

Natural history of CAVC

Heart failure occurs within the first one to two months of birth in most infants with CAVC defects. Prognosis in unrepaired disease is poor, with most dying before the age of three years and others developing pulmonary arterial hypertension within the first year. For this reason, surgical repair in infancy is recommended. Usually, complete repair is recommended as an initial strategy. Pulmonary artery banding as a palliative first step is reserved for patients with complex valve leaflet attachments and mild ventricular size discrepancies. Unbalanced CAVC defects usually require a staged surgical approach to a Fontan procedure in which the common ventricle is used as the systemic pump and the systemic venous return is directed passively to the lungs.

Partial anomalous pulmonary venous return

Partial anomalous pulmonary venous return (PAPVR), as an isolated lesion, occurs in approximately 1% of all CHD

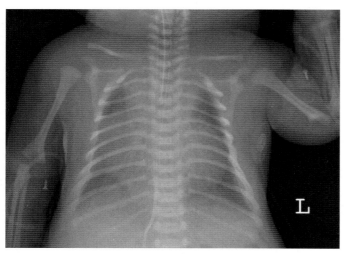

Figure 3.24 Common atrioventricular canal defect – chest X-ray. Anteroposterior CXR in a newborn with a common atrioventricular canal defect reveals cardiomegaly of all four chambers as well as increased pulmonary vascular markings.

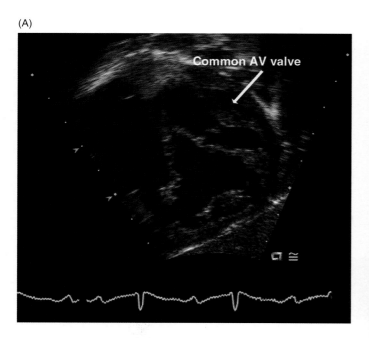

(A)

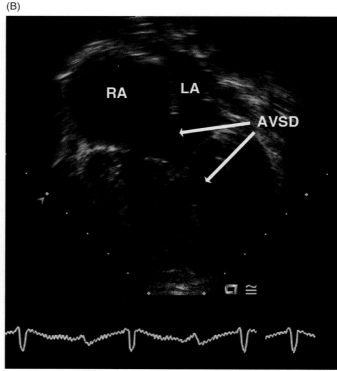

(B)

Figure 3.25 Common atrioventricular canal defect – echocardiogram. (A) Echocardiogram in the parasternal short-axis view demonstrates a common atrioventricular (AV) valve. (B) The apical four-chamber view demonstrates the atrial and ventricular septal defects (AVSD) associated with a common atrioventricular canal defect.

(A)

(B)

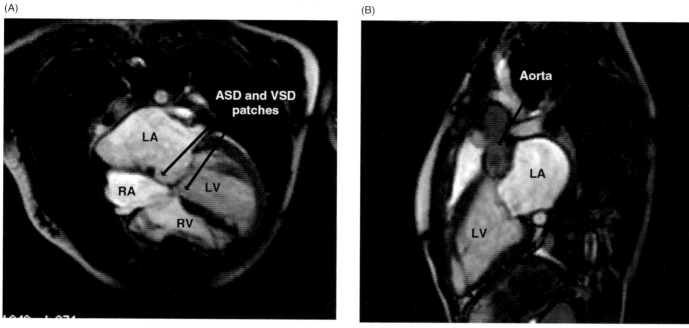

Figure 3.26 Common atrioventricular canal defect – MRI. Common atrioventricular canal defect following repair. (A) Four-chamber cine image demonstrates the attachments of the atrioventricular valves at the same level, which is typical post-repair. (B) Three-chamber cine image demonstrates crowding of the left ventricular outflow tract, commonly referred to as the "gooseneck deformity", which is the result of the anterior displacement of the aorta and main pulmonary artery given the arrested formation of the atrioventricular canal.

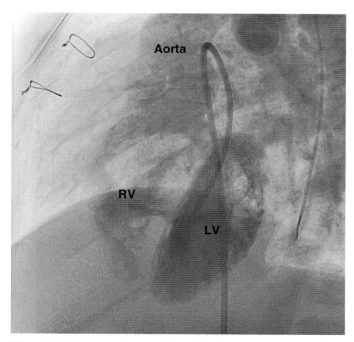

Figure 3.27 Common atrioventricular canal defect – angiography. Depicted is a lateral angiogram via a catheter in the left ventricle (the catheter course is IVC to RA through ASD into LV). The common atrioventricular valve is visualized. The large ventricular septal defect component of the endocardial cushion defect allows opacification of the right ventricle and aorta (transposed great vessels). The pulmonary artery is opacified, but does not arise from either ventricle (pulmonary atresia with a shunt).

(Figure 3.28). The pathology is the persistence of fetal pulmonary venous drainage into the right atrium directly or via the systemic veins. Right-sided PAPVR is more common than left-sided PAPVR (2 : 1). The right pulmonary veins can drain either into the superior vena cava (SVC) or inferior vena cava (IVC). PAPVR to the SVC is often associated with a sinus venosus defect (intra-atrial communication). PAPVR to the IVC is associated with Scimitar syndrome. The other components of Scimitar syndrome include intact atrial septum, hypoplasia of the right lung, and bronchopulmonary sequestration. The left pulmonary veins can drain into the innominate vein or coronary sinus.

Physiology of PAPVR

The physiology of PAPVR is that of a left-to-right shunt with right-sided chamber enlargement. The degree of shunt is determined by the amount of lung that the anomalous veins are draining and the presence (or absence) of an associated atrial-level shunt.

Imaging diagnosis

Chest X-rays may reveal cardiomegaly and an increased pulmonary vascularity. Echocardiography may show an unexplained right ventricular enlargement. In this case, MRI is commonly requested to evaluate for partial anomalous

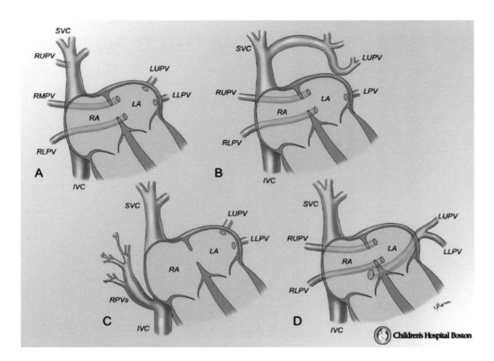

Figure 3.28 Partial anomalous pulmonary venous return – diagram. Different types of partial anomalous pulmonary venous return (PAPVR) are presented in this diagram. (A) Drainage of the right upper pulmonary vein (RUPV) to the superior vena cava. (B) Drainage of the left upper pulmonary vein (LUPV) via a vertical vein to the innominate vein. (C) Drainage of the right pulmonary veins (RPVs) to the inferior vena cava (Scimitar syndrome). (D) Drainage of the left upper pulmonary vein and left lower pulmonary vein (LLPV) into the coronary sinus. RLPV = right lower pulmonary vein; LPV = left pulmonary vein; RMPV = right medial pulmonary vein. *From the Multimedia Library of Congenital Heart Disease, Children's Hospital, Boston, MA, editor Robert Geggel, MD,* www.childrenshospital.org/mml/cvp *with permission.*

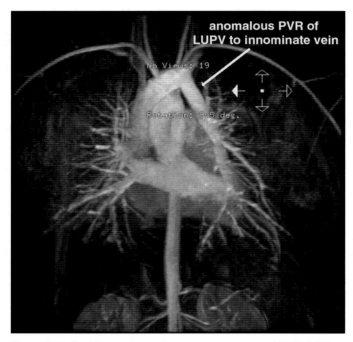

Figure 3.29 Partial anomalous pulmonary venous return – MRI. Gadolinium-enhanced 3D MIP MRA image of PAPVR of the left upper pulmonary vein (LUPV) to the left innominate vein. MRI is commonly requested to identify partial anomalous pulmonary venous return in the setting of unexplained right ventricular enlargement by echocardiogram.

pulmonary venous return (Figure 3.29). Sometimes, a PAPVR may be diagnosed as an incidental finding on a CT which has been performed for other reasons (Figure 3.30). In the case of a Scimitar syndrome, chest X-rays may demonstrate a hypoplastic right hemithorax with shift of the mediastinum to the right, as well as a curvilinear density, extending from the right hilum inferiorly, which represents the "scimitar" vein and drains below the diaphragm (Figure 3.31). Cross-sectional imaging studies can confirm this diagnosis (Figures 3.32, 3.33).

Natural history of PAPVR

The degree of right-sided enlargement is a function of the amount of left-to-right shunt. In the absence of an intra-atrial communication, the degree of shunt is fixed. However, in the presence of an ASD, the shunt can progress over time as the compliance of the left ventricle decreases with aging (as is seen in other ASD lesions). PAPVR is usually asymptomatic in infancy and childhood. The development of pulmonary arterial hypertension is rare. Pulmonary infections can occur in patients with Scimitar syndrome. Surgical repair is recommended if the degree of shunt (Qp : Qs) is greater than 1.5 in uncomplicated lesions and greater than 2 in complicated lesions.

Repair of PAPVR

The surgical approach to the repair of PAPVR varies depending on the nature of the connections. Left-sided PAPVR to the innominate vein is usually easily repaired by connecting the anomalous veins to the left atrial appendage, and can be done without bypass surgery. Right-sided PAPVRs, such as those associated with a sinus venosus defect or Scimitar syndrome, are more complicated and often require complex baffling of the veins. Postoperative complications with venous obstruction are more common following repair of these lesions.

(A)

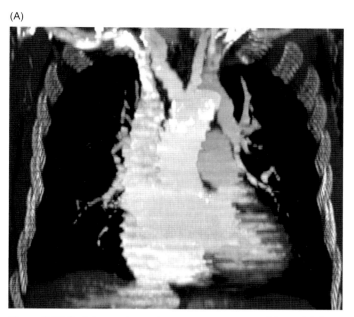

(B)

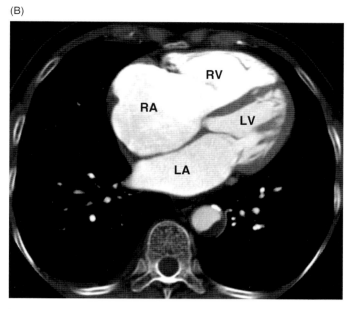

Figure 3.30 Partial anomalous pulmonary venous return – CT scan. (A) Contrast-enhanced CT Scan of a patient with PAPVR diagnosed at age 76 during a CT scan performed for other reasons; not an uncommon scenario. (B) CT scan demonstrating right ventricular enlargement in the same patient.

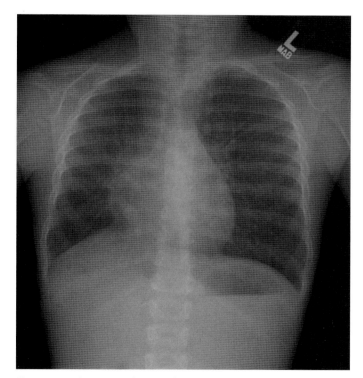

Figure 3.31 Scimitar syndrome – chest X-ray. CXR in a young woman with Scimitar syndrome demonstrates the classic "scimitar" appearance of the right pulmonary veins draining into the inferior vena cava. Hypoplastic right lung is also visualized.

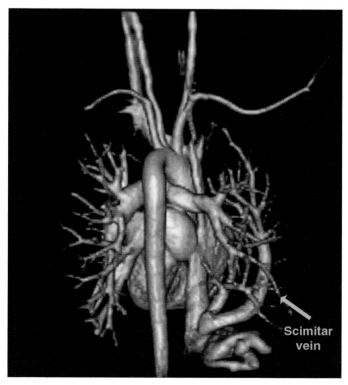

Figure 3.32 Scimitar syndrome – MRI. Gadolinium-enhanced 3D MRA reconstruction of Scimitar syndrome in which all of the right pulmonary veins drain into the right inferior vena cava just below the junction of the inferior vena cava and right atrium.

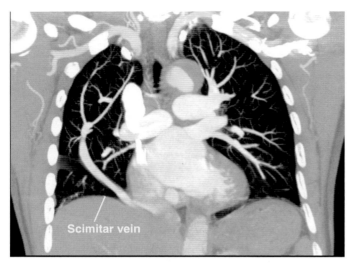

Figure 3.33 Scimitar syndrome – CT scan. Contrast-enhanced CT scan in the coronal reconstruction reveals a Scimitar vein.

Obstructive lesions

Coarctation of the aorta

Coarctation (CoA) occurs in 8–10% of all CHD. Around 30% of patients with Turner syndrome have CoA and thus should be screened carefully. Bicuspid aortic valve (BAV) is commonly associated with CoA; in fact, 50–70% of all CoA patients will have a BAV. CoA is also commonly associated with other CHD lesions including aortic arch hypoplasia, VSD, and mitral valve abnormalities.

CoA always occurs at the aortic isthmus, the site of attachment of the ductus arteriosus during fetal life (Figure 3.34). The pathology is as follows. The ductal tissue is oxygen dependent. Constriction of the duct occurs once newborns take their first breaths. In CoA, the ductal tissue migrates abnormally around the circumference of isthmus of the descending aorta; thus, with ductal constriction, the aorta is cinched down by this tissue like a noose.

Physiology of CoA

The physiology of a CoA is that of systemic outflow obstruction, leading to increased afterload on the left heart and diminished perfusion of the systemic vasculature in severe cases.

Imaging diagnosis

Imaging studies may show localized or diffuse types of CoA. The localized type, also termed the adult, postductal, or juxtaductal type, is much more common and characterized by a narrow, discrete coarctation just beyond the left subclavian artery at the level of the ductus. Radiographically, left ventricular enlargement may be evident and the transverse portion of the thoracic aorta may be dilated. Instead of a

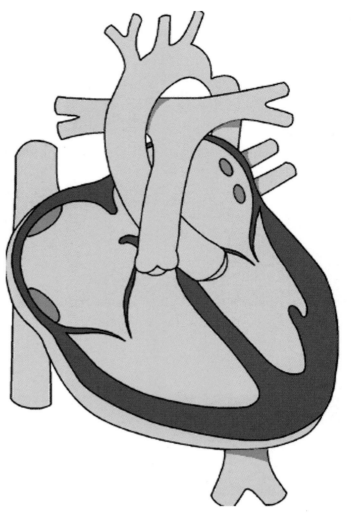

Figure 3.34 Coarctation of the aorta – diagram. Anatomical drawing depicting discrete coarctation of the aorta (CoA). The aorta is narrowed distal to the origin of the left subclavian artery at the attachment site of the previous ductus arteriosus. *From the Multimedia Library of Congenital Heart Disease, Children's Hospital, Boston, MA, editor Robert Geggel, MD,* www.childrenshospital.org/mml/cvp *with permission.*

smooth, curvilinear contour to the proximal descending aorta, a notch is present. The contour of the aorta at this level may resemble the number 3; the upper portion of the 3 is due to the dilated proximal left subclavian artery and aorta proximal to the coarctation; the middle portion of the 3 is due to the coarctation itself; and the lower portion of the 3 is due to poststenotic dilatation of the descending aorta (Figure 3.35). A reverse-3 sign can be seen on barium esophagograms as a result of the same anomaly. Rib notching may be present and is due to pressure erosion caused by dilated intercostal arteries, which serve as collateral vessels between the internal mammary arteries and the descending aorta. The first, second and third ribs are not notched, since their intercostal arteries arise from the thyrocervical trunk, which originates from the aorta above the coarctation. Echocardiography, MRI and angiography may evaluate the associated hemodynamics and detect possible postsurgical complications, such as aneurysms at the previous repair site (Figures 3.36–3.40).

The diffuse type, also known as the infantile, tubular hypoplastic, or preductal type, is characterized by a long segment of aortic narrowing that extends from just distal to the subclavian artery to the ductus. Intracardiac defects (VSD, ASD, deformed mitral valve) are present in half of the patients with the diffuse type of coarctation, and the ductus is almost always patent.

Natural history of CoA

Simple CoA can range from mild narrowing of the isthmus, often presenting later in life with a murmur and systemic

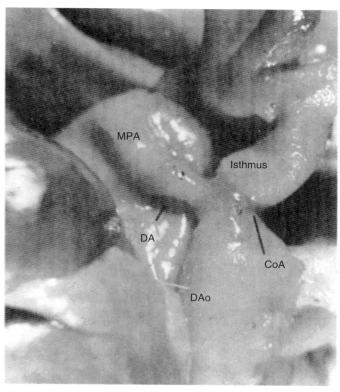

Figure 3.37 Coarctation of the aorta – pathology. Pathological specimen of coarctation of the aorta in a newborn. DA = ductus arteriosus; MPA = main pulmonary artery. DAo = descending aorta.

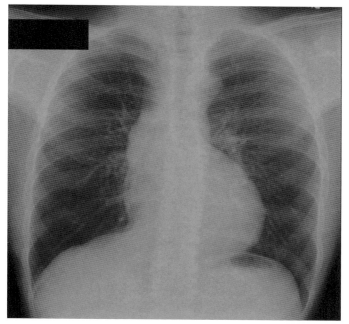

Figure 3.35 Coarctation of the aorta – chest X-ray. Anteroposterior CXR in an adolescent with unrepaired coarctation of the aorta demonstrates the characteristic "3 sign" and rib notching.

(A)

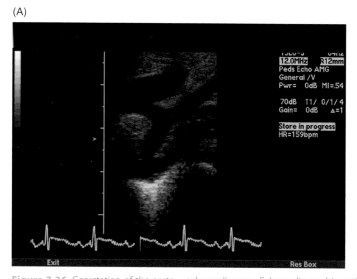

(B)

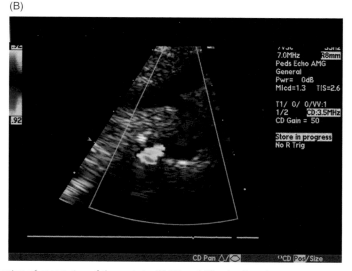

Figure 3.36 Coarctation of the aorta – echocardiogram. Echocardiographic evaluation of coarctation of the aorta in (A) 2D and (B) color Doppler.

(A)

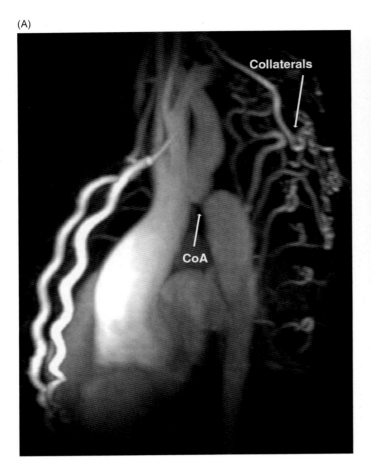

(B)

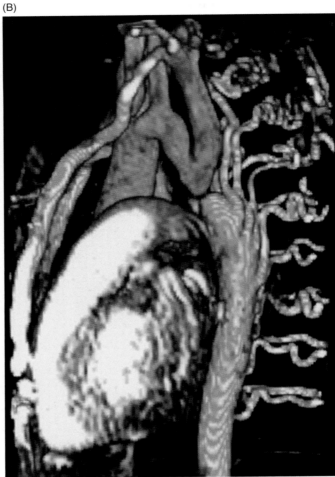

Figure 3.38 Coarctation of the aorta – MRI. (A) Gadolinium-enhanced 3D MIP MRA image and (B) gadolinium-enhanced 3D MRA reconstruction of coarctation of the aorta demonstrates a tight discrete narrowing at the isthmus with multiple collaterals responsible for providing flow to the descending aorta distal to the obstruction.

hypertension, to severe obstruction presenting with congestive heart failure and/or absence of pulses in the neonatal period.

Long-term complications of unrepaired CoA vary depending on the severity of obstruction. Death from poor perfusion and/or congestive heart failure in the newborn period occurs if the obstruction is severe. If the obstruction is less severe, complications later in life include chronic systemic hypertension, aortic dissection and rupture, cerebral berry aneurysms, premature coronary artery disease, and heart failure. Once repaired, patients need to be followed for recurrent or residual obstruction at the repair site, particularly if surgical repair was performed in infancy. In addition, aneurysms can occur at the repair site. Chronic systemic hypertension and premature coronary artery disease can also occur late, even if the repair is successful. Finally, if there is an associated BAV, the development of an ascending aortic aneurysm can occur and needs to be screened for with serial imaging.

Repair of CoA

In infancy, surgical repair is preferred. There are (and have been) a number of different surgical approaches to the surgical repair of CoA. If possible, surgical resection of the CoA and end-to-end anastomosis is the preferred approach. In the past, left subclavian artery flap procedure was often performed. In the present day, patch aortoplasty is preferred if additional tissue is needed to complete the repair. If CoA presents later in life, percutaneous balloon angioplasty and/or stent placement are a desirable alternative to surgery.

Cyanotic congenital heart lesions

Tetralogy of Fallot

Tetralogy of Fallot (TOF) occurs in 10% of all CHD and is the most common form of cyanotic CHD. The tetralogy – large VSD, right ventricular outflow tract (RVOT) obstruction, large overriding aorta, and RV hypertrophy – are all the result of

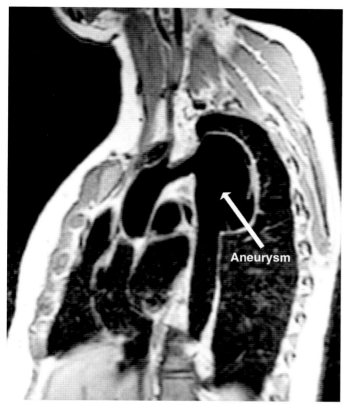

Figure 3.39 Coarctation of the aorta – MRI. Sagittal oblique black blood MR image of the aorta reveals an aneurysm at the site of previous coarctation repair; not an uncommon complication, one that needs careful monitoring with imaging. Also note the hypoplastic aortic arch in this patient.

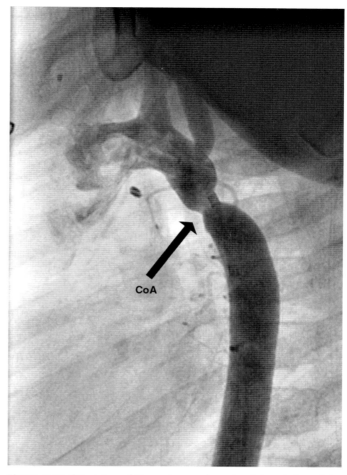

Figure 3.40 Coarctation of the aorta – angiography. A lateral view of the aortic arch and descending aorta reveals a discrete coarctation.

one single abnormality in cardiac morphogenesis. This abnormality is the malalignment of the infundibular septum anteriorly during the division of the common great vessel into the aorta and main pulmonary artery. The RVOT obstruction is the result of subvalvar (infundibular) crowding and hypoplasia of the pulmonary valve.

There is a spectrum of severity of TOF (Figures 3.41–3.43). On the severe end of the spectrum is TOF with pulmonary atresia (PA), in which infundibular crowding eliminates the outflow from the right ventricle and the pulmonary valve does not form. In this type of TOF, the branch pulmonary arteries may be discontinuous, receiving blood supply only from the ductus arteriosus (70%) or aortopulmonary collaterals (30%).

TOF with absent pulmonary valve (APV) is a rare and serious form of TOF. It is associated with an absent or severely dysplastic pulmonary valve and aneurysmally dilated branch pulmonary arteries. The pathology of this disease is thought to be the result of absence of the ductus arteriosus in fetal life. In the absence of a fetal ductus, there is no escape for blood being ejected from the right ventricle and the large forward stroke volume regurgitates back into the right ventricle. This large forward and backward stroke volume leads to malformation

of the pulmonary valve and aneurysmal stretch of the branch pulmonary arteries.

Physiology of TOF

Patients with TOF are cyanotic secondary to obstruction to pulmonary blood flow and mixing of oxygenated and deoxygenated blood at the ventricular level. The severity of cyanosis depends on the degree of RVOT obstruction and anatomy of the pulmonary vascular bed. Rarely, patients with TOF and PA are ductal dependent and require intervention in the newborn period. Right ventricular hypertrophy is the result of an unrestrictive VSD. As a result, the right ventricle remains at systemic pressure until repair.

Imaging of TOF

Chest X-rays show the characteristic "boot-shaped heart" secondary to right ventricular hypertrophy, and a concave main pulmonary artery segment due to pulmonary atresia (Figure 3.44). Echocardiography demonstrates infundibular malalignment, ventricular septal defect and the overriding aorta (Figure 3.45). MRI can help to further define the specific

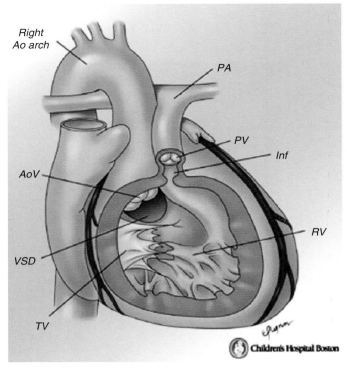

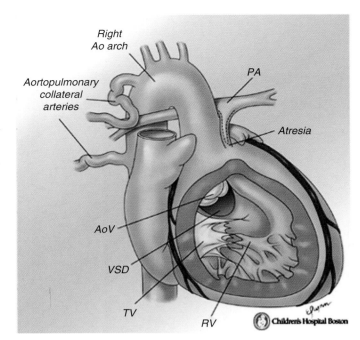

Figure 3.41 Tetralogy of Fallot – diagram. Right ventricular view of cardiac anatomy of tetralogy of Fallot (TOF) with pulmonary stenosis. The aortic valve (AoV) can be seen through the ventricular septal defect (VSD). There is infundibular stenosis (Inf) in the subpulmonary valve region, hypoplastic pulmonary valve (PV) and hypoplastic pulmonary arteries (PA). A right aortic arch is present in approximately 25% of patients. TV = tricuspid valve. *From the Multimedia Library of Congenital Heart Disease, Children's Hospital, Boston, MA, editor Robert Geggel, MD, www.childrenshospital.org/mml/cvp with permission.*

Figure 3.42 Tetralogy of Fallot with pulmonary atresia – diagram. Right ventricular view of tetralogy of Fallot (TOF) associated with pulmonary atresia. There is atresia of the right ventricular outflow tract and hypoplasia of the pulmonary arteries (PA). Aortopulmonary collateral arteries are quite common in this defect. AoV = aortic valve; TV = tricuspid valve; VSD = ventricular septal defect. *From the Multimedia Library of Congenital Heart Disease, Children's Hospital, Boston, MA, editor Robert Geggel, MD, www.childrenshospital.org/mml/cvp with permission.*

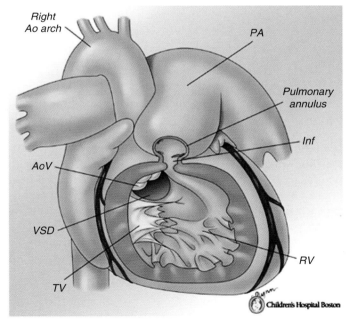

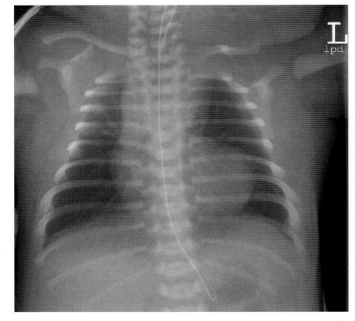

Figure 3.43 Tetralogy of Fallot with absent pulmonary valve – diagram. Right ventricular view of tetralogy of Fallot (TOF) associated with absent pulmonary valve. There is infundibular stenosis (Inf). The absent or nearly absent pulmonary valve leaflets are associated with severe pulmonary regurgitation, which leads to the development of markedly dilated pulmonary arteries (PA). AoV = aortic valve; TV = tricuspid valve; VSD = ventricular septal defect. *From the Multimedia Library of Congenital Heart Disease, Children's Hospital, Boston, MA, editor Robert Geggel, MD, www.childrenshospital.org/mml/cvp with permission.*

Figure 3.44 Tetralogy of Fallot – chest X-ray. Anteroposterior CXR of a newborn with tetralogy of Fallot reveals the characteristic "boot-shaped heart" secondary to right ventricular hypertrophy and concave main pulmonary artery segment.

type of TOF, as described above (Figures 3.46–48). Longitudinal MRI studies can help to monitor right ventricular dilatation, hypertrophy and function (Figure 3.49).

Natural history of TOF

As mentioned above, the severity of cyanosis depends on the degree of RVOT obstruction and anatomy of the pulmonary vascular bed. Complete obstruction to pulmonary blood flow can occur ("Tet spell"). Such events are now rare since surgical repair in early infancy is the standard of care at most institutions. Palliative shunts in the newborn period were previously employed to augment pulmonary blood flow, but these are less commonly performed as neonatal surgical repair is possible.

Repair of TOF

The goal of surgical repair is to close the VSD (usually with a patch) and relieve RVOT obstruction. Relief of outflow tract

obstruction is accomplished by resection of infundibular muscle and widening of the RVOT with a patch. In the setting of severe obstruction, the patch is extended as a transannular patch, destroying pulmonary valve competence.

TOF with PA remains a severe form of TOF that is difficult to repair. In the setting of confluent branch pulmonary

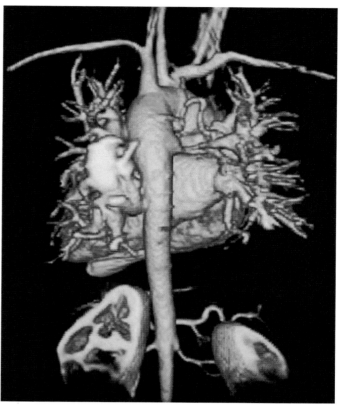

Figure 3.47 Tetralogy of Fallot – MRI. Gadolinium-enhanced 3D MRA reconstruction of the anatomy in a patient with tetralogy of Fallot and pulmonary atresia with multiple aortopulmonary collateral arteries. This is the most severe form of this disease and is characterized by the pulmonary blood flow arising entirely from collaterals from the aorta.

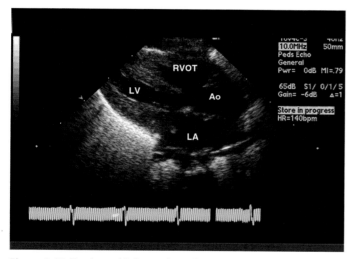

Figure 3.45 Tetralogy of Fallot – echocardiogram. Parasternal long-axis echocardiogram of a newborn with tetralogy of Fallot. Notice the infundibular malalignment, ventricular septal defect and the overriding aorta (Ao). RVOT = right ventricular outflow tract.

(A) (B)

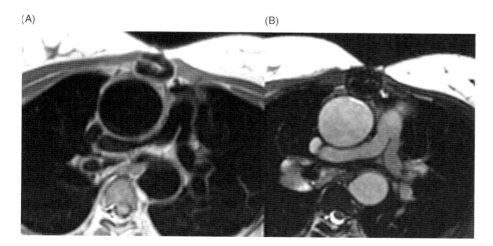

Figure 3.46 Tetralogy of Fallot – MRI. (A) Axial black blood MR image and (B) axial cine MR image of the branch pulmonary arteries in a patient with tetralogy of Fallot and severe pulmonary stenosis, repaired with placement of an RV-to-PA conduit. The large ascending aorta is typical of this disease as there is unequal division of the great vessels. The hypoplastic branch pulmonary arteries are also typical of TOF, particularly if there is severe pulmonary stenosis or pulmonary atresia.

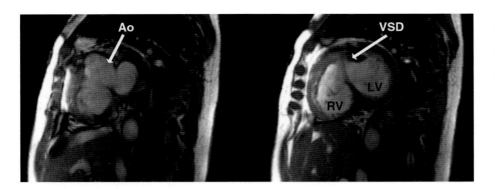

Figure 3.48 Tetralogy of Fallot – MRI. Two contiguous slices in the short axis through the right and left ventricle near the base of the heart in an adult patient with unrepaired tetralogy of Fallot and pulmonary atresia. The right ventricle is hypertrophied, consistent with it being chronically pressure overloaded. There is a large malalignment ventricular septal defect (VSD) with override of the aorta (Ao) over both ventricles. There is no evidence of a pulmonary valve or main pulmonary artery.

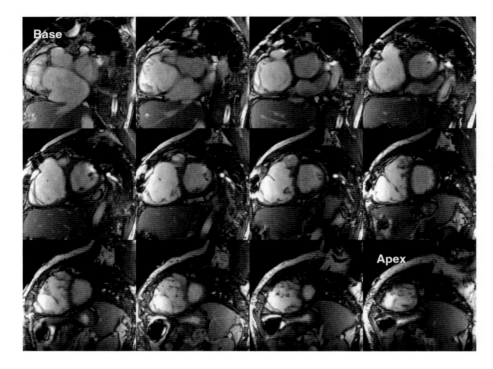

Figure 3.49 Tetralogy of Fallot – MRI. Shown are multiple slices through the short axis of the ventricles in a patient with repaired tetralogy of Fallot. One time point in the cardiac cycle is represented; however, this sequence is able to collect multiple time points throughout the cardiac cycle. Because of chronic pulmonary insufficiency, this patient has developed right ventricular dilatation and dysfunction. Tracing the right and left ventricular endocardial surfaces at end systole and end diastole allows determination of end systolic and end diastolic volumes as well as ejection fraction. Once the right ventricle reaches a certain degree of dilatation and dysfunction, pulmonary valve replacement is recommended.

arteries, a homograft can be placed from the RV to the confluence of the branch pulmonary arteries. In the setting of discontinuous pulmonary arteries and/or aortopulmonary collaterals, a staged unifocalization procedure is usually performed in which pulmonary arteries and collaterals are ultimately connected to a conduit arising from the RV. Timing of VSD closure is dependent on the anatomy and caliber of the pulmonary arterial bed.

TOF with APV also remains a severe form of TOF with high morbidity and mortality. In early life these complications are the result of airway obstruction by the aneurysmally dilated branch pulmonary arteries. Surgical repair necessitates early pulmonary arterioplasty.

Although many patients with surgically repaired TOF will do well through childhood and young adulthood, morbidity and mortality increase later in adulthood, including progressive exercise intolerance, right ventricular failure, atrial and ventricular arrhythmias and sudden death. Most

of these complications are the result of chronic pulmonary insufficiency leading to right ventricular dilatation and dysfunction. Pulmonary valve replacement in adolescence and young adulthood is thought to mitigate some of these complications.

All TOF patients have abnormal pulmonary vascular beds; not only the TOF with PA or APV. Many will need percutaneous or surgical address of focal obstructions before and/or after repair.

Truncus arteriosus

Truncus arteriosus (TA) accounts for approximately 2% of all CHD. It is characterized by a single arterial trunk arising from the normally formed ventricles via a single semilunar valve: the truncal valve. In addition, the pulmonary arteries arise from the common trunk. There is nearly always an associated ventricular septal defect (Figure 3.50). There are two different classification

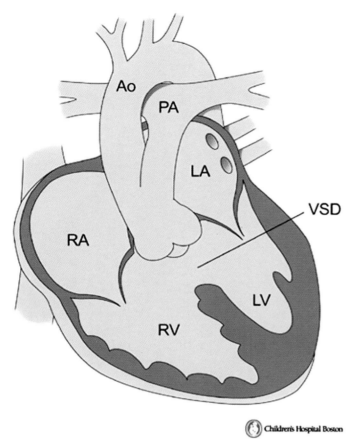

Figure 3.50 Truncus arteriosus – diagram. Type I truncus arteriosus (TA) is depicted. There is one common great vessel arising from the heart, the ascending portion of which supplies the aorta (Ao), coronary arteries and pulmonary arteries (PA). A ventricular septal defect (VSD) is nearly universally associated with this defect. *From the Multimedia Library of Congenital Heart Disease, Children's Hospital, Boston, MA, editor Robert Geggel, MD, www.childrenshospital.org/mml/cvp with permission.*

schemes (Figure 3.51); both based on the location of the origins of the pulmonary arteries from the common arterial trunk.
In the Collett and Edwards scheme:

Type I. Characterized by the origin of a main pulmonary artery from the left lateral aspect of the ascending common trunk.

Type II. Characterized by separate but proximate origins of the right and left pulmonary arteries from the posterior aspect of the ascending common trunk.

Type III. Characterized by separate origins of the branch pulmonary arteries laterally from the common trunk.

Type IV. Characterized by separate origins of the branch pulmonary arteries from the descending aorta.

In the Van Praagh scheme:

Type A1. Identical to Collett and Edwards type I.

Type A2. Includes both Collett and Edwards type II and III.

Type A3. Characterized by the right pulmonary artery arising from the right lateral aspect of the ascending trunk while the left pulmonary artery is atretic and blood flow to the left lung is via collateral arteries.

Type A4. Characterized by the association with interrupted aortic arch.

Physiology of TA

The physiology in patients with TA is similar to TOF with pulmonary atresia. Cyanosis is usually seen shortly after birth and congestive heart failure occurs early.

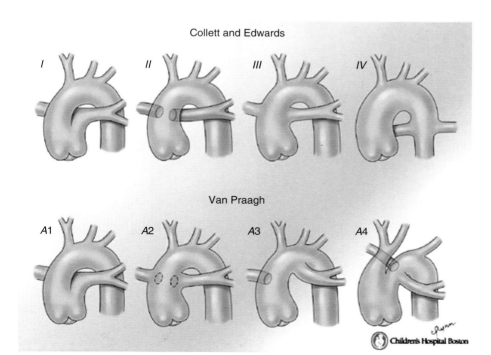

Collett and Edwards

Van Praagh

Figure 3.51 Classification of truncus arteriosus types. Collett and Edwards (types I–IV) and Van Praagh (types A1–A4) classifications of truncus arteriosus (TA) are presented. **Collett and Edwards** type I: origin of a main pulmonary artery from the left lateral aspect of the ascending common trunk. Type II: separate but proximate origins of the right and left pulmonary arteries from the posterior aspect of the ascending common trunk. Type III: separate origins of the branch pulmonary arteries laterally from the common trunk. Type IV: separate origins of the branch pulmonary arteries from the descending aorta. **Van Praagh** type A1: identical to Collett and Edwards type I. Type A2: includes Collett and Edwards type II and III. Type A3: origin of right pulmonary artery from the right lateral aspect of the ascending trunk with atretic left pulmonary artery (blood flow to the left lung via collateral arteries). Type A4: associated with interrupted aortic arch. *From the Multimedia Library of Congenital Heart Disease, Children's Hospital, Boston, MA, editor Robert Geggel, MD, www.childrenshospital.org/mml/cvp with permission.*

Imaging of TA

Chest radiographs may show cardiomegaly, a concave pulmonary artery segment and normal to reduced pulmonary vascularity. Echocardiography and MRI demonstrate a truncal valve giving rise to an ascending aorta and a main pulmonary artery, as well as a large ventricular septal defect (Figures 3.52, 3.53).

Repair of TA

Definitive surgical repair in a patient with TA includes closure of the ventricular septal defect to direct flow of blood from the left ventricle to the truncus arteriosus (which becomes

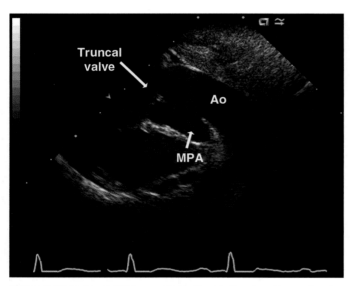

Figure 3.52 Truncus arteriosus – echocardiogram. Parasternal long-axis echocardiographic views of the truncus arteriosus demonstrating a truncal valve giving rise to an ascending aorta (Ao) and a main pulmonary artery (MPA).

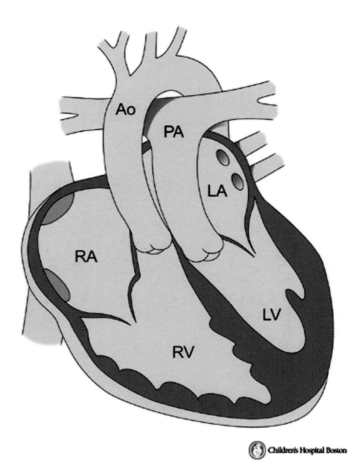

Figure 3.54 D-transposition of the great arteries (D-TGA) – diagram. The atria are normally positioned, the ventricles looped properly and are concordant with the atria, but the great vessels are transposed such that the aorta arises from the right ventricle and the pulmonary artery (PA) arises from the left ventricle. The aorta (Ao) is to the right and anterior relative to the pulmonary artery. *From the Multimedia Library of Congenital Heart Disease, Children's Hospital, Boston, MA, editor Robert Geggel, MD, www.childrenshospital.org/mml/cvp with permission.*

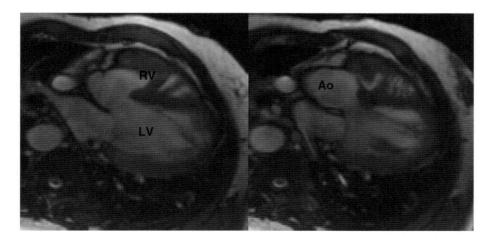

Figure 3.53 Truncus arteriosus – MRI. Cine MRI in an adult patient with truncus arteriosus. The aorta (Ao) arises off both ventricles, and the ventricles communicate via a large ventricular septal defect.

then the neo-aorta). The right ventricle is then attached to the pulmonary arteries via an RV-to-PA conduit. The development of truncal valve stenosis or insufficiency is not uncommon and often needs to be surgically addressed. The RV-to-PA conduit similarly can become regurgitant and stenotic requiring readdress.

D-transposition of the great arteries

D-transposition of the great arteries (D-TGA) accounts for approximately 5% of all CHD. In this defect, the atria are normally positioned and the ventricles loop normally; however, the aorta arises from the right ventricle anteriorly and to the right of the pulmonary artery which arises from the left ventricle (Figure 3.54). In D-TGA there is usually a subaortic conus or infundibulum (with absence of subpulmonary conus). In D-TGA, an associated VSD occurs in 30–40% of patients. In these patients, other lesions are commonly associated including coarctation of the aorta, interrupted aortic arch, pulmonary atresia and overriding atrioventricular valves.

Physiology of D-TGA

Deoxygenated blood is circulated through the body and oxygenated blood is circulated through the lungs. Associated defects permitting mixing (ASD, PDA, VSD) are required for survival in the newborn period.

Natural history of D-TGA

Unrepaired, patients with D-TGA will develop rapidly progressive hypoxemia, congestive heart failure and death, usually before six months of age. Patients without a VSD and only a small ASD require a percutaneous balloon atrial septostomy (Rashkind procedure) at birth. Early repair is necessary to prevent pulmonary arterial hypertension (Figure 3.55).

Imaging of D-TGA

Chest X-rays typically show a narrow superior mediastinum, cardiomegaly, an egg-shaped and enlarged heart silhouette, as well as an increased pulmonary vascularity (Figure 3.56). Echocardiography demonstrates the aortic and pulmonic valves in the same plane with the aorta (anterior) and main

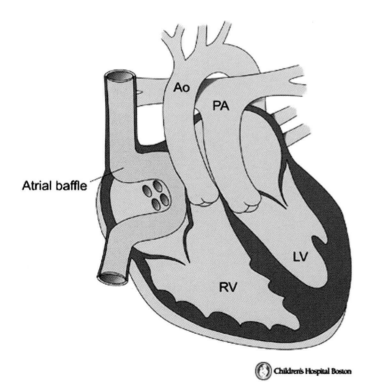

Figure 3.55 D-transposition of the great arteries following atrial switch – diagram. Diagram detailing the anatomy of D-TGA after an atrial switch procedure. A baffle is placed in the atria so that blood returning via the inferior and superior vena cavae is directed via a baffle to the left ventricle and then to the pulmonary artery (PA). The pulmonary venous blood courses around the baffle to reach the right ventricle and then to the aorta (Ao). *From the Multimedia Library of Congenital Heart Disease, Children's Hospital, Boston, MA, editor Robert Geggel, MD*, www.childrenshospital.org/mml/cvp *with permission.*

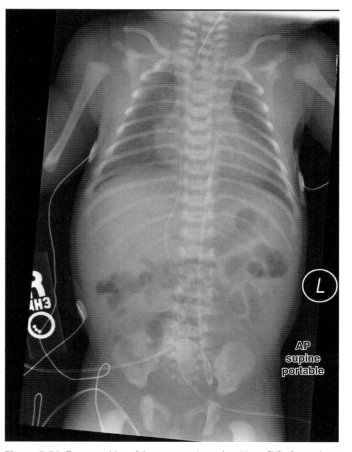

Figure 3.56 D-transposition of the great arteries – chest X-ray. CXR of a newborn with D-transposition of the great arteries. Cardiomegaly, increased pulmonary vascularity, an egg-shaped heart and a narrow superior mediastinum are characteristic.

pulmonary artery (posterior) running parallel to each other (Figure 3.57). MRI is useful in preoperative evaluations and postoperative longitudinal monitoring of systemic and pulmonary venous pathways (Figures 3.58, 3.59).

Repair of D-TGA

In 1950, Blalock and Hanlon performed the first palliative procedure which consisted of surgical resection of the atrial septum. In 1957, Senning performed the first corrective procedure involving redirection of blood flow at the atrial level using atrial septal tissue to create intra-atrial baffles. In 1963, Mustard performed a similar procedure using artificial material to create the intra-atrial baffles. In 1979, Jatene was finally able to successfully perform an arterial switch. Until this time, the translocation of the coronary arteries had been the stumbling block to performing this procedure.

Patients following atrial switch suffer from a number of residual hemodynamic lesions. Most importantly, they have a right ventricle as the systemic pumping chamber. Ultimately, right ventricular dilatation and dysfunction ensue. Tricuspid regurgitation can result from right ventricular dilatation and can worsen the progression of enlargement. Systemic venous baffle obstruction is not uncommon, particularly after transvenous pacemaker lead placement. Pulmonary venous baffle obstruction is less common, but serious, in that it can result in pulmonary arterial hypertension. Atrial arrhythmias and

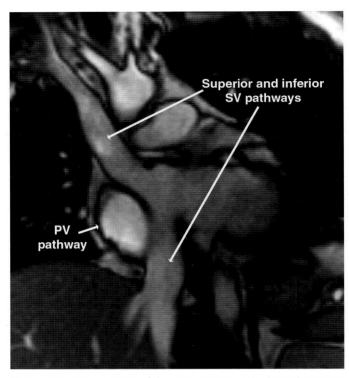

Figure 3.58 D-transposition of the great arteries – MRI. Cine MR image in coronal oblique plane demonstrates the systemic venous (SV) and pulmonary venous (PV) pathways in a patient with D-transposition of the great arteries following an atrial switch procedure.

(A)

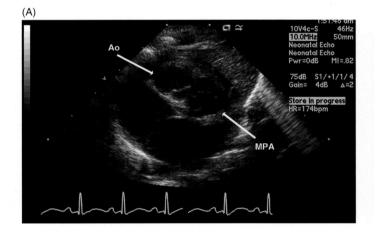

(B)

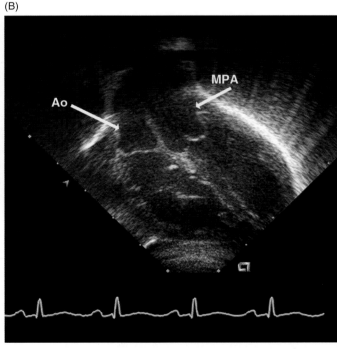

Figure 3.57 D-transposition of the great arteries – echocardiogram. Shown are (A) parasternal short-axis and (B) subcostal views in patient with D-transposition of the great arteries. The aortic and pulmonic valves are in the same plane and the aorta (Ao; anterior) and main pulmonary artery (MPA; posterior) run parallel to each other.

(A)

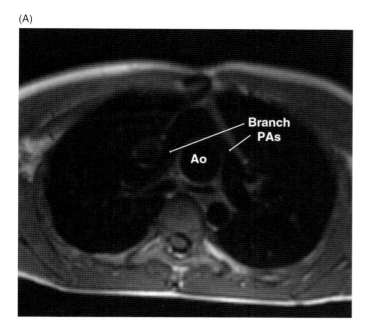

(B)

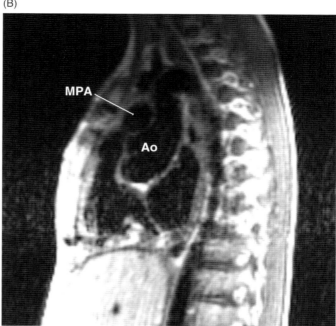

Figure 3.59 D-transposition of the great arteries – MRI. (A) Axial black blood MR image of the appearance of the pulmonary arteries (PAs) as they drape across the ascending aorta (Ao) in a patient with D-transposition of the great arteries following arterial switch procedure. (B) Sagittal black blood MR image showing posterior displacement of the ascending aorta by the main pulmonary artery (MPA) after the arterial switch procedure.

sinus node dysfunction can result from surgical scar. Rapidly conducted atrial arrhythmias are thought to be the primary cause of sudden death in this population.

Patients following arterial switch suffer pathology as well. Coronary artery obstruction can result from translocation of these vessels. In addition, supravalvar aortic and branch pulmonary artery obstruction can occur.

L-transposition of the great arteries

L-transposition of the great arteries (L-TGA) is not a cyanotic heart lesion; however, discussion of this lesion following D-TGA seems appropriate. It is a rare lesion occurring in less than 1% of all patients with CHD. In this defect, the atria are normally positioned; the right ventricle loops leftward and sits posterior and leftward of the left ventricle. The great vessels are transposed: the aorta arises from the right ventricle (left and anterior), and the main pulmonary artery arises from the left ventricle (right and posterior). The resultant flow of blood is normal in that deoxygenated blood is directed to the lungs and oxygenated blood is directed to the body.

Although there is theoretically no functional abnormality, this circulation is not normal. First and foremost, the right ventricle is the systemic pumping chamber; a task the right ventricle is not morphologically prepared to do. In addition, more than 80% of these patients will have an associated lesion including VSD (80%), valvar and subvalvar pulmonary stenosis or atresia (50%), Ebstein's anomaly of the tricuspid valve, and AV nodal conduction disturbances.

Natural history of L-TGA

The natural history of L-TGA is variable depending on the presence of associated lesions. Occasionally, patients without associated lesions can be asymptomatic into adulthood. In the presence of a large VSD and resultant torrential pulmonary blood flow, newborns need either palliation (pulmonary arterial band), or repair (definitive VSD closure or atrial and arterial switch procedures termed a "double switch"). In the presence of pulmonary stenosis or atresia and insufficient pulmonary blood flow, newborns need either palliation with a systemic to pulmonary artery shunt, or repair with either RV outflow tract reconstruction or, in the setting of a suitable VSD, Rastelli procedure and atrial switch. In the presence of a dysplastic or Ebstein's tricuspid valve, tricuspid (systemic atrioventricular valve) regurgitation develops in upwards of 30% of patients. Progressive AV nodal block also occurs in up to 30% of patients, usually requiring pacemaker placement.

Total anomalous pulmonary venous return

Total anomalous pulmonary venous return (TAPVR) is a rare lesion accounting for approximately 1% of all CHD. There are four types of TAPVR including supracardiac (50%), cardiac (20%), infracardiac (20%) and mixed (10%) (Figures 3.60–3.63).

In supracardiac TAPVR, the common confluence of the pulmonary veins drains via the vertical vein into the left innominate vein. Chest X-rays show the characteristic snowman sign (Figure 3.61). In cardiac TAPVR, the common

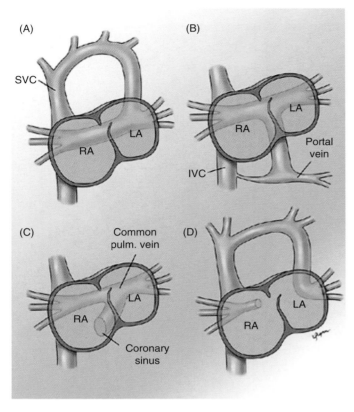

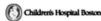

Figure 3.60 Total anomalous pulmonary venous return – diagram. Different types of total anomalous pulmonary venous return (TAPVR) are depicted in this diagram. There is always an atrial communication enabling blood to reach the left side of the heart. (A) Supracardiac TAPVR – right and left pulmonary veins join in a confluence posterior to the left atrium and are connected via an ascending vertical vein to the innominate vein. (B) Infradiaphragmatic TAPVR – the confluence of pulmonary veins drains via a descending vertical vein to the portal venous system. (C) Coronary sinus TAPVR – right and left pulmonary veins drain into the coronary sinus. (D) Mixed TAPVR – left pulmonary veins drain via a vertical vein to the innominate vein and right pulmonary veins connect directly to the right atrium. IVC = inferior vena cava; SVC = superior vena cava. *From the Multimedia Library of Congenital Heart Disease, Children's Hospital, Boston, MA, editor Robert Geggel, MD,* www.childrenshospital.org/mml/cvp *with permission.*

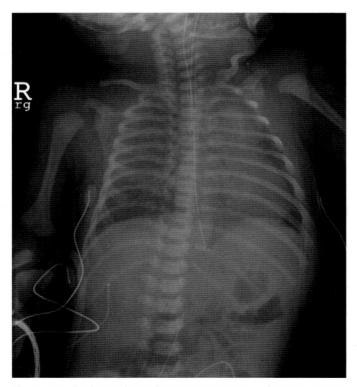

Figure 3.61 Total anomalous pulmonary venous return – chest X-ray. Antero-posterior CXR in infant with supracardiac TAPVR reveals the characteristic snowman sign.

confluence of the pulmonary veins drains into either the coronary sinus or directly into the back of the right atrium. In infracardiac (subdiaphragmatic) TAPVR, the common confluence of the pulmonary veins passes through the diaphragm via the esophageal hiatus and then drains into the portal vein, ductus venosus, hepatic vein, or the inferior vena cava directly (Figure 3.63). The mixed type of TAPVR is a combination of the aforementioned types (Figure 3.62).

Natural history of TAPVR

The natural history of this lesion is dependent on whether there is obstruction to pulmonary venous drainage. If there is no obstruction, newborns will have mild cyanosis secondary to complete mixing of oxygenated and deoxygenated blood. Congestive heart failure is common in newborns as there is usually torrential pulmonary blood flow. Unrepaired, two-thirds will die before one year of age. In contrast, obstructed TAPVR is usually a surgical emergency; without repair death ensues in days to months.

Univentricular heart

Univentricular physiology occurs in a number of congenital heart defects and is defined by the absence or hypoplasia of one ventricle. This physiology occurs in double inlet right

(A)

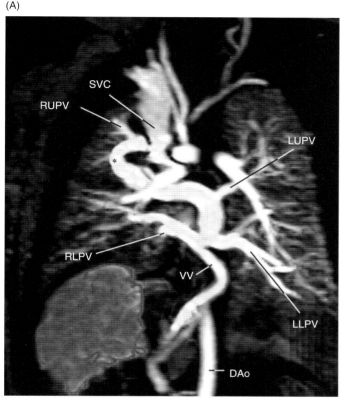

(B)

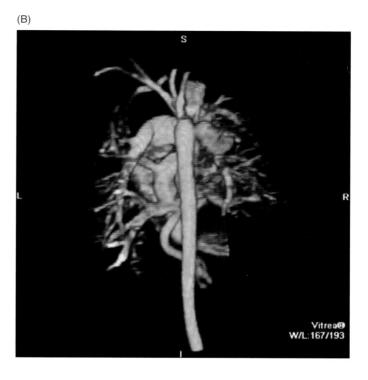

Figure 3.62 Total anomalous pulmonary venous return – MRI. (A) Gadolinium-enhanced 3D MIP MRA image and (B) gadolinium-enhanced 3D MRA reconstruction of the anatomy in a newborn with mixed-type total anomalous pulmonary venous return and coarctation of the aorta. DAo = descending aorta; SVC = superior vena cava; RUPV = right upper pulmonary vein; LUPV = left upper pulmonary vein; RLPV = right lower pulmonary vein; LLPV = left lower pulmonary vein; VV = vertical vein.

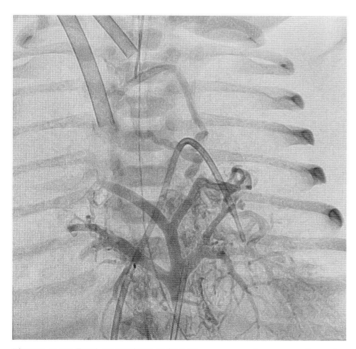

Figure 3.63 Total anomalous pulmonary venous return – angiography. "Upside down Christmas tree" appearance of the four pulmonary veins draining into a vertical vein that travels below the diaphragm.

or left ventricle, absence of one atrioventricular connection such as mitral atresia or tricuspid atresia (Figures 3.64–3.66), common AV canal communicating preferentially with only one ventricle (unbalanced AVC), or severe stenosis or atresia of a semilunar valve, such as pulmonary atresia with intact ventricular septum or critical aortic stenosis or aortic atresia (hypoplastic left heart syndrome, Figures 3.67–3.70). This list is not exhaustive.

Natural history of patients with univentricular physiology

As a whole, patients with unrepaired univentricular hearts have a poor prognosis. In the largest series of unoperated single-ventricle patients ($N = 83$), 70% of patients with well-formed left ventricles died before the age of 16, with an annual attrition rate of 4.8%, and 50% of patients with well-formed right ventricles died within four years of diagnosis. In a series of palliated single-ventricle patients there was 30% and 46% mortality within five years of diagnosis for single left and single right ventricles, respectively. Of note, these results likely represent a significant underestimation of mortality as they reflect only patients who survived the neonatal period.

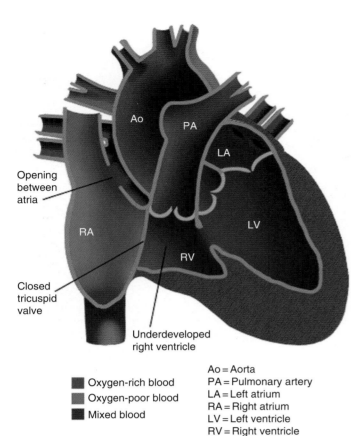

Opening
between
atria

Closed
tricuspid
valve

Underdeveloped
right ventricle

■ Oxygen-rich blood
■ Oxygen-poor blood
■ Mixed blood

Ao = Aorta
PA = Pulmonary artery
LA = Left atrium
RA = Right atrium
LV = Left ventricle
RV = Right ventricle

Figure 3.64 Tricuspid atresia – diagram. Diagram depicts tricuspid atresia type Ic. There is absence of the tricuspid valve and hypoplasia of the right ventricle. The different types include: type I – normally related great arteries; type II – D-transposed great arteries; type III – other great artery relationships; type IV – persistent truncus arteriosus. The different subtypes include: subtype a – pulmonary atresia; subtype b – pulmonary stenosis; subtype c – no obstruction to pulmonary flow. *From the Multimedia Library of Congenital Heart Disease, Children's Hospital, Boston, MA, editor Robert Geggel, MD, www.childrenshospital. org/mml/cvp with permission.*

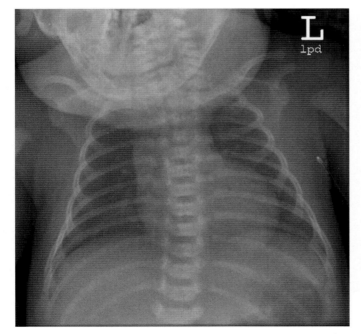

Figure 3.65 Tricuspid atresia – chest X-ray. Anteroposterior CXR in an infant with tricuspid atresia, normally related great arteries and pulmonary stenosis reveals normal chamber size and a concave main pulmonary artery segment giving a boot-shaped appearance. There is a paucity of pulmonary blood flow.

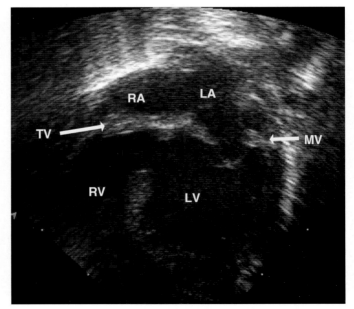

Figure 3.66 Tricuspid atresia – echocardiogram. Apical four-chamber view of the heart in an infant with tricuspid atresia. There is a plate where the tricuspid valve (TV) should be, the right ventricle is hypoplastic, and there is a large ventricular septal defect. MV = mitral valve.

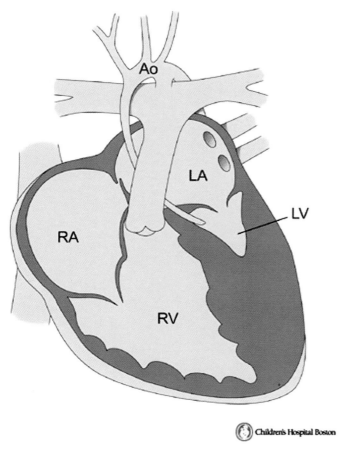

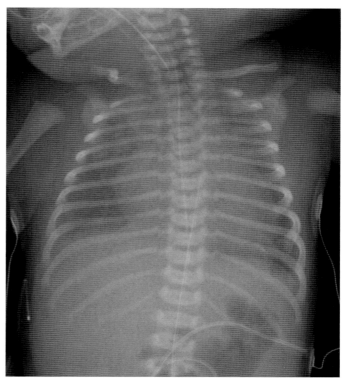

Figure 3.68 Hypoplastic left heart syndrome – chest X-ray. Anteroposterior CXR in a newborn with hypoplastic left heart syndrome reveals an enlarged heart with increased pulmonary vascular markings and pulmonary edema.

Figure 3.67 Hypoplastic left heart syndrome – diagram. Hypoplastic left heart associated with aortic atresia is presented in this diagram. The left ventricle is hypoplastic and hypertrophied. The ascending aorta (Ao) is severely hypoplastic. Blood flows to the ascending aorta retrograde from the patent ductus arteriosus. *From the Multimedia Library of Congenital Heart Disease, Children's Hospital, Boston, MA, editor Robert Geggel, MD,* www.childrenshospital.org/mml/cvp *with permission.*

Physiology in the single ventricle

To understand the variable presenting physiology of patients with univentricular hearts, one must first recognize that these patients have a single ventricle pumping to two circulations in parallel. How they present depends on the presence or absence of obstruction to systemic or pulmonary flow. Of note, they all present with cyanosis, the degree of which is also variable.

- *Unobstructed systemic blood flow with unobstructed pulmonary blood flow.* Patients with single ventricles, unobstructed systemic blood flow and unobstructed pulmonary blood flow have torrential pulmonary blood flow and present with congestive heart failure. They are minimally cyanotic initially because, despite a complete mixing lesion, they have tremendous pulmonary blood flow. As a result of excessive pulmonary blood flow, however, they quickly develop pulmonary edema and thus pulmonary venous desaturation and progressive

cyanosis. These patients often require a palliative procedure to limit pulmonary blood flow, such as a pulmonary arterial band. If left unrepaired, they will develop Eisenmenger physiology.

- *Unobstructed systemic blood flow with obstructed pulmonary blood flow.* Patients with single ventricles, unobstructed systemic blood flow and obstructed pulmonary blood flow present with significant cyanosis. They will often require a systemic-to-pulmonary arterial shunt as a palliative procedure to provide adequate pulmonary blood flow in preparation for a definitive repair at a later date.

- *Obstructed systemic blood flow with unobstructed pulmonary blood flow.* Patients with single ventricles, obstructed systemic blood flow and unobstructed pulmonary blood flow require a palliative procedure in infancy to provide adequate systemic blood flow and limit pulmonary blood flow. Only in the past two decades have we been able to provide such a palliation; previously these patients died within hours to months.

Repair of the single ventricle: the Fontan procedure

In the modern era, patients with single ventricles will ultimately undergo a Fontan procedure (Figure 3.71). The goal of

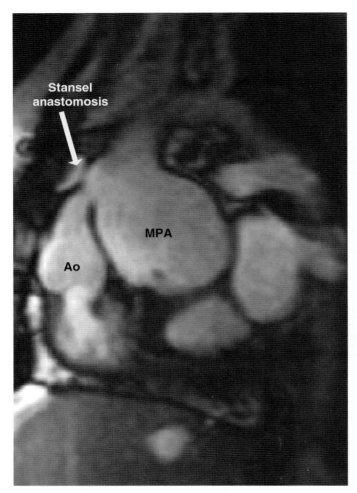

Figure 3.69 Hypoplastic left heart syndrome – MR. Cine MR image depicts the Damus-Kaye-Stansel anastomosis, an anastomosis between the main pulmonary artery (MPA) and the ascending aorta (Ao). This anastomosis is necessary for establishing stable systemic arterial flow.

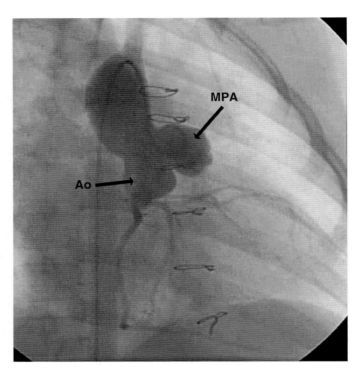

Figure 3.70 Hypoplastic left heart syndrome – angiography. With a catheter in the ascending aorta, an injection opacifies the Damus-Kaye-Stansel anastomosis, an anastomosis between the main pulmonary artery (MPA) and the ascending aorta (Ao). This anastomosis is necessary for establishing stable systemic arterial flow.

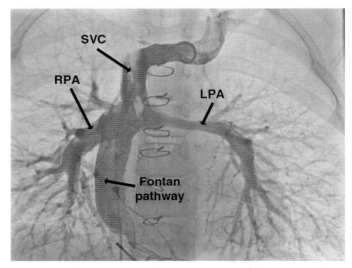

Figure 3.71 Fontan – angiography. An ap angiogram of the Fontan pathway (lateral tunnel). Opacified is the innominate vein draining into the right superior vena cava (SVC), which is connected to the pulmonary arteries (RPA, LPA) via a right bidirectional cavopulmonary (Glenn) anastomosis. The inferior vena cava is connected to this Fontan pathway via an intra-atrial baffle (lateral tunnel) to the undersurface of the branch pulmonary arteries.

this procedure is to separate the systemic and pulmonary circulations by using the single ventricle as the systemic pumping chamber and allowing systemic venous blood to flow passively to the pulmonary circulation. Although this procedure has allowed many children to survive childhood and live relatively normal early lives, they ultimately suffer many complications including chronic systemic venous hypertension, hepatic dysfunction, arrhythmias, thromboembolic complications, protein-losing enteropathy, progressive cyanosis, and low cardiac output state.

Rings and slings
Aortic arch abnormalities and pulmonary artery sling

Vascular rings represent a group of abnormalities of the aortic arch, many of which cause respiratory and feeding difficulties.

They are either complete vascular rings that entirely encircle the trachea and esophagus (double aortic arch and right aortic arch with left ligamentum arteriosum) or incomplete vascular

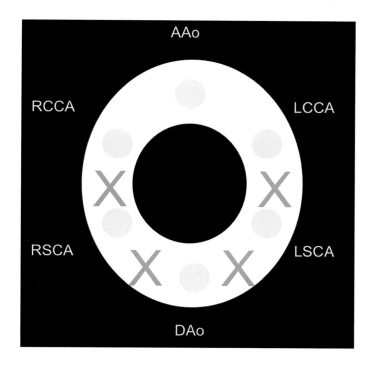

Figure 3.72 Vascular rings – diagram. Depicted is a graphic of the double aortic arch that is present during fetal development. If the arch divides between the right common carotid (RCCA) and the right subclavian (RSCA) arteries, there is a left aortic arch with aberrant right subclavian. If the arch divides between the right subclavian artery and the descending aorta (DAo), there is a left aortic arch with normal branching. If the arch divides between the left subclavian artery (LSCA) and the descending aorta, there is a right aortic arch with mirror image branching. If the arch divides between the left common carotid (LCCA) and left subclavian arteries, there is a right aortic arch with aberrant left subclavian. AAo = ascending aorta.

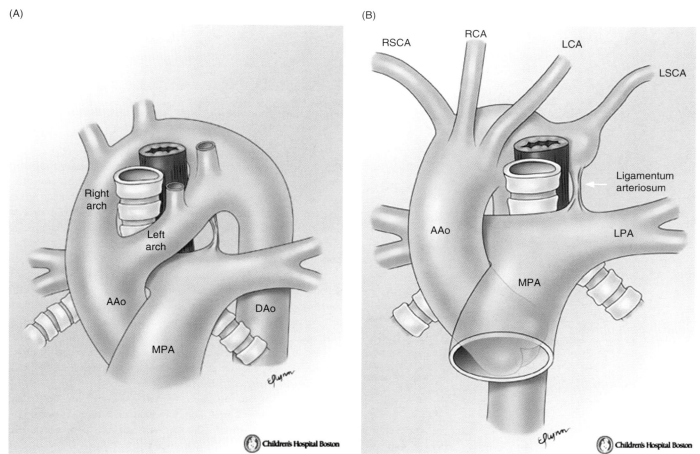

Figure 3.73 Vascular rings – diagram. (A) Double aortic arch in which the ascending aorta (AAo) leads to an anterior left arch and posterior right arch that join to form the descending aorta (DAo). The arches encircle the posterior esophagus and anterior trachea. The ligamentum arteriosum joins the left arch to the pulmonary artery. (B) Right aortic arch with an aberrant origin of the left subclavian artery (LSCA), in which the aortic arch crosses over the right bronchus and the order of origin of brachiocephalic arteries arising from the aorta is: right subclavian artery (RSCA), right carotid artery (RCA), left carotid artery (LCA) and left subclavian artery (LSCA). The posterior esophagus and anterior trachea are encircled by a vascular ring that is completed by the ligamentum arteriosum. In this figure there is an outpouching at the base of the left subclavian artery that is termed a diverticulum of Kommerell. MPA = main pulmonary artery; LPA = left pulmonary artery. *From the Multimedia Library of Congenital Heart Disease, Children's Hospital, Boston, MA, editor Robert Geggel, MD, www.childrenshospital.org/mml/cvp with permission.*

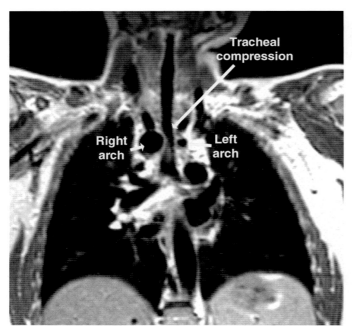

Figure 3.74 Double aortic arch – MRI. Coronal black blood MR image in a four-year-old with a double aortic arch. The right (dominant) arch is seen to compress the trachea laterally.

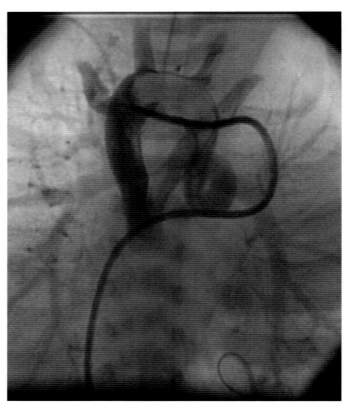

Figure 3.75 Double aortic arch – angiography. A catheter is positioned in the right aortic arch near the right subclavian artery (the catheter course is IVC to RA to RV to MPA to PDA to aorta). Angiography reveals a double aortic arch.

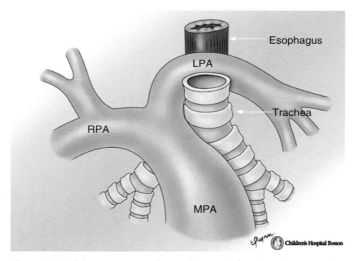

Figure 3.76 Pulmonary artery sling – diagram. Left pulmonary artery sling is depicted, in which the left pulmonary artery (LPA) arises from the right pulmonary artery (RPA) and courses between the posterior esophagus and anterior trachea. MPA = main pulmonary artery. *From the Multimedia Library of Congenital Heart Disease, Children's Hospital, Boston, MA, editor Robert Geggel, MD, www.childrenshospital.org/mml/cvp with permission.*

rings that do not entirely encircle but do compress the trachea and esophagus (anomalous innominate artery, aberrant right subclavian artery and anomalous left pulmonary artery; Figures 3.72, 3.73).

Double aortic arch is the most common vascular ring (40%; Figures 3.72, 3.74, 3.75). This lesion consists of patent right and left aortic arches that surround the trachea and esophagus. The right arch gives rise to the right common carotid and right subclavian artery, and the left arch gives rise to the left common carotid and the left subclavian artery. The right arch is usually the larger of the two. It is usually an isolated defect, although it can be associated with other congenital heart defects.

Right aortic arch with left ligamentum arteriosus is the second most common vascular ring (30%; Figure 3.73). The right aortic arch usually has mirror image branching (left innominate artery, right common carotid artery, right subclavian artery). The ligamentum arteriosus usually arises from the left subclavian artery. This ring is almost always associated with more complex CHD; particularly the conotruncal abnormalities such as TOF and truncus arteriosus.

Anomalous innominate artery is less common, occurring in 10% of vascular rings. The defect consists of an innominate artery that arises more distally than normal from the aortic arch and can cause tracheal compression.

Aberrant right subclavian artery occurs in 20% of all known vascular rings; however, this may be an underestimation as it is often asymptomatic. In this lesion, the right subclavian artery arises from the descending aorta and travels

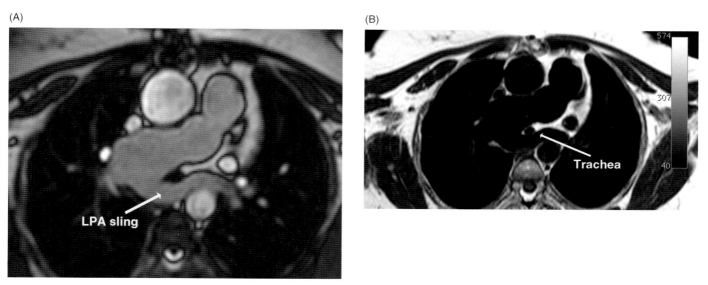

Figure 3.77 Pulmonary artery sling – MRI. (A) Axial cine image of the branch pulmonary arteries in a patient with a pulmonary artery sling. (B) Axial black blood imaging in the same plane, demonstrating tracheal compression. LPA = left pulmonary artery.

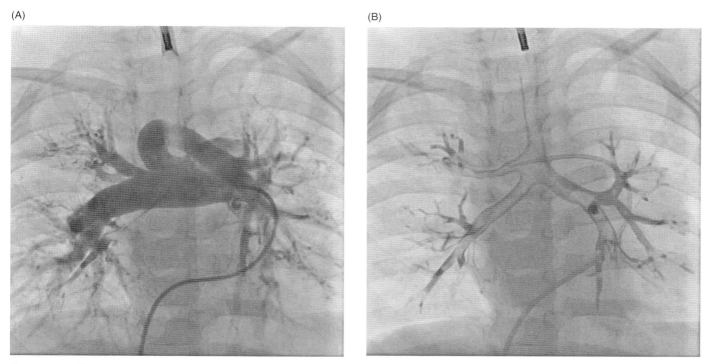

Figure 3.78 Pulmonary artery sling – angiography and bronchogram. (A) Anteroposterior angiogram with injection in the main pulmonary artery reveals a pulmonary artery sling with left pulmonary artery from the right pulmonary artery. (B) Bronchogram in the same patient reveals right lateral compression of the trachea by the sling.

posterior to the esophagus. This can occasionally cause mild feeding difficulties.

Anomalous left pulmonary artery or pulmonary artery sling is quite rare. In this lesion, the left pulmonary artery arises from the right pulmonary artery and courses behind the trachea and in front of the esophagus causing compression of both (Figures 3.76–78). This defect is associated with other CHD 50% of the time.

Further reading

Bandettini WP, Arai AE (2008) Advances in clinical applications of cardiovascular magnetic resonance imaging. *Heart* **94**, 1485–95.

Chan FP (2008) MR and CT imaging of the pediatric patient with structural heart disease. *Semin Thorac Cardiovasc Surg* **20**, 393–9.

Chan FP (2009) MR and CT imaging of the pediatric patient with structural heart disease. *Semin Thorac Cardiovasc Surg Pediatr Card Surg Annu* **12**, 99–105.

Dae MW (2007) Pediatric nuclear cardiology. *Semin Nucl Med* **37**, 382–90.

Dillman JR, Hernandez RJ (2009) Role of CT in the evaluation of congenital cardiovascular disease in children. *Am J Roentgenol* **192**, 1219–31.

Franklin RC, Jacobs JP, Krogmann ON *et al.* (2008) Nomenclature for congenital and pediatric cardiac disease: historical perspectives and The International Pediatric and Congenital Cardiac Code. *Cardiol Young* **18**(Suppl. 2), 70–80.

Gaca AM, Jaggers JJ, Dudley LT, Bisset GS 3rd (2008) Repair of congenital heart disease: a primer—part 1. *Radiology* **247**, 617–31.

Gaca AM, Jaggers JJ, Dudley LT, Bisset GS 3rd (2008) Repair of congenital heart disease: a primer—part 2. *Radiology* **248**, 44–60.

Gutiérrez FR, Ho ML, Siegel MJ (2008) Practical applications of magnetic resonance in congenital heart disease. *Magn Reson Imaging Clin N Am* **16**, 403–35.

Jone PN, Schowengerdt KO Jr (2009) Prenatal diagnosis of congenital heart disease. *Pediatr Clin North Am* **56**, 709–15. Review.

Kellenberger CJ, Yoo SJ, Büchel ER (2007) Cardiovascular MR imaging in neonates and infants with congenital heart disease. *Radiographics* **27**, 5–18.

Krishnamurthy R (2009) The role of MRI and CT in congenital heart disease. *Pediatr Radiol* **39**(Suppl. 2), S196–204.

Lopez L (2009) Advances in echocardiography. *Curr Opin Pediatr* **21**, 579–84.

Marcotte F, Poirier N, Pressacco J *et al.* (2009) Evaluation of adult congenital heart disease by cardiac magnetic resonance imaging. *Congenit Heart Dis* **4**, 216–30.

McLaren CA, Elliott MJ, Roebuck DJ (2008) Vascular compression of the airway in children. *Paediatr Respir Rev* **9**, 85–94.

Mertens L, Friedberg MK (2009) The gold standard for noninvasive imaging in congenital heart disease: echocardiography. *Curr Opin Cardiol* **24**, 119–24.

Mertens L, Ganame J, Eyskens B (2008) What is new in pediatric cardiac imaging? *Eur J Pediatr* **167**, 1–8.

Simonetti OP, Cook S (2006) Technical aspects of pediatric CMR. *J Cardiovasc Magn Reson* **8**, 581–93.

Spevak PJ, Johnson PT, Fishman EK (2008) Surgically corrected congenital heart disease: utility of 64-MDCT. *Am J Roentgenol* **191**, 854–61.

Tanous D, Benson LN, Horlick EM (2009) Coarctation of the aorta: evaluation and management. *Curr Opin Cardiol*, in press.

Tsai IC, Chen MC, Jan SL *et al.* (2008) Neonatal cardiac multidetector row CT: why and how we do it. *Pediatr Radiol* **38**, 438–51.

Turner CG, Tworetzky W, Wilkins-Haug LE, Jennings RW (2009) Cardiac anomalies in the fetus. *Clin Perinatol* **36**, 439–49, xi. Review.

Warnes CA (2006) Transposition of the great arteries. *Circulation* **114**, 2699–709.

Weber OM, Higgins CB (2006) MR evaluation of cardiovascular physiology in congenital heart disease: flow and function. *J Cardiovasc Magn Reson* **8**, 607–17.

Wiant A, Nyberg E, Gilkeson RC (2009) CT evaluation of congenital heart disease in adults. *Am J Roentgenol* **193**, 388–96. Review.

Pediatric trauma

Sandra Wootton-Gorges

Head trauma

Pediatric head trauma is the leading cause of death in the pediatric population. The mechanism of injury varies based upon the age of the child: non-accidental trauma falls predominate in the child under two, while motor-vehicle accidents and bicycle injuries predominate in the older child. As one would suppose, the greater biomechanical forces generally produce more significant injuries; the type of force determines the particular type of associated injury.

Computed tomography of the head is a rapid and sensitive test for identifying intracranial injury, but must be used judiciously. Clinical features which may be associated with an increased risk of intracranial injury after blunt head trauma include altered mental status, short term memory loss, vomiting, headache, post-traumatic seizure, clinical evidence of skull fracture, and scalp hematoma in children less than two years of age. Magnetic resonance imaging is more sensitive for both non-hemorrhagic intra-axial lesions and subtle extra-axial hematomas. Advanced MR imaging techniques such as susceptibility-weighted imaging, spectroscopy, diffusion-weighted imaging (DWI) and diffusion tensor imaging may provide further characterization in traumatic brain injury. For example, susceptibility-weighted imaging is useful in detecting small hemorrhagic lesions often associated with diffuse axonal injury (Figure 4.1), while diffusion-weighted imaging is useful in the detection of ischemic injury (Figure 4.2).

Skull fractures

Compared with adults, the calvarium in a child is softer and thinner, and, in children under four, the calvarium is unilaminar and lacks diploe. Children are thus more likely to suffer skull fracture (Figure 4.3) from minor trauma, and children with skull fracture are at increased risk of intracranial injury. Basilar, depressed (Figure 4.4) or stellate fractures require greater impact than simple linear fractures. Scalp hematomas are common with skull fracture.

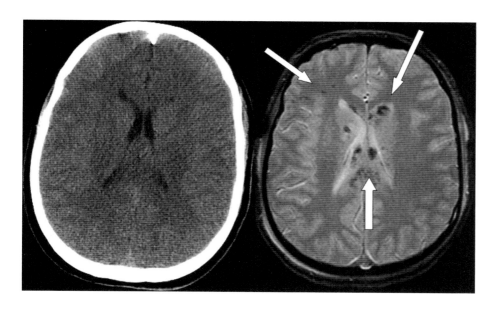

Figure 4.1 Axial CT and GRE (gradient echo) images of a 16-year-old motor-vehicle accident victim. While the CT does not show any abnormality, the GRE shows multiple low-intensity foci (arrows) within punctate parenchymal hemorrhagic axonal injury in the basal ganglia, right frontal white matter and corpus callosum, and left frontal intraventricular hemorrhage.

Essentials of Pediatric Radiology, ed. Heike E. Daldrup-Link and Charles A. Gooding. Published by Cambridge University Press.
© Cambridge University Press 2010.

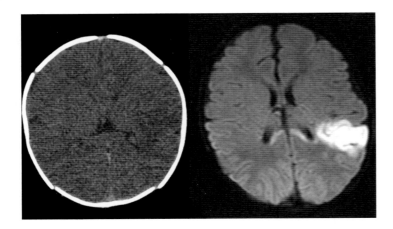

Figure 4.2 Unenhanced CT and DWI axial images of a seven-day-old. While no abnormality is seen by CT, the DWI clearly shows hyperintense left temporal cytotoxic edema/infarction which extends into the splenium of the corpus callosum.

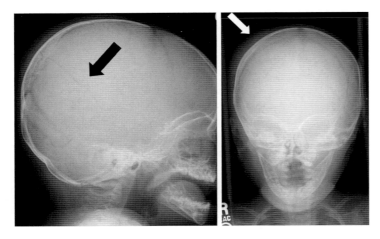

Figure 4.3 Lateral and frontal skull radiographs show a scalp hematoma (white arrow) adjacent to a linear right parietal skull fracture (black arrow) in this eight-month-old baby.

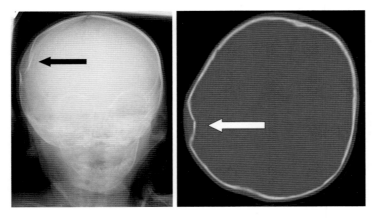

Figure 4.4 Frontal skull radiograph and axial CT bone window images demonstrating a depressed right parietal skull fracture (arrows).

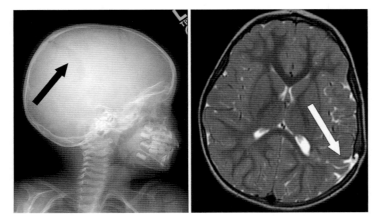

Figure 4.5 Lateral skull radiograph showing a growing skull fracture (black arrow) in a two-year-old. The accompanying T2-weighted MRI image shows the meninges bulging into the fracture line (white arrow).

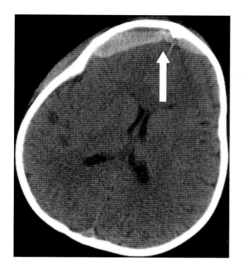

Figure 4.6 Axial unenhanced CT showing an acute, high-density right epidural hemorrhage crossing the midline anterior to the falx.

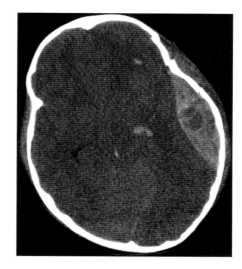

Figure 4.7 Unenhanced CT of a two-year-old, showing an inhomogeneous left temporoparietal EDH, suggesting continuing hemorrhage, and punctate left frontal and left thalamic intraparenchymal hemorrhage, hemorrhage in the aqueduct of Sylvius, left frontal skull fracture, diffuse cerebral edema with cisternal effacement, and midline shift to the right.

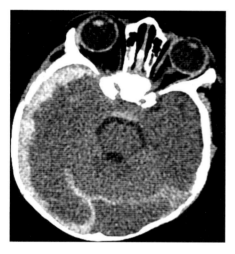

Figure 4.8 CT of a four-month-old boy after minor head trauma. There is an extensive right-sided subdural high-density hematoma that extends onto the tentorium and crosses to the left. After clinical evaluation, it was found that this infant has hemophilia.

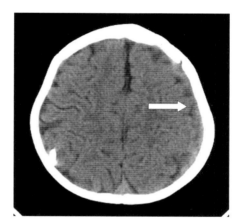

Figure 4.9 This 15-month-old has an isodense left subdural hematoma (arrow) which displaces the brain. There is a subdural shunt on the opposite side.

Complications of skull fracture may include meningitis (especially with basilar fracture) and leptomeningeal cyst, or growing fracture (Figure 4.5). Growing fractures result from interposition of torn meninges within the fracture fragments. With time, CSF pulsations widen the fracture site. Leptomeningeal cysts are most common under three years of age and in the parietal and frontal bones.

Epidural hematoma

Epidural hematomas (EDHs) are less common in children than in adults. They occur between the skull and the outer dura, and are limited by the sutures. However, they can cross the midline as they are extradural (Figure 4.6). They are typically biconvex, high-attenuation fluid collections by CT; inhomogeneity should suggest continuing hemorrhage (Figure 4.7). Associated adjacent skull fracture is less commonly seen in children than in adults. In fact, many epidural

hematomas in children are venous due to dural tear or diploic hemorrhage, and evolve more slowly than arterial hemorrhage.

Subdural hematoma

Subdural hematomas (SDHs) occur between the arachnoid and inner dura, usually from tearing of cortical bridging veins. They may occur after accidental or non-accidental trauma, and are more commonly associated with underlying parenchymal injury than EDHs. Pediatric subdural hematomas have no consistent relationship to skull fracture. Unlike adults, in children SDHs may be bilateral in up to 80% of cases and frequently extend onto the tentorium or into the interhemispheric fissure (Figure 4.8). The lack of dural adhesions in children may allow extensive spread of the SDH to involve the temporal, frontal and parietal regions. Acute (<3 days) SDHs are crescentic, high-density collections by CT, and are limited by dural attachments. Accidental SDHs are more frequently homogeneous than those due to non-accidental trauma. Over the ensuing one to three weeks, the SDH becomes isodense (Figure 4.9), and then hypodense with respect to the brain. By MR, the appearance of the SDH depends upon its age (Table 4.1).

The "big black brain" is profound brain injury which occurs in infants with acute subdural hematoma (both traumatic and non-accidental) (Figure 4.10). With this entity, the hemisphere is hypodense, with loss of gray–white differentiation; the thalami may or may not be involved. It may be unilateral or bilateral, and it crosses multiple vascular territories. The involved brain goes on to sustain rapid and profound atrophic change, and mortality is high. The exact pathophysiology of this lesion is not yet understood, and may represent a combination of hypoxic-ischemic injury, perfusion–demand mismatch, increased metabolic demand from seizures, hypercarbia and other factors that exceed the ability of the infant brain to compensate.

Subarachnoid hemorrhage

Acute post-traumatic subarachnoid hemorrhage (SAH) is not uncommon. It is seen by CT as high-density blood within the sulci, sylvian fissure and interpeduncular cistern (Figure 4.11). SAH in isolation, or if disproportionately severe, should suggest a vascular injury. FLAIR sequences are more sensitive in detecting SAH than other routine MR sequences, with the SAH appearing hyperintense (normal CSF would be hypointense).

Table 4.1 Dating of subdural hematomas

Age	T1W	T2W	FLAIR
Acute	Isointense	Bright	Bright
Early subacute (3–7 day)	Bright	Isointense	Bright
Late subacute (3 week)	Bright	Bright	Bright
Old (4 month)	Dark	Bright	Isointense

Reproduced with permission from Duhem et al. (2006).

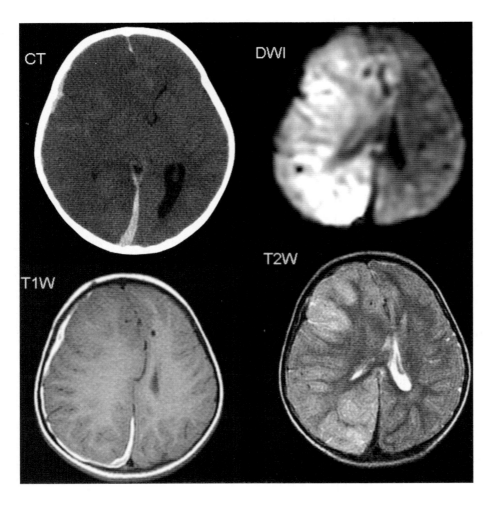

Figure 4.10 "Big black brain" is seen in the right cerebral hemisphere in this 17-month-old victim of non-accidental trauma. The CT shows marked midline shift to the left, effacement of the right lateral ventricle and trapping of the left trigone, a rim of hyperdense acute SDH (arrow) which extends into the posterior interhemispheric fissure, and SAH into the sulci. By DWI, the hemisphere, both cortex and white matter, shows cytotoxic edema/infarction. On T1W (T1-weighted) images, the SDH is bright, while on T2W images it is isointense, suggesting early subacute hemorrhage.

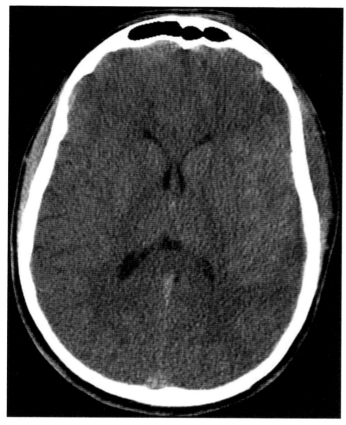

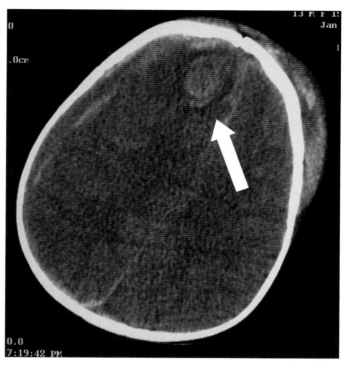

Figure 4.12 Hemorrhagic contusion (arrow) in a 13-month-old who suffered a fall from the second story of a building. The right frontal lesion is a coup-type lesion, seen just below a frontal fracture. There is associated hyperacute SDH. There is also midline shift to the left.

Figure 4.11 Subarachnoid hemorrhage is seen as high density filling the sulci in the left temporal region, in this teenager who was involved in a motor-vehicle accident. There is an adjacent scalp hematoma.

Table 4.2 Dating of intraparenchymal hemorrhage

Age	T1W	T2W	FLAIR
Acute	Isointense	Dark	Dark
Early subacute (3–7 day)	Isointense	Dark	Dark
Late subacute (3 week)	Bright	Bright	Bright
Old (4 month)	Dark	Dark	Dark

Reproduced with permission from Duhem *et al.* (2006).

Intraparenchymal injury

Parenchymal injuries may include contusions, diffuse axonal injury, and parenchymal hematomas. The differentiation between a contusion and parenchymal hematoma is somewhat arbitrary in the setting of trauma: if the lesion contains more than two-thirds blood, it is considered a hematoma.

Contusions (Figure 4.12) may occur in the brain just below the point of impact (coup lesion) or opposite the impact site (contracoup lesion), and account for about half of all intra-axial injuries. Contusions in the frontal or temporal lobes may occur as the parenchyma slides over the rough floor of the frontal and middle cranial fossae. They usually involve the gray matter and spare the white matter, and appear acutely as ill-defined high-attenuation lesions by CT. Over the first four to six days after injury the contusion may swell, and surrounding edema may develop. Thus, close monitoring of these patients is necessary, as resulting neurological deterioration and/or herniation may occur. MRI is more sensitive in detecting non-hemorrhagic contusions, while gradient echo sequences are helpful in detecting hemorrhagic lesions.

Parenchymal hematomas occur most frequently in the frontal lobes and basal ganglia. The appearance of intraparenchymal

hemorrhage by MRI varies based upon its age and the location and oxygenation state of the hemoglobin within the hematoma (Table 4.2).

Diffuse axonal injury (DAI) results from angular or rotational shearing forces which tear axons. These occur most commonly at the gray–white matter junction, splenium of the corpus callosum, dorsolateral brain stem and internal capsule. CT may be normal in DAI, or may show punctate hemorrhages with high attenuation. MRI is more sensitive in the diagnosis of DAI (Figure 4.1). The lesions are punctate round or elliptical hypointense foci, which parallel the axonal tracts by susceptibility MR (GRE – gradient echo) sequences. Typical clinical findings include unconsciousness, posturing and hypertension.

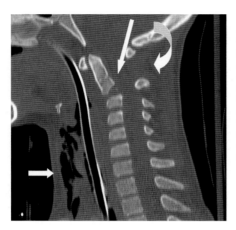

Figure 4.13 Twelve-year-old boy. Sagittal reformatted cervical spine CT image shows a C2 fracture (long arrow) along with widening of the C1–2 interspace, indicating posterior ligamentous disruption (curved arrow) resulting from flexion injury. There is also a tracheal fracture (short arrow) with subcutaneous emphysema in the anterior neck.

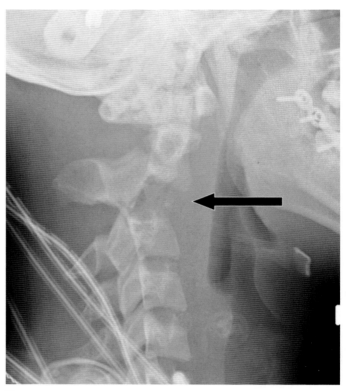

Figure 4.14 Lateral c-spine radiograph showing perched facets at the C2–3 level (arrow) in this child with cervical spine dislocation (and C2 endplate fracture). There is associated prevertebral soft tissue swelling.

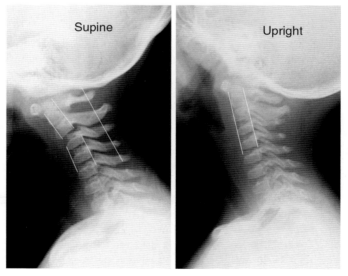

Figure 4.15 Lateral spine radiographs in a three-year-old. The supine examination shows pseudosubluxation at C2–3. This is due to the relatively large occiput in children, and cervical spine ligamentous laxity. While there appears to be offset at C2–3 along the anterior and posterior vertebral body lines, the spinous process line appears intact. When the patient is placed upright, the spinal alignment is normal at C2–3.

Cervical spine trauma

Cervical spine injuries are relatively uncommon in pediatric trauma patients, and most commonly result from motor-vehicle accidents. Other causes include sports-related activities, falls and child abuse. The relatively larger head in children, underdeveloped neck muscles, incomplete vertebral ossification, immature vertebral configuration, and ligamentous laxity account for a different injury pattern in the cervical spine in the pediatric population when compared with adults. Injuries may include fractures (Figure 4.13), dislocations (Figure 4.14) (with or without fractures) or SCIWORA (spinal cord injury without radiographic abnormality). Upper cervical spine (C1–C4) injuries predominate, especially in the child under eight years, while, in older children, injury may also occur in the lower cervical spine. In motor-vehicle trauma, cervical spine injury is usually associated with other (especially head) injuries.

SCIWORA injuries predominate in sports-related injuries (except diving injuries), in motor-vehicle accidents in the very young child, and at the C1–4 level. MRI is very useful in this diagnosis, and may show ligamentous tear or hemorrhage, disc hemorrhage, spinal cord edema, hemorrhage, or disruption.

The cervical spine radiograph (Figure 4.15) is the mainstay in the diagnosis of cervical spine injury in children, but flexion-extension radiographs have not proved useful in the pediatric patients with normal static cervical spine radiographs. Helical CT with multiplanar reconstruction has become an important tool in the diagnosis of cervical trauma in the pediatric population as it is extremely accurate, though the radiation risk raises concern. MRI is useful in defining cord and nerve injury in those patients with neurological symptoms (Figure 4.16).

Atlanto-occipital dislocation (AOD) is a highly unstable and often fatal injury. However, with improved on-scene resuscitation, more patients are surviving this injury. There is usually associated head injury in these patients, which may mask the cervical injury. Initial lateral cervical radiographs usually define AOD (Figure 4.17). The normal basion–dens interval

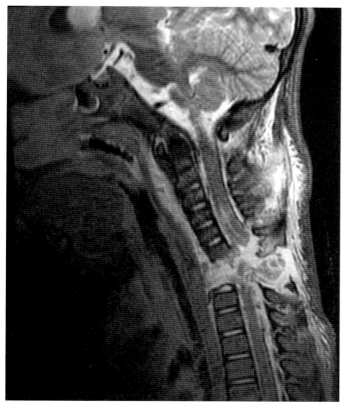

Figure 4.16 This T2-weighted MR image clearly defines the devastating cervical spine injury in this child. There is complete cord transsection at the C6–7 level with gross distraction at the C6 vertebral body endplate fracture. There is central cord edema just above this level. Complete ligamentous disruption is seen posteriorly. There is marked prevertebral soft tissue swelling anteriorly, and subcutaneous soft tissue edema posteriorly.

is less than 12 mm, and the basion should be no more than 12 mm anterior to the posterior axial line in children. If there is deviation from these measurements, then AOD should be suspected, and CT with multiplanar reconstruction and MRI to assess for ligamentous and cord injury may further define the injury.

Chest trauma

Chest injuries are second only to head injury as the cause of death in pediatric blunt trauma. Clinical predictors for intrathoracic injury after pediatric blunt trauma include hypotension, GCS (Glasgow Coma Scale) score <15, abnormal chest examination or auscultation, tachypnea, and femur fracture.

Chest radiography is still the mainstay in the diagnosis of pediatric chest trauma, with CT reserved for selected cases. Pulmonary contusion (Figure 4.18), rib fractures (Figure 4.19), pneumothorax (Figure 4.20) and hemothorax are the most common injuries seen. Other more serious but less common injuries may include cardiac, vascular (Figure 4.21) or diaphragmatic injury, or sternal fracture (Figure 4.22). Bronchial injuries are rare in children. Half of patients will have multiple thoracic injuries.

Abdominal trauma

Most abdominal trauma in children is blunt, including motor-vehicle accidents, bicycle, skateboard, motorcycle and ATV (all terrain vehicle) accidents, falls, assault and non-accidental trauma.

CT is the standard imaging modality utilized in the evaluation of pediatric abdominal trauma. Its role is to obtain accurate delineation of the extent and type of intra-abdominal injury. While FAST (focused abdominal sonography for trauma) scanning is a useful screening test in the adult population, it has not proven to be as useful in the pediatric population, as children

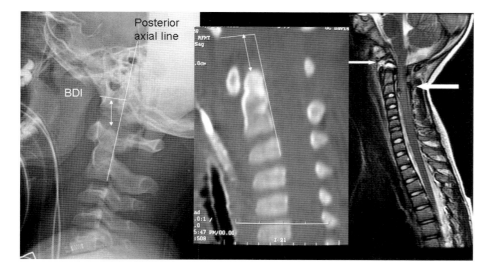

Figure 4.17 Atlanto-occipital disassociation in a six-year-old. The basion–dens interval (BDI) is increased both on the c-spine radiograph and on the CT reformatted image. The basion should not be more than 12 mm anterior to the posterior axial line. Note the prevertebral soft tissue swelling as well. T2-weighted MRI on another patient with AOD shows the associated ligamentous injury (small arrow) and cord edema and hematoma (larger arrow).

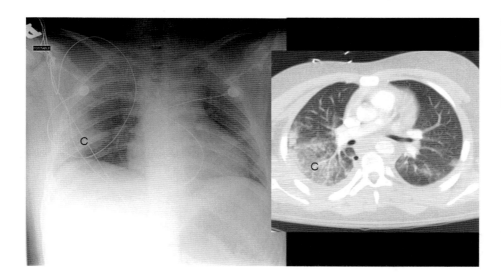

Figure 4.18 Fifteen-year-old involved in a motor-vehicle accident. Chest radiograph and CT show airspace opacity due to pulmonary contusion in the right lateral lung base (C). The mediastinum is also widened in this patient, who did have a mediastinal hematoma and aortic injury. Bilateral small pleural effusions/hemorrhage are better seen by CT.

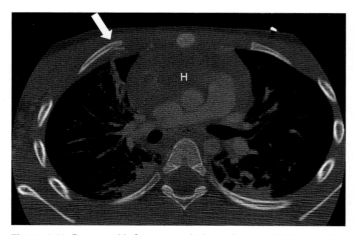

Figure 4.19 Five-year-old after motor-vehicle accident. Axial CT image of the chest shows an anterior right third rib fracture (arrow). The patient also had a large mediastinal hematoma (H) due to venous bleeding.

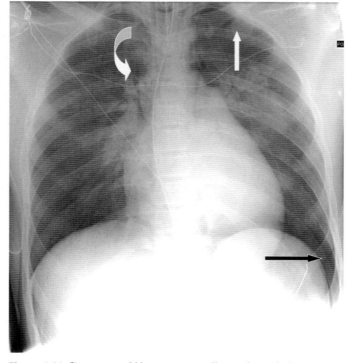

Figure 4.20 Sixteen-year-old hanging victim. Chest radiograph demonstrates both a pneumomediastinum (curved arrow), and left pneumothorax (straight arrows) in this intubated patient. There is a nice example of a deep sulcus sign (black arrow).

with solid organ injury may not have free fluid present, and FAST scan will miss retroperitoneal injury.

Strict attention to technical details is very important in CT for pediatric abdominal trauma. First, strategies which minimize radiation dose must be utilized, as CT radiation-induced cancer remains a significant concern for the pediatric population. Children are more radiosensitive than adults, and have a longer life expectancy in which to manifest radiation-induced cancer. The milliamperage, kilovoltage, and pitch, etc. need to be adjusted based on the patient size. Intravenous contrast, typically at a dose of 2.0 ml kg^{-1}, is necessary to improve differentiation between normal and pathological parenchyma. Oral contrast is usually not given for CT evaluation for blunt trauma in children.

There is considerable debate as to the indication for CT examination in children after trauma. Since children are often unable to verbalize their symptoms, and localization of their pain can be difficult, CT is often used as a screening tool to detect intra-abdominal injury. However, certain indications have been associated with a high risk of intra-abdominal injury, including: more than three clinical indications (such as abdominal abrasions, contusions, ecchymoses, distension, absence of bowel sounds, tenderness, presence of blood per rectum or per nasogastric tube, hematuria, dropping or low hematocrit), gross hematuria, abdominal tenderness, trauma score ≤12, bicycle accident as the mechanism of injury, and

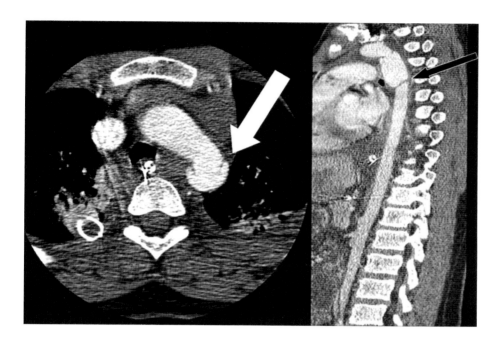

Figure 4.21 Twelve-year-old with aortic tear. CTs in axial and sagittal planes show the flap (black arrow) and pseudoaneurysm (white arrow).

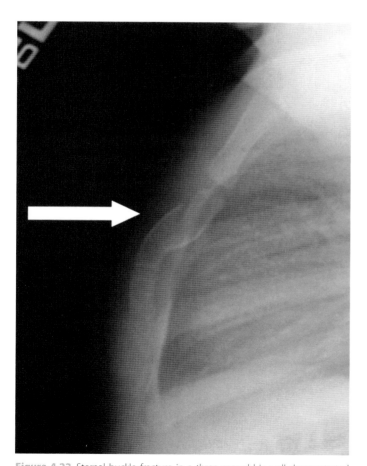

Figure 4.22 Sternal buckle fracture in a three-year-old is well demonstrated on this lateral radiograph.

Table 4.3 Liver injury scale

Grade	Injury description
I	Subcapsular hematoma, <10% surface area Capsular laceration, <1 cm parenchymal depth
II	Subcapsular hematoma, 10–50% surface area Intraparenchymal hematoma <10 cm in diameter Capsular laceration, 1–3 cm parenchymal depth, <10 cm in length
III	Subcapsular hematoma, >50% surface area or expanding Ruptured subcapsular or parenchymal hematoma Intraparenchymal hematoma >10 cm or expanding Laceration >3 cm parenchymal depth
IV	Parenchymal disruption 25–75% of hepatic lobe or 1–3 Couinaud's segments within a single lobe
V	Parenchymal disruption >75% of hepatic lobe or >3 Couinaud's segments in a single lobe Juxtahepatic venous injury Hepatic avulsion

Reproduced from Moore *et al.* (1995), with permission from Elsevier.

evidence of lap-belt injury. Neurological impairment without concurrent abdominal signs is a low-yield indicator of underlying abdominal injury.

Liver and spleen

The thinner abdominal wall and the relatively larger exposure of the spleen and liver below the ribcage in children make these organs more likely to be injured after blunt trauma than in adults.

Children with hepatic injuries typically present with abdominal pain and elevated hepatic enzyme levels. Injuries are characterized according to type of injury (Table 4.3) and site of

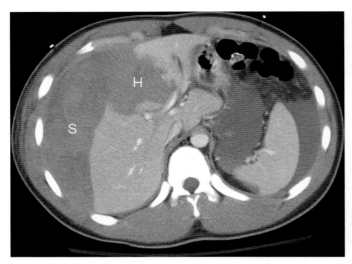

Figure 4.23 Contiguous liver parenchymal hematomas (H) and subcapsular hematoma (S) (grade III injury) in a 16-year-old. The inhomogeneous nature of the hematomas suggests continuing hemorrhage. There is also a large amount of blood in the peritoneal cavity.

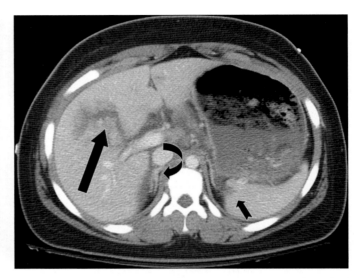

Figure 4.24 Fourteen-year-old girl who was run over by a car. Enhanced CT examination of the abdomen shows a liver laceration (arrow) and periportal edema/hemorrhage. There is also a small medial splenic contusion or hematoma noted (arrowhead). The right adrenal gland is compressed by a component of retroperitoneal hemorrhage (curved arrow).

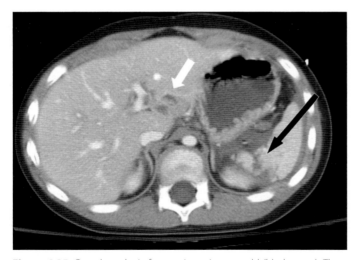

Figure 4.25 Complex splenic fracture in a nine-year-old (black arrow). There are also small liver hematomas noted (white arrow).

Table 4.4 Splenic injury scale

Grade	Injury description
I	Subcapsular hematoma, <10% surface area Capsular laceration, <1 cm parenchymal depth
II	Subcapsular hematomas, 10–50% surface area Intraparenchymal hematoma <5 cm in diameter Capsular laceration, 1–3 cm parenchymal depth which does not involve trabecular vessel
III	Subcapsular hematoma, >50% surface area or expanding Ruptured subcapsular or parenchymal hematoma Intraparenchymal hematoma >5 cm or expanding Laceration >3 cm parenchymal depth or involving trabecular vessels
IV	Laceration involving segmental or hilar vessels with >25% devascularization of spleen
V	Completely shattered spleen Hilar vascular injury which devascularizes spleen

Reproduced from Moore *et al.* (1995), with permission from Elsevier.

involvement. Injuries include subcapsular and parenchymal hematomas, lacerations and fractures. The right lobe is the most commonly injured. Parenchymal hematomas (Figure 4.23) are oval or rounded collections of blood, whereas lacerations (Figure 4.24) are linear or branching. A fracture extends completely through the parenchyma, dividing it into two or more fragments. If the laceration or fracture extends through the biliary tree, a bile leak may develop. About 70% of patients with hepatic injury will have free intraperitoneal fluid, most commonly in the pelvis. The amount of fluid increases with the injury grade.

Splenic injuries likewise include subcapsular or parenchymal hematomas, lacerations, fractures (Figure 4.25), and splenic pedicle injuries. These injuries may be described both by position and by severity (Table 4.4).

Pancreas

Pancreatic injury (Table 4.5), which results from compression of the pancreas against the spine, may include laceration (Figure 4.26), hematomas, contusion, transaction, or clinical pancreatitis. The pancreatic body is the most frequently injured area of the pancreas. The presence of peripancreatic fluid, especially fluid in the lesser sac, in the absence of abdominal visceral injury should strongly suggest pancreatic injury. It also suggests injury

Table 4.5 Pancreatic injury scale

Grade	Injury description
I	Minor contusion or superficial laceration without duct injury
II	Major contusion or laceration without duct injury or tissue loss
III	Distal transaction or parenchymal injury with duct injury
IV	Proximal transection or parenchymal injury involving ampulla
V	Massive disruption of pancreatic head

Reproduced from Moore *et al.* (1995), with permission from Elsevier.

to the main pancreatic duct. Pseudocysts may develop in about one-third of children with pancreatic injury.

Adrenal gland

Post-traumatic adrenal hemorrhage is seen in only about 3% of children after blunt trauma; it is rarely seen as an isolated injury. Hemorrhage is usually unilateral and right sided, but may be bilateral. The enlarged gland may be oval or triangular, and will be of lower density than the adjacent enhanced liver or spleen on enhanced CT (Figure 4.27). Adjacent diaphragmatic crural thickening, as well as associated ipsilateral intrathoracic and/or intra-abdominal injuries, is frequent.

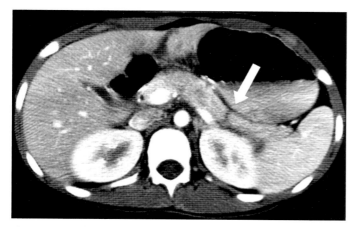

Figure 4.26 Enhanced CT image showing a distal body pancreatic fracture (arrow) in this teenage girl involved in a motor-vehicle accident.

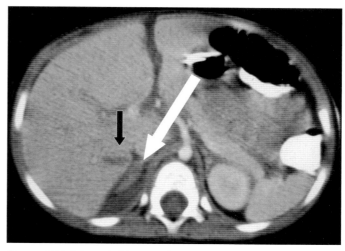

Figure 4.27 Enhanced CT image shows an enlarged, hypodense adrenal gland hemorrhage (white arrow) with surrounding retroperitoneal hemorrhage, along with a small liver laceration (black arrow) in a pediatric patient.

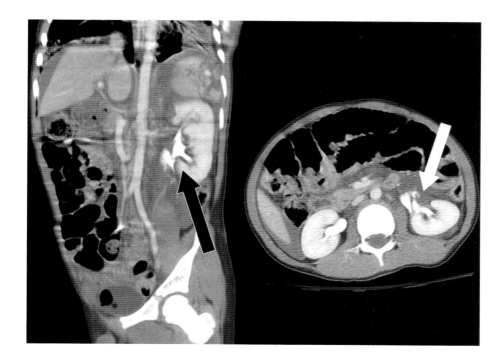

Figure 4.28 Enhanced CT images show a renal laceration with ureteropelvic junction tear and contrast extravasation (arrows). There is an associated perirenal hematoma/urinoma. The patient also has a splenic laceration and free intraperitoneal fluid.

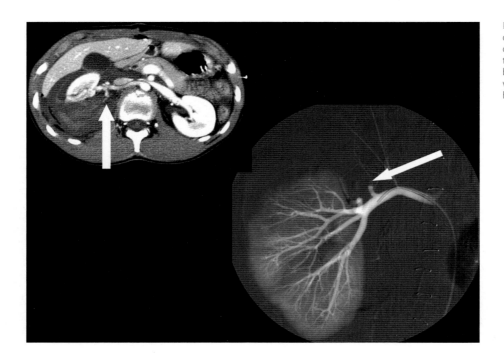

Figure 4.29 Sixteen-year-old in motorcycle accident. There is right upper pole renal laceration with devascularization and perirenal hemorrhage. The truncated right upper pole artery can be seen by both CT and angiography (arrow). The patient went on to embolization because of continuing hemorrhage from the torn artery.

Table 4.6 Kidney injury scale

Grade	Injury description
I	Contusion (hematuria with normal imaging studies) Nonexpanding subcapsular hematoma
II	Nonexpanding perirenal retroperitoneal hematoma Laceration <1 cm parenchymal depth without urinary extravasation
III	Laceration >1 cm parenchymal depth without collecting system rupture or urinary extravasation
IV	Parenchymal laceration extending through the renal cortex, medulla and collecting system Main renal artery or vein injury with contained hemorrhage
V	Shattered kidney Renal hilum avulsion with devascularization

Reproduced from Moore *et al.* (1995), with permission from Elsevier.

Genitourinary

The relatively larger size, low position, and mobility of the pediatric kidney, as well as the paucity of perirenal fat in children, make the kidney susceptible to injury following abdominal trauma. Renal injuries include renal contusions, hematomas, lacerations (with or without collecting system involvement) (Figure 4.28), and vascular injury (Figure 4.29) or avulsion (Table 4.6). They are frequently seen in association with other intra-abdominal injuries, and may be found in the absence of hematuria. Most children with blunt grade

I–IV injuries are managed conservatively, while grade V injury frequently requires nephrectomy. In contrast, most with penetrating injuries of grade II–V require operative management.

As the bladder is located deep within the bony pelvis, bladder injury or rupture after trauma is uncommon in children, and is usually associated with gross hematuria. CT is accurate in the diagnosis of bladder rupture if performed with the bladder distended with contrast. The distribution of contrast extravasation will define the rupture as intraperitoneal or extraperitoneal (Figure 4.30). In addition, a sentinel clot adjacent to the dome of the bladder is frequently seen with intraperitoneal rupture.

Bladder injury may be associated with pelvic fracture(s). CT is more sensitive than plain radiography in detection of pelvic fractures in children.

Bowel

Bowel injury after blunt abdominal trauma in children is relatively infrequent. A specific history of lap-belt injury, bicycle handlebar injury or child abuse should heighten suspicion. Pneumoperitoneum, retroperitoneal air, free intraperitoneal fluid, bowel wall thickening, bowel wall defect, focal hematomas, mesenteric stranding, fluid at the mesenteric root, and active hemorrhage may be used to suggest this bowel injury. If oral contrast material is given during the exam, extraluminal oral contrast material is a specific sign of bowel perforation, but this finding is quite uncommon (Figure 4.31). Most institutions, however, do not give oral contrast in the setting of trauma.

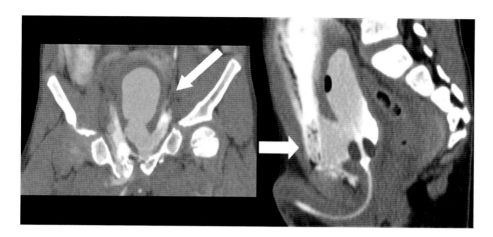

Figure 4.30 Extraperitoneal bladder rupture in a seven-year-old hit by a car. Reformatted CT images of a CT cystogram demonstrate a large defect in the anterior bladder wall which communicates with a large extraperitoneal collection of contrast (arrows). The patient has multiple pelvic fractures. Retrograde urethrography (not shown) did not show a urethral tear.

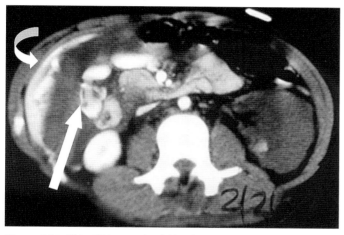

Figure 4.31 Older CT image of a child with a duodenal rupture. The patient had received oral contrast prior to the CT exam, and a large amount of this contrast is located in the right abdomen (curved arrow). Irregularity of the duodenal lumen is seen at the site of rupture (arrow). Other CT windows demonstrated free intraperitoneal air. Note the naked facet sign in this patient also with a Chance fracture.

The hypoperfusion complex, or "shock bowel," consists of diffuse dilatation of the intestine with fluid, thickening and intense contrast enhancement of the bowel wall, intense enhancement of the mesentery, kidneys and/or pancreas, and decreased caliber of the aorta and inferior vena cava, along with moderate to larger peritoneal fluid collections.

Lap-belt injury complex

The lap-belt injury complex results from acute flexion of the abdomen over a lap belt during rapid deceleration. The abdominal viscera are compressed and the spine is flexed over the fulcrum of the belt. Chance or compression fracture of the thoracolumbar junction and/or hollow viscus (bowel or bladder) injury may result (Figure 4.32). Solid organ injury (liver, spleen, pancreas) and mesenteric injury may also occur. Rarely there may be injury to the abdominal aorta. Clues to

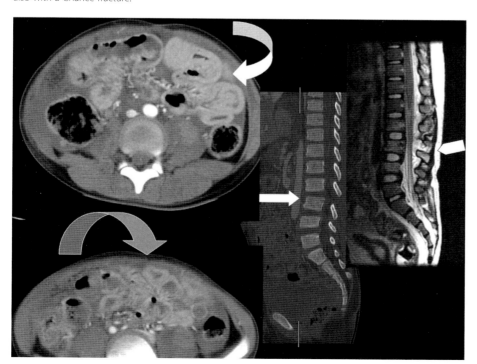

Figure 4.32 Seven-year-old restrained back-seat motor-vehicle passenger involved in auto accident. Axial CT images show bowel wall thickening and enhancement consistent with bowel wall injury (curved arrows), along with free intraperitoneal fluid. Jejunal rupture was found at surgery. There is a lap-belt ecchymosis (gray arrow). Sagittal reformatted CT image defines the Chance fracture at L2–3 (white arrow) with widening of the intraspinous distance, and endplate fracture at the superior endplate of L3. The T2-weighted MR image shows the associated ligamentous damage (arrowhead).

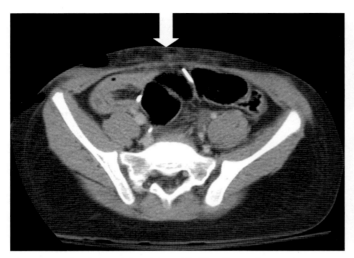

Figure 4.33 Lap-belt ecchymosis in a girl with a Chance fracture. A transverse band of edema/subcutaneous hemorrhage is seen in the anterior abdominal wall (arrow). There is an associated laceration at the right lateral anterior abdomen.

the diagnosis of lap-belt injury complex include a transverse abdominal linear ecchymosis (Figure 4.33) and unexplained intraperitoneal fluid.

A Chance fracture (Figure 4.32) is an unstable flexion–distraction transverse fracture of the spine through the posterior elements and into the vertebral body. It typically occurs at the T12–L2 level. Sagittal reformatted CT images are very useful in this diagnosis. Fortunately, associated spinal cord injury is rare.

While most patients with a lap-belt injury complex present immediately after their injury, occasionally one may see a delayed presentation with intestinal stricture developing a few weeks after lap-belt injury. This probably results from ischemia of the bowel from mesenteric injury or hematomas with subsequent healing and fibrosis.

Common pediatric fractures

Fractures in pediatric patients differ from adults. Pediatric bone is more porous and tolerates greater deformation than adult bone. The open physis is the weakest part of the bone. Children's fractures heal more rapidly than adults, and remodeling usually restores normal alignment in the plane of adjacent joint motion. Nonunion is rare. A few of the fractures commonly seen in the pediatric population are discussed below.

Bowing fractures (Figure 4.34), most common in the forearm, result from acute deformation of the bone in response to longitudinal compression, such as a fall on an outstretched arm. Microfractures occur on the concave side of the bone, and bowing results.

Greenstick fractures (Figure 4.35) result when the bone is angulated beyond its limits of bowing. This incomplete fracture

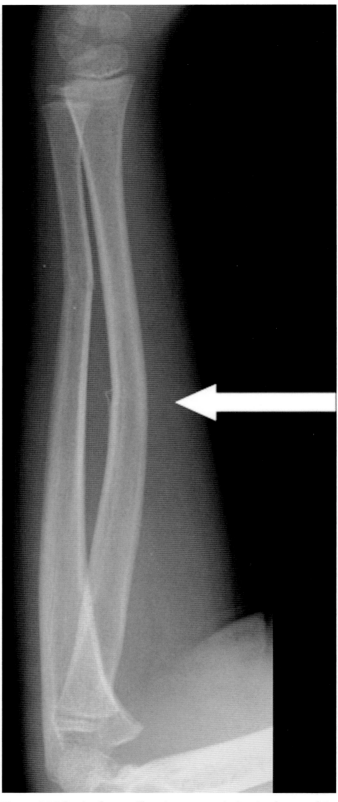

Figure 4.34 Bowing fracture. There is an apex volar bowing fracture of the radial diaphysis (arrow), along with a greenstick fracture of the distal ulnar diaphysis.

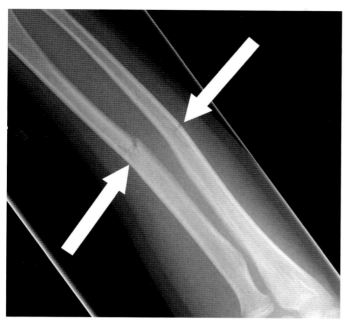

Figure 4.35 Greenstick fractures of the mid-radius and ulna (arrows). These are incomplete fractures, here resulting from a fall on an outstretched arm.

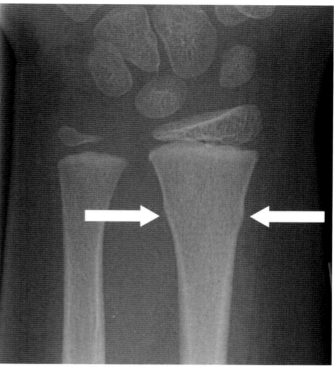

Figure 4.36 Subtle distal radial torus (or buckle) fracture (arrows). This fracture typically occurs at the diametaphysis, as this is where the cortical bone is the thinnest. The cortex buckles outward, and one can also note disruption of the trabecular pattern at the fracture site.

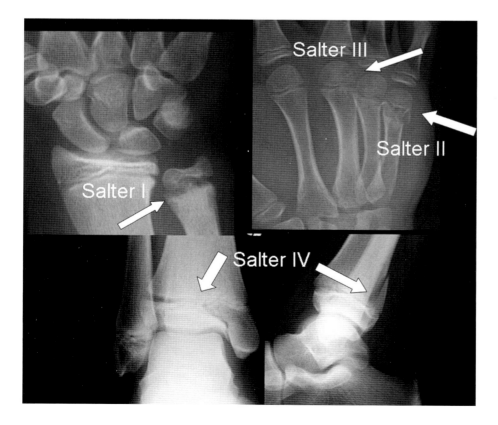

Figure 4.37 Salter fractures. Salter I fractures are fractures through the physis, or growth plate. Salter II fractures involve the metaphysis and physis. Salter III fractures extend through the physis and epiphysis. Salter IV fractures involve the physis, metaphysis and epiphysis. Salter V fractures (not pictured) are crush injuries of the physis.

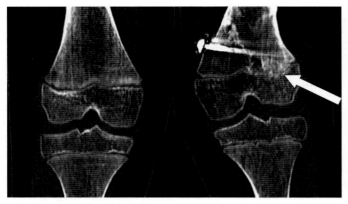

Figure 4.38 Coronal CT reformatted images in a child who suffered a Salter II fracture of his distal femur. There is growth arrest across the lateral distal femoral physis (arrow) with resultant valgus angulation distally.

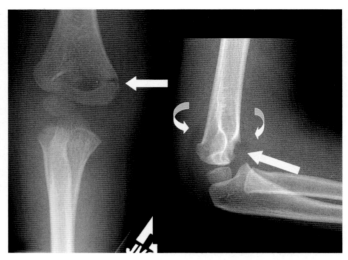

Figure 4.39 Supracondylar fractures result from a fall on an outstretched arm. Here we can see an elbow joint effusion (curved arrows) as well as the fracture line (arrows). There is mild posterior displacement of the distal fracture fragment.

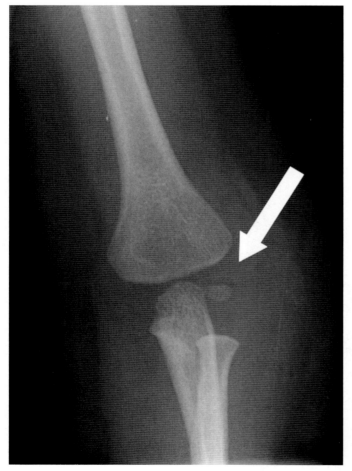

Figure 4.40 Two-year-old with lateral condylar fracture. There is soft tissue swelling seen laterally. In addition, a sliver of bone from the lateral condyle (arrow) is seen above the capitellum, pulled distally by the forearm musculature.

occurs on the tension side of the bone, with bending seen on the compression side of the bone.

Torus fracture (Figure 4.36), or buckle fracture, results from compression failure. Outward cortical buckling occurs usually near the metaphysis, where the cortex is thinnest. This fracture is most commonly seen at the distal radius after a fall on an outstretched arm.

Physeal fractures account for up to 20% of pediatric fractures. These are most common in the distal radius, and between ages 10 and 16. These fractures occur through the zone of hypertrophying cartilage within the physis (Figure 4.37). Resulting growth arrest is relatively uncommon (Figure 4.38).

The clavicle is a commonly fractured bone in childhood. It usually fractures at its midshaft and heals without sequelae.

Supracondylar fractures (Figure 4.39) result from hyperextension at the elbow. Lateral and medial condylar fractures result from varus or valgus stress at the elbow, respectively (Figure 4.40, Figure 4.41). The forearm extensor and flexor musculature attach at these sites, and will pull the fractured fragments distally (Figure 4.42).

Slipped capital femoral epiphysis (SCFE; Figure 4.43) is a Salter I fracture of the capital femoral physis. Most are idiopathic and are seen in 12–15-year-old patients who are typically overweight and tall for their age but with delayed bony maturation. SCFE is more common in boys. SCFE has also been associated with hypothyroidism, hypopituitarism, renal osteodystrophy and prior irradiation for malignancy.

Toddler fractures (Figure 4.44) are non-displaced spiral or oblique fractures of the tibial diaphysis which occur in toddlers between approximately nine months and three

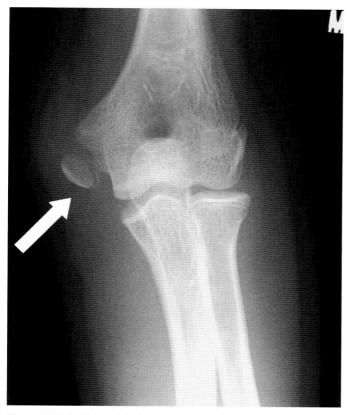

Figure 4.41 Medial condylar fracture. There is soft tissue swelling adjacent to this minimally displaced Salter-II-type fracture of the medial condyle (arrow).

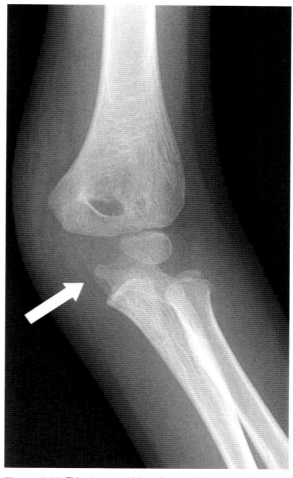

Figure 4.42 This six-year-old boy has a displaced medial condylar fracture. The medial epicondylar ossification center has been pulled distally (arrow) by the forearm flexor musculature to overlie the elbow joint. This should not be mistaken for the trochlear ossification center. There is medial elbow soft tissue swelling. (Compare normal elbow in Chapter 1, Figure 1.17.)

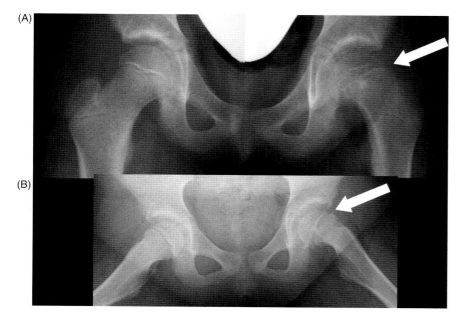

(A)

(B)

Figure 4.43 Slipped capital femoral epiphysis. Two different boys with left SCFE are shown. (A) Widening of the physis, as well as posterior medial positioning of the femoral head (arrow) are demonstrated. A frog lateral (B) better shows the posterior medial positioning of the femoral head on the left (arrow).

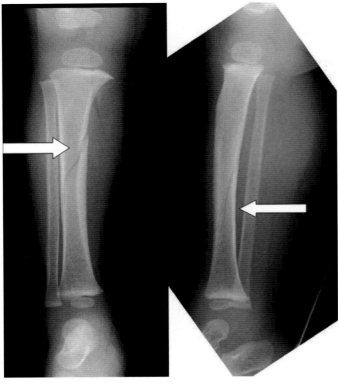

Figure 4.44 Toddler fracture, or a non-displaced spiral fracture of the tibia, is seen in the nine-month to three-year-old age range and results from an (often minor) twisting injury.

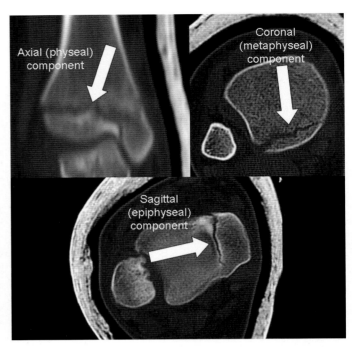

Figure 4.45 Triplane fracture. CT examination demonstrates the sagittal, coronal and axial fracture lines of this Salter IV fracture. Note the medial aspect of the distal tibial physis is closed, but the lateral aspect is open. This is the same patient as shown in Figure 4.37.

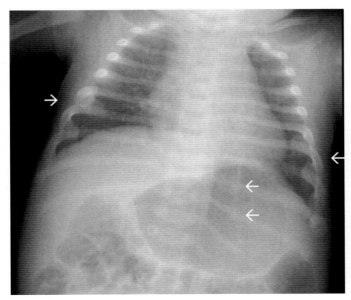

Figure 4.46 Multiple bilateral rib fractures from non-accidental trauma. This infant has subacute right lateral sixth and seventh, left lateral sixth through ninth, and left posterior ninth and tenth healing rib fractures (arrows) with callus formation.

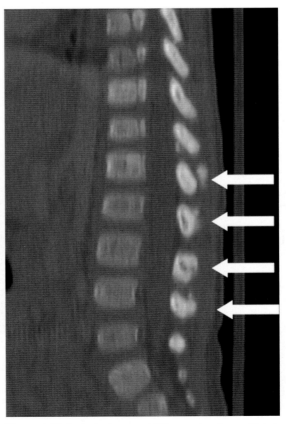

Figure 4.47 Sagittal reformatted CT image showing multiple healing spinous process fractures resulting from non-accidental trauma to this infant.

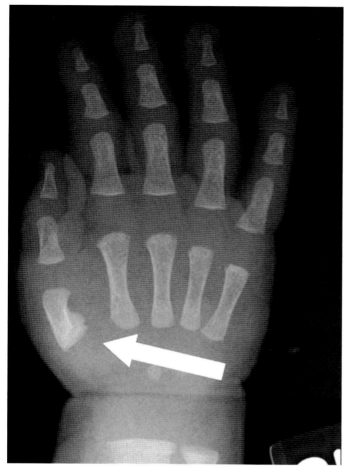

Figure 4.48 Three-month-old abused baby with a healing first metacarpal fracture (arrow).

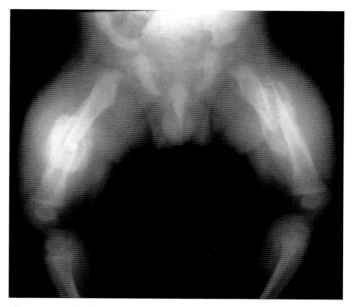

Figure 4.49 This five-month-old has exuberant callus formation at healing bilateral femoral fractures resulting from non-accidental trauma.

years of age. This twisting injury may occur after minimal trauma.

The unique closure of the distal tibial physis, beginning at "Kump's bump" (the anteromedial distal tibial physis), progressing posteromedially then anterolaterally, results in complex fractures which occur near the completion of growth (girls 12–14 years old; boys 13–14 years old). The Tillaux fracture is a Salter III fracture extending through the epiphysis and lateral physis of the distal tibia. Triplane fractures (Figure 4.45) are Salter IV fractures which extend in all three planes. The axial part of this fracture occurs through the physis, the sagittal through the epiphysis, and coronal through the metaphysis.

Non-accidental trauma

Physical abuse of children results in up to 5000 deaths each year, and accounts for 10% of pediatric emergency-room visits in the USA. The role of the radiologist is to discover, describe and document skeletal, visceral and intracranial abusive injuries.

Skeletal survey is useful to define fractures in children under the age of two years. Up to half of the fractures seen by skeletal survey in abused infants are clinically occult. Fractures with a high specificity for inflicted injury include rib fractures (Figure 4.46) in children under one year (especially posterior), the classic metaphyseal lesion (CML; also known as corner fracture or bucket-handle fracture) and spiral fracture of the femur. The "s" fractures – sternum, spinous process (Figure 4.47) and scapula – are also high-specificity fractures for child abuse. Digital fractures (Figure 4.48), bilateral fractures (Figure 4.49), multiple fractures at various ages of healing, vertebral body fractures and epiphyseal separation fractures (Figure 4.50) also should raise suspicion for non-accidental trauma.

The CML (Figure 4.51) results from a twisting injury. It is a subepiphyseal planar fracture through the immature primary spongiosa of the metaphysis of the long bone, especially the femur, tibia and humerus. The appearance of the CML is affected by the radiographic projection, as well as the degree of separation of the fracture. If viewed tangentially, a discrete fragment (or corner fracture) will be seen. If viewed obliquely, one will see a bucket-handle fracture.

Head injuries are the leading cause of death in abused infants. They may result from shaking or from impact. Skull fractures in abused children are more often multiple, bilateral, complex and may cross the midline (Figure 4.52). Intracranial injuries may include subdural hematoma, parenchymal contusion/hematoma, shear injury and cerebral

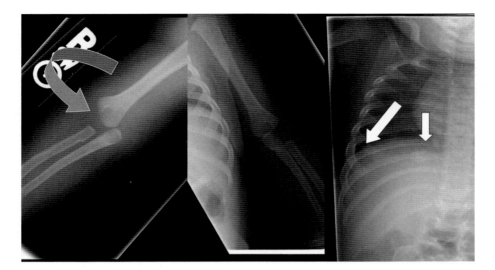

Figure 4.50 Seven-month-old victim of child abuse. There is a right distal humeral epiphyseal separation fracture (curved arrow) recognized because the radius does not properly align with the distal humeral shaft. (The normal left side is shown for comparison). This fracture is actually a Salter-type injury through the distal humerus, which is still cartilaginous, with displacement of the distal humerus and elbow structures together (not an elbow dislocation). There are also acute lateral sixth to eighth right and subacute right ninth rib fractures (arrows).

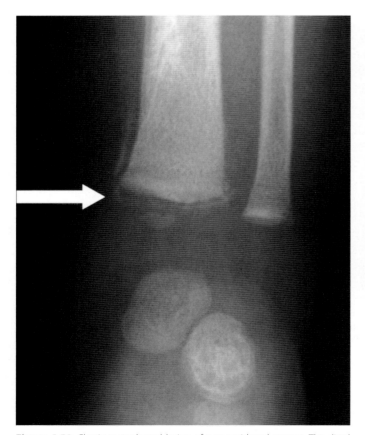

Figure 4.51 Classic metaphyseal lesion of non-accidental trauma. The distal tibial fracture appears with the "bucket-handle" appearance, while the distal fibular lesion appears with the "corner-fracture" appearance.

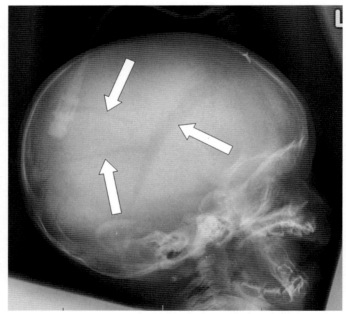

Figure 4.52 Multiple skull fractures are seen (arrows) in this two-month-old abused infant.

edema. SDH is more commonly due to non-accidental trauma than accidental trauma in children under two years. SDH resulting from non-accidental trauma is commonly seen posteriorly along the interhemispheric fissure and parieto-occipital region (Figure 4.53). Inhomogeneous SDH may represent hyperacute hemorrhage with unclotted as well as clotted blood, or arachnoid tear with CSF extending into the subdural hemorrhage. Retinal hemorrhages are seen with shaking injuries.

Up to 20% of abused children suffer visceral injury, and visceral injury is responsible for 12% of all abuse-related deaths. Duodenal or proximal jejunal hematomas, laceration,

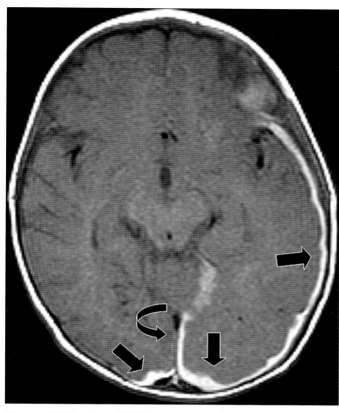

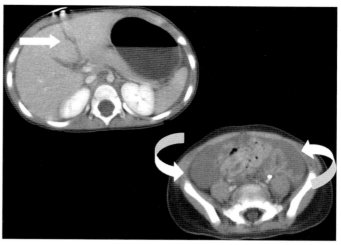

Figure 4.54 CT of liver laceration (arrow) with intraperitoneal hemorrhage (curved arrows) resulting from non-accidental trauma.

Figure 4.53 T1-weighted MRI demonstrating subacute, high intensity subdural hematomas at the posterior interhemispheric fissure, bilateral occipital and left parietal regions in this abused infant.

or mesenteric injury are most common, along with pancreatic injury. However, any solid organ injury may also occur (Figure 4.54).

Summary

Trauma is the leading cause of death in the pediatric population. Injury patterns in the pediatric patient differ from that of the adult. Thus, the radiologist caring for children needs to be knowledgeable about these injury patterns to offer optimal imaging care to these young patients.

Further reading

Head trauma

Ashwal S, Holshouser BA, Tong KA (2006) Use of advanced neuroimaging techniques in the evaluation of pediatric traumatic brain injury. *Dev Neurosci* **28**, 309–26.

Duhaime AC, Durham S (2007) Traumatic brain injury in infants: the phenomenon of subdural hemorrhage with hemispheric hypodensity ("big black brain"). *Prog Brain Res* **161**, 293–302.

Duhaime AC, Alario AJ, Lewander WJ et al. (1992) Head injury in very young children: mechanisms, injury types, and ophthalmologic findings in 100 hospitalized patients younger than 2 years of age. *Pediatrics* **90**, 179–85.

Duhem R, Vinchon M, Tonnelle V, Soto-Ares G, Leclerc X (2006) Main temporal aspects of the MRI signal of subdural hematomas and practical contribution to dating head injury. *Neurochirurgie* **52**, 93–104.

Gean A *Imaging of Head Trauma* (New York: Raven Press, 1994) pp. 368–426.

Haydel MJ, Shembekar AD (2003) Prediction of intracranial injury in children aged five years and older with loss of consciousness after minor head injury due to nontrivial mechanisms. *Ann Emerg Med* **42**, 507–14.

Khoshyomn S, Tranmer BI (2004) Diagnosis and management of pediatric closed head injury. *Sem Pediatr Surg* **13**, 80–6.

Noguchi K, Ogawa T, Inugami A et al. (1995) Acute subarachnoid hemorrhage: MR imaging with fluid-attenuated inversion recovery pulse sequences. *Radiology* **196**, 773–7.

Palchak MJ, Holmes JF, Vance CW et al. (2003) A decision rule for identifying children at low risk for brain injuries after blunt head trauma. *Ann Emerg Med* **42**, 492–506.

Poussaint TY, Moeller KK (2002) Imaging of pediatric head trauma. *Neuroimag Clin N Am* **12**, 271–94.

Schutzman SA, Greenes DS (2001) Pediatric minor head trauma. *Ann Emerg Med* **37**, 65–74.

Tung GA, Kumar M, Richardson RC, Jenny C, Brown WI (2006) Comparison of accidental and nonaccidental traumatic head injury in children on noncontrast computed tomography. *Pediatrics* **118**, 626–33.

Woodcock RJ, Davis PC, Hopkins KL (2001) Imaging of head trauma in infancy and childhood. *Sem Ultrasound CT MR* **22**, 162–82.

Zimmerman RA, Bilaniuk LT (1994) Pediatric head trauma. *Neuroimaging Clin N Am* **4**, 349–66.

Cervical spine trauma

Brown RL, Brunn MA, Garcia VF (2001) Cervical spine injuries in children: a review of 103 patients treated consecutively at a level 1 pediatric trauma center. *J Pediatr Surg* **36**, 1107–14.

Dwek JR, Chung CCB (2000) Radiography of cervical injury in children: are flexion-extension radiographs useful for acute trauma. *AJR Am J Roentgenol* 174, 1617–19.

Eleraky MA, Theodore N, Adams M, Rekate HL, Sonntag VKH (2000) Pediatric cervical spine injuries: report of 102 cases and review of the literature. *J Neurosurg* 92, 12–17.

Hanson JA, Blackmore CC, Mann Fa, Wilson AJ (2000) Cervical spine injury: a clinical decision rule to identify high-risk patients for helical CT screening. *AJR Am J Roentgenol* 174, 713–17.

Harris JH, Carson GC, Wagner LK (1994) Radiologic diagnosis of traumatic occipitovertebral dissociation: 1. Normal occipitovertebral relationships on lateral radiographs of supine subjects. *AJR Am J Roentgenol* 162, 881–6.

Jimenez RR, DeGuzman MA, Shiran S, Karrellas A, Lorenzo RL (2008) CT versus plain radiographs for evaluation of c-spine injury in young children: do benefits outweigh risks? *Pediatr Radiol* 38, 635–44.

Pang D (2004) Spinal cord injury without radiographic abnormality in children, 2 decades later. *Neurosurgery* 55, 1325–42.

Platzer P, Jaindl M, Thalhammer G et al. (2007) Cervical spine injuries in pediatric patients. *J Trauma* 62, 389–96.

Slack SE, Clancy MJ (2004) Clearing the cervical spine of paediatric trauma patients. *Emerg Med J* 21, 189–93.

Steinmetz MP, Lechner RM, Anderson JS (2003) Atlantooccipital dislocation in children: presentation, diagnosis, and management. *Neurosurg Focus* 14, 1–7.

Chest trauma

Cooper A, Barlow B, DiScala C, String D (1994) Mortality and truncal injury: the pediatric perspective. *J Pediatr Surg* 29, 33–8.

Holmes JF, Sokolove PE, Brant WE, Kuppermann N (2002) A clinical decision rule for identifying children with thoracic injuries after blunt torso trauma. *Ann Emerg Med* 39, 492–9.

Renton J, Kincaid S, Ehrlich PF (2003) Should helical CT scanning of the thoracic cavity replace the conventional chest X-ray as a primary assessment tool in pediatric trauma? An efficacy and cost analysis. *J Pediatr Surg* 38, 793–7.

Abdominal trauma

Angus LD, Tachmes L, Kahn S et al. (1993) Surgical management of pediatric renal trauma: an urban experience. *Am Surg* 59, 388–94.

Benya EC, Lim-Dunham JE, Landrum O, Statter M (2000) Abdominal sonography in examination of children with blunt abdominal trauma. *AJR Am J Roentgenol* 174, 1613–16.

Bernstein MP, Mirvis SE, Shanmuganathan K (2006) Chance-type fractures of the thoracolumbar spine: imaging analysis in 53 patients. *AJR Am J Roentgenol* 187, 859–68.

Brenner DJ, Elliston CD, Hall EJ, Berdon WE (2001) Estimated risks of radiation-induced fatal cancer from pediatric CT. *AJR Am J Roentgenol* 176, 289–96.

Bulas DI, Taylor GA, Eichelberger MR (1989) The value of CT in detecting bowel perforation in children after blunt abdominal trauma. *AJR Am J Roentgenol* 153, 561–4.

Capaccio E, Magnano GM, Valle M, Derchi LE (2006) Traumatic lesions of the adrenal glands in paediatrics: about three cases. *Radiol Med* 111, 906–10.

Chan DPN, Abujudeh HH, Cushing GL, Novelline RA (2006) CT cystography with multiplanar reformation for suspected bladder rupture: experience in 234 cases. *AJR Am J Roentgenol* 187, 1296–1302.

Choit RL, Tredwell SJ, Leblanc JG, Reilly CW, Mulpuri K (2006) Abdominal aortic injuries associated with Chance fractures in pediatric patients. *J Pediatr Surg* 41, 1184–90.

Durbin DR, Arbogast KB, Moll EK (2001) Seat-belt syndrome in children: a case report and review of the literature. *Pediatr Emerg Care* 17, 474–7.

Federle MP, Griffiths B, Minagi H, Jeffrey RB (1987) Splenic trauma: evaluation with CT. *Radiology* 162, 69–71.

Guillamondegui OD, Mahboubi S, Stafford PW, Nance ML (2003) The utility of the pelvic radiograph in the assessment of pediatric pelvic fractures. *J Trauma* 55, 236–40.

Hall EJ (2002) Lessons we have learned from our children: cancer risks from diagnostic radiology. *Pediatr Radiol* 32, 700–6.

Hennes HM, Smith DS, Schneider K et al. (1990) Elevated liver transaminase levels in children with blunt abdominal trauma: a predictor of liver injury. *Pediatrics* 86, 87–90.

Moore EE, Cogbill TH, Malangni MA et al. (1995) Organ injury scaling. *Surg Clin North Am* 75, 293–303.

Mutabagani KJ, Coley BD, Zumberge N et al. (1999) Preliminary experience with focused abdominal sonography for trauma (FAST) in children: is it useful? *J Pediatr Surg* 24, 48–54.

Nance ML, Mahboubi S, Wickstrom J, Prendergast F, Stafford PW (2002) Pattern of abdominal free fluid following isolated blunt spleen or liver injury in the pediatric patient. *J Trauma* 52, 85–7.

Nguyen MM, Das S (2002) Pediatric renal trauma. *Urology* 59, 762–6.

Shalaby-Rana E, Eichelberger M, Kerzner B, Kapur S (1992) Intestinal stricture due to lap-belt injury. *AJR Am J Roentgenol* 158, 63–4.

Shin SS, Jeong YY, Chung TW et al. (2007) The sentinel clot sign: a useful CT finding for the evaluation of intraperitoneal bladder rupture following blunt trauma. *Korean J Radiol* 8, 492–7.

Siegel MJ The child with abdominal trauma. In *Practical Pediatric Radiology*, 3rd edn., ed. SvW Hilton, DK Edwards (Philadelphia: Saunders Elsevier, 2006) Chapter 10, pp. 351–73.

Sivit CJ, Cutting JP, Eichelberger MR (1995) CT diagnosis and localization of rupture of the bladder in children with blunt abdominal trauma: significance of contrast material extravasation in the pelvis. *AJR Am J Roentgenol* 164, 1243–6.

Sivit CJ, Taylor GA, Newman KD et al. (1991) Safety-belt injuries in children with lap-belt ecchymosis: CT findings in 61 patients. *AJR Am J Roentgenol* 157, 111–14.

Sivit CJ, Eichelberger MR, Taylor GA et al. (1992) Blunt pancreatic trauma in children: CT diagnosis. *AJR Am J Roentgenol* 158, 1097–100.

Sivit CJ, Ingram JD, Taylor GA et al. (1992) Posttraumatic adrenal hemorrhage in children: CT findings in 34 patients. *AJR Am J Roentgenol* 158, 1299–302.

Sivit CJ, Taylor GA, Bulas DI et al. (1992) Posttraumatic shock in children: CT findings associated with hemodynamic instability. *Radiology* 182, 723–6.

Stalker HP, Kaufman RA, Towbin R (1986) Patterns of liver injury in childhood: CT analysis. *AJR Am J Roentgenol* 147, 1199–205.

Strouse PJ, Close BJ, Marshall KW, Cywes R (1999) CT of bowel and mesenteric trauma in children. *Radiographics* 19, 1237–50.

Taylor GA, Eichelberger MR (1989) Abdominal CT in children with neurologic impairment following blunt trauma. *Ann Surg* **210**, 229–33.

Taylor GA, Fallat ME, Eichelberger MR (1987) Hypovolemic shock in children: abdominal CT manifestations. *Radiology* **164**, 479–81.

Taylor GA, Eichelberger MR, O'Donnell R, Bowman L (1991) Indications for computed tomography in children with blunt abdominal trauma. *Ann Surg* **213**, 24–30.

Fractures

Laor T, Jaramillo D, Oestreich AE Musculoskeletal system. In *Practical Pediatric Imaging: Diagnostic Radiology of Infants and Children*, 3rd edn., ed. DR Kirks (Philadelphia: Lippincott-Raven, 1998) Chapter 5, pp. l415–47.

Ozonoff MB Skeletal trauma. In *Pediatric Orthopedic Radiology*, 2nd edn., ed. MB Ozonoff (Philadelphia: WB Saunders Co., 1992) Chapter 8, pp. 604–89.

Non-accidental trauma

Barnes PD, Robson CD (2000) CT findings in hyperacute nonaccidental brain injury. *Pediatr Radiol* **30**, 74–81.

Duhaime AC, Alario AJ, Lewander WJ *et al.* (1992) Head injury in very young children: mechanisms, injury types and ophthalmologic findings in 100 hospitalized patients younger than 2 years of age. *Pediatrics* **90**, 179–85.

Hilton SvW Differentiating the accidentally injured from the physically abused child. In *Practical Pediatric Radiology*, 3rd edn., ed. SvW Hilton, DK Edwards (Philadelphia: Saunders Elsevier, 2006) Chapter 17, pp. 576–629.

Kleinman PK (1990) Diagnostic imaging in infant abuse. *AJR Am J Roentgenol* **155**, 703–12.

Kleinman PK, Marks SC, Blackbourne B (1986) The metaphyseal lesion in abused infants: a radiologic-histopathologic study. *AJR Am J Roentgenol* **146**, 895–905.

Lonergan GJ, Baker AM, Morey MK, Boos SC (2003) Child abuse: radiological-pathological correlation. *Radiographics* **23**, 811–45.

Nimkin K, Kleinman PK (1997) Imaging of child abuse. *Pediatr Clin North Am* **44**, 615–35.

Sivit CJ, Taylor GA, Eichelberger MR (1989) Visceral injury in battered children: a changing perspective. *Radiology* **173**, 659–61.

Society for Pediatric Radiology, National Association of Medical Examiners (2004) Post-mortem radiography in the evaluation of unexpected death in children less than 2 years of age whose death is suspicious for fatal abuse. *Pediatr Radiol* **34**, 675–7. DOI 10.1007/s00247-004-1235-3.

Zimmerman RA, Bilaniuk LT, Bruce D *et al.* (1978) Interhemispheric acute subdural hematomas: a computed tomographic manifestation of child abuse by shaking. *Neuroradiology* **16**, 39–40.

Chapter 5

Nontraumatic pediatric emergencies

Harvey Teo and David Stringer

Respiratory system

Croup

Croup, or acute laryngotracheobronchitis, is the commonest cause of acute stridor in infants and young children under two years of age. The peak incidence is in the second year of life. The commonest organism is the parainfluenza virus, although other viruses are also known to cause the condition. Pathologically, subglottic tracheal narrowing occurs due to edema accumulating within the loose attachment of the mucosa in this region. The symptoms range from mild cough to severe life-threatening respiratory obstruction.

The diagnosis of croup is based on clinical findings, and there is no evidence that other investigations or radiographs are useful in the diagnosis of this condition. If radiographs are performed, the ap view may show an inverted V-shaped narrowing of the subglottic region which extends below the level of the lower margins of the pyriform sinuses and appears more marked in inspiration (Figure 5.1). This is also known as the "steeple-sign," but this sign may be absent in up to 50% of cases and may be present in the absence of croup. The narrowing in the subglottic region is less pronounced on the lateral view than the ap view, as the narrowing occurs primarily laterally. Hypopharyngeal distension, indistinctness and thickening of the vocal cords may also be seen. The epiglottis is normal.

Epiglottitis

Acute epiglottitis or membranous croup is a bacterial infection of the epiglottis and aryepiglottic folds. *Haemophilus influenzae* type B (Hib) is the commonest organism causing acute epiglottitis, but since the widespread implementation of a conjugate vaccine for Hib, the incidence of epiglottitis has significantly declined in children. Sporadic cases still occur due to vaccine failure. The age group of patients with acute epiglottitis is three to five years. The clinical onset and presence of systemic symptoms are more rapid and severe than croup. The clinical triad of drooling, dysphagia and distress is a classic presentation. A viral prodrome and cough are seldom observed with acute epiglottitis and are more often witnessed

in association with croup. Acute epiglottitis is a medical emergency, and imaging and other investigations should be postponed until the airway is secure. The lateral neck radiograph may show the epiglottis and aryepiglottic folds to be swollen and rounded (Figure 5.2). Hypopharyngeal distension may also be present. On the ap neck radiograph, there may be subglottic narrowing resembling croup. The poor sensitivity (38%) and specificity (78%) of plain films limits their utility, especially since the larynx can be safely and accurately visualized with flexible laryngoscopy in most modern institutions.

The wheezing child

Wheezing is defined as a high-pitch, whistling sound occurring during the expiratory phase of respiration. It is caused by airway

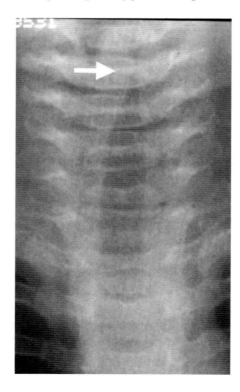

Figure 5.1 One-year-old boy with stridor. The frontal view of the neck shows steeple-shaped narrowing of the subglottic region (arrow) suggestive of croup.

Essentials of Pediatric Radiology, ed. Heike E. Daldrup-Link and Charles A. Gooding. Published by Cambridge University Press.
© Cambridge University Press 2010.

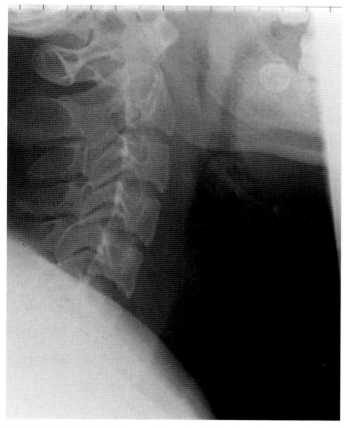

Figure 5.2 Two-year-old boy with acute stridor. Lateral neck radiograph shows swelling of the epiglottis and aryepiglottic folds consistent with the diagnosis of acute epiglottitis.

obstruction beyond the carina. The causes of wheezing differ depending on the age of the patient. These are listed in Table 5.1.

Foreign bodies

Foreign-body inhalation in children is commonest between the ages of six months to four years. A high index of suspicion is often required to diagnose this condition because children are often unable to give an accurate history of foreign-body inhalation, and symptoms may mimic other conditions such as reactive airway disease and pulmonary or upper respiratory tract infections.

The sudden inhalation of a foreign body may result in acute respiratory compromise, infection, atelectasis and death. In a study of 132 patients, a history of foreign-body inhalation was given in only 53.8% of patients. Other patients presented with recurrent chest infection, difficulty in breathing, cough and stridor. Clinical examination revealed rhonchi, decreased breath sounds and intercostal retractions on the affected side. Peanuts and food accounted for more than 60% of the ingested foreign bodies.

The history and clinical symptoms should guide imaging evaluation. Lateral views of the neck are advised if stridor is present. If the foreign body is suspected in the lower airway, inspiratory and expiratory views of the chest may detect air-trapping on the side of the foreign body (Figure 5.3). This air-trapping is due to a ball-valve effect of the foreign body within the main bronchus of the affected lung. Normal radiographic findings do not exclude foreign bodies, and atypical radiographs such as bilateral emphysema, atelectasis or pneumonia may also be seen. Decubitus views of the chest or fluoroscopy can help with the differential diagnosis by demonstrating air-trapping or mediastinal shift.

Table 5.1 Causes of wheezing in a child, by age

Age	Pathology	Key imaging findings
Newborn and infants	1. Pneumonia	Focal, lobar or diffuse distribution of airspace infiltrates, interstitial pattern or dense consolidation
	2. Aspiration	Airspace infiltrates involving the dependent lobes, usually the right upper lobe after aspiration in supine position, and the right lower lobe after aspiration in an upright position.
	3. Cardiac edema	Cardiac enlargement, bilateral increased interstitial markings and prominent vasculature, diffuse airspace shadowing in later stage
3–6 years	1. Viral pneumonia	Parahilar–peribronchial infiltrates, hyperexpansion, segmental or lobar atelectasis, and hilar adenopathy
	2. Bacterial pneumonia	Unilateral or lobar airspace infiltrates, dense consolidation, cavitation, pneumatocele formation and pleural effusion
	3. Foreign-body aspiration	Unilateral hyperinflation due to air-trapping on the side of the foreign body, best appreciated on inspiratory–expiratory views or fluoroscopy
	4. Asthma	Bronchial wall thickening with prominent central lung markings, air-trapping, atelectasis, superimposed infection, airleak complications
>6 years	1. Atypical pneumonia (mycoplasm)	Peribronchial and perivascular interstitial infiltrates, patchy consolidation and homogeneous ground-glass acinar consolidation predominantly involving the lower lobes. Hilar adenopathy is commonly seen
	2. Bacterial pneumonia	Unilateral or lobar airspace infiltrates, dense consolidation, cavitation, pneumatocele formation and pleural effusion
	3. Asthma	Bronchial wall thickening with prominent central lung markings, air-trapping, atelectasis, superimposed infection, airleak complications

(A)

(B)

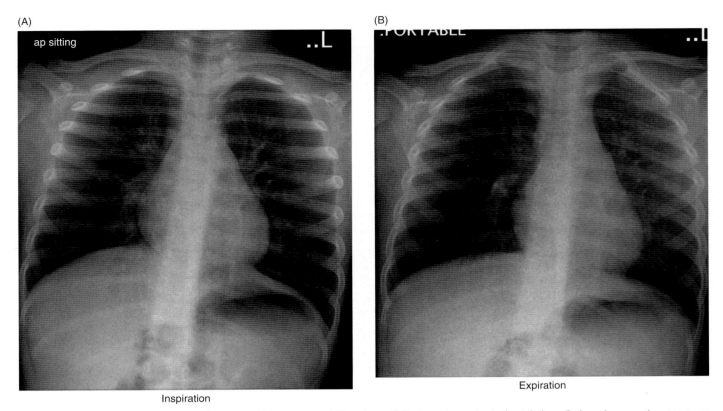

Inspiration

Expiration

Figure 5.3 Four-year-old boy who aspirated a peanut. (A) Inspiratory and (B) expiratory CXRs show air-trapping in the right lung. On bronchoscopy, the peanut was found in the right main bronchus.

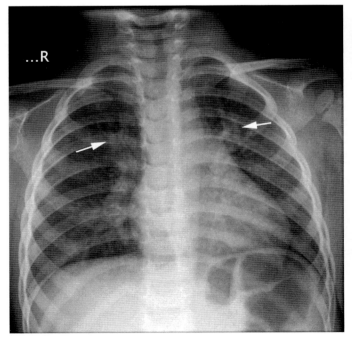

Figure 5.4 Eighteen-month-old girl with reactive airway disease due to a bout of bronchiolitis. Anteroposterior radiograph shows the presence of bronchial wall thickening with prominent central lung markings (arrows).

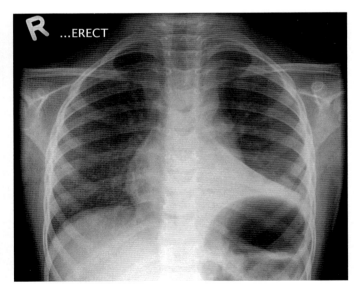

Figure 5.5 Six-year-old boy with acute exacerbation of reactive airway disease. CXR shows the presence of a left lower lobe collapse likely due to mucoid secretions obstructing the left lower lobe bronchus. Follow-up CXR (not shown) performed a few days later following treatment shows complete clearance of the collapse.

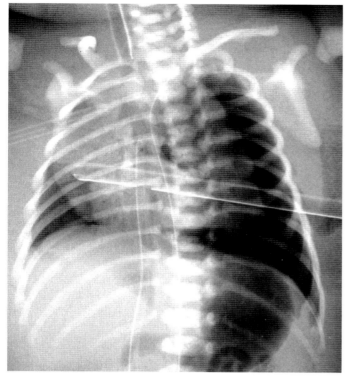

Figure 5.6 Premature neonate with several tubes and line *in situ*. This slightly rotated radiograph shows the presence of a left tension pneumothorax compressing the left lung and displacing the left hemidiaphragm downwards.

Reactive airway disease

Reactive airway disease (RAD) results from airway inflammation and hyperresponsiveness to allergens, pollutants and/or irritants. In response to these stimulants, mediators such as cytokines, eosinophils, heparin, histamine, interleukins, leukotrienes, lymphocytes and tryptase are released, which result in excessive mucous secretion, bronchospasm and pulmonary impairment. Death may occur in severe cases.

More than 50% of children with asthma develop their first attack before two years of age, and 25% develop their first wheeze before the age of one year. The peak age of reactive airway disease in children is between 6 and 12 years. The condition is 1.5 times more common in boys than in girls.

Symptoms include wheezing, fever, tachycardia, tachypnea and coughing. In severe cases, flaring of the nasal alae, intercostal retractions, cyanosis and respiratory collapse may occur. Differentiation between RAD and acute viral bronchiolitis is often difficult to determine on clinical grounds, and a child's first attack may occur during a bout of acute bronchiolitis.

Chest radiographs may be normal in children with asthma. The commonest finding is bronchial wall thickening with prominent central lung markings (Figure 5.4). Air-trapping and atelectasis are commonly noted (Figure 5.5). Superimposed infection or airleak complications may be seen.

Airleaks

Airleak problems in the chest include pneumothorax, pneumomediastinum, pneumopericardium and pulmonary interstitial emphysema. Pneumothorax is the condition where there is air in the pleural space, and may be life-threatening if not recognized early. There is an increased risk of spontaneous

(A)

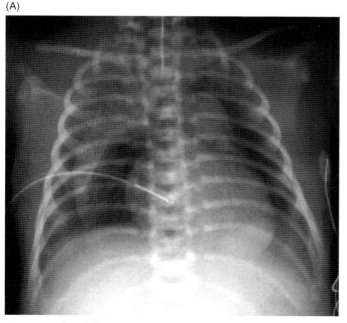

(B)

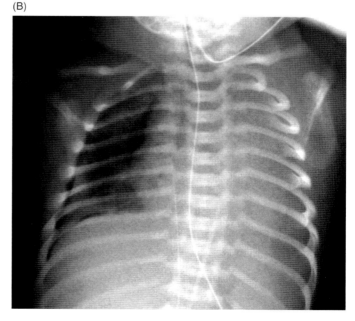

Figure 5.7 Two different neonates with airleak complications. (A) A pneumomediastinum is noted elevating the right side of the thymus away from the mediastinum. (B) Another neonate with a right pneumothorax. Air can be seen outlining the right lung. The thymus is not lifted away from the mediastinum.

<header>

Chapter 5: Nontraumatic pediatric emergencies

</header>

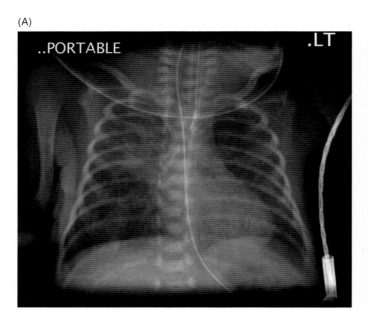

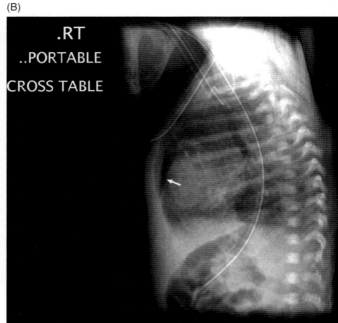

Figure 5.8 Premature neonate with several tubes and lines *in situ*. (A) Anteroposterior view shows a vague lucency in the lower lobe of the right lung, possibly due to a small pneumothorax. (B) A cross-table lateral horizontal beam radiograph shows the presence of lucency in the retrosternal region consistent with a small pneumothorax (arrow).

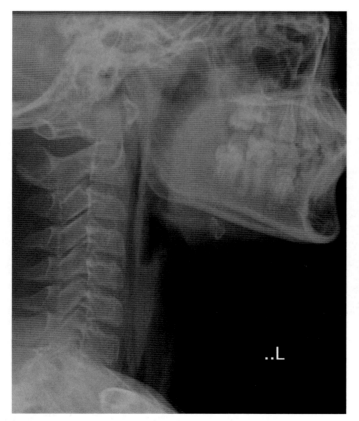

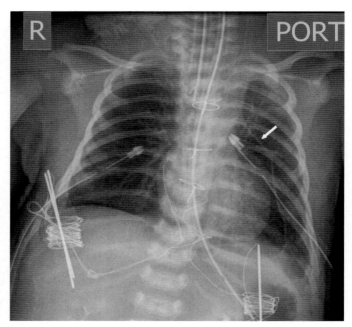

Figure 5.10 Three-week-old neonate immediately post-cardiac surgery shows the presence of air surrounding the heart within the pericardium, known as a pneumopericardium. Note that the air does not go above the level of the great vessels because the pericardium does not extend above this point (arrow).

Figure 5.9 Thirteen-year-old boy with sudden onset of neck and chest pain. Lateral neck X-ray shows the presence of gas tracking up from the chest into the retropharyngeal region due to pneumomediastinum. The pneumomediastinum could not be visualized on the CXR (not shown). Further evaluation with CT and upper GI series did not reveal a cause of the pneumomediastinum.

pneumothorax in patients with Marfan syndrome and cystic fibrosis. In premature newborns, pneumothorax is often seen as a complication of intubation and positive pressure ventilation. Nontraumatic causes of airleaks include asthma, chest infection, pneumatoceles and foreign bodies. Often there is no known cause. A tension pneumothorax is an emergency which occurs when there is substantial mass effect on the underlying lung and shift of the mediastinum towards the opposite side. If untreated, this leads to a decrease in the venous return and cardiac output which, in turn, may lead to shock.

Patients with pneumothorax may present with pleuritic chest pain, dyspnea, tachypnea and cyanosis. On physical examination there are decreased breath sounds and hyperresonance to percussion on the affected side.

Pneumothoraces may have different appearances on chest radiographs in children. They are commonly seen as a peripherally situated lucent zone without noticeable vessels. The lung "falls" towards the hilar region. A tension pneumothorax is recognized when there is shift of the mediastinum to the contralateral side with depression of the ipsilateral hemidiaphragm (Figure 5.6). Neonates are generally supine, and pleural air accumulates anteriorly and medially. This appears as a lucent "stripe" next to the diaphragm and mediastinum. This may sometimes be confused with a pneumomediastinum. However, a pneumomediastinum usually outlines and elevates the thymus, whereas a pneumothorax compresses the thymus against the mediastinal structures (Figure 5.7). A horizontal beam view may be helpful in doubtful cases, by delineating the pneumothorax beneath the retrosternal region (Figure 5.8). Pneumomediastinum may track up into the retropharyngeal soft tissue (Figure 5.9). A pneumopericardium is an airleak where air collects within the pericardium surrounding the heart. It is limited superiorly by the reflection of the pericardium over the great vessels (Figure 5.10).

Gastrointestinal

Nontraumatic pediatric gastrointestinal emergencies are listed in Table 5.2. Of note, some of the pathologies listed in these tables are explained in more detail in Chapter 2.

Table 5.2 Nontraumatic gastrointestinal pediatric emergencies

Age	Pathology	Key imaging findings
Newborn	1. Bowel atresia	Duodenal atresia – "double-bubble" sign, jejunal and ileal atresia – nonspecific bowel dilatation. The more dilated bowel loops are noted, the more distal the point of atresia. Unused microcolon
	2. Meconium ileus	Plain radiographs show bowel dilatation with a bubbly appearance in the right lower quadrant with distal low bowel obstruction. Contrast enema shows a microcolon with a distended ileum containing filling defects due to inspissated meconium
	3. Hirschsprung disease	Plain radiographs show a low distal obstruction. Contrast enema shows irregular contractions in the rectum and a transition zone, i.e. the point of transition between dilated normal ganglionated bowel and non-dilated abnormal non-ganglionated bowel
	4. Meconium plug	Plain radiographs show a distal obstruction. Enema with hypertonic contrast agent demonstrates meconium as filling defects in the distal colon and rectum. Possible small, immature, left colon
Infants	1. Intussusception	Plain radiographs show a soft tissue mass, distal small bowel obstruction and nonvisualization of gas in the ascending colon. Sonographically, a "target sign" is seen as a hypoechoic ring with an echogenic center on transverse sections, and a "pseudokidney sign" with hypoechoic bowel wall extending along a hyperechoic mucosa on longitudinal sections
	2. Midgut volvulus	Plain radiographs may show a "double-bubble" appearance but are usually normal. An upper gastrointestinal series using radiographic contrast shows the position of the duodenojejunal junction to be abnormal (normally it should be at the left of the spine, at or nearly at, the same level as the duodenal cap and lies posterior in location). In volvulus the jejunum is twisted below the duodenojejunal junction, producing a corkscrew appearance
	3. Obstructed hernia	Plain radiographs show numerous loops of dilated small bowel, and an air-filled bowel loop may be seen in the inguinal canal or scrotum. US can confirm the diagnosis
>3 years	1. Appendicitis	Plain radiographs may show bowel distension, air–fluid levels or appendicolith. Ultrasound shows an inflamed, swollen, noncompressible, blind-ending tubular appendix with an outer wall diameter of 6 mm or more, an appendicolith, and increased echogenicity of the surrounding inflamed mesentery, ileus and intraperitoneal collections if perforated. CT shows a swollen appendix with an outer diameter of more than 6 mm, a "target sign" due to appendiceal wall thickening, an appendicolith, pericecal fat stranding, thickening of the adjacent bowel walls, free peritoneal fluid, lymphadenopathy, phlegmons and abscesses
	2. Hennoch-Schönlein purpura	An upper GI series, ultrasound or CT scan of the abdomen may show bowel wall thickening and increased vascularity on Doppler imaging predominantly involving the proximal small bowel. Echogenic hematomas may be seen on US becoming hypoechoic over time. Ileus, bowel dilatation, ascites and intussusception may be seen
	3. Chole(docho)-lithiasis	Ultrasound shows echogenic foci in the gallbladder with posterior acoustic shadowing. Gallbladder wall thickening and tenderness may be elicited during scanning (positive ultrasound Murphy's sign). Biliary duct dilatation may be present

Table 5.3 Common causes of intestinal obstruction in children, in order of frequency

Hypertrophic pyloric stenosis (HPS)

Intussusception

Intestinal atresia

Incarcerated hernia

Imperforate anus

Hirschsprung disease

Adhesion

Malrotation

Meconium plug

Meconium ileus

Annular pancreas

Meckel's diverticulum

Adapted from Janik et al. (1981).

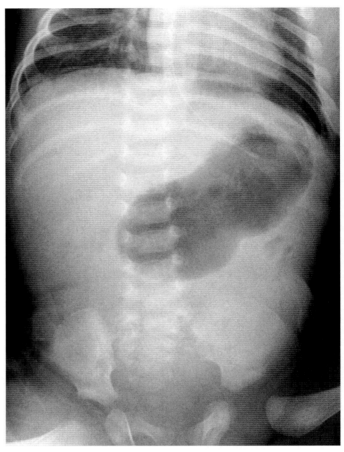

Figure 5.11 Hypertrophic pylorus stenosis. Four-week-old boy with recurrent vomiting. Hyperperistalsis of the stomach was noted clinically. Supine abdominal radiograph shows the presence of a dilated stomach with a "waist" due to peristalsis. No gas is seen in the intestines, indicating the presence of gastric outlet obstruction.

Intestinal obstruction may be functional or mechanical (Table 5.3). Functional obstruction, also known as paralytic ileus, is due to a hypomotility of the bowel. The commonest causes are postoperation, gastroenteritis, ischemia, sepsis and hypokalemia. The condition can usually be diagnosed from the clinical history and examination. The plain abdominal radiograph shows multiple, generalized, dilated loops of bowel (see Figure 5.29). Air–fluid levels may be seen on the erect or horizontal beam images. Causes of mechanical bowel obstructions can be diagnosed based on specific imaging findings.

Hypertrophic pyloric stenosis

Hypertrophic pyloric stenosis (HPS) is a condition where hypertrophy of the circular muscle of the pylorus leads to gastric outlet obstruction. It usually occurs in infants between three to six weeks of age, and is three times more common in boys than in girls. Some rare cases run in families and some countries have more cases than others (e.g. Sweden has three times more than North America).

Clinically, the children present with nonbilious, classically projectile, vomiting a few weeks after birth. If left untreated, loss of weight develops. On physical examination, peristaltic waves of gastric contraction may be visualized, known as the "caterpillar sign." A "pyloric tumor" may also be palpated.

Plain films may show absence of air distal to the pylorus. The "caterpillar sign" may be seen on radiographs (Figure 5.11). There has been an increasing reliance on ultrasound, which has become the preferential modality for investigation. The study should be dynamic and is best performed in conjunction with a clear fluid feed (e.g. 10% dextrose water) to enable peristalsis of the stomach to be assessed, along with gastric emptying. A high frequency linear transducer is required.

The hypertrophied pyloric muscle appears relatively hypoechoic on ultrasound. The normal pylorus should have

a length of <16 mm and one muscle wall should have a thickness of <4 mm. Measurements exceeding these numbers indicate HPS. Length measurements are overall more accurate than diameter (Figure 5.12). The pylorus may fail to open and passage of gastric contents through the pylorus may not be seen. Active gastric peristalsis may also be demonstrated on ultrasound.

In rare cases, when a US is not possible, an upper GI series may be performed, which will demonstrate elongation of the pyloric canal ("string sign"), the "double track sign" due to folding of the compressed mucosa, the "shoulder sign" (aka mushroom or umbrella sign) where the pyloric muscle bulges into the distal antrum and base of the duodenal cap, and the "pyloric-tit sign" where the pyloric mass indents on the lesser curvature of the stomach (Figure 5.13).

Diagnosis may be difficult in early stages when the entity is evolving. Close clinical follow-up and repeat imaging is important in establishing the diagnosis in such cases (Figure 5.14). Associated gastroesophageal reflux may be assessed via ultrasound or fluoroscopy. Possible differential diagnoses of gastric outlet obstruction are listed in Table 5.4.

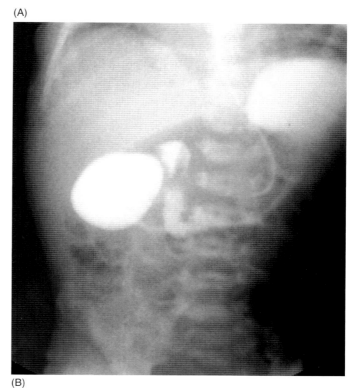

(A)

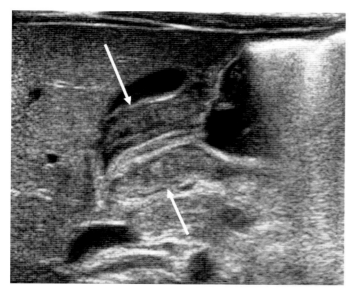

Figure 5.12 Hypertrophied pylorus stenosis. Same patient as Figure 5.11. Longitudinal US image of the pylorus shows it to be hypertrophic, measuring 18 mm in length and each wall measuring 7 mm in thickness (arrows).

(B)

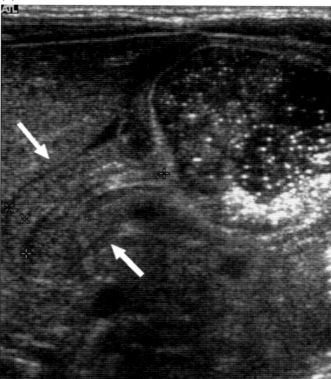

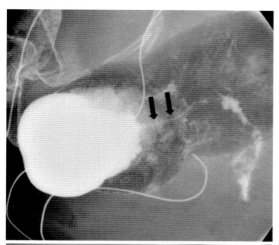

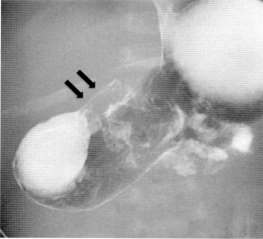

Figure 5.13 Six-week-old child with vomiting. Upper GI series shows the presence of an elongated pylorus with a thin sliver of contrast passing through it, consistent with HPS (arrows).

Figure 5.14 Three-week-old boy with vomiting. (A) Upper GI series shows a normal pylorus with good flow of contrast into the duodenum without delay. (B) Repeat US was performed after the symptoms worsened over six days, and shows unequivocal HPS.

Table 5.4 Causes of gastric outlet obstruction

Pathology	Key imaging findings
Hypertrophic pyloric stenosis	Plain films may show the "caterpillar sign," absence of air distal to the pylorus or a distended stomach
	Sonographically, the hypertrophied pyloric muscle appears hypoechoic, with wall thickness ≥ 4 mm and length ≥ 16 mm. Pylorus remains closed with no passage of gastric contents. Active gastric peristalsis may be seen
	Upper GI series demonstrates the "string sign," "double track sign," "shoulder sign" and the "pyloric-tit sign"
Pylorospasm	Pyloric muscle appears normal on ultrasound with wall thickness ≤ 4 mm and length ≤ 16 mm. Gastric emptying may be delayed but eventually occurs with normal pyloric peristalsis
Paralytic ileus	Generalized bowel distension
Gastric volvulus	Gas–fluid level in the fundus and antrum of the stomach. Upper GI series – mesenteroaxial volvulus: stomach upright with pylorus above the gastroesophageal junction; organoaxial volvulus: stomach in horizontal position with pylorus facing downwards
Gastric antral web	Gastric distension, upper GI series – gastric obstruction, pylorus not demonstrated
Duodenal atresia/web/stenosis/ annular pancreas	Gastric distension, upper GI series – "windsock," duodenal web/diaphragm may be seen

Volvulus of the stomach

Gastric volvulus is an uncommon but potentially life-threatening condition where the stomach is abnormally twisted, resulting in a compromised blood supply. This can result in incarceration, gangrene and death. Volvulus of the stomach may be mesenteroaxial or organoaxial. The less common mesenteroaxial volvulus occurs when the stomach twists around its short axis, that is, an axis from lesser to greater curvature, perpendicular to the luminal (long) axis of the stomach. The more common organoaxial volvulus occurs when the stomach rotates around its long axis, that is, the axis between the esophagogastric junction and the pylorus. The normal stomach is fixed and prevented from abnormal rotation by the four gastric ligaments – the gastrohepatic, gastrosplenic, gastrocolic and gastrophrenic. Patients are predisposed to gastric volvulus when these ligaments are abnormally loose or absent. Pyloric obstruction leading to chronic gastric dilatation, hiatus hernia, diaphragmatic hernias, eventration of diaphragm and adhesions also serve as predisposing factors for volvulus of stomach. A tight wrap after Nissen's fundoplication is also known to predispose to gastric volvulus.

Patients may present acutely or with recurrent abdominal pain. Acutely, the child presents with sudden onset of abdominal distension, pain and vomiting. Occasionally, chest pain may be experienced when the distended stomach compresses on structures within the chest. In chronic or recurrent volvulus, symptoms are nonspecific abdominal pain.

Plain radiographs may show a gas–fluid level in the fundus and antrum of the stomach. Mesenteroaxial volvulus is diagnosed when the stomach is upright in position with a pylorus above the gastroesophageal junction (Figure 5.15). The organoaxial type shows a stomach in horizontal position with a pylorus facing downward (Figure 5.16). Hence, the greater curvature is seen higher than the lesser curvature and in front of the lower portion of the esophagus.

Malrotation and midgut volvulus

Malrotation is a congenital failure of bowel rotation between the 5th and 11th weeks of gestation. The normal bowel rotates 290° counterclockwise during embryological development. The term "malrotation" describes a partial or complete absence of this normal rotation. Table 5.5 lists the various types of malrotation. The type IIIA malrotation is most likely to lead to a midgut volvulus and occurs when the duodenum fails to rotate the final 90° and fixes at 180° rotation. This leads to a location of the duodenojejunal junction below the level of the pylorus and a high location of the cecum in the right upper or mid-abdomen. The mesenteric attachments of the bowel loops are very short and centralized around the superior mesenteric artery and vein. This predisposes to twisting of the small bowel around the mesenteric axis, called midgut volvulus. Up to three rotations may be asymptomatic, but further rotations usually lead to major compression of the mesenteric vessels, anoxia and gangrene of the small bowel, a life-threatening emergency which warrants immediate diagnosis and surgical intervention.

The majority of patients present with bilious vomiting; 75% within the first month of life and 90% within the first year of life. There is a high mortality rate if the diagnosis of

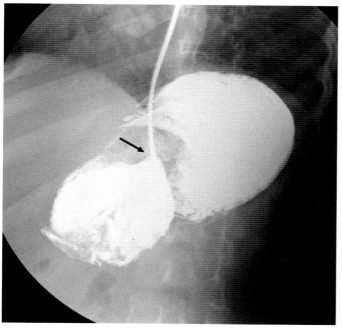

Figure 5.15 Mesenteroaxial volvulus of the stomach. Six-year-old boy with acute vomiting. Single contrast barium meal shows the presence of the gastro-esophageal junction to lie inferiorly (arrow). Contrast could not pass through the pylorus into the small bowel, indicating the presence of obstruction.

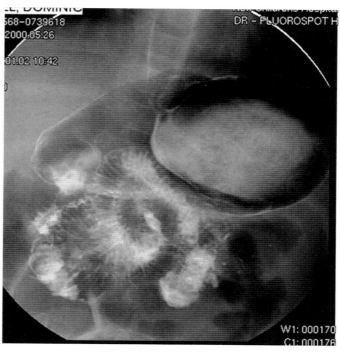

Figure 5.16 Organoaxial volvulus of the stomach. Eight-year-old boy with acute abdominal pain and vomiting. Single contrast upper GI series shows the greater curvature of the stomach lying superior to the lesser curvature.

Table 5.5 Types of malrotation

Type	Key imaging findings
I Nonrotation	Small bowel on the right of the abdomen, large bowel on the left
IIA Duodenal malrotation	Duodenum is nonrotated and situated on the right. Colon is normally rotated and in normal position
IIB Reversed rotation	SMA behind duodenum, colon behind SMA
IIC Reversed rotation	SMA behind duodenum, colon in front of SMA and duodenum (a form of internal hernia)
IIIA Classical malrotation	Duodenum lies to the right of midline and the cecum is high riding – may result in volvulus
IIIB Ladd's bands	Duodenum lies to the right of midline, cecum in normal position in the right iliac fossa but Ladd's bands run from the hepatic flexure downwards, resulting in obstruction
IIIC Mobile cecum (normal variant)	Cecum is high riding but the duodenum is normal in fixation
IIID Others	Paraduodenal hernia

SMA = superior mesenteric artery.
Adapted from Snyder and Chaffin (1954).

a midgut volvulus is delayed. The clinical diagnosis can be difficult in the very young child where abdominal pain is difficult to assess. A small percentage of patients present with clinical shock and ischemic bowel.

A malrotation may be suspected based on plain films if bowel loops are found in an unusual position, such as multiple gas-filled loops of small bowel located in the right abdominal quadrant with significantly less or absent bowel gas in the left abdominal quadrant. A midgut volvulus may present as a duodenal obstruction with a "double-bubble" appearance or, rarely, a "corkscrew" appearance of proximal gas-filled loops of bowel with a paucity of bowel gas more distally (Figure 5.17).

An upper GI fluoroscopy is the best modality to evaluate for suspected malrotation and midgut volvulus. The most important sign to look for is the position of the duodenojejunal junction, which is normally located to the left of the spine, at, or nearly at, the same level as the pylorus (Figure 5.18). In patients with malrotation, the duodenojejunal junction is located below the level of the pylorus and projects on the spine or to the right of the spine. In young infants, the duodenojejunal junction may sometimes be displaced by a much distended stomach, by a feeding tube or by some other mass lesion. Care should be taken in this age group to not "over-diagnose" malrotations, and other signs of malrotation, such as abnormal position of proximal small bowel and cecum, should be always carefully evaluated.

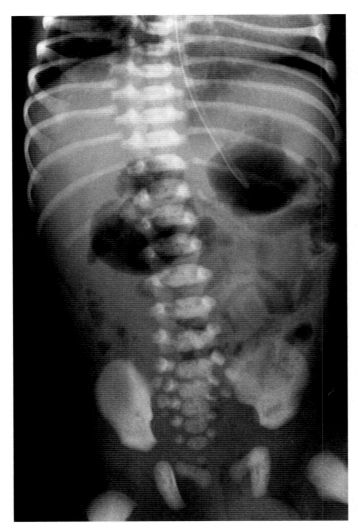

Figure 5.17 Two-week-old neonate with recurrent vomiting due to malrotation and midgut volvulus. Plain abdominal radiograph shows air in the fundus of the stomach and proximal duodenum consistent with a "double-bubble" appearance.

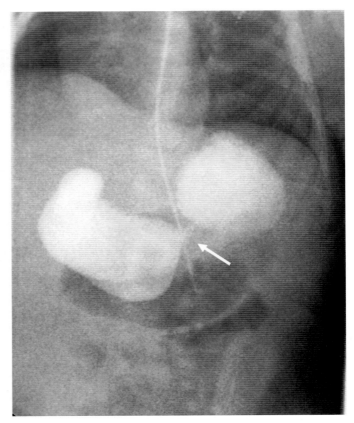

Figure 5.18 Three-week-old neonate with malrotation and midgut volvulus. A spot image from the upper GI series shows complete obstruction at the D3 level (arrow) with dilatation of the duodenum proximal to the obstruction.

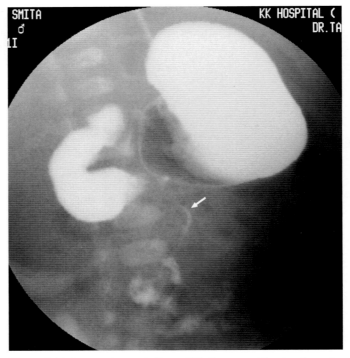

Figure 5.19 Same patient as in Figure 5.17. The upper GI series shows the presence of a corkscrew appearance in the distal duodenum due to malrotation and small bowel volvulus (arrow).

In case of a midgut volvulus, signs of malrotation are noted in conjunction with signs of "twisted bowel." The proximal duodenum may be dilated, the second or third portion of the duodenum may show a typical "beak sign" and the proximal jejunum may show a corkscrew appearance (Figure 5.19).

Ultrasound studies may demonstrate duodenal dilatation as well as abnormal positions of the superior mesenteric artery and vein in the axial section (Figure 5.20). Doppler studies may show clockwise twisting of the mesenteric vessels known as the "whirlpool" sign. In complete volvulus, an inversion of the superior mesenteric artery (SMA) and vein (SMV) may be seen with the artery situated to the right of the vein. The SMA is normally situated to the left of the SMV. However, a normal US does not exclude malrotation, and patients with suspected

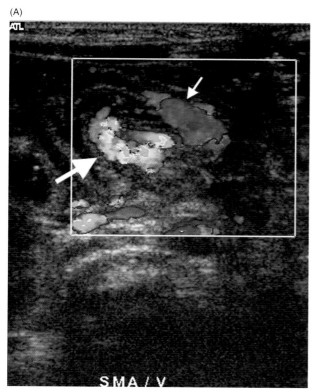

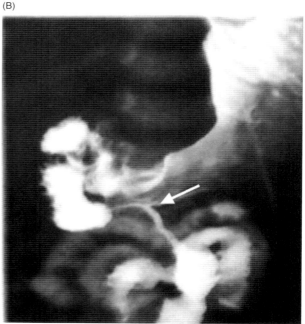

Figure 5.20 Three-year-old boy with bilious vomiting and midgut volvulus. (A) US shows the superior mesenteric artery (large arrow) on the right of the superior mesenteric vein (small arrow). The vessels are also twisting around one another giving rise to the "whirlpool" image. (B) Upper GI series shows a duodenal obstruction with the duodenojejunal junction to be situated lower than its expected position confirming the diagonsis of midgut volvulus and malrotation.

midgut volvulus should have an immediate barium meal to confirm the diagnosis.

Intussusception

An intussusception occurs when a segment of intestine prolapses into a more distal bowel segment. These segments are termed the intussusceptum and the intussuscipiens, respectively. Intussusception is most commonly ileo–colic. Ileo–ileo–colic and small bowel–small bowel intussusception form the bulk of the remainder. Intussusception may lead to bowel necrosis, perforation and obstruction. Children are most commonly affected in the first two years of life, but idiopathic intussusceptions up to four years of age are not uncommon. These patients often have a history of gastrointestinal infection, with inflammatory nodes causing the lead point for an intussusception. In young babies, other possible lead points are Meckel's diverticulum or duplication cysts, while in children over four years of age, a lymphoma or polyp may also be an underlying cause.

The classical triad of colicky abdominal pain, vomiting and bloody ("redcurrant") jelly stools is seen in less than 25% of cases. Physical examination is usually unremarkable, but occasionally the intussusception may be palpable.

Plain abdominal radiographs may show the presence of a curvilinear soft tissue mass within the colon, or the absence of bowel gas in the ascending colon (Figure 5.21). However, these signs are present in less than 50% of plain radiographs. A left lateral decubitus view has been shown to increase the ability to diagnose patients with an indeterminate supine view.

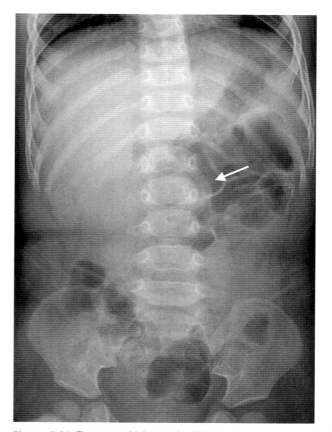

Figure 5.21 Three-year-old boy with abdominal pain and lower GI tract bleeding. Plain abdominal radiograph shows the presence of a soft tissue mass in the central abdomen outlined on its left side by air within the large bowel (arrow). This finding is suspicious for an intussusception.

(A)

(B)

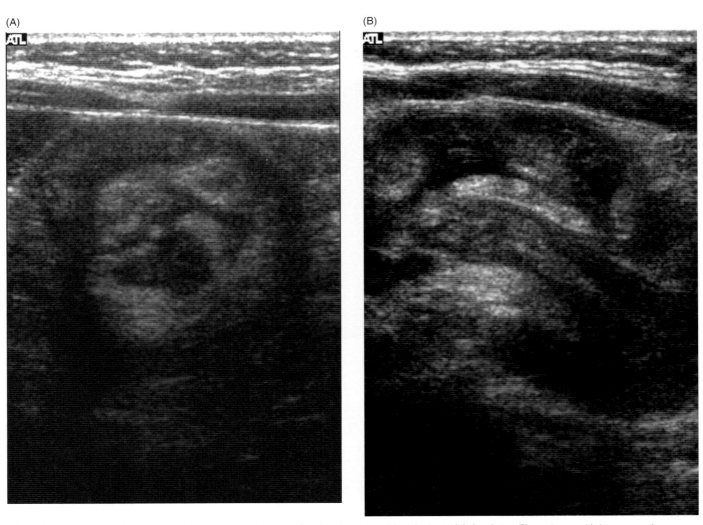

Figure 5.22 Same patient as Figure 5.21. US shows the presence of a "doughnut" sign (A) and a "pseudokidney" sign (B) consistent with intussusception.

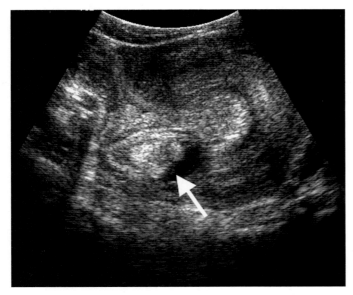

Figure 5.23 Ten-year-old boy with abdominal pain. US shows the presence of an intussusception with a stalk leading to an echogenic nodule (arrow) and a small amount of surrounding fluid in the intussusception. A lead point was suspected and air-enema reduction was not attempted. A Meckel's diverticulum was found at surgery.

Rarely, a target sign due to a lucent mesenteric "ring" in the intussusceptum may be seen on X-rays.

Ultrasound has become the modality of choice to diagnose an intussusception. The characteristic finding of an ileo–colic intussusception is a "target sign," i.e. a hypoechoic ring with an echogenic center on transverse US sections, and a "pseudokidney sign" with hypoechoic bowel wall extending along a hyper-echoic mucosa (Figure 5.22). Sometimes a lead point may be suspected if a stalk can be visualized (Figures 5.23, 5.24). Occasionally concentric rings may be seen. The appearance is more complex when there is an ileo–ileo–colic intussusception, as there is more than one loop of bowel within the colon (Figure 5.25).

CT is not used in the diagnosis of patients with suspected ileo–colic intussusceptions but small bowel intussusceptions may be detected incidentally. The latter usually occur in older children or adults, are usually transient short-segment small bowel–small bowel intussusceptions and show no evidence of intestinal obstruction. These incidental intussusceptions resolve spontaneously and are clinically insignificant.

Once the diagnosis has been made the surgeon has to be involved/informed, as radiological treatment by reduction has

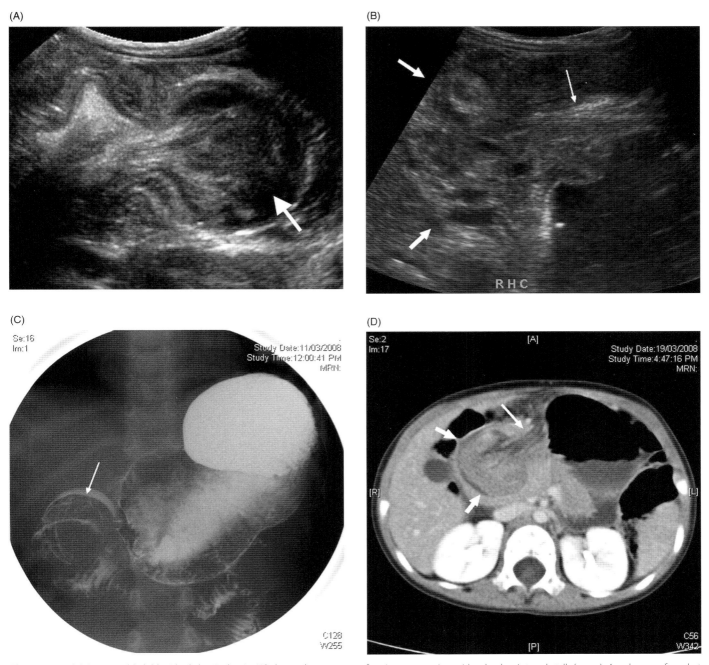

Figure 5.24 (A) Six-year-old child with abdominal pain. US shows the presence of an intussusception with a lead point and stalk (arrow). A polyp was found at surgery. (B) Another patient; a four-year-old boy with epigastric pain. US shows the presence of a polypoidal mass in the duodenum (white arrows). The stalk of the polyp can be seen (small arrow). (C) Upper GI series shows the presence of a filling defect in the duodenum. (D) CT shows the presence of the polyp (arrows) in the upper duodenum with the stalk (small arrow) originating from the stomach.

a small but definite risk of perforation and the surgeon needs to be available in case of complications with an imaging-guided intussusception reduction.

Intussusception reduction

Radiology plays an important role in the management of children with intussusception. Image-guided liquid or air

reduction of intussusception is the treatment of choice unless the child has peritonitis or free intraperitoneal gas due to perforation, or is in shock or sepsis (Figure 5.26). The relative advantages of air vs. barium or Hypaque (sodium amidotrizoate) enema reduction of intussusception has been widely discussed in the literature, and the choice between one method and the other depends on the radiologist's or institution's

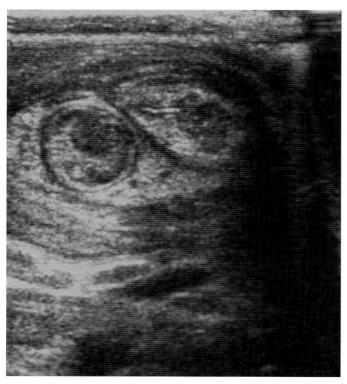

Figure 5.25 US image shows an intussusception with more than one bowel loop within the intussuscipiens, consistent with an ileo–ileo–colic intussusception.

experience and practice. Most radiologists prefer to use air, and this is now generally accepted as the technique of choice. A gas pressure between 80 mm and 120 mm of mercury should be used. These limits are equivalent to pressures that would be generated by a barium enema with a bag positioned approximately 3 ft (0.9 m) and 6 ft (1.8 m) respectively above the patient. The air is run in and quickly fills the bowel and outlines the head of the intussusception. Typically, intussusception reduction is confirmed when air is seen to pass rapidly into the small bowel. There is often some delay when the intussusception has been reduced to the ileocecal valve as this may be edematous. Persistence at this time is important to ensure that a total reduction has occurred (Figure 5.27).

The literature suggests that fluoroscopically guided air enema reduction has a lower perforation rate, lower radiation exposure and a higher reduction rate than barium enemas. Recently, ultrasound-guided reductions have also been described.

Intussusceptions may reoccur in approximately 10% of cases post-reduction. There is no contraindication to reducing the intussusception with an enema procedure again. There is no limit to the number of reductions one can perform. However, many centers refer the patients to surgery after more than three recurrences in order to evaluate for underlying lead points.

Complications

Perforation rates with air enema vary between 0.14% and 2.8%. The latter was reported in an early study using high pressures. Perforation rate in experienced hands should be much less than 1%. Chronic perforation is a more serious complication and occurs in a very small percentage, often related to areas of necrosis in the bowel. Perforation will require immediate surgical management. If a perforation does occur, it has been shown that perforations that occur with air enemas are smaller and produce much less contamination of the peritoneum compared to liquid enemas, and hence have a better recovery rate from surgery.

Intestinal hernias

Intestinal hernias are abnormal protrusions of intestines through a defect or weakness of the abdominal wall or internally within the abdomen. The different types of hernias described include indirect inguinal, direct inguinal, femoral, umbilical, incisional, internal and spigelian hernias, amongst others. Incarcerated or irreducible hernias predispose to obstruction and should be treated urgently because complications such as intestinal obstruction, gangrene and sepsis may develop. Indirect and umbilical hernias are the commonest hernias in children. Internal hernias are rare but important because they have a high mortality rate when not recognized. There are several types of internal hernias, with the paraduodenal type being the commonest. The other, much rarer types include transmesenteric, supra- and/or perivesical, intersigmoid, foramen of Winslow, mesocolic and, rarely, omental hernias.

Indirect inguinal hernias occur because of failure of closure of the processus vaginalis during embryological development. The processus vaginalis is an out-pouching of peritoneum that accompanies the testis on its descent from the abdomen down into the scrotum. The processus vaginalis should close after the testis has descended into the scrotum. Failure to do so gives rise to a condition called a patent processus vaginalis, and this defect predisposes to the formation of inguinal hernias. The incidence is 10–20 per 1000 live births and is much more common in boys than girls. Occasionally an ovary may herniate through a patent processus vaginalis, or an undescended testis may lie within one.

Umbilical hernias occur through failure of closure of the umbilicus and are common in children less than two years of age (Figure 5.28). More than 80% heal spontaneously between three and five years, without treatment.

Unobstructed indirect inguinal hernias may be asymptomatic or present as a lump in the inguinal region which may or may not extend into the scrotum. Incarcerated or irreducible hernias present as painful, irreducible lumps and, when obstructed, symptoms such as vomiting, pain and abdominal distension occur. Internal hernias are difficult to diagnose clinically because they present with nonspecific symptoms of

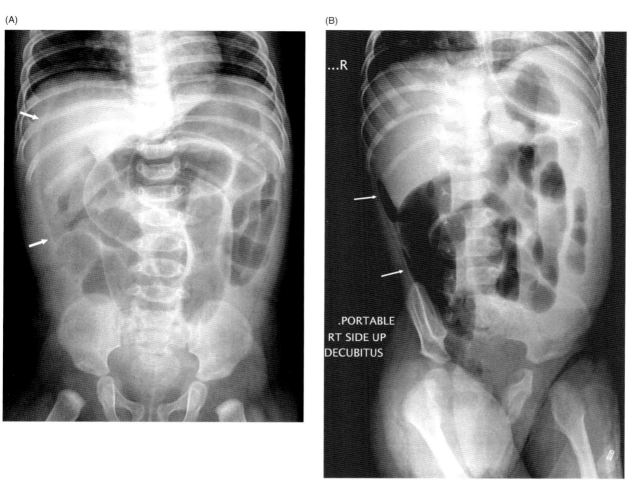

Figure 5.26 Eight-month-old child brought to the Children's Emergency department with vomiting, marked abdominal distension and almost in cardio-respiratory collapse. Plain abdominal radiographs in the (A) supine and (B) left lateral decubitus position show the presence of free intraperitoneal gas (arrows). An intussusception was found to be the cause of perforation at surgery.

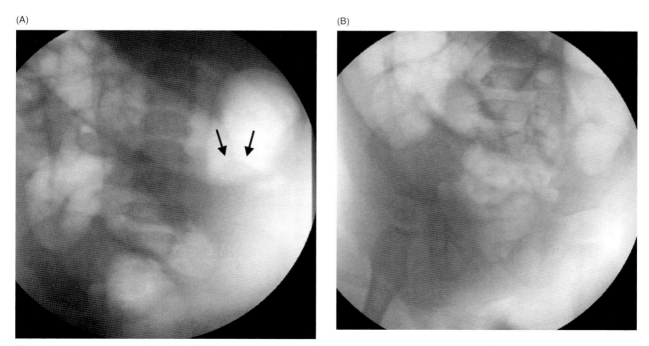

Figure 5.27 Same patient as Figure 5.21. (A) Spot image taken during air enema reduction shows the presence of the intussusception in the ascending colon (arrows); the patient is in the prone position. (B) Another spot image after reduction shows abundant air in the small bowel, indicating successful reduction of the intussusception.

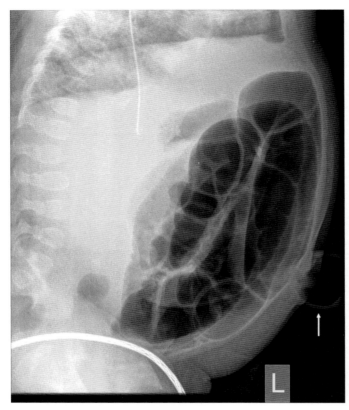

Figure 5.28 Six-month-old previously premature baby with marked bowel dilatation of uncertain cause. A lateral abdominal radiograph shows the presence of an umbilical hernia (arrow).

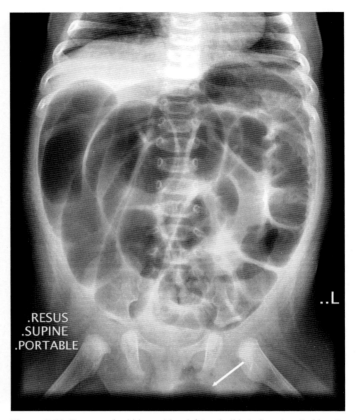

Figure 5.29 Four-month-old boy with a left irreducible indirect inguinal hernia. Supine abdominal radiograph shows the presence multiple dilated loops of bowel, consistent with intestinal obstruction. Air can be seen in the left inguinal hernia (arrow).

intestinal obstruction. Umbilical hernias are obvious clinically but seldom cause obstruction.

Plain abdominal radiographs show numerous loops of dilated small bowel in patients with obstructed indirect inguinal hernias, and air may be seen in the inguinal hernia (Figure 5.29). Ultrasound is able to detect the obstructed loop of bowel in the inguinal region or scrotum (Figure 5.30). US is useful in the assessment of these patients who present with pain and swelling in the inguinal region, because it is possible to distinguish an obstructed inguinal hernia from other differentials such as lymphadenitis and to assess the opposite side for the presence or absence of a patent processus vaginalis. Color Doppler imaging is also useful in documenting blood flow to the bowel loop. Further imaging is usually not required.

In obstructed internal hernias, plain abdominal radiographs show nonspecific features of intestinal obstruction. Previously, internal hernias were assessed with upper GI series. Findings include apparently encapsulated distended bowel loops in an abnormal location, arrangement or crowding of small bowel loops within the hernial sac, and evidence of intestinal obstruction with segmental dilatation and stasis. On dynamic fluoroscopic evaluation, apparent fixation and reversed peristalsis may be visualized (Figure 5.31).

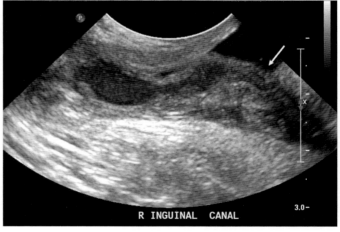

Figure 5.30 Same patient as in Figure 5.29. US of the left inguinal region shows a loop of bowel, with normal peristalsis, herniating into the left scrotum (arrow).

CT has been reported to be useful in the diagnosis of these patients because of its availability, speed and multiplanar reformatting capabilities. Findings such as apparent encapsulation of distended bowel loops in an abnormal location, arrangement or crowding of small bowel loops within the

(A)

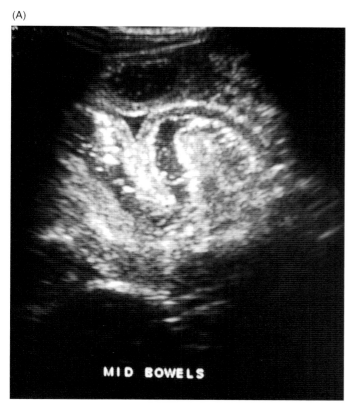

MID BOWELS

(B)

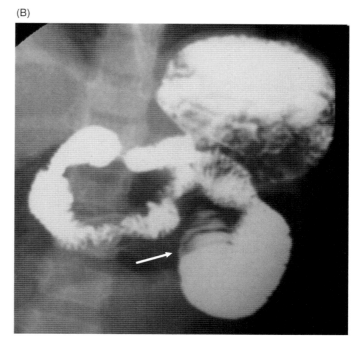

Figure 5.31 Six-year-old boy with abdominal pain and vomiting. (A) Initial US shows the presence of dilated, fluid-filled loops of bowel in the epigastric region. Reversed peristalsis was seen on real-time imaging. (B) Upper GI series shows a dilated obstructed loop of bowel in the proximal jejunum. A paraduodenal hernia was found at surgery.

sac, evidence of segmental obstruction, and mesenteric vessel abnormalities with engorgement, crowding, twisting and stretching of these vessels suggest the diagnosis of internal hernias (Figures 5.32, 5.33).

Gastrointestinal bleeding

Gastrointestinal tract (GIT) bleeding is uncommon in children. However, it has been reported in 6.4% of ICU (intensive care) patients in one prospective study. GIT bleeding can generally be divided into upper GIT and lower GIT causes (Tables 5.6 and 5.7), although overlaps are noted.

A thorough history and complete physical examination can narrow the differential diagnosis significantly. The age of the patient is a key factor because some conditions such as necrotizing enterocolitis and cow's milk allergy present during the neonatal and early infancy period respectively. Drug ingestion such as NSAIDs is also important. Observing the characteristics of the bleeding may also point to the correct diagnosis in many cases.

Imaging has a limited role in the evaluation of most cases of GIT bleeding in children. Plain radiographs are useful in detecting radiopaque foreign bodies, bowel perforation or obstruction. Intramural gas, free intraperitoneal gas, portal venous gas and fixed dilated loops of bowel in an ill, premature

neonate points to necrotizing enterocolitis. Barium studies may diagnose gastric ulcers, erosive gastritis, inflammatory bowel disease and juvenile polyps. Ultrasound, CT and MRI may detect liver disease and varices in patients with portal hypertension (Figure 5.34) and vascular malformations that may give rise to GIT bleeding. Technetium 99m pertechnetate scans are used to detect ectopic gastric tissue within a Meckel's diverticulum or duplication cyst (Figure 5.35). Technetium 99m-labeled red blood cells have been used to identify occult sites of slow, ongoing bleeds. Angiography is reserved for cases of profuse bleeding. CT has been shown to be able to detect occult GIT hemorrhage in children (Figure 5.36).

Foreign-body ingestion

Foreign-body ingestion in children is a common occurrence. Most ingested foreign bodies are excreted harmlessly without complications. Foreign bodies may be harmful when they are poisonous, or cause obstruction and even perforation to the gastrointestinal tract. Foreign bodies that become stuck in the GI system most commonly lodge at the level of the cricopharyngeus muscle (Figure 5.37), mid-esophagus level where the aortic arch and carina overlap, lower gastroesophageal junction and ileocecal valve.

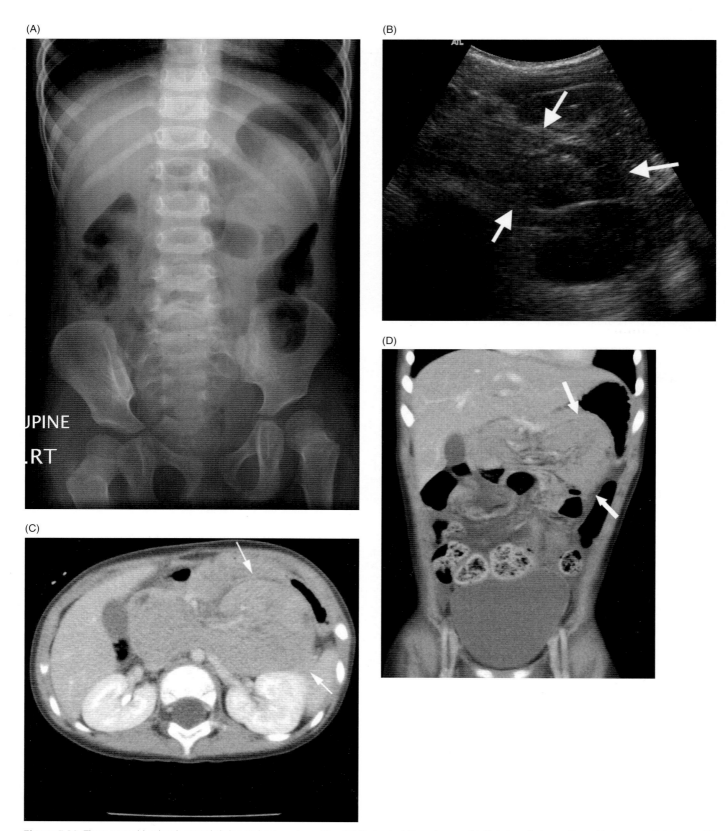

Figure 5.32 Three-year-old girl with central abdominal pain and vomiting. (A) Abdominal X-ray shows mild dilatation of a loop of bowel in the central abdomen. (B) US shows the presence of dilated fluid-filled loop of bowel in the central abdomen (arrows), anterior to the kidney and crossing the midline. An internal hernia was suspected and a CT was performed. (C) Axial and (D) coronal reconstructions show the presence of a fluid-filled loop of dilated bowel in the central abdomen suspicious for an internal hernia (arrows). A mesocolic hernia was confirmed at surgery. A defect was noted in the mesocolon with small bowel herniating into the defect. Congenital fibrous adhesion bands were also noted encircling the small bowel and mesentery. The blood supply to the bowel was preserved.

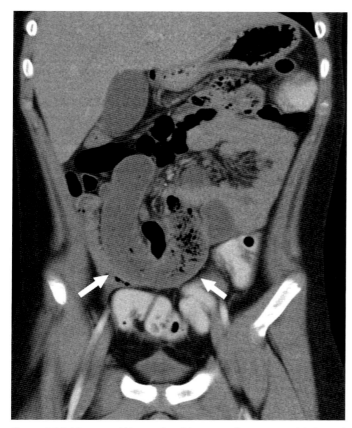

Figure 5.33 Nine-year-old boy with sudden onset of severe central abdominal pain and vomiting. Coronal reconstruction section from a multislice CT shows the presence of a dilated loop of bowel situated in the central abdomen. At surgery a Meckel's diverticulum with an adhesion band causing an internal hernia was found.

Table 5.6 Causes of upper GIT bleeding

Pathology	Key imaging findings
Mallory-Weiss	Best diagnosed on endoscopy
Varices	Upper GI series shows multiple serpiginous filling defects involving the lower third of the esophagus. Cross-sectional imaging shows the varices as slow-flowing serpiginous vascular structures
Esophagitis	Upper GI series shows irregular ulcerations and nodules due to granulations and thickened mucosal folds. CT shows nonspecific thickening of the esophageal wall
Ulcer and gastritis	Upper GI series shows focal contrast collections (ulcer crater) with surrounding filling defect (halo) due to edema
Arteriovenous malformations	Angiography shows an abnormal tangle of vessels with a supplying artery and an early draining vein
GIT duplications	Ultrasound shows fluid-filled cystic mass with echogenic mucosal lining and an outer hypoechoic wall or muscle. Technetium 99m pertechnetate shows uptake within the ectopic gastric tissue if present
Henoch-Schönlein purpura	Upper GI series, ultrasound or CT scan of the abdomen may reveal bowel wall thickening and increased vascularity on Doppler imaging, predominantly involving the proximal small bowel. Ileus, bowel dilatation, intussusception and ascites may be present
Foreign-body injury	Plain ap radiographs should localize the foreign body if it is radiopaque

Table 5.7 Causes of lower GIT bleeding

Pathology	Key imaging findings
0–3 years	
Necrotizing enterocolitis	Plain X-ray – intramural gas, portal venous gas or free intraperitoneal gas, paralytic ileus and persistent bowel distension
Allergic colitis	Plain X-ray – intramural gas, toxic megacolon, bowel perforation Contrast enema – narrowing and mucosal irregularity of the rectum with an abnormal rectosigmoid index – similar to Hirschsprung disease
Anal fissure	None – clinical diagnosis
Intussusception	See Table 5.2
Above 3 years	
Infectious gastroenteritis	Ultrasound and barium enema – nonspecific bowel fold thickening
Meckel's diverticulum	Technetium 99m pertechnetate shows uptake within the ectopic gastric tissue present with the diverticulum at the same time as uptake is seen in the gastric mucosa. Tracer may be seen traveling down the intestinal lumen if active bleeding is present
Juvenile polyps	Barium enema – polypoidal filling defect, may be multiple in polyposis syndromes
Ulcerative colitis	Barium enema – fine granularity of the colonic mucosa, stippling, shallow ulceration, pseudopolyps, fibrotic shortening Cross-sectional imaging – bowel wall thickening
Crohn's disease	Barium enema – deep ulcerations, cobblestone pattern, fistula formation

(A)

(B)

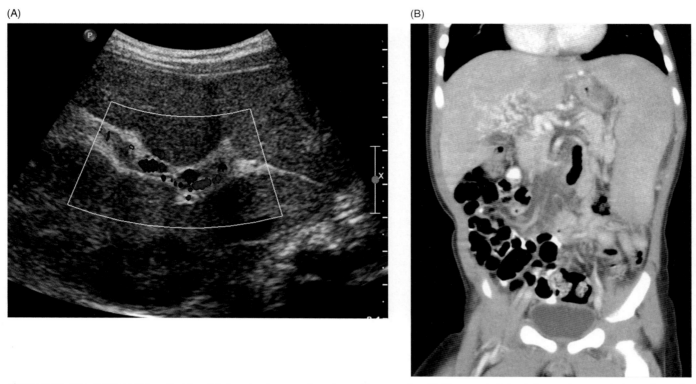

Figure 5.34 Nine-month-old boy with idiopathic hepatosplenomegaly and portal hypertension. (A) Ultrasound of the abdomen shows multiple small vessels in the region of the porta hepatis and a normal portal vein could not be visualized. Cavernous transformation of the portal vein was suspected due to portal hypertension. (B) Coronally reconstructed image from a multislice CT confirms the presence of cavernous transformation of the portal vein with varices. Splenomegaly is also noted.

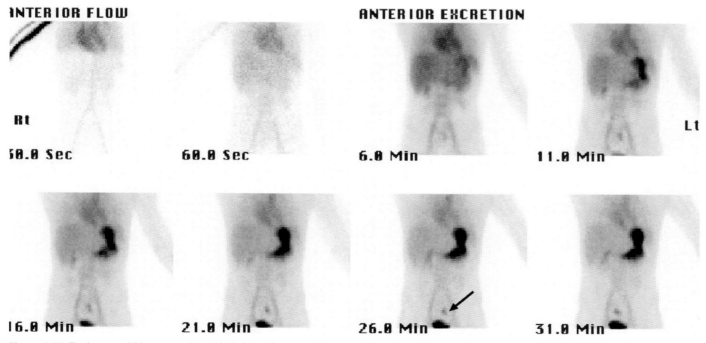

Figure 5.35 Twelve-year-old boy presenting with abdominal pain and gastrointestinal bleeding. A technetium 99m pertechnetate scan shows the presence of a focus of tracer uptake in the pelvis (arrow) appearing at the same time as the stomach. This finding is highly suspicious for ectopic tissue in a Meckel's diverticulum, which was confirmed at surgery.

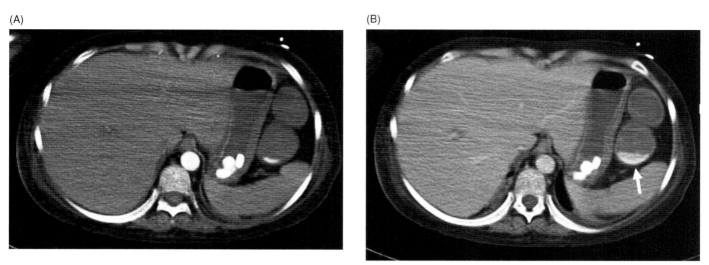

Figure 5.36 Patient with acute lymphoblastic leukemia after bone marrow transplantation, now with graft-versus-host disease, presented with gastrointestinal bleeding. Intravenous contrast-enhanced CT performed in the (A) arterial and (B) portal venous phases shows the presence of contrast extravasating into the small bowel in the left upper quadrant of the abdomen (arrow). Tablets are noted in the stomach.

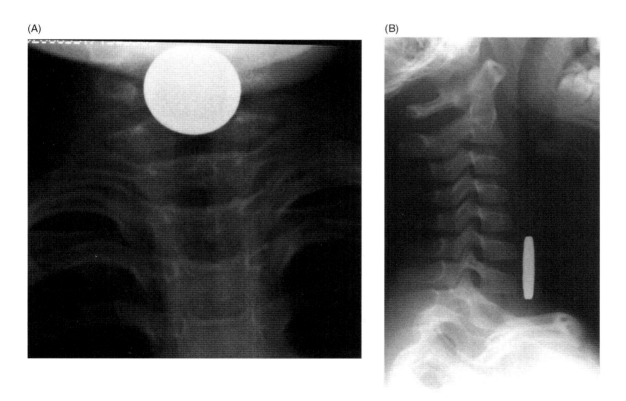

Figure 5.37 Four-year-old boy who swallowed a coin. (A) Anteroposterior and (B) lateral views show the presence of the radiopaque coin situated just anterior to the C6 vertebral body which is the level of the cricopharyngeus muscle.

The caregiver is often able to give a history of foreign-body ingestion. Occasionally patients may present with symptoms secondary to the complications of foreign-body ingestion, such as bleeding and perforation.

Plain ap radiographs showing the neck, chest, abdomen and pelvis (mouth through anus) should localize the foreign body if it is radiopaque (Figure 5.38). Coins in the esophagus appear in a coronal orientation, whereas coins in the trachea appear

(A)

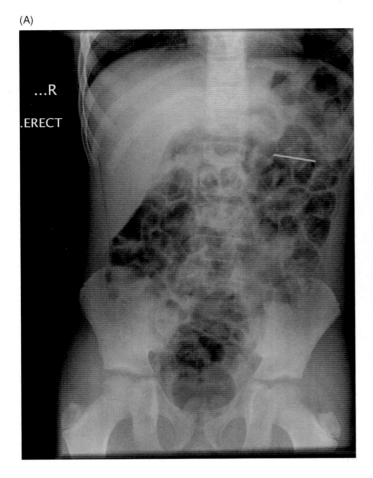

(B)

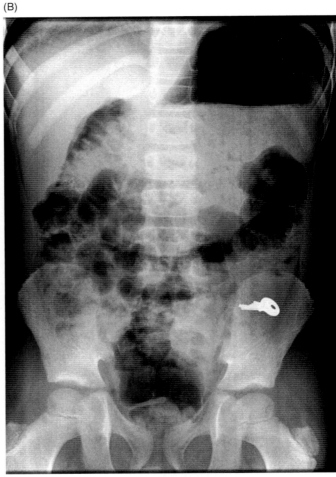

Figure 5.38 Six-year-old boy who swallowed a key. (A) Initial abdominal radiograph shows the presence of a linear metallic foreign body in the left side of the abdomen. There was some concern that this was a sharp object. A repeat radiograph (B) confirms the object to be a key which was subsequently passed out naturally without intervention.

in the sagittal orientation on ap or pa chest radiographs, allowing for their exact anatomical localization (Figure 5.37). The nature of the foreign body should be stated because large, sharp or potentially dangerous foreign bodies may necessitate laparoscopic or surgical removal. In general, foreign bodies above the gastroesophageal junction are endoscopically or bronchoscopically retrieved due to potential respiratory compromise, while most foreign bodies in or beyond the stomach are harmless and find their natural exit. Exceptions are large or very sharp foreign bodies, potentially toxic foreign bodies (e.g. certain flat batteries) and multiple mini-magnets (which may cause bowel ischemia or disruption).

Henoch-Schönlein purpura

Henoch-Schönlein purpura (HSP), an anaphylactoid purpura, is a nonthrombocytopenic purpura with a vasculitic etiology. It affects blood vessels throughout the body, including the bowel. The etiology of HSP is unknown but a preceding upper respiratory tract infection is seen in about 50% of cases. Most children are between the ages of 2 and 11 years old and there is a 2 : 1 ratio of boys to girls.

Symptoms of HSP include rash on the legs, subcutaneous edema, abdominal pain, bloody stools, vomiting, joint pains and scrotal edema. Physical examination reveals a purpuric rash, distributed predominantly in the buttocks and lower limbs; edema of the hands, feet, and scalp; an arthritis involving the knees and ankles; abdominal tenderness; and scrotal edema. In these clinical scenarios, the diagnosis does not need additional imaging tests. However, in about 10%, the initial presentation is with abdominal pain alone and the radiologist may be the first to diagnose the condition.

Plain radiographs of the abdomen are often unremarkable. An upper GI series, ultrasound or CT scan of the abdomen may reveal bowel wall thickening and increased vascularity on Doppler imaging, predominantly involving the proximal small bowel (Figures 5.39, 5.40). The bowel thickening is caused by hemorrhage and edema. Hematomas may be seen, initially

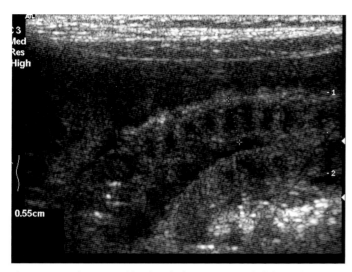

Figure 5.39 Three-year-old girl with skin purpura and abdominal pain. US shows the presence of a markedly thickened loop of bowel in the epigastric region, consistent with HSP duodenitis.

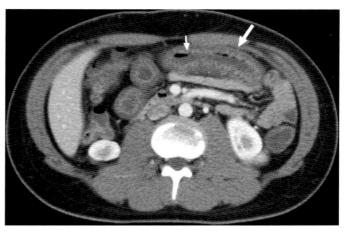

Figure 5.40 Fifteen-year-old boy with HSP presented with severe abdominal pain. CT shows the presence of several loops of thick-walled small bowel (large arrow) with enhancing mucosa (small arrow) consistent with HSP enteritis.

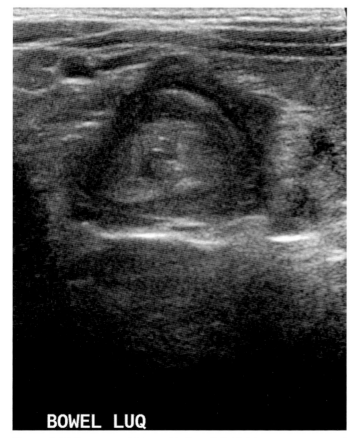

BOWEL LUQ

Figure 5.41 Seven-year-old boy with Henoch-Schönlein purpura presented with abdominal pain. US shows the presence of a small bowel–small bowel intussusception in the epigastric region. The wall of the small bowel is thickened consistent with HSP bowel. The patient recovered without treatment of the intussusception.

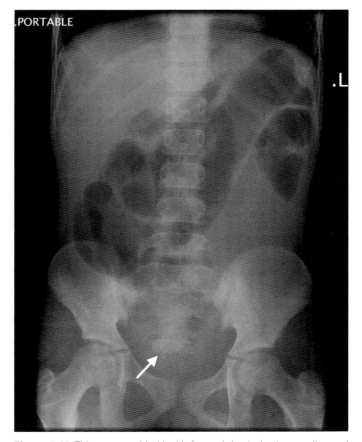

Figure 5.42 Thirteen-year-old girl with fever, abdominal pain, guarding and rebound tenderness. Abdominal radiograph shows the presence of an ovoid fecolith in the pelvis (arrow). Ileus is also seen. A ruptured appendix with the appendicolith situated in the pelvic abscess was found.

(A)

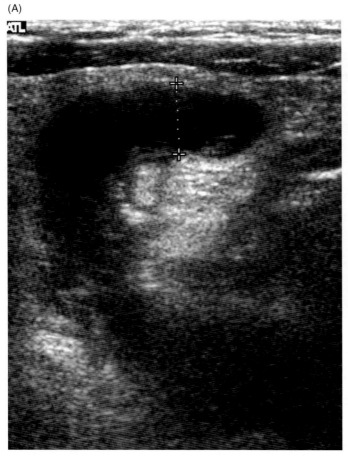

(B)

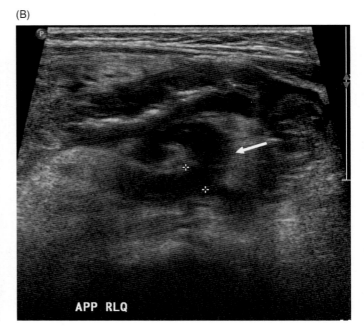

Figure 5.43 (A) Ten-year-old girl with right-sided abdominal pain. US shows the presence of a blind-ending tubular structure with an outer-wall to outer-wall diameter of approximately 8 mm, consistent with an inflamed appendix. (B) Two-year-old girl with right-sided abdominal pain and guarding. US shows the presence of an inflamed appendix (arrow) with surrounding increased echogenicity of the mesentery consistent with mesenteric inflammation. The appendix is situated posterior to the thick-walled cecum. A ruptured retrocecal appendix was found at surgery.

being echogenic on US but with time becoming hypoechoic as they are absorbed. Ileus, bowel dilatation and ascites may also be seen. Intussusception may be present (Figure 5.41), and perforation is an uncommon but serious complication. Serial ultrasound may be used in the follow-up patients with bowel involvement by HSP.

Appendicitis

Acute appendicitis is the most common cause for abdominal surgery in children. The incidence of acute appendicitis is highest at age 10–19 years, ranging from 75 to 233 per 100 000 per year in different countries.

The symptoms of acute appendicitis may vary widely, but most children will have some degree of abdominal pain with or without fever. On physical examination, rebound tenderness and guarding may be present. Abdominal distension due to ileus may also be seen.

Plain radiographs have limited value in the diagnosis of acute appendicitis but may reveal nonspecific findings such as bowel distension or air–fluid levels. An appendicolith

identified in a patient suspected of having acute appendicitis, however, is considered diagnostic (Figure 5.42). Ultrasound is the modality of choice for use in children with suspected appendicitis because it is accurate, has no radiation and is cheaper than CT scans. Signs of appendicitis on ultrasound are an inflamed, swollen, noncompressible appendix with an outer wall diameter of 6 mm or more, detection of an appendicolith, increased echogenicity of the surrounding mesentery consistent with inflammation, ileus of the bowel and, in cases of perforation, intraperitoneal collections (Figure 5.43). CT scans should be reserved for patients with an elevated body mass index, in cases where ultrasound is not diagnostic or inconclusive or in uncooperative patients. CT scan protocols differ and institutions may perform CT with or without bowel, rectal and intravenous contrast. Signs of appendicitis on CT include a swollen appendix with an outer diameter of more than 6 mm, an appendix appearing in cross-section as a "target sign" due to appendiceal wall thickening, an appendicolith, pericecal fat stranding, thickening of the adjacent bowel walls, free peritoneal fluid, lymphadenopathy, phlegmons and

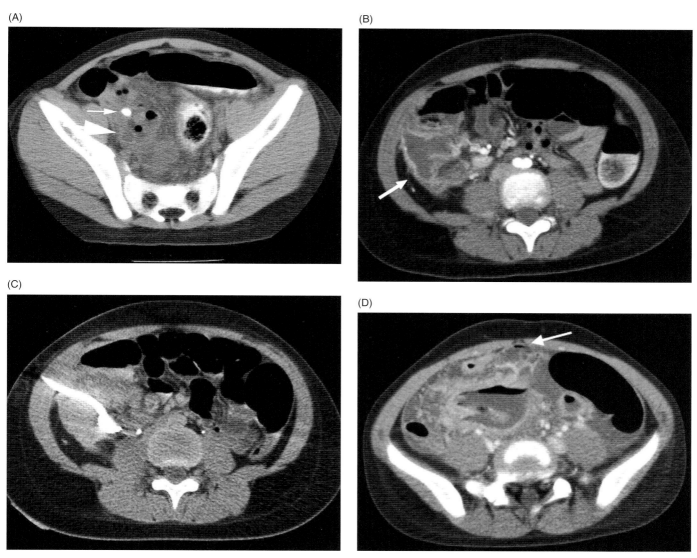

Figure 5.44 (A) Six-year-old girl with right-sided abdominal pain. US examination was suboptimal because the patient was very tender in the right lower quadrant of the abdomen with rebound tenderness. CT performed with rectal contrast but without intravenous contrast shows the presence of an appendicolith in the right side of the pelvis (small arrow) with surrounding abscesses (large arrow) due to a ruptured appendix. This was confirmed at surgery. (B) Nine-year-old boy with right-sided abdominal pain. CT shows the presence of a rim-enhancing abscess in the right lower quadrant of the abdomen consistent with a ruptured appendix, confirmed at surgery (arrow). (C) Same patient as in (B). The abscess was drained percutaneously immediately after the diagnostic scan. A drainage catheter is noted within the abscess cavity which has largely been evacuated. (D) Six-year-old boy presenting with clinical features of peritonitis. CT shows the presence of a rim-enhancing lesion in the right side of the lower abdomen with an air–fluid level. An unusually abundant amount of fluid can be seen within the peritoneal cavity. Free gas is also noted (arrow). Surgery revealed ruptured appendicitis.

abscesses (Figure 5.44). An appendix is normal if its outer-wall diameter is less than 6 mm or if it is completely filled with air or bowel contrast, if this is used in the examination. CT may help in providing guidance for percutaneous drainage of an appendiceal abscess prior to elective delayed appendectomy (Figure 5.44C).

Cholelithiasis

Gallstones are relatively rare in children and generally fall into three types. Gallstones can occur in infancy, most often in premature neonates who are undergoing parenteral therapy. Their

gallbladders are not contracting well and they accumulate biliary sludge which can aggregate into sludge balls and hence progress to malleable gall "stones." These very rarely cause a clinical problem and are found during routine ultrasound examination. These usually disappear when nutrition and the general status of the infant improves. Very rarely they can be displaced into the common bile duct and so may cause obstruction requiring removal.

In infants after the neonatal period, most gallstones are found in association with a choledochal cyst. After infancy, there is a very low rate of gallstones, which slightly increases with increasing age. In adolescents, gallstones may be associated with hemolytic disorders. Gallstones are also seen with some types of cholecystitis. Table 5.8 lists the causes of gallstones in older children.

Many gallstones may remain asymptomatic and are found during evaluation of other abnormalities. If they enter the bile ducts they can cause biliary colics and obstruction. Biliary colic is different from renal colic in that the pain develops over an hour or two and then subsides slowly.

A calcified gallstone on a plain film in children is exceedingly rare. More commonly, it may be found on ultrasound examination or as an incidental finding on a CT or MRI.

The appearance on ultrasound will depend on the amount of calcification (Figure 5.45). If calcified, there will be dense shadowing beyond; otherwise, gallstones appear as focal densities, most often within the gallbladder.

Genitourinary
Acute scrotal pain

The causes of acute scrotal pain are listed in Table 5.9. Ultrasound is now the modality of choice for evaluation of scrotal

Table 5.8 Causes of gallstones in older children

Hemolytic anemia

Cystic fibrosis

Choledochal cyst

Ileal disease such as Crohn's disease or post-resection

Metachromatic leukodystrophy

Wilson's disease

pain because it is readily available, quick and accurate in the differential diagnosis of underlying pathologies. MRI and scintigraphy are other modalities that have been used in the case of equivocal US findings.

Testicular torsion

Testicular torsion has a bimodal frequency of occurrence with extra-vaginal torsion occurring in the neonatal age group and intra-vaginal torsion occurring in an older age group. In intra-vaginal testicular torsion, patients have an abnormally high attachment of the tunica vaginalis, allowing the testis to rotate freely on the spermatic cord. This is known as the bell-clapper deformity. The twisting of the testis causes venous occlusion and engorgement, with arterial ischemia resulting in testicular infarction. In extra-vaginal testicular torsion, the testis is mobile because it has not yet descended into the scrotum, where it attaches to the tunica vaginalis. This predisposes to testicular torsion.

Testicular pain, swelling and tenderness are the chief complaints in testicular torsion. Systemic symptoms such as nausea and vomiting may be present. Scrotal skin redness is also usually seen.

A patient presenting with clinical features suspicious for testicular torsion should undergo surgery without delay. In patients with equivocal signs and symptoms, ultrasound is useful in establishing the diagnosis. In early testicular torsion, the affected testis may be slightly enlarged, with normal or decreased echogenicity. In cases presenting after 24 hours, the testis becomes heterogeneous in echotexture, the epididymal head may be enlarged and hydroceles are frequently seen (Figure 5.46). Unilateral decreased or absent

(A)

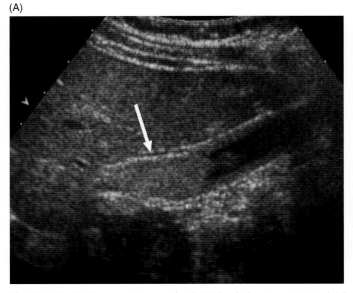

(B)

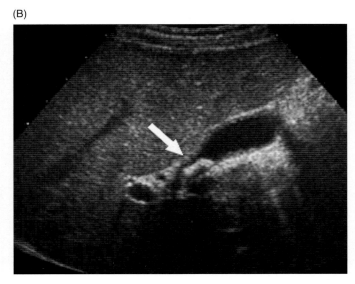

Figure 5.45 (A) Ultrasound image of gallbladder sludge in a patient who had fasted overnight. (B) Fourteen-year-old girl with thalassemia major. US shows the presence of an echogenic gallstone.

Table 5.9 Causes of acute scrotal pain

Testicular torsion

Torsion of a testicular appendage

Epididymo-orchitis

Incarcerated hernia

Trauma

Tumor

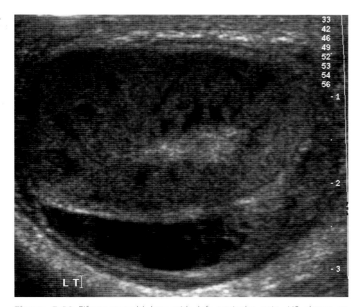

Figure 5.46 Fifteen-year-old boy with left testicular pain. US shows an enlarged left testis with heterogeneous echoes and a small hydrocele. Color Doppler imaging (not shown) shows no flow within the left testis. Testicular torsion was found at surgery.

flow is an accurate sign of testicular torsion, but the presence of blood flow does not exclude torsion because torsions may be intermittent or incomplete. Twisting of the spermatic cord may also be seen with color Doppler imaging. Doppler flow may be difficult to demonstrate in young children with a normal testis.

Torsion of the testicular appendage

The two most frequent testicular appendages giving rise to torsion are the appendix testis, a remnant of the paramesonephric (müllerian) duct, and the appendix epididymis, a remnant of the mesonephric (wolffian) duct. These appendages are pedunculated and may undergo torsion. This condition is considered benign but often presents clinically with acute scrotal pain, indistinguishable from testicular torsion. It is often difficult to distinguish the causes of acute scrotal pain on clinical grounds, but occasionally torsion of the testicular appendage can be diagnosed when a small, hard nodule is palpated over the upper pole of the testis and a "blue" spot is observed through the scrotal skin. Classically, systemic symptoms are not present in cases of testicular appendage torsion.

Ultrasound of torsion of the testicular appendage shows a hyperechoic nodule adjacent to the testis or epididymis with blood flow within the testis preserved (Figure 5.47).

Epididymo-orchitis

Epididymo-orchitis is inflammation of the epididymis and testis. It is frequently caused by mumps and coxsackie viruses, *Escherichia coli*, *Neisseria gonorrhoeae*, *Chlamydia trachomatis* and other coliforms. It is often associated with urinary tract infection.

The ultrasound features of epididymitis are a swollen epididymis with increased blood flow. The epididymis may be of varying echogenicity. When the infection spreads to the testis it

(A)   (B)

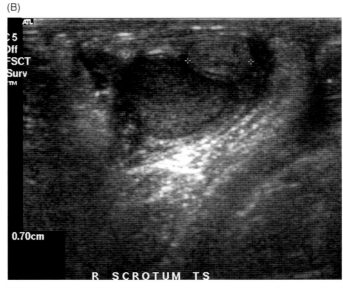

Figure 5.47 Ten-year-old boy with right testicular pain. US of the right testis in the (A) longitudinal and (B) transverse sections shows the presence of a well-defined echogenic nodular structure adjacent to the testis. Color Doppler imaging of the testis (not shown) shows normal vascularity. No vascularity could be demonstrated within the nodule. This finding is consistent with a torsed testicular appendage, which was confirmed at surgery.

(A)

(B)

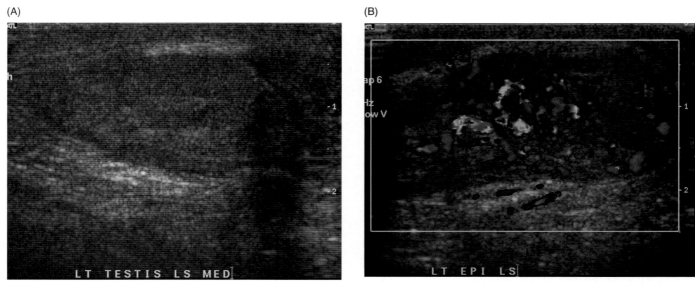

Figure 5.48 Four-year-old boy with left testicular pain, swelling and redness over the scrotum. (A) Testicular US shows marked heterogeneity in the testis with a swollen epididymis. (B) Color Doppler US shows marked increased vascularity in the testis. These findings are consistent with a diagnosis of epididymo-orchitis.

appears diffusely or focally enlarged and may return varying echo-texture. Color Doppler signals are also increased (Figure 5.48).

Renal calculi

Renal calculi are responsible for 1 in 1000 to 1 in 7600 pediatric hospital admissions annually in the United States. Renal calculi are 50 times more common in adults than in children. Most affected children have an identifiable predisposition to stone formation, including metabolic risk factors, structural urinary tract abnormalities and urinary tract infection. Boys are more frequently affected than girls with a male-to-female ratio of 1.4 : 1 to 2.1 : 1.

The clinical presentation in adolescents is similar to that of adults with loin to groin pain. Younger children present more commonly with hematuria and urinary infection.

Plain radiographs may detect large radiopaque renal calculi (Figure 5.49). Ultrasound is more sensitive and is also able to detect non-radiopaque calculi in addition to providing more detailed information, such as accompanying hydronephrosis or underlying structural defects (Figure 5.50). An intravenous urogram (IVU) is now rarely used in the evaluation of stone disease. In cases where US findings are inconclusive, a nonenhanced helical CT scan has a high sensitivity and specificity (96–98%), but is associated with radiation exposure. CT may detect small stones not detectable on US and has a greater potential to identify alternative diagnoses if a stone is not present (Figure 5.51).

Ovarian cysts and torsion of ovary

Ovarian cysts can occur at any age in childhood, but are commonest after puberty. In the younger child they rarely measure more than 1 cm in diameter and they usually wax and wane over time. Occasionally, a neonate may present with a very large simple ovarian cyst, probably related to maternal hormones.

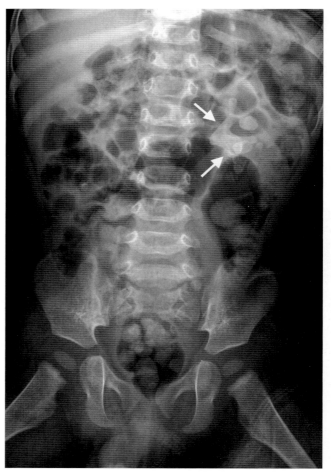

Figure 5.49 Two-year-old boy with left-sided loin pain. Abdominal radiograph shows the presence of a left staghorn calculus (arrows). The cause of the calculus is unknown.

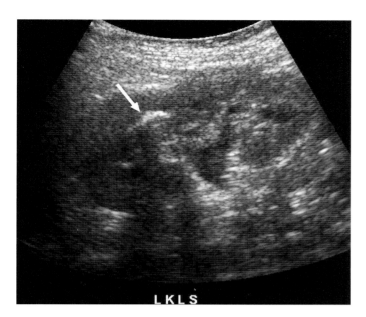

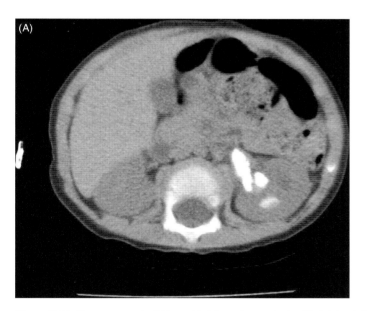

Figure 5.50 Same patient as Figure 5.49. The US after ESWL (extracorporeal shock-wave lithotripsy) shows only a remnant small calculus in the upper pole of the kidney. Minimal calyceal dilatation in the lower pole is evident.

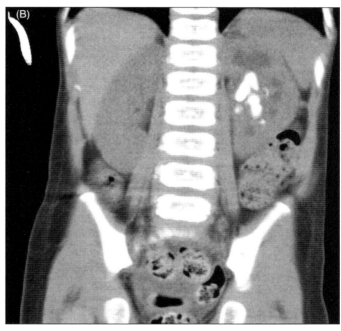

Figure 5.51 Nineteen-month-old boy with left staghorn calculus. (A) Axial and (B) coronal reconstruction CT images show the calculus in the left kidney.

These can fill a large portion of the abdomen. The diagnosis is made by ultrasound. Small cysts require no treatment. Very large cysts require decompression as they are at risk of torsion. The decompression of large cysts is an easy percutaneous procedure under ultrasound control. The differential diagnosis of cysts in the abdomen and pelvis are listed in Table 5.10.

After puberty more follicular cysts are seen and these also wax and wane, according to the menstrual cycle. These follicular cysts become larger in the first half of the menstrual cycle until one dominant follicle becomes even larger, up to 3 cm in size. This Graafian follicle ruptures during ovulation, at which point the other follicles involute. This Graafian follicle matures into the corpus luteum. This is a normal cycle and requires no treatment. Physiological cysts are usually asymptomatic. However some cysts, especially if large, may undergo torsion, which often also involves other adnexal structures. The torsion compromises vascular and lymphatic drainage and can lead to infarction. This is uncommon in childhood and occurs more commonly in the older child.

Although torsion may occur in normal ovaries, it is more likely to occur in abnormally enlarged ovaries with ovarian cysts and teratomas.

When ovaries undergo torsion, presenting symptoms include sudden onset of lower abdominal or pelvic pain. Occasionally systemic symptoms of nausea and vomiting may be present.

Table 5.10 Differential diagnosis of cysts in the abdomen and pelvis

Ovarian cysts

Duplication cysts

Choledochal cysts

Mesenteric cysts

Cystic hygroma

Table 5.11 Differential diagnosis of torsion of the ovary

Acute appendicitis

Gastroenteritis

Renal colic

Pelvic inflammatory disease

Ectopic pregnancy

Physical examination may reveal a pelvic mass. Table 5.11 lists the differential diagnoses of ovarian torsion in children.

On ultrasound, physiological cysts are seen as clear, anechoic, thin-walled cysts usually less than 1 cm in size. The most suggestive grayscale appearance of ovarian torsion on ultrasound is a unilaterally enlarged ovary with multiple peripheral follicles measuring 8–12 mm. Solid cysts with low-level echoes and complex lesions with septations or debris may also be seen. Occasionally, an underlying ovarian lesion such as a teratoma may cause the ovary to undergo torsion (Figure 5.52). Color and spectral Doppler imaging findings are also variable, but venous flow tracings are particularly important because, in early or milder degrees of torsion, venous flow is compromised before arterial flow decreases. The presence of arterial and venous flow does not exclude torsion, however. Laparoscopy should still be performed in any patient in whom there is high clinical suspicion for ovarian torsion.

CT or MRI may occasionally diagnose ovarian torsion. Findings include a twisted vascular pedicle, fallopian tube thickening, smooth wall thickening of an ovarian cystic mass, ascites, and deviation of the uterus to the affected side. Blood products can be identified within the tube, adnexal mass, and peritoneum. Post-contrast MRI can be helpful in identifying nonvascularized ovaries suggestive of infarction.

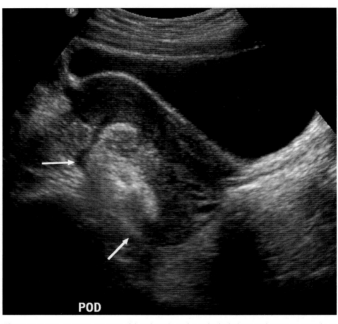

Figure 5.52 Fourteen-year-old girl with right-sided abdominal pain. Sagittal US image shows the presence of an echogenic lesion situated in the pouch of Douglas (arrows) with no vascularity demonstrated. A normal left ovary was visualized but a normal right ovary could not be seen. A diagnosis of right ovarian torsion with an underlying teratoma was made, which was confirmed at surgery.

Hydronephrosis

A hydronephrosis is defined as an abnormal uni- or bilateral dilatation of the renal collecting system. Hydronephrosis is often asymptomatic, but may rarely present with pain and gross hematuria. Potential differential diagnoses are listed in Table 5.12. Many cases are diagnosed during prenatal US. All cases should be assessed with a postnatal US performed, ideally, one week after birth. However, it is acceptable to perform this earlier if urgent management is necessary, such as in cases of high-grade obstruction or posterior urethral valves (PUVs). An imaging workflow for the investigation of hydronephrosis is shown in Flowchart 1.

A voiding cystourethrography (VCUG) should be performed to assess for vesicoureteric reflux (VUR), and for PUV in boys, should hydronephrosis still be detected on postnatal US. If VUR is present, a dimercaptosuccinic acid (DMSA) scan may be performed to assess for renal scarring and renal function compromise, particularly if the VUR is severe. If VUR is absent, a Lasix (furosemide) mercaptylacetyltriglycine (MAG3) scan may be performed to assess the split renal function and severity of obstruction (Flowchart 1). This should be done when the child is at least one month old, when the kidneys are more mature. This imaging protocol is generally accepted, but some individual and local adaptations may be necessary. For example, the VCUG may not be required so urgently if a ureteropelvic junction obstruction (UPJO) seems to be the likely cause of hydronephrosis on the initial US scan.

Vesicoureteric reflux

Vesicoureteric reflux (VUR) is defined as retrograde flow of urine from the urinary bladder into the ureter. Primarily this is caused by incompetence of the ureterovesical junction. Secondary causes include neuropathic bladder and posterior urethral valves (PUVs). VUR is thought to be a benign condition without urinary tract infection (UTI), but in the presence of UTI it may cause renal scarring. The International Classification of VUR is listed in Table 5.12 and is graded based on VCUG findings (Figure 5.53). Recently, VUR has been assessed using US with US contrast media in some institutions. Follow-up may be

Table 5.12 Hydronephrosis

Primary VUR	VUR on VCUG is detected and graded as follows: Grade I reflux: reflux into the ureter Grade II reflux: reflux into a non-dilated pelvicalyceal system Grade III reflux: reflux into a mildly dilated pelvicalyceal system with mild ureteric tortuosity Grade IV reflux: reflux into a moderately dilated pelvicalyceal system with moderate ureteric tortuosity Grade V reflux: reflux into a severely dilated pelvicalyceal system with marked ureteric tortuosity

Secondary VUR
  1. Neuropathic bladder
  2. Posterior urethral valves
	In addition to the above findings:
	  Cone-shaped bladder with trabeculation of the bladder wall
	  Dilatation of the posterior (prostatic) urethra with bladder wall trabeculation

Primary ureteric obstruction
  1. Ureteropelvic junction obstruction
 	
  2. Ureterovesical junction obstruction
	US shows pelvicalyceal dilatation of the kidney, renal cortical thinning in severe cases and no dilatation of the ureter. ^{99m}Tc MAG3 scan shows prolonged $t_{1/2}$ and a drainage curve which shows persistent uptrend. In severe cases, renal function is compromised
	US shows megaureter (ureteric dilatation >1 cm). VCUG is performed to determine the presence of VUR. ^{99m}Tc MAG3, IVP, CT or MR show obstruction at the ureterovesical junction

Secondary ureteric obstruction
  1. Intrinsic (stone)
 	
  2. Extrinsic (tumor)
	Calculus – usually visible on plain radiographs. US is useful for detecting non-radiopaque renal calculi, and CT is sensitive for ureteric calculi
	IVU or CT shows an irregular ureteric stricture

Ureterocele	US shows a dilated distal ureter, protruding into the bladder, and often associated with a hydroureter. Simple ureterocele = orthotopic insertion. Ectopic ureterocele = ectopic insertion into the bladder and almost always associated with a duplicated collecting system. VCUG may demonstrate the ureterocele as a filling defect
Ectopic ureter	The orifice of an ectopic ureter may insert ectopically into the bladder, the urethra or the vagina. US may show an obstructed, dilated upper pole ureter of a duplicated collecting system. IVU or MRU is often needed to show the site of ectopic insertion

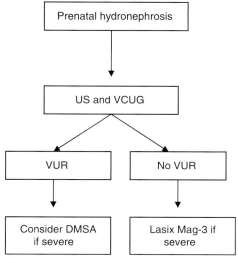

Flowchart 1 Imaging algorithm for prenatal hydronephrosis.

performed using radionuclide VCUG in children with documented reflux. The advantage of radionuclide VCUG is that it provides much lower radiation doses compared to a standard VCUG, which allows for a prolonged examination, thus increasing its sensitivity. Disadvantages of the radionuclide study include difficulty in the grading of the reflux and in not providing the anatomical detail that is provided by a contrast VCUG.

Posterior urethral valves

Posterior urethral valves (PUVs) are congenital mucosal folds in the posterior urethra resulting in different grades of bladder outlet obstruction and proximal urinary tract dilatation. US findings suggestive of PUVs include an enlarged, trabeculated, thick-walled bladder with posterior urethral dilation and unilateral or bilateral hydronephrosis. These findings are confirmed by a VCUG showing severe VUR in addition to the above findings (Figure 5.54). PUVs are treated with surgical ablation and follow-up imaging is necessary to confirm relief of the obstruction, bladder emptying and upper tract dilatation.

Ureteropelvic junction obstruction

Ureteropelvic junction obstruction (UPJO) is most commonly caused by an adynamic ureteral segment at the junction between the ureter and the renal pelvis. Extrinsic compression

(A)

(B)

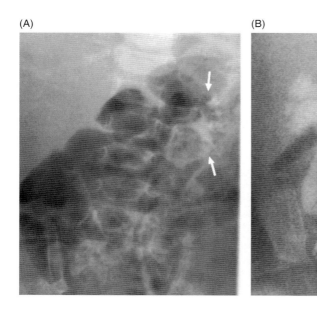

Figure 5.53 VUR is graded on the VCUG findings. (A) Grade II VUR. VCUG shows reflux of contrast into the left pelvicalyceal system. The calyces of the kidney are sharp and not blunted, consistent with grade II VUR (arrow). (B) Grade III and VI VUR. VCUG shows bilateral VUR with blunting of the calyces of the left kidney consistent with grade III VUR. The right VUR shows a greater degree of blunting of the calyces and tortuosity of the ureter consistent with grade V VUR.

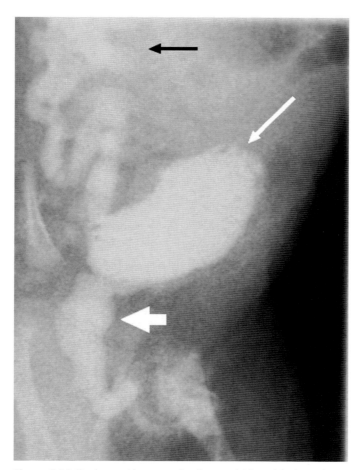

Figure 5.54 Newborn with antenatally diagnosed bilateral hydronephrosis. VCUG shows a dilated posterior urethra (large arrow) with a trabeculated bladder (small arrow) and right grade V VUR (black arrow). These findings are diagnostic of PUV.

of the proximal ureter by the presence of accessory lower pole renal vessels is very uncommon in children. Obstruction to urine outflow at this point may cause hydronephrosis. US shows the presence of hydronephrosis to varying degrees depending on the severity of the obstruction (Figure 5.55A). A dilated ureter distal to the UPJO is not visualized. The severity of obstruction in a ^{99m}Tc MAG3 scan is assessed by the $t_{1/2}$ (the time it takes for half of the radionuclide to leave the renal collecting system), the drainage curve and the split renal function. A $t_{1/2}$ of less than 10 minutes is normal, more than 20 minutes is abnormal and between 10 and 20 minutes is indeterminate. A drainage curve showing a persistent upward trend and a renal function of less than 40% of total renal function are abnormal findings (Figure 5.55B–D). Surgical correction is indicated in the presence of symptoms, declining renal function on renal scan, and increasing hydronephrosis on ultrasound.

Megaureter

Megaureter is defined as ureteral dilatation with a diameter of more than 1 cm. It may be classified as primary or secondary, and as refluxing, refluxing obstructive, or nonrefluxing nonobstructive megaureter. Imaging should include US, VCUG, and ^{99m}Tc MAG3 renal scan to confirm the diagnosis and to determine if obstruction is present (Figure 5.56).

Ureterocele

A ureterocele is a cystic dilatation of the distal ureter in the bladder wall. Most cases are associated with ureteral duplication causing obstruction of the upper pole moiety in a duplicated collecting system. US often shows the ureterocele as an anechoic cystic lesion in the bladder wall, usually associated with a hydroureter and hydronephrosis of the upper moiety of a duplicated system (Figure 5.57). The renal parenchyma

(A)

(B)

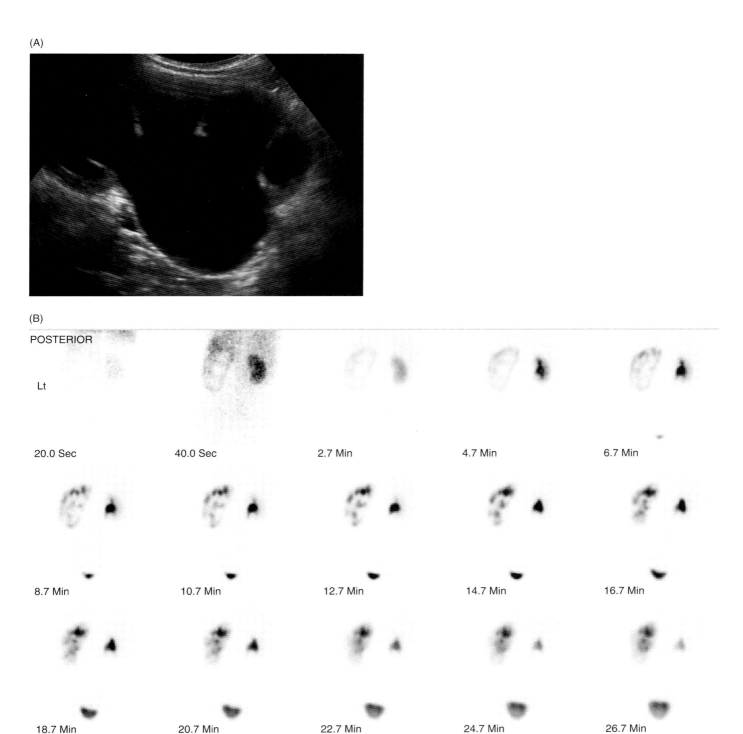

Figure 5.55 Seven-year-old boy with incidentally detected hydronephrosis. (A) Longitudinal US image of the left kidney shows hydronephrosis involving the kidney, with no evidence of ureteric dilatation, suggestive of UPJO. (B) Serial images from a ^{99m}Tc MAG3 examination obtained over a period of 26.7 minutes show normal uptake, excretion and clearance of the tracer from the right kidney. Over the same period of time, there is gradual accumulation of tracer in the initially photopenic central areas of the left kidney corresponding to the dilated pelvicalyceal system. There is no clearance of tracer from the left pelvicalyceal system, indicating that obstruction is present. (C) The drainage curve of the right kidney is normal as shown by the downward gradient over 29 minutes. The drainage curve of the left kidney is consistent with complete obstruction as shown by the persistent upward gradient and plateau with no downward gradient over 29 minutes. (D) An additional image obtained 90 minutes after initial injection of the tracer still shows accumulation of tracer in the hydronephrotic left kidney.

(C)

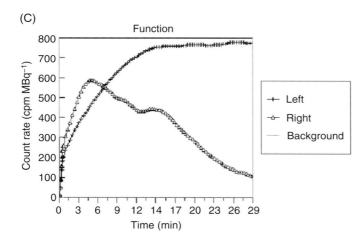

(D)

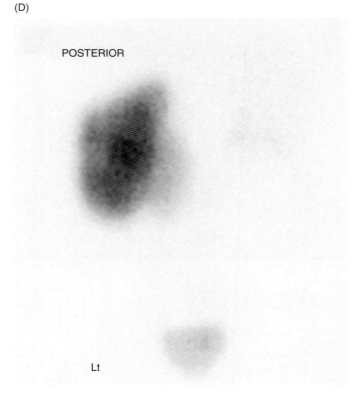

Figure 5.55 (Cont.)

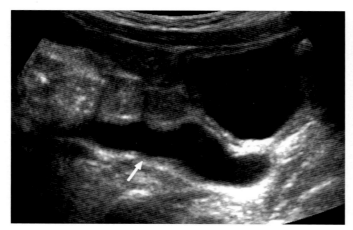

Figure 5.56 One-year-old boy with nonobstructive, nonrefluxing megaureter. Sagittal US image shows dilatation of the distal portion of the right ureter (arrow). No reflux was detected on VCUG and no obstruction was demonstrated on ^{99m}Tc MAG3 scan.

overlying the dilated collecting system is often very thin with poor function. Occasionally, large ureteroceles may cause bladder outlet obstruction.

Ectopic ureter

Ectopic ureters are often associated with the upper pole moiety in a duplicated kidney. The Weigert-Meyer rule applies to completely duplicated systems where the ureter associated with the upper moiety inserts distal and medial to the ureter associated with the lower moiety. The ectopic upper pole

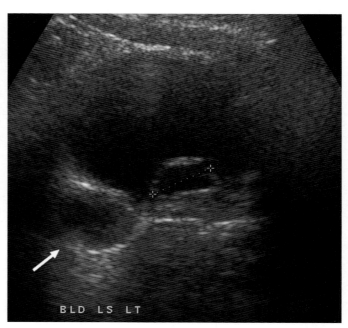

Figure 5.57 Two-year-old boy with a duplex left kidney. US image shows the presence of a ureterocele (measured between the cursors) in the bladder associated with a left hydroureter (arrow) from the upper moiety of the kidney.

ureter may be obstructed and associated with a ureterocele. The lower pole ureter inserts orthotopically, but may be prone to VUR. In girls, the ectopic ureter may insert in the bladder neck or vagina, leading to incontinence. In boys, the most common site of insertion is the posterior urethra. The dilated ureter and upper moiety pelvicalyceal dilatation can be visualized on ultrasound. The site of the distal ectopic insertion can be visualized on IVU, or more recently MR urogram (MRU) has been used (Figure 5.58). ^{99m}Tc MAG3 has been used to indicate the degree of obstruction. Surgery is the definitive treatment for ectopic ureters.

Musculoskeletal

Radiological approach to the child with an acute limp

The imaging evaluation of a child with an acute limp should be guided by the clinical findings. Knee or pelvic pain may

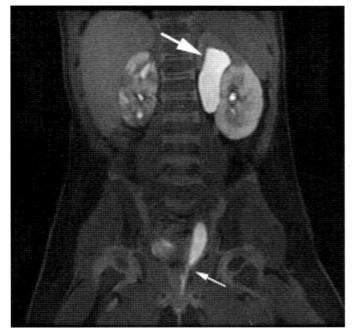

Figure 5.58 Three-year-old girl with urinary incontinence. Dynamic coronal MRU image post-contrast shows the left kidney to be a duplex kidney with a dilatation of the collecting system of the upper moiety (large arrow). The ureter associated with the upper moiety inserts in the vagina (small arrow).

mimic hip pain, and these areas should be excluded. Plain radiographs are usually the first investigation performed. Ultrasound is useful in imaging joint effusions and guiding interventional drainage procedures. Cross-sectional modalities such as CT or MR may be performed to image areas not easily accessed by plain radiographs, such as the sacroiliac joint, acetabulum and the spine.

Transient synovitis

Transient synovitis is the commonest cause of hip pain in children aged between 3 and 10 years of age and is due to nonspecific inflammation and hypertrophy of the synovium. It may affect other joints as well. The main diagnostic issue with transient synovitis is distinguishing this entity from septic arthritis.

Patients will present with subacute pain of the affected joint. Systemic signs are mild or nonexistent. Distinguishing from septic arthritis may be possible based on fever (an oral temperature >38.5 °C), refusal to bear weight, an elevated C-reactive protein level, erythrocyte sedimentation rate and serum white blood-cell count. Patients make a full recovery.

Plain radiography is usually normal although joint effusion may occasionally be present. Ultrasound is useful in detecting an effusion and guiding aspiration procedures if necessary. Distinguishing septic from transient synovitis is not possible based on ultrasound findings alone (Figure 5.59). MR findings of transient synovitis include joint effusion, synovial enhancement, contralateral joint effusion, synovial thickening, and signal intensity alterations and enhancement in surrounding soft tissue. Contralateral (asymptomatic) joint effusions are more commonly seen in transient synovitis compared to septic arthritis, while signal intensity alterations in bone marrow and contrast enhancement of the soft tissues are more commonly seen in septic arthritis. Ipsilateral effusion and synovial thickening and enhancement are present in both diseases. Decreased perfusion of the femoral epiphysis on fat-suppressed gadolinium-enhanced coronal T1-weighted MRI has also been reported as being useful for differentiating septic arthritis from transient synovitis.

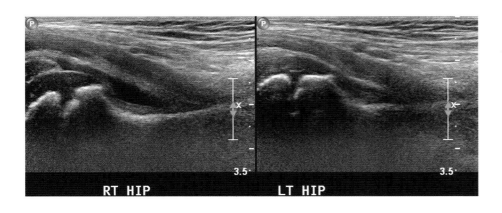

Figure 5.59 Three-year-old boy with left hip pain. Longitudinal images of the right and left hips show the presence of a right hip effusion. The patient was well clinically with no signs of sepsis. A diagnosis of transient synovitis was made and the patient made a full recovery.

Legg-Calvé-Perthes disease

Legg-Calvé-Perthes disease (LCP) is a condition where there is idiopathic avascular necrosis of the femoral head. Boys are more commonly affected than girls and the peak age of occurrence is between four to eight years. Bilateral disease can occur but is usually asymmetrical. Hip pain and limping is the main presenting symptom, but referred pain to the knee may also be encountered.

Plain radiographs may be normal for three to six months after the onset of symptoms. In the initial stage, the epiphysis appears smaller than its opposite counterpart on plain radiographs (Figure 5.60). Lateral subluxation of the femoral head and a subcortical fracture may be present. Sclerosis, impaction and fragmentation of the epiphysis then occur. This stage of the disease occurs over a period of 18 months. Focal metaphyseal lucencies, which are small masses of cartilage, may persist for several years. In the regenerative phase, there is further widening of the femoral neck, re-ossification and incomplete containment of the femoral head by the acetabulum.

MRI is useful in detecting early cases when the radiograph is normal. In such cases, MR shows low signal intensity on T1-weighted images and high signal intensity on T2-weighted images with lack of gadolinium enhancement. MRI can also determine and assess the extent of physeal and marrow involvement, the preoperative femoral head coverage and articular integrity.

Radionuclide bone scans may be useful in diagnosis by detecting lack of tracer uptake in the femoral epiphysis, but MRI is more sensitive and provides better anatomical depiction.

Most patients do well without treatment. There is evidence that the prognosis is related to the degree of involvement of the femoral head. The prognosis is poorer in patients with more than half the femoral head involved compared to those with less than half the head involved.

Slipped capital femoral epiphysis

Slipped capital femoral epiphysis (SCFE) is a condition where there is posterior and medial displacement of the femoral head relative to the femoral neck. It occurs more commonly in males than females. In males it usually occurs between the ages of 13 and 16 years, and in females it occurs between the ages of 11 and 14 years. Affected patients are usually overweight. Mechanical forces are thought to cause shear stresses on the physis, resulting in displacement of the femoral head. SCFE is bilateral and asymmetric in 20–32% of cases. Complications of SCFE include chondrolysis and avascular necrosis, which may result in premature fusion of the epiphyseal plate, femoral neck shortening and degenerative arthritis.

The commonest presenting complaint is pain in the groin, hip or knee, and limping. Avascular necrosis is the most serious complication of slipped capital femoral epiphysis, and patients with avascular necrosis exhibit a more rapid arthritic deterioration of the hip. Chondrolysis occurs in 5–7% of all children, and the incidence increases as the severity of the slipped capital femoral epiphysis increases. Patients present

(A)

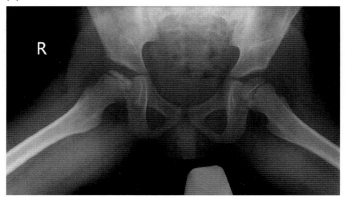

(B)

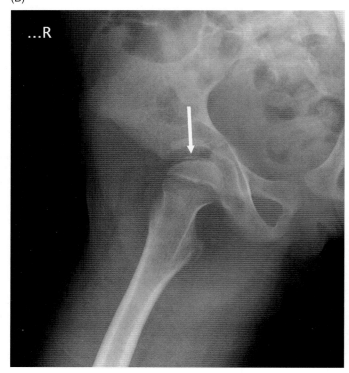

(C)

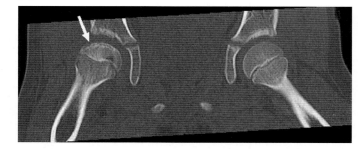

Figure 5.60 Six-year-old boy with right hip pain. (A) Frog-leg lateral view shows a flattened, sclerotic right femoral head with early fragmentation consistent with avascular necrosis. Seven-year-old girl with right hip pain. (B) Frog-leg lateral view cropped to show only the right hip illustrates a subcortical fracture of the femoral head. (C) CT was performed to assess the congruency of the acetabulum and confirms the presence of the subcortical fracture. The acetabulum is normal.

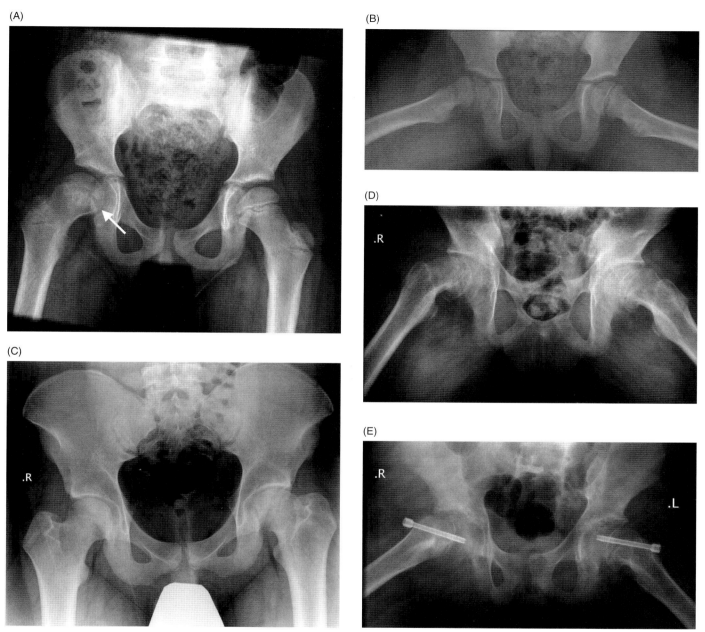

Figure 5.61 Six-year-old boy with right hip pain. (A) Anteroposterior radiograph of the pelvis shows widening of the right epiphyseal plate (arrow) with sclerosis of the femoral neck consistent with SCFE. The diagnosis is confirmed on (B) the frog-leg lateral view which shows posteromedial displacement of the femoral head relative to the femoral neck. (C) Fourteen-year-old boy with chronic SCFE of the left hip. Anteroposterior radiograph of the pelvis shows SCFE involving the left hip. The epiphyseal plate has fused and the SCFE is now stable. Anteroposterior radiograph performed three years prior (not shown) shows no change in the degree of the slippage. (D) Twelve-year-old boy with bilateral hip pain. Frog-leg lateral radiograph shows bilateral SCFE with the right side more severely affected than the left. (E) Postoperative radiograph shows the presence of screws transfixing the SCFE bilaterally.

with pain and loss of hip motion out of proportion to the severity of the slipped epiphysis.

Radiographically, the earliest sign may be mild widening and blurring of the epiphysis on the ap view (Figure 5.61). On the normal radiograph, one-sixth of the epiphysis usually lies laterally to a line drawn tangentially to the lateral margin of the neck of the femur. This line is known as Klein's line. In SCFE, there may be no intersection between this line and the femoral

head. There is also an apparent reduction in the epiphyseal height. The frog-lateral view is important because the displacement of the femoral head is perpendicular to the X-ray beam, making posterior displacement easier to detect. However, the view may be difficult to obtain because of pain. A loss of articular cartilage width can be seen on radiographs in children with chondrolysis. On MRI, synovitis, periphyseal edema and joint effusion are regular features of SCFE.

Further reading

Croup

Everard ML (2009) Acute bronchiolitis and croup. *Pediatr Clin North Am* **56**(1), 119–33, x–xi.

Stroud RH, Friedman NR (2001) An update on inflammatory disorders of the pediatric airway: epiglottitis, croup, and tracheitis. *Am J Otolaryngol* **22**, 268–75.

Swischuk LE Nasal passages, mandible and upper airway. In *Imaging of the Newborn, Infant and Young Child*, 4th edn., ed. LE Swischuk (Philadelphia: Williams and Wilkins, 1997) pp. 159–98.

Swischuk LE, Smith PC, Fagan CJ (1974) Abnormalities of the pharynx and larynx in childhood. *Semin Roentgenol* **9**, 283–300.

Acute epiglottitis

Sobol SE, Zapata S (2008) Epiglottitis and croup. *Otolaryngol Clin North Am* **41**(3), 551–66, ix.

Foreign bodies

Yadav SP, Singh J, Aggarwal N, Goel A (2007) Airway foreign bodies in children: experience of 132 cases. *Singapore Med J* **48**(9), 850–3.

Zerella JT, Dimler M, McGill LC, Pippus KJ (1998) Foreign body aspiration in children: value of radiography and complications of bronchoscopy. *J Pediatr Surg* **33**, 1651–4.

Airleaks

O'Lone E, Elphick HE, Robinson PJ (2008) Spontaneous pneumothorax in children: when is invasive treatment indicated? *Pediatr Pulmonol* **43**(1), 41–6.

Swischuk LE (1988) Two lesser known but useful signs of neonatal pneumothorax. *AJR Am J Roentgenol* **151**, 135–7.

The wheezing child

McNichol KN, Williams HB (1973) Spectrum of asthma in children. I. Clinical and physiological components. *Br Med J* **4**, 7.

Tal A, Bavilski C, Yohai D *et al.* (1983) Dexamethasone and salbutamol in the treatment of acute wheezing in infants. *Pediatrics* **71**, 13.

Yawn BP, Wollan P, Kurland M, Scanlon P (2002) A longitudinal study of the prevalence of asthma in a community population of school-age children. *J Pediatr* **140**(5), 576–81.

Gastrointestinal

Janik JS, Ein SH, Filler RM *et al.* (1981) An assessment of the surgical treatment of adhesive small bowel obstruction in infants and children. *J Pediatr Surg* **16**, 225–9.

Hypertrophic pyloric stenosis

Blickman JG *Pediatric Radiology* (St. Louis: Mosby, 1994) pp. 57–110.

Hutson JM, Beastley SW, Woodward AA (eds.) *Jones' Clinical Paediatric Surgery*, 4th edn. (Melbourne: Blackwell Scientific Publication, 1992) pp. 121–32.

John SD, Swischuck LE Pediatric gastrointestinal tract. In *Diagnostic Ultrasound*, 2nd edn., ed. CM Rumack, CM Wilson, JW Charboneau (St. Louis: Mosby, 1998) pp. 1717–47.

Laney DW, Balistreri WF The gastrointestinal tract and liver. In *Rudolph's Fundamentals of Pediatrics*, ed. AM Rudolph, RK Kamei (Stamford: Appleton and Lange, 1998) pp. 395–417.

Stringer DA, Babyn P *Pediatric Gastrointestinal Imaging and Intervention* (Toronto: BC Decker, 2000) pp. 275–81.

Volvulus of the stomach

Blickman JG *Pediatric Radiology* (St. Louis: Mosby, 1994) pp. 57–110.

Darani A, Mendoza-Sagaon M, Reinberg O (2005) Gastric volvulus in children. *J Pediatr Surg* **40**(5), 855–8.

Stringer DA, Babyn P *Pediatric Gastrointestinal Imaging and Intervention* (Toronto: BC Decker, 2000) pp. 298–9.

Malrotation

Dufour D, Delaet MH, Dassonville M, Cadranel S, Perlmutter N (1992) Midgut malrotation, the reliability of sonographic diagnosis. *Pediatr Radiol* **22**(1), 21–3.

McAlister WH, Kronemer KA (1996) Emergency gastrointestinal radiology of the newborn. *Radiol Clin North Am* **34**(4), 819–44.

Snyder WH, Chaffin L (1954) Embryology of the intestinal tract: presentation of 10 cases of malrotation. *Ann Surg* **140**, 368–80.

Stringer DA, Babyn P *Pediatric Gastrointestinal Imaging and Intervention* (Toronto: BC Decker, 2000) pp. 311–32.

Intussusception

Applegate KE (2008) Intussusception in children: imaging choices. *Semin Roentgenol* **43**(1), 15–21.

Del-Pozo G, Gonzalez-Spinola J, Gomez-Anson B *et al.* (1996) Intussusception: trapped peritoneal fluid detected with US—relationship to reducibility and ischemia. *Radiology* **201**, 379–83.

Hooker RL, Hernanz-Schulman M, Yu C, Kan JH (2008) Radiographic evaluation of intussusception: utility of left-side-down decubitus view. *Radiology* **248**(3), 987–94.

Peh WC, Khong PL, Chan KL *et al.* (1996) Sonographically guided hydrostatic reduction of childhood intussusception using Hartmann's solution. *AJR Am J Roentgenol* **167**(5), 1237–41.

Stringer DA, Babyn P *Pediatric Gastrointestinal Imaging and Intervention* (Toronto: BC Decker, 2000) pp. 421–34.

Strouse PJ, DiPietro MA, Saez F (2003) Transient small-bowel intussusception in children on CT. *Pediatr Radiol* **33**, 316–20.

Intestinal hernias

Erez I, Rathause V, Vacian I *et al.* (2002) Preoperative ultrasound and intraoperative findings of inguinal hernias in children: A prospective study of 642 children. *J Pediatr Surg* **37**(6), 865–8.

Graf JL, Caty MG, Martin DJ, Glick PL (2002) Pediatric hernias. *Semin Ultrasound CT MR* **23**(2), 197–200.

Martin LC, Merkle EM, Thompson WM (2006) Review of internal hernias: radiographic and clinical findings. *AJR Am J Roentgenol* **186**(3), 703–17.

GIT bleeding

Donnelly LF, Frush DP, O'Hara SM, Johnson ND, Bisset GS 3rd (1998) CT appearance of clinically occult abdominal hemorrhage in children. *AJR Am J Roentgenol* **170**(4), 1073–6.

Fox VL (2000) Gastrointestinal bleeding in infancy and childhood. *Gastroenterol Clin North Am* **29**(1), 37–66.

Leung AK, Wong AL (2002) Lower gastrointestinal bleeding in children. *Pediatr Emerg Care* **18**(4), 319–23.

Foreign-body ingestion

O'Hara SM (1997) Acute gastrointestinal bleeding. *Radiol Clin North Am* **35**(4), 879–95.

Stringer DA, Babyn P *Pediatric Gastrointestinal Imaging and Intervention* (Toronto: BC Decker, 2000) pp. 210–13.

Henoch-Schönlein purpura

Chang WL, Yang YH, Lin YT, Chiang BL (2004) Gastrointestinal manifestations in Henoch-Schönlein purpura: a review of 261 patients. *Acta Paediatr* **93**(11), 1427–31.

Connolly B, O'Halpin D (1994) Sonographic evaluation of the abdomen in Henoch-Schönlein purpura. *Clin Radiol* **49**(5), 320–3.

Stringer DA, Babyn P *Pediatric Gastrointestinal Imaging and Intervention* (Toronto: BC Decker, 2000) pp. 406–8.

Appendicitis

Puig S, Staudenherz A, Felder-Puig R, Paya K (2008) Imaging of appendicitis in children and adolescents: useful or useless? A comparison of imaging techniques and a critical review of the current literature. *Semin Roentgenol* **43**(1), 22–8.

Rosendahl K, Aukland SM, Fosse K (2004) Imaging strategies in children with suspected appendicitis. *Eur Radiol* **14**(Suppl. 4), L138–L145.

Stringer DA, Babyn P *Pediatric Gastrointestinal Imaging and Intervention* (Toronto: BC Decker, 2000) pp. 520–4.

Cholelithiasis

Stringer DA, Babyn P *Pediatric Gastrointestinal Imaging and Intervention* (Toronto: BC Decker, 2000) pp. 553–5.

Genitourinary imaging: testicular torsion

Gunther P, Schenk JP, Wunsch R *et al.* (2006) Acute testicular torsion in children: the role of sonography in the diagnostic workup. *Eur Radiol* **16**(11), 2527–32.

Leslie JA, Cain MP (2006) Pediatric urologic emergencies and urgencies. *Pediatr Clin North Am* **53**(3), 513–27.

Lin EP, Bhatt S, Rubens DJ, Dogra VS (2007) Testicular torsion: twists and turns. *Semin Ultrasound CT MR* **28**(4), 317–28.

Pearl MS, Hill MC (2007) Ultrasound of the scrotum. *Semin Ultrasound CT MR* **28**(4), 225–48.

Renal calculi

Nicoletta JA, Lande MB (2006) Medical evaluation and treatment of urolithiasis. *Pediatr Clin North Am* **53**(3), 479–91, vii.

Ovarian cysts and ovarian torsion

Kamaya A, Shin L, Chen B, Desser TS (2008) Emergency gynecologic imaging. *Semin Ultrasound CT MR* **29**(5), 353–68.

Rousseau V, Massicot R, Darwish AA *et al.* (2008) Emergency management and conservative surgery of ovarian torsion in children: a report of 40 cases. *J Pediatr Adolesc Gynecol* **21**(4), 201–6.

Hydronephrosis

Fefer S, Ellsworth P (2006) Prenatal hydronephrosis. *Pediatr Clin North Am* **53**(3), 429–47.

Riccabona M, Avni FE, Blickman JG *et al.* (2009) Imaging recommendations in paediatric uroradiology. Minutes of the ESPR uroradiology task force session on childhood obstructive uropathy, high-grade fetal hydronephrosis, childhood haematuria, and urolithiasis in childhood. ESPR Annual Congress, Edinburgh, UK, June 2008. *Pediatr Radiol* **39**(8), 891–8.

Musculoskeletal imaging: transient synovitis

Caird MS, Flynn JM, Leung YL *et al.* (2006) Factors distinguishing septic arthritis from transient synovitis of the hip in children. A prospective study. *J Bone Joint Surg Am* **88**(6), 1251–7.

Kwack KS, Cho JH, Lee JH *et al.* (2007) Septic arthritis versus transient synovitis of the hip: gadolinium-enhanced MRI finding of decreased perfusion at the femoral epiphysis. *AJR Am J Roentgenol* **189**(2), 437–45.

Uziel Y, Butbul-Aviel Y, Barash J *et al.* (2006) Recurrent transient synovitis of the hip in childhood. Longterm outcome among 39 patients. *J Rheumatol* **33**(4), 810–11.

Yang WJ, Im SA, Lim GY *et al.* (2006) MR imaging of transient synovitis: differentiation from septic arthritis. *Pediatr Radiol* **36**(11), 1154–8.

Zamzam MM (2006) The role of ultrasound in differentiating septic arthritis from transient synovitis of the hip in children. *J Pediatr Orthop B* **15**(6), 418–22.

Perthes disease

Sebag G, Ducou Le Pointe H, Klein I *et al.* (1997) Dynamic gadolinium enhanced subtraction MR imaging. A simple technique for the early diagnosis of Legg-Calvé-Perthes disease: Preliminary results. *Pediatr Radiol* **27**, 216–20.

Uno A, Hattori T, Noritake K, Suda H (1995) Legg-Calvé-Perthes disease in the evolutionary period: comparison of magnetic resonance imaging with bone scintigraphy. *J Pediatr Orthop* **15**(3), 362–7.

Wall EJ (1999) Legg-Calvé-Perthes' disease. *Curr Opin Pediatr* **11**(1), 76–9.

Slipped capital femoral epiphysis

Loder RT (1996) The demographics of slipped capital femoral epiphysis. An international multicenter study. *Clin Orthop Relat Res* **322**, 8–27.

Loder RT (1998) Slipped capital femoral epiphysis. *Am Fam Physician* **57**(9), 2135–42, 2148–50.

Tins B, Cassar-Pullicino V, McCall I (2009) The role of pre-treatment MRI in established cases of slipped capital femoral epiphysis. *Eur J Radiol* **70**(3), 570–8.

Chapter 6

Infections, inflammations and HIV

Kate M. Park and Catherine M. Owens

Congenital infections

The imaging features of congenital infections (sometimes called the STORCH or TORCH infections: Syphilis, Toxoplasmosis, Other, Rubella, Cytomegalovirus and Herpes simplex) differ from those seen in older children and adults as the insult occurs while the nervous system is still developing. The manifestations largely depend on the fetal age at the time of infection and the severity of the infection. Generally, infections within the first two trimesters lead to congenital malformations, and those in the third trimester lead to destructive lesions.

Viral infections are usually transmitted transplacentally but can be acquired from the birth canal at birth. Bacterial infections usually ascend from the cervix.

Syphilis

Treponema pallidum infection is acquired transplacentally, usually in the second or third trimester. Most neonates are asymptomatic in the first few weeks of life and, of these asymptomatic neonates, 20% will have metaphyseal abnormalities on plain film.

Neurological symptoms may develop within the first two years of life. The main neuropathological finding is an inflammatory infiltration of the leptomeninges, which is seen as enhancement of the affected leptomeninges on imaging studies. The infiltrate may extend into the cerebral parenchyma and appear as an enhancing parenchymal mass or cause arterial narrowing which can lead to cerebral infarction.

Toxoplasmosis

Toxoplasma gondii is a protozoan usually acquired by pregnant women through ingestion of oocytes in undercooked meat. One in 1000–3500 live births are affected. The majority of neonates are asymptomatic at birth, and the infection may be generalized or purely nervous system related. The prognosis without treatment is poor. Neuropathologically, there is diffuse inflammatory infiltration of the meninges and hydrocephalus is common.

Severe infections in the second trimester can lead to hydranencephaly or porencephaly, but cortical malformations such as polymicrogyria are uncommon, unlike in cytomegalovirus infection.

The imaging features vary widely, with more severe abnormalities seen in cases of earlier insult. Cross-sectional imaging commonly demonstrates calcification, usually affecting the basal ganglia, periventricular regions and cerebral cortex, microcephaly, large ventricles and hydrocephalus. The calcification may resorb with appropriate treatment.

Other: varicella-zoster virus, lymphocytic choriomeningitis virus, human immunodeficiency virus

Varicella-zoster virus (VZV)

VZV is rare in pregnancy, and in the majority of cases no significant harm comes to the fetus. Infection prior to 20 weeks gestation may lead to spontaneous abortion. Reported MRI features include hydrocephalus and cerebellar aplasia or destruction of the temporal and occipital lobes with ventricular dilatation and normal cerebellum, basal ganglia and parietal lobes.

Lymphocytic choriomeningitis virus (LCM)

LCM is an arenavirus found throughout temperate regions of Europe and North America. Infection is either through contact with affected rodents or via infected pets. The incidence is unknown and probably underrecognized. Infection in the first trimester leads to spontaneous abortion. Infection in the second and third trimesters leads to a clinical and imaging picture resembling those in toxoplasmosis and CMV.

Human immunodeficiency virus (HIV)

In untreated HIV-positive mothers, the perinatal infection rate is 30%, compared with 2% when treated with maternal antiretrovirals and cesarean section with avoidance of breastfeeding. CNS disease is seen in 20–60% of infected children. Neurological

Essentials of Pediatric Radiology, ed. Heike E. Daldrup-Link and Charles A. Gooding. Published by Cambridge University Press.
© Cambridge University Press 2010.

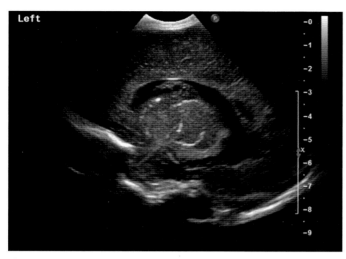

Figure 6.1 Sagittal ultrasound in a neonate shows lenticulostriate vasculopathy, a nonspecific finding seen in a number of conditions including the TORCH infections.

symptoms are rare in the neonatal period, with onset generally seen between two months and five years of age, and are discussed further in the section on HIV below.

Rubella

Congenital rubella infection is rare in western countries because of screening and vaccination programs. Infection in the third trimester has little effect on the fetus. Ocular, cardiac and neurological defects are seen in fetuses infected in the first two months of gestation, and neurological symptoms usually develop by four months of age.

Ultrasound may demonstrate the fairly nonspecific finding of branching curvilinear hyperechogenicity in the basal ganglia and the walls of the lateral ventricles, "lenticulostriate vasculopathy" (Figure 6.1). Neuroimaging findings include ventriculomegaly and multifocal regions of abnormal signal throughout the white matter, often with associated periventricular calcification and cysts, and basal ganglia calcification (Figure 6.2). Cortical calcification can also occur. In addition, MRI may demonstrate delayed myelination.

High resolution CT of the temporal bones may show malformation of the inner ear structures, associated with congenital deafness.

Cytomegalovirus (CMV)

Cytomegalovirus is the most common serious viral infection among newborns in the USA, affecting approximately 1% of all births, and over half will be classified as having severe permanent neurological sequelae.

As in other TORCH infections, ultrasound may demonstrate lenticulostriate vasculopathy.

In early infection (first half of the second trimester), CT and MRI features include lissencephaly with thinning of the

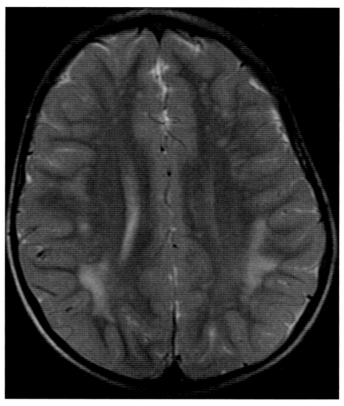

Figure 6.2 Axial T2-weighted MR in a four-year-old shows multiple areas of abnormal high signal in the deep and subcortical white matter of both cerebral hemispheres, consistent with congenital rubella infection.

cortex, hypoplastic cerebellum, delayed myelination, ventriculomegaly and periventricular calcification.

Infection in the middle of the second trimester leads to the more typical appearance of polymicrogyria, with less ventricular dilatation and less consistent cerebellar hypoplasia. Diffuse or multifocal white matter abnormalities may be associated with enlargement of the anterior part of the temporal horn of the lateral ventricle. The cortical malformations are best demonstrated on T2-weighted images. Alternatively, there may be a lack of gyral anomalies but multiple white matter lesions in the deep white matter with sparing of the immediate periventricular and subcortical white matter (Figure 6.3).

In infants infected postnatally or in late gestation, the gyral pattern is normal with mild ventricular and sulcal prominence, and damaged periventricular or subcortical white matter, with scattered periventricular calcification or hemorrhage.

Herpes simplex virus (HSV)

"Congenital" HSV is acquired through exposure to type II herpetic genital lesions at birth. The incidence is 1 in 2000–5000 deliveries per year, with involvement of the brain in 30% of cases. Presentation is usually within the first two to four weeks with either visceral disease or CNS meningoencephalitis, and outcome is poor.

139

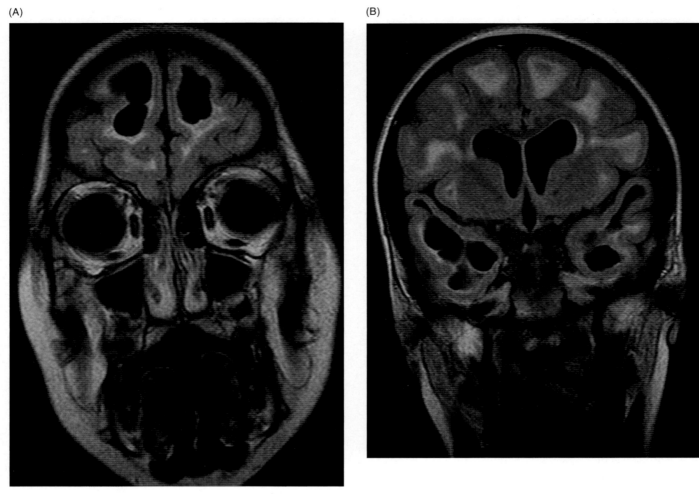

Figure 6.3 (A), (B) Coronal FLAIR MR in an eight-year-old shows extensive white matter changes involving the subcortical and deep white matter and sparing the periventricular white matter, with cystic change in the frontal and temporal lobes consistent with congenital CMV infection.

Initial ultrasound findings are subtle with diffuse hyperechogenicity, which gradually increases and is associated with ventricular compression. There is rapid loss of brain substance, which can occur as early as the second week. As encephalomalacia develops, the ventricles enlarge.

Early in the disease, diffusion-weighted MR imaging reveals reduced perfusion. Subtle hyperintensity may be seen on concurrent T2-weighted images.

After one to two days, CT and MR will show patchy areas of abnormal signal (hypodense on CT, hypointense on T1WSE [T1-weighted spin echo] and hyperintense on T2WSE), primarily within the white matter, which progress rapidly in both prominence and size. Post-contrast scans may show minimal enhancement in a meningeal pattern. There is cerebellar involvement in 50% of affected patients.

Chronic findings are of a severe, diffuse cerebral atrophy with profound cortical thinning, encephalomalacia of the white matter (which is often multicystic) and punctate or gyriform calcification (Figure 6.4).

Other central nervous system infections

Meningitis

Meningitis is the most common central nervous system (CNS) infection in children, occurring more frequently in the first few months of life than in older children. Presentation varies with age and may be very nonspecific in young children.

Two-thirds of neonatal cases in the USA are due to group B *Streptococcus* and *Escherichia coli* (*E. coli*). Most cases (in normal infants of over one month) are due to *Haemophilus influenzae* type b, *Streptococcus pneumoniae* or *Neisseria meningitides*, with *E. coli* also remaining an important pathogen.

Diagnosis is not made by imaging (which is often normal in uncomplicated purulent meningitis), but can be very useful when looking for complications. Meningeal enhancement and/or enhancement over the cerebral convexities may be seen post-contrast on CT or MRI in uncomplicated cases.

The complications which may be demonstrated on imaging include hydrocephalus, venous thrombosis, cavernous sinus thrombosis, venous or arterial infarction, subdural effusions and empyemas, cerebritis, abscess and ventriculitis (Figure 6.5).

Tuberculous meningitis

Presentation of tuberculous (TB) meningitis can be very non-specific, and neurological symptoms may only become apparent at one to two weeks. Without prompt diagnosis and treatment, devastating damage to the brain and ultimately death occur in an average of three weeks.

Hydrocephalus is common, and on noncontrast CT and T1-weighted MR images, soft tissue density may be seen filling the cisterns with marked cisternal enhancement post-contrast. Most patients develop basal ganglia and thalamic infarcts in the subacute phase, with cortical infarcts less common (Figure 6.6).

Tuberculomas, which are of high-density on pre-contrast CT, are seen at the gray–white matter junction as single or multiple punctate or ring-enhancing foci. Durally based lesions are less common. On T1-weighted MRI, a central area of isointensity is surrounded by a rim of high signal, and then a further complete or partial rim of hypointensity (Figure 6.7). On T2W images they are hypointense.

Calcification and surrounding vasogenic edema are uncommon. Occasionally, the central caseous portion of a granuloma may liquefy and form a tuberculous abscess. These are generally larger than tuberculomas, with more vasogenic edema and central hyperintensity on T2.

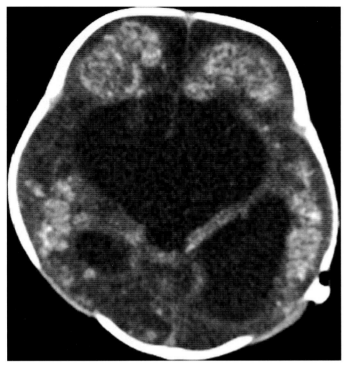

Figure 6.4 Axial CT in a three-month-old shows marked ventriculomegaly and extensive parenchymal calcification, consistent with congenital herpes simplex infection.

(A)

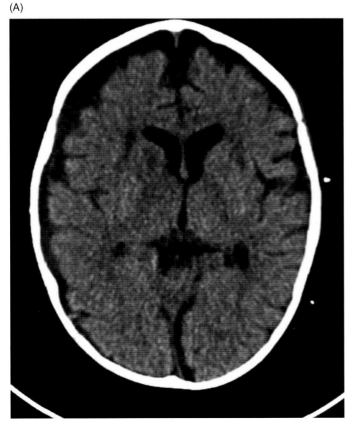

(B)

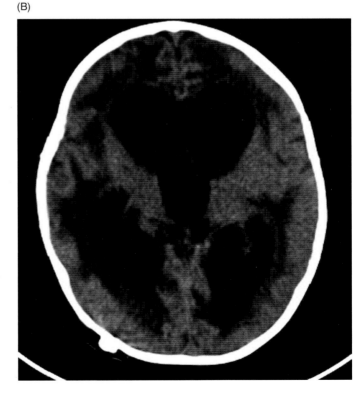

Figure 6.5 (A) Axial CT scan in a nine-month-old with pneumococcal meningitis shows bilateral subdural effusions and bilateral low density basal ganglia infarcts. (B) A later axial CT scan shows development of marked hydrocephalus with transependymal edema.

(A)

(B)

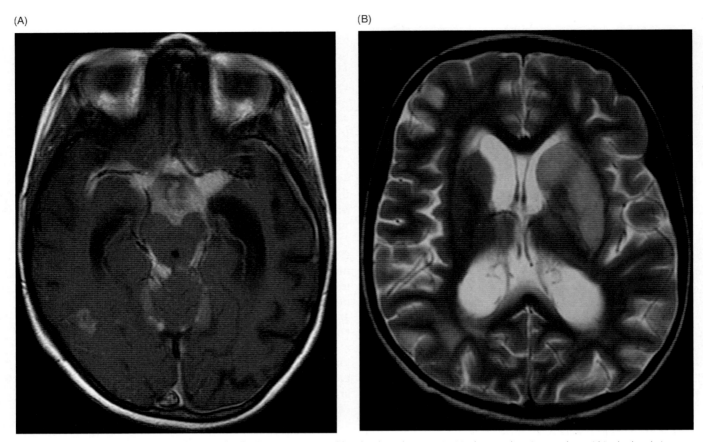

Figure 6.6 (A) Contrast-enhanced axial T1-weighted MR in a seven-year-old with tuberculous meningitis shows enhancing exudate within the basal cisterns and around the brainstem, leptomeningeal lesions and developing hydrocephalus. (B) Axial T2-weighted MR shows an associated left middle cerebral artery infarct.

(A)

(B)

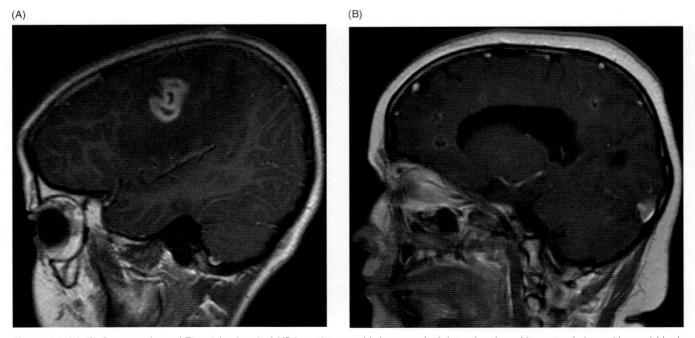

Figure 6.7 (A), (B) Contrast-enhanced T1-weighted sagittal MR in a nine-year-old shows cerebral ring-enhancing white matter lesions with a variable degree of surrounding edema consistent with tuberculomas.

Bacterial cerebritis and brain abscess

Cerebritis is the earliest stage of a purulent brain infection. It may be either focal or multifocal and resolve or progress to abscess formation. The infective organism reaches the brain via hematogenous spread, extension of a contiguous infection, secondary to a penetrating wound or in association with cardiopulmonary pathology.

In early cerebritis, CT and MR will show evidence of edema in the affected brain, with ill-defined areas of abnormal signal which may enhance post-contrast (Figure 6.8). Diffusion-weighted imaging demonstrates reduced perfusion. There is usually associated mild-to-moderate mass effect. Serial imaging is essential to assess response to treatment, with unsuccessful treatment of cerebritis leading to abscess formation. In infants and newborns abscesses are relatively large, with relatively poor capsule formation and rapid enlargement. They usually originate in the periventricular white matter and may rupture into the adjacent lateral ventricle. In older children, the subcortical white matter and basal ganglia are more common locations.

On ultrasound, abscesses are seen as regions of low echogenicity often with hyperechoic rims. Echogenic debris may be seen in the dependent portion of the cavity.

On unenhanced CT, abscesses are of low density with a thin wall of slightly increased density. Post-contrast, a ring of enhancing tissue surrounds the low attenuation center. It is most commonly located at or near the gray–white matter junction with a ring of edema around it. The inner margin of the ring tends to be smooth and regular.

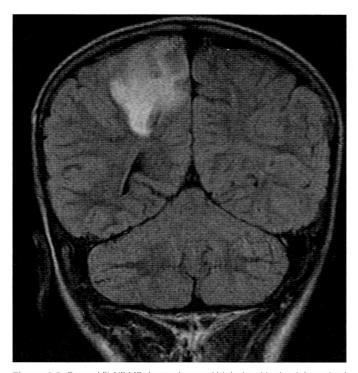

Figure 6.8 Coronal FLAIR MR shows abnormal high signal in the right parietal lobe consistent with a focal cerebritis.

On MR, the abscess walls are hyperintense on T1, hypointense on T2 and enhance post-contrast. The center of the abscess is hypointense on T1 and hyperintense on T2 (Figure 6.9). Diffusion-weighted imaging (DWI) is the best method for differentiating an abscess from a cystic or necrotic tumor. Abscesses usually show hyperintensity or reduced diffusion on DWI, whereas cystic or necrotic tumors typically demonstrate increased diffusion.

Lyme disease

Lyme disease is a systemic disorder caused by *Borrelia burgdorferi*, a tick-borne spirochete. Neurological involvement occurs in about 20% of affected children. The most common presentations are with fever, headache, behavioral change and facial palsy, and a chronic form has also been described.

CT scans are usually normal in Lyme disease. MR imaging is positive in 25%, showing focal regions of high intensity in the white matter on T2. In children with cranial neuropathies, leptomeningeal enhancement can be seen with or without enhancement of the affected cranial nerve.

Periventricular hyperintensity can be seen on T2 and FLAIR images in the chronic form. There may be spinal cord involvement.

Rocky Mountain spotted fever

Rocky Mountain spotted fever is a tick-borne rickettsial infection caused by *Rickettsia rickettsii*. Presentation is typically with abrupt onset of fever, headache and rash, usually two to eight days after the tick bite. There is CNS involvement in 75% of patients, characterized by altered consciousness, confusion, hallucinations, seizures and meningism, secondary to a destructive vasculitis in the brain with multiple small infarctions.

CT demonstrates discrete or confluent foci of low density in the cerebral white matter which, on MR, are seen as punctate foci of high intensity on T2. Following treatment, there is complete resolution of the changes.

Viral infections

Viral spread to the CNS usually occurs via the hematogenous route, although a few viral pathogens spread via the peripheral nerves. Although some viruses have predilections for specific areas of the brain, most viruses can produce a number of different clinical syndromes depending on the part of the brain affected, and therefore the clinical and imaging findings of different viral infections can show marked overlap.

Early imaging in viral encephalitis demonstrates edema in the affected areas, seen as patchy areas of hyperechogenicity on ultrasound, low density on CT, low signal on T1 and high signal on T2 and FLAIR images (Figures 6.10 and 6.11). Diffusion-weighted images show the early changes most clearly with reduced diffusion in the affected areas.

Herpes simplex encephalitis

Over the age of six months, infection is caused by the herpes simplex 1 virus with herpes simplex 2 virus causing congenital or perinatally acquired herpes.

(A)

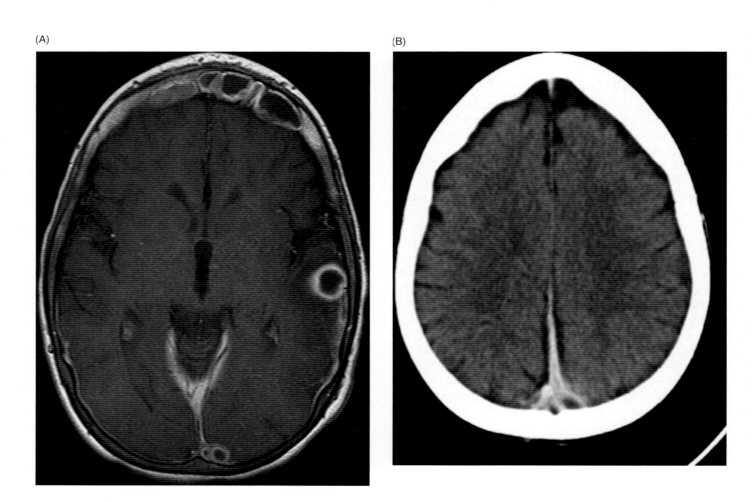

(B)

(C)

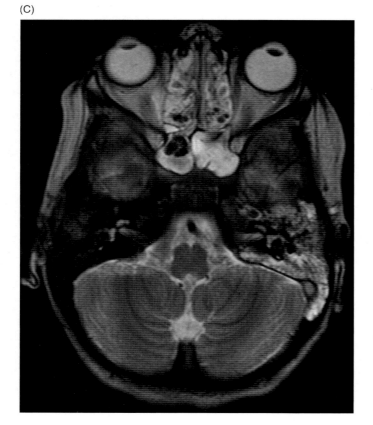

Figure 6.9 (A) Axial contrast-enhanced T1-weighted MR in seven-year-old shows a left temporal lobe abscess with surrounding edema, a subdural collection over the left cerebral convexity and thrombosis of the superior sagittal sinus which is split (normal variant); also seen on (B) axial contrast-enhanced CT. (C) Axial T2-weighted MR shows paranasal sinus and left mastoid air cell fluid/soft tissue which may be the source of infection.

(A)

(B)

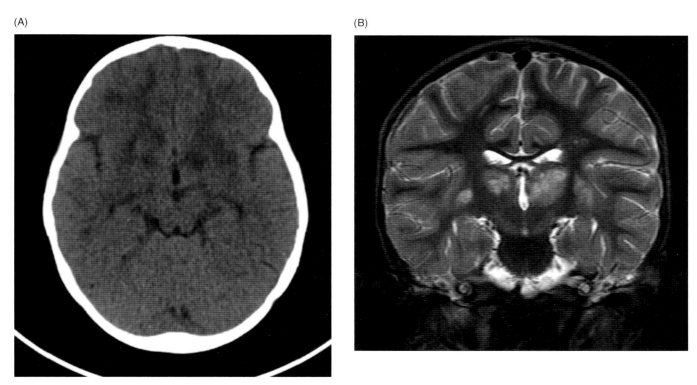

Figure 6.10 (A) Axial CT and (B) coronal T2-weighted MR in a 16-month-old show bilateral asymmetrical swelling and abnormal signal within the hypothalamus, mesial temporal lobes and basal ganglia, with scattered lesions within the centrum semiovale consistent with a viral encephalitis.

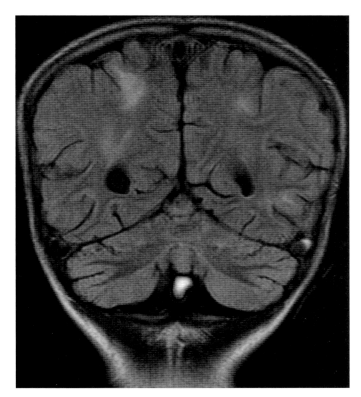

Figure 6.11 Coronal FLAIR MR in a four-year-old shows high signal in the cortex and subcortical white matter of the posterior parietal lobes, left temporal lobe and cerebellar hemispheres consistent with a viral encephalitis.

Imaging, particularly CT, is fairly insensitive early on in the course of the disease. Diffusion-weighted MR images will be the first to show abnormality, with reduced diffusion in the affected regions. After intravenous contrast, mild enhancement of the leptomeninges, cortex and subcortical white matter is seen.

Towards the end of the first week of the disease, areas of both increased and decreased diffusion may be seen in different regions of the brain. On T2 and FLAIR images, the affected areas appear hyperintense, particularly in the medial temporal lobe, insular cortex, and orbital surfaces of the frontal lobe (Figure 6.12). Areas of both T1 and T2 shortening may develop secondary to hemorrhage or calcification.

Involvement is usually unilateral, but bilateral disease is not uncommon. Rapid progression to the frontal and parietal lobes can occur. The disease eventually becomes well demarcated, and multicystic encephalomalacia often ensues.

Varicella-zoster encephalitis

The majority of cases of chicken pox occur in children under the age of 10, and central nervous system complications are seen in less than 0.1%. The most common manifestation is of acute cerebellar ataxia which develops within 10 days of the onset of the rash.

MR studies may show acute cerebellar swelling and hyperintensity and lesions of varying size at the gray–white matter junction in the cerebral cortex and basal ganglia.

145

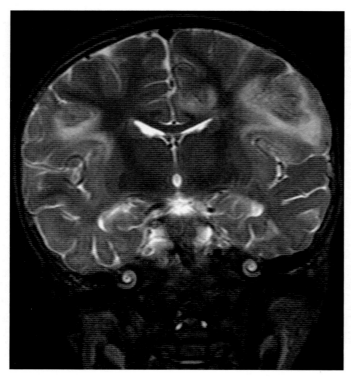

Figure 6.12 Coronal T2-weighted MR in an eight-month-old shows bilateral asymmetric abnormal high signal in the frontotemporal cortices and subcortical white matter consistent with herpes encephalitis.

In rare cases, children may present with acute onset hemiplegia one to four months after chickenpox. Imaging typically shows acute basal ganglia infarction with a variable amount of cerebral cortex infarction in the distribution of the middle cerebral artery.

Measles encephalitis

Involvement of the CNS following measles infection can manifest in one of three ways:

Acute postinfectious encephalitis is thought to be an autoimmune disorder; neurological symptoms begin 4–14 days after the appearance of the rash in 0.1% of cases of measles.

Imaging shows involvement of the basal ganglia and cerebral cortex with high intensity on T2 and reduced diffusion acutely. Scattered foci of high intensity may develop in the white matter with disease evolution and, ultimately, high intensity on T1 and atrophy may occur.

In progressive infectious encephalitis, patients exhibit progressive neurological deterioration from three to six months after the illness. The imaging findings have not been described.

Subacute sclerosing panencephalitis (SSPE) is an illness caused by reactivation of the measles virus a number of years after the initial infection. It is characterized by a progressive mental deterioration and neurological symptoms and leads to death within three years.

CT findings are nonspecific, with diffuse atrophy and multifocal areas of low density in the periventricular and subcortical white matter.

MR images may be normal in the first three to four months after the onset of symptoms. This is followed by the development of high signal in the cerebral cortex and subcortical white matter on T2 and FLAIR, usually bilaterally and asymmetrically in the parietal and temporal lobes. With disease progression, the high signal extends into the periventricular white matter and corpus callosum and finally into the brainstem. Diffuse atrophy develops in the latter stages. Basal ganglia involvement is seen in about a third of patients.

Enterovirus infections

The enteroviruses are rarely seen in western countries. Neurological complications are seen in up to 50% of cases and have distinctive imaging findings.

Spinal poliomyelitis is the most common form of neurological presentation. Patients develop headache, vomiting, meningism and muscle pain followed by a flaccid paralysis one to two days later.

MRI demonstrates high signal in the ventral horns of the spinal cord on T2 with or without enhancement of the ventral horns post-contrast.

Bulbar polio/rhombencephalitis is less common and typically affects the 9th to 11th cranial nerves, leading to hoarseness, difficulty in swallowing or airway obstruction.

MRI demonstrates high signal in the brainstem on T2, particularly in the dorsal medulla and pons, which may extend posteriorly or superiorly.

Cerebral encephalitis gives nonspecific high signal on T2, affecting the cerebral hemispheres.

Fungal infections

Fungal infection of the nervous system is uncommon in the pediatric population. Infection can occur in an immunocompetent child or as an opportunistic infection in an immunocompromised child. The manifestations of fungal infections are identical to those in adults and will not be discussed further here.

Upper respiratory tract infections

Pharyngitis/tonsillitis

The diagnosis of pyogenic infection of the pharyngeal wall or tonsillar fossa can generally be made clinically on direct inspection without the need for radiological input. If peritonsillar abscess is suspected, however, imaging may be indicated.

In uncomplicated tonsillitis, contrast-enhanced CT demonstrates enlarged tonsils with stranding of the adjacent parapharyngeal fat. If a peritonsillar abscess has developed, it is more common to see a central hypodensity with rim enhancement.

Studies in young adults also suggest that perioral ultrasound scans can be useful in differentiating peritonsillar abscess from cellulitis. This may be technically more difficult in the pediatric population.

Retropharyngeal cellulitis and abscess

Retropharyngeal cellulitis is a pyogenic infection of the retro-pharyngeal space that usually follows recent pharyngitis or upper respiratory tract infection. Presentation is with sudden-onset fever, neck stiffness, dysphagia and occasionally stridor. More than 50% of cases occur in children between 6 and 12 months of age.

Thickening of the retropharyngeal soft tissues is seen on lateral radiograph. In a normal infant or young child, the distance from the anterior aspect of the vertebral column to the air column of the posterior pharyngeal wall should be no greater than the diameter of the vertebral body at C6. However, particularly in infants who have relatively short necks and are difficult to position, it is common to see "pseudothickening" of the tissues. The neck must be well extended and, if possible, the film taken in inspiration. Anterior convexity of the retropharyngeal soft tissues suggests true widening of the soft tissues. There may also be loss or reversal of the normal cervical lordosis.

Differentiation of cellulitis from abscess is only possible on plain films if gas can be seen within the soft tissues. Otherwise, suspicious cases require contrast-enhanced CT. Uncommon differential diagnoses for thickened retropharyngeal tissues include hemorrhage, neuroblastoma and anterior myelomeningocele.

Epiglottitis

Epiglottitis is a life-threatening bacterial cellulitis of the supra-glottic structures that affects the lingual surface of the epiglottis and aryepiglottic folds. It is characterized by sudden-onset acute respiratory obstruction, stridor, high fever and dysphagia. Most cases are secondary to *Hemophilus influenzae* (Hib), and the incidence has decreased dramatically since the introduction of the Hib vaccine. Peak age of presentation is three to six years old, and diagnosis is generally made clinically under direct inspection.

If imaging is required, the child must be accompanied by a physician able to intubate or perform a tracheostomy. A lateral radiograph in the upright position shows thickening and rounding of the epiglottis with loss of the vallecular air space. The aryepiglottic folds are also thickened, and there may be distension of the hypopharynx. Imaging usually makes the diagnosis apparent, but the differential includes croup, foreign-body aspiration and retropharyngeal abscess.

Acute laryngotracheobronchitis (croup)

Croup is the leading cause of upper airway obstruction in young children. It commonly occurs between six months and three years of age and is usually viral in etiology. Presentation is with a short history of upper respiratory tract infection (URTI) and a harsh "barking" cough, hoarseness and intermittent inspiratory stridor. The insidious onset distinguishes it from epiglottitis.

In classic cases, radiological investigation is unnecessary, but can be useful to exclude other causes of respiratory distress which may require intervention, such as foreign-body aspiration.

The radiographic findings are characteristic. There is edema of the subglottic mucosa, which causes narrowing of the tracheal air column for 5–10 mm or more below the level of the vocal cords and loss of the normal shoulders of the subglottic trachea. Normal tracheal width is then resumed. This symmetric upward tapering has been likened to a "church steeple." There may be no radiographic abnormalities in up to 50% of patients. The subglottic narrowing is milder on the lateral view but, in contrast to epiglottitis, the supraglottic structures appear normal.

The differential diagnosis includes subglottic and proximal tracheal stenosis or a radiolucent foreign body lodged in the subglottic mucosa.

Bacterial tracheitis

Bacterial tracheitis, also known as exudative tracheitis, membranous croup or membranous laryngotracheobronchitis, is a rare but potentially life-threatening purulent infection of the trachea in which exudative plaques form along the tracheal wall. It is more common in autumn and winter and is most common in children of six months to eight years old. A number of bacteria have been implicated. It is unclear whether the infection is primary or a secondary bacterial infection following damage to the respiratory mucosa from a viral infection. There is often a several-day history of viral URTI or croup-type symptoms followed by a high fever and respiratory distress. Concurrent sites of infection, particularly pneumonia, are common.

The lateral radiograph may demonstrate the "steeple sign" of croup, but the tracheal air column can appear diffusely hazy with multiple luminal soft tissue irregularities indicating pseudomembrane detachment.

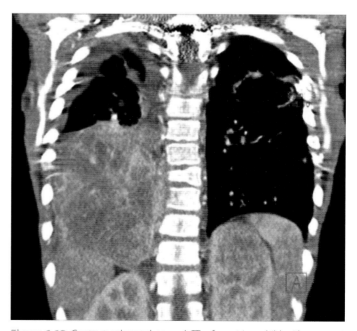

Figure 6.13 Contrast-enhanced coronal CT reformat in a child with recurrent respiratory papillomatosis shows a large heterogeneously enhancing squamous cell carcinoma in the right lower hemithorax, with associated involvement and partial collapse of the T7 vertebral body.

(A)

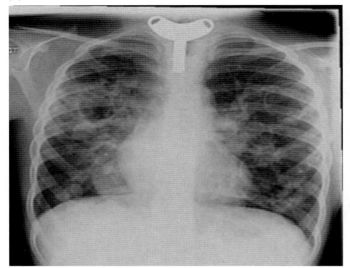

(B)

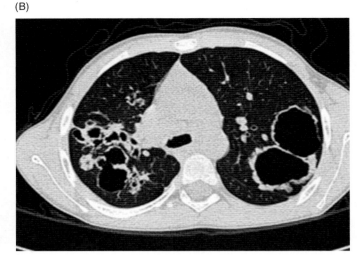

(C)

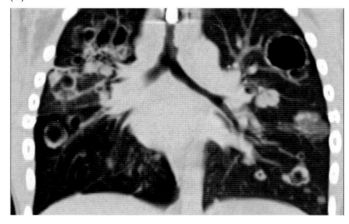

Figure 6.14 (A) Chest radiograph, (B) axial CT and (C) coronal MIP in a child with recurrent respiratory papillomatosis show a tracheostomy, multiple bilateral cavitating nodules and irregularity of the trachea and bronchi consistent with recurrent respiratory papillomatosis.

Recurrent respiratory papillomatosis

Recurrent respiratory papillomatosis (RRP) is a chronic disease caused by human papillomavirus (HPV) types 6 and 11, characterized by the proliferation of benign squamous papillomas within the aerodigestive tract. Although benign, RRP tends to be more aggressive in children than adults and can be fatal due to recurrence and spread throughout the respiratory tract. There is also a malignant potential, with 10% of adult patients developing squamous cell carcinoma (Figure 6.13). There is no known cure. Vertical transmission occurring during delivery through an infected birth canal is presumed to be the major mode of transmitting infection to children.

Children present with hoarseness, as laryngeal papillomas are the most common manifestation. In very young children, hoarseness may go unnoticed and stridor may be the presenting complaint.

The course of the disease is varied and unpredictable, ranging from spontaneous remission to aggressive disease. Spread to the trachea, bronchi or even alveoli is seen.

Plain films may demonstrate focal or diffuse nodular narrowing of the airways with nodules arising from the mucosal surface. Airway obstruction can lead to atelectasis, air-trapping, post-obstructive infection and bronchiectasis. Cavitating parenchymal nodules are seen with distal spread. These changes may be demonstrated on CXR; however, both the intraluminal extent of the disease and the more distal sequelae are better evaluated with CT (Figure 6.14).

Bronchiolitis and pneumonia

Neonatal pneumonia

Pneumonia occurs in less than 1% of newborn infants and is more common in premature infants than term. It can result from a large number of infectious agents, the majority of which produce a radiographic appearance of patchy, asymmetric perihilar densities and hyperinflation.

The most common pathogen, group B *Streptococcus*, gives a slightly different radiological picture with bilateral granular

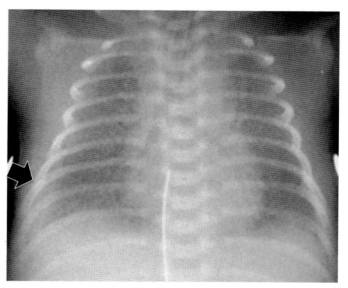

Figure 6.15 Chest radiograph of a neonate with group B streptococcal pneumonia shows bilateral granular opacities and a right-sided effusion (arrow).

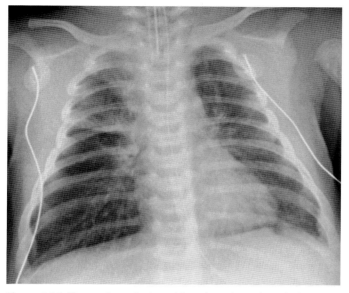

Figure 6.16 Chest radiograph shows bilateral streaky peribronchial opacities radiating from the hila, with peribronchial wall thickening, early right upper lobe collapse and flattening of the diaphragm due to hyperinflation consistent with bronchiolitis.

opacities and low lung volumes similar to the changes seen relating to hyaline membrane disease (HMD) (Figure 6.15). However, the presence of pleural effusions may be a helpful differentiating factor as they are uncommon in HMD but seen in two-thirds of patients with group B streptococcal pneumonia.

Chlamydial pneumonia may be acquired from the mother by direct contact during vaginal delivery. Pneumonia develops between two weeks and three months of age, and radiographic abnormalities include hyperinflation and patchy, asymmetric interstitial and alveolar opacities. Pleural effusions are uncommon.

Bronchiolitis and viral pneumonia

Bronchiolitis is an acute, viral, inflammatory disease of the upper and lower respiratory tract that may result in obstruction of the small airways. It can occur in all age groups, but because older children have larger airways they can better accommodate mucosal edema and therefore severe respiratory symptoms are much more common in young infants. Respiratory syncytial virus (RSV) can be cultured from a third of outpatients and 80% of hospitalized children presenting with wheeze-associated respiratory disease at less than six months of age. Overall mortality from RSV bronchiolitis is estimated at 0.2–7%. Many infants who have been hospitalized for bronchiolitis in infancy continue to have bronchial hyperreactivity for a number of years. There is a clinical and radiological overlap of bronchiolitis and bronchopneumonia.

In all age groups, viral lower respiratory tract infections (LRTIs) are much more common than bacterial infections. In four-month to five-year-olds, 95% of LRTIs are viral, with a decreasing proportion seen in school children. RSV, parainfluenza and influenza viruses and adenovirus are the most common pathogens.

In bronchiolitis, chest radiography is most useful for excluding congenital anomalies or other conditions. It usually shows hyperinflation and 20–30% will also show lobar infiltrates or atelectasis.

On chest radiograph, the latter is seen as increased peribronchial opacities that are symmetric, coarse markings radiating from the hila into the lung. Associated small airway occlusion may lead to areas of both hyperinflation and subsegmental collapse, more common in the middle and lower portions of the lung (Figure 6.16).

Bacterial pneumonia

Streptococcus pneumoniae is the most common bacterial pathogen in both pre-school and older children, with *Mycoplasma pneumoniae* and *Chlamydia pneumoniae* seen more frequently in children over five years of age and adolescents. Infection occurs secondary to inhalation of the infection agent into the airspaces resulting in inflammation within the acini, leading to consolidation.

Presentation, particularly in younger children, may be nonspecific, and findings on physical examination are also often less reliable than those in adults.

Chest radiographs may demonstrate localized airspace opacification with air bronchograms. Typically, the distribution is lobar or segmental. Associated pleural effusions are not uncommon. In children less than eight years old, the consolidation may appear as a "round" mass-like lesion (Figure 6.17). This is most commonly seen in *Streptococcus pneumoniae* infection and is thought to relate to poor development of collateral pathways of ventilation.

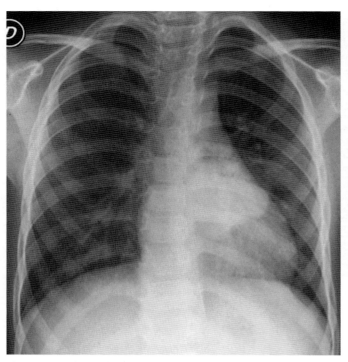

Figure 6.17 Chest radiograph shows a round mass-like lesion behind the heart consistent with a "round" pneumonia.

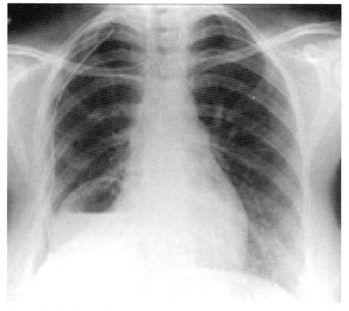

Figure 6.19 Chest radiograph shows a lung abscess in the right lower lobe with an air–fluid level. A chest drain has been inserted for an associated empyema.

The radiographic changes of pneumonia may persist for up to four weeks, and repeat chest radiograph is not usually required in an otherwise healthy child whose symptoms resolve.

Causes of failure of suspected pneumonia to resolve include: infected developmental lesions, bronchial obstruction,

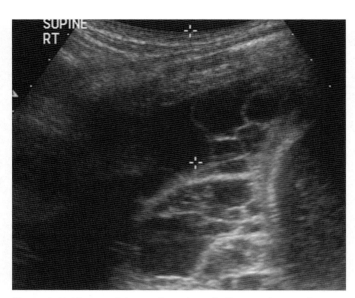

Figure 6.18 Ultrasound shows a "complicated" effusion with septae between areas of both anechoic and echogenic fluid.

gastroesophageal reflux and aspiration and underlying systemic disorders.

Complications of pneumonia
Parapneumonic effusions

Chest ultrasound (US) is the initial investigation of choice in suspected pleural effusion or empyema. There is no radiation involved and, due to the high spatial and contrast resolution of ultrasound, it can also differentiate "complicated" effusions, those with loculations and/or echogenic fluid, from "simple" effusions, those which are anechoic and unseptated, which may impact on management (Figure 6.18). However, it is important to note that in the setting of a parapneumonic effusion, no imaging modality can accurately differentiate between infected and reactive effusions, as even pus can appear anechoic on ultrasound. Studies suggest CT is no better at differentiating "simple" effusion from empyema with pleural enhancement seen in almost all cases of parapneumonic effusion, infected or not. CT should therefore be reserved for the more complicated cases.

Lung parenchyma complications

Complications such as cavitation or abscess formation may be demonstrated on chest radiograph, but are often more clearly depicted on CT (Figure 6.19). Noncompromised consolidated lung parenchyma enhances diffusely on post-contrast CT (Figure 6.20). Areas of decreased or absent enhancement indicate underlying parenchymal ischemia or infarction. A spectrum of suppurative parenchymal complications can be seen, including cavitatory necrosis, lung abscess, pneumatocele, bronchopleural fistula and pulmonary gangrene.

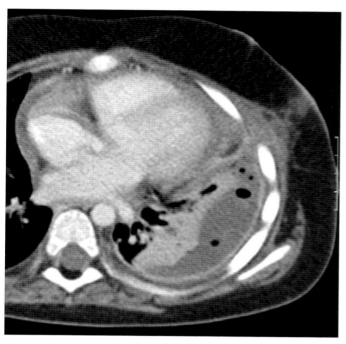

Figure 6.20 Axial contrast-enhanced CT shows enhancing consolidated lung and pleura with an associated empyema containing gas.

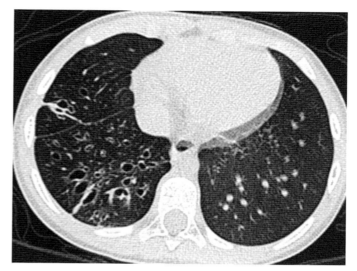

Figure 6.21 Axial HRCT shows bronchiectasis affecting the right lung as a complication of previous bacterial pneumonia.

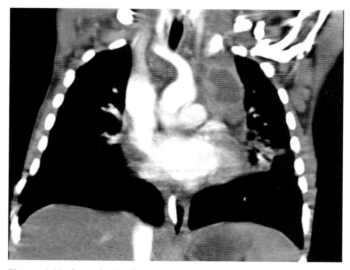

Figure 6.22 Coronal MIP of a contrast-enhanced CT shows left axillary and mediastinal lymphadenopathy, with evidence of necrosis, and left-sided consolidation consistent with the known diagnosis of pulmonary tuberculosis.

On CT, an abscess is seen as a fluid and/or gas-filled cavity with enhancing walls. A pneumatocele is a thin-walled cyst and may represent resolving or healing necrosis.

Cavitory necrosis describes a dominant area of necrosis within a consolidated lobe. CT findings include loss of normal lung architecture, decreased parenchymal enhancement, loss of the lung–pleural margin and multiple thick-walled cavities containing air or fluid but without an enhancing border. Unlike adults, cavitatory necrosis in children can often be managed medically without the need for surgical intervention, and follow-up imaging may reveal only minimal scarring.

Chronic complications of pneumonia

Bronchiectasis is dilatation and thickening of the bronchi related to damage to the bronchial wall. It is best seen on high-resolution CT (HRCT; Figure 6.21).

Swyer-James syndrome is a manifestation of obliterative bronchiolitis characterized by unilateral lung hyperlucency, thought to be secondary to abnormal growth of the affected portion of the lung following a viral infection. Radiography demonstrates a hyperlucent lung of normal or small volume with a small but present hilum due to diminished pulmonary arterial flow. Air-trapping is seen on expiratory films.

Pulmonary tuberculosis

Childhood tuberculosis (TB) is more commonly primary than reactive. Radiographic and CT features include parenchymal consolidation, mediastinal and hilar lymphadenopathy and pleural effusion. Affected lymph nodes often demonstrate central low density on CT due to necrosis (Figure 6.22).

Reactive TB typically affects the apical and posterior segments of the upper lobes and the superior segments of the lower lobes. It appears as patchy areas of consolidation, and cavitation is common (Figure 6.23).

Miliary TB occurs secondary to diffuse hematogenous dissemination and can occur any time after the primary infection. On both radiograph and CT, multiple, small (<1 cm) reticulonodular opacities are seen evenly spread throughout both lungs (Figure 6.24).

(A)

(B)

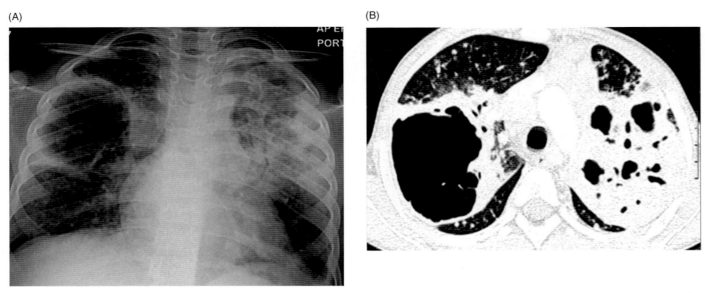

Figure 6.23 Reactive Tuberculosis (A) Chest radiograph shows bilateral patchy consolidation with a cavitating lesion in the right hemithorax. (B) Axial CT in the same patient demonstrates bilateral cavitating upper lobe lesions and consolidation.

(A)

(B)

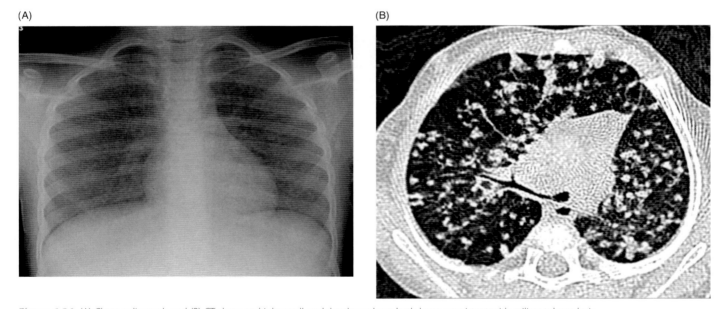

Figure 6.24 (A) Chest radiograph and (B) CT show multiple small nodules throughout both lungs consistent with miliary tuberculosis.

Pulmonary histoplasmosis

Histoplasmosis is a fungal infection endemic in parts of the United States. Acute imaging findings include bilateral non-segmental areas of airspace opacification, nodular opacities and hilar and/or mediastinal lymphadenopathy. Dissemination of the disease is uncommon unless the host is immunocompromised. Both lung nodules and lymph nodes may calcify with resolution of the infection.

Complications include broncholiths, caused by calcified lymph nodes eroding into a bronchus, and fibrosing mediastinitis, caused by large lymph nodes encasing and narrowing mediastinal structures.

Pulmonary aspergillosis

Aspergillus occurs in individuals with an underlying structural abnormality such as a cavity, or in those with atopy or immunodeficiency.

The most common appearance of the infection is with an aspergilloma or fungal ball, which develops in a preexisting lung cavity or cyst. Classic imaging findings are those of

(A)

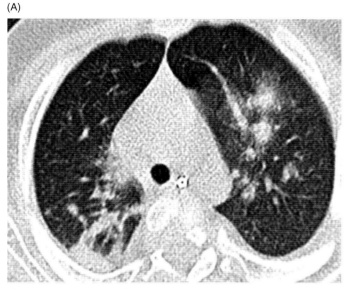

(B)

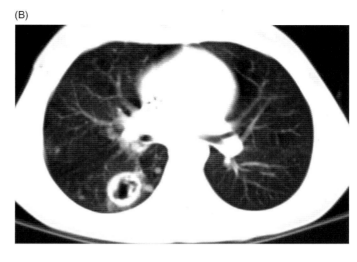

Figure 6.25 (A) Axial CT shows multiple bilateral nodular opacities with surrounding ground-glass "halo" consistent with invasive aspergillosis. (B) Axial CT in a different patient with invasive aspergillosis shows multiple nodules within the right lung, the largest of which is cavitating.

a discrete intracavitory mass with an air crescent between the mass and the cavity wall. The mass may be shown to be mobile, with change in position following change in patient position.

Allergic bronchopulmonary aspergillosis is a hypersensitivity disorder that occurs predominantly in patients with asthma or cystic fibrosis. Imaging demonstrates bronchiectactic change with impacted mucus often with distal air-trapping. Mucus-plugging of the small airways may also be seen on CT ("tree-in-bud").

In immunocompromised patients, particularly those with severe neutropenia, angioinvasive aspergillosis can occur. There is invasion of the blood vessels causing pulmonary infarction and necrotizing pneumonia. Plain films and CT findings include nodular opacities and rounded areas of parenchymal consolidation. The nodules may cavitate, and on CT a "halo" of irregular ground-glass opacification may be seen surrounding the nodule secondary to hemorrhage in the adjacent lung (Figure 6.25).

Gastrointestinal tract infections
Esophageal inflammation
Epidermolysis bullosa dystrophica
Epidermolysis bullosa dystrophica (EBD) is a rare skin disease characterized by marked mechanical fragility of epithelial tissues and the formation of skin blisters and ulcers. One of the most common sites of extracutaneous injury in inherited EBD is the gastrointestinal tract. Painful blisters and erosions may develop within the oral cavity, esophagus, small and large intestines, rectum and anus. Severe blistering can then lead to stricture formation. Rectal strictures may result in chronic constipation and even megacolon.

Imaging of the upper intestinal tract with a contrast study may be preferable to endoscopy, which can be technically difficult due to oral or esophageal deformities. The esophagus tends to be affected at the sites of maximal trauma by ingested material, the very proximal and distal ends and at the level of the carina. The bullae may resolve or ulcerate and bleed and scarring may lead to stricture formation of varying lengths.

Infective esophagitis
Infective esophagitis is very rare in the immunocompetent population and is further discussed in the section below on human immunodeficiency virus.

Gastritis
Infectious gastritis
Helicobacter pylori infection is prevalent worldwide and is often asymptomatic. However, although less common in children than adults, gastritis and gastric and duodenal ulcers are described, and rates of recurrence in children shown to be markedly reduced following successful eradication of *H. pylori*.

Contrast studies may demonstrate thickened mucosal folds, particularly in the body and antropyloric regions, and ulceration. Infectious gastritis is also seen in HIV-infected patients and is discussed briefly in the section on human immunodeficiency virus, below.

Chronic granulomatous disease of childhood
Chronic granulomatous disease (CGD) of childhood is a syndrome of recurrent infection whose underlying pathophysiology

(A)

(B)

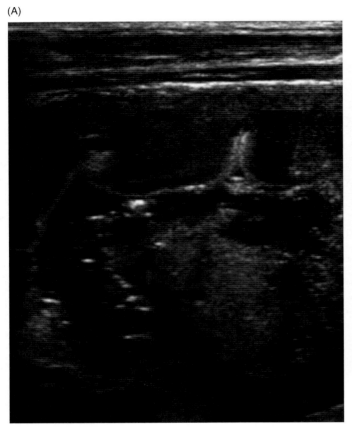
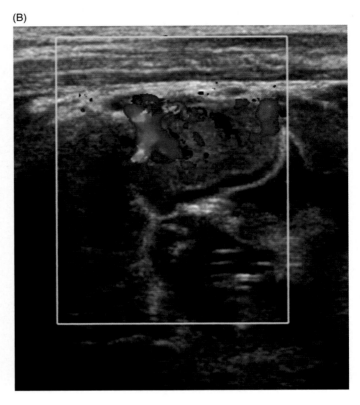

Figure 6.26 Ultrasound in a patient with chronic granulomatous disease shows (A) mucosal thickening and (B) hypervascularity on Doppler in the fundus of the stomach.

is one of disordered phagocytosis. The most common GI manifestation is chronic antral gastritis.

Sonographically, there is abnormal thickening of the stomach wall, most commonly in the antropyloric region, which may be demonstrated on ultrasound (Figure 6.26). An upper GI series shows narrowing of the antropyloric lumen secondary to chronic inflammation and fibrosis. The proximal duodenum may also be involved.

Inflammatory bowel disease

The incidence of pediatric inflammatory bowel disease (IBD) is rising. Etiologically, a complex interaction of environmental, genetic and immune factors is thought to be involved, with the majority of new cases being nonfamilial. Approximately 20% of newly diagnosed ulcerative colitis (UC) and 25–30% of newly diagnosed Crohn's disease (CD) presents in under-20-year-olds, with the median age of onset in the pediatric age group of 12 years.

Presentation can be very nonspecific and depends on the site and extent of mucosal inflammation. UC most commonly presents with diarrhea and blood per rectum, abdominal pain and weight loss. CD may present with similar features or have a delayed presentation with symptoms including recurrent abdominal pain, fatigue, anorexia, weight loss and anemia.

Differentiating CD and UC can be difficult in some pediatric cases. The gold standard for diagnosis is endoscopy and biopsy, with imaging playing an important complementary role. More recently, wireless capsule endoscopy (WCE) has begun to play an increasing role in both diagnosis and follow-up of small bowel pathology in children, and has been shown to be safe and well tolerated and more sensitive than radiological and standard endoscopic modalities.

In CD there is transmural inflammatory change, which can affect any part of the GI tract, often with skip lesions. In children, proximal bowel involvement in, for example, the duodenum and jejunum is more common than in adults (Figure 6.27). Chronic inflammation and fibrosis lead to thickened, stenotic bowel loops, and transmural extension predisposes to fistula, sinus or abscess formation.

In UC, disease extends from the rectum proximally, and inflammation is usually limited to the mucosa. There is bowel wall thickening and inflammatory polyp formation.

Imaging can be helpful as a diagnostic tool and for assessing disease extent and complications.

Plain films can show complications such as perforation, obstruction, distended bowel loops and toxic megacolon. In colitis, there may be haustral or bowel wall thickening or loss of the normal haustral markings. Symmetric haustral

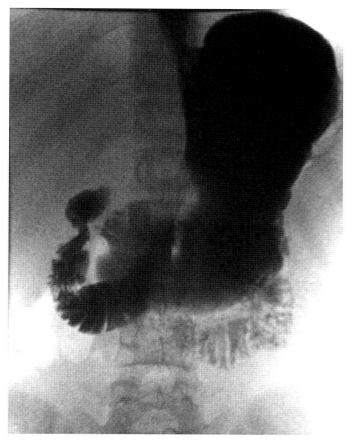

Figure 6.27 Small bowel follow-through in a child with Crohn's disease shows a stricture in the second part of the duodenum.

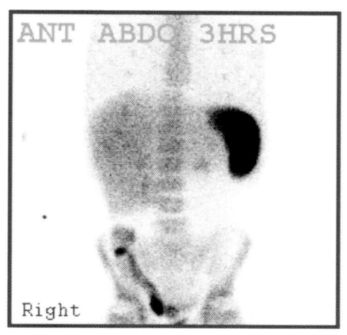

Figure 6.28 Technetium-labeled white blood-cell scan in a child with suspected Crohn's disease shows increased uptake in the region of the terminal ileum and cecal pole.

thickening and "thumbprinting" are more common in UC than CD.

Technetium-labeled white blood-cell scans can be a useful tool in the evaluation of inflammatory bowel disease, being noninvasive and able to image the large and small bowel simultaneously (Figure 6.28). False negatives can be a problem.

Ultrasound is often performed as an early investigation for unexplained abdominal pain or in known disease to look for progression, remission and complications such as abscess formation. In active disease, the bowel wall is thickened with a narrow or collapsed lumen and increased vascularity on Doppler settings (Figure 6.29).

In CD, there is decreased peristalsis in affected loops of small bowel. A "target sign" with central echogenicity and surrounding hypoechogenicity may be seen in transverse section. Early in the disease, the five alternating hyper- and hypoechogenic layers of bowel wall are generally preserved unless inflammation is very severe. The inflamed mesentery is thickened and echoic with hypoechoic enlarged lymph nodes seen within it.

Chronically, the bowel becomes fibrosed with loss of the layered echopattern leaving thickened, hypoechoic bowel with loss of colonic haustra and fixed loops secondary to mesenteric

fatty fibroproliferation. Ultrasound may also demonstrate stenoses with a fixed narrow lumen and prestenotic dilatation and peristalsis. Mildly inflamed regions of bowel can be missed on ultrasound.

Contrast studies, particularly of the small bowel, are a long-standing part of both diagnosis and follow-up in inflammatory bowel disease, and are still relied upon. However they may be supplanted by WCE, CT and MRI in the future. A small bowel follow-through (SBFT) should include assessment of the esophagus, stomach and small bowel. Findings in CD include: mucosal nodularity or thickening; aphthous ulceration; the "string sign," a thin, irregular channel of barium in the lumen of a circumferentially inflamed loop of bowel; bowel loop separation; stenosis with prestenotic dilatation or pseudodiverticulosis (Figure 6.30). Deep linear ulceration surrounding edematous mucosa can give a "cobblestone" appearance. Contrast enema is not required if satisfactory ileocolonoscopic views are obtained, and is poorly tolerated if there is fulminant rectal or perianal disease.

In UC, a double contrast enema may show granular mucosa and ulceration, which has a "collar-button" appearance with barium in the ulcer crevice and pseudopolyps of interposed mucosa and granulation tissue between the ulcer margins.

In more chronic cases, there is narrowing of the colonic luminal caliber, and the colon becomes shortened, featureless and noncompliant. Contrast enema is contraindicated in acute colitis, perforation or toxic megacolon.

Multidetector computed tomography (MDCT) is well tolerated and is especially useful for assessing extraluminal disease. Ideally, intravenous contrast should be given for better detection of areas of inflammation, and intraluminal contrast

(A)

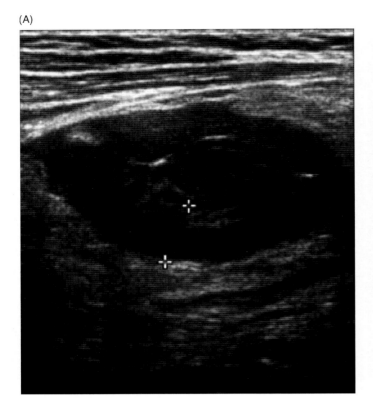

(B)

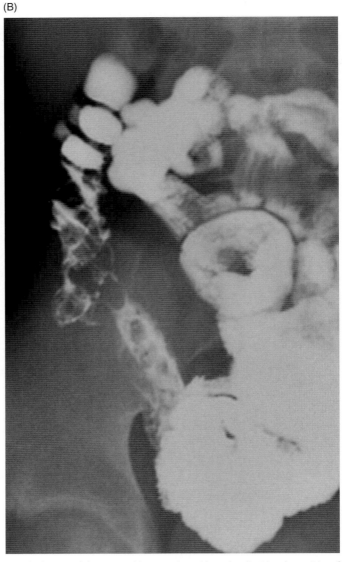

Figure 6.29 (A) Ultrasound in a child with suspected inflammatory bowel disease shows thickening of the terminal ileum and cecal bowel wall with echogenicity of the surrounding mesentery. (B) Small bowel follow-through in the same child shows bowel loop separation around the terminal ileum and cecum with terminal ileal mucosal irregularity and narrowing.

with adequate bowel distension is essential. The disadvantages include the need for IV access, and the radiation burden.

CD and UC have many common features, but extraluminal manifestations are more common in CD, with UC largely demonstrating mucosal change. Wall thickening in UC is generally more uniform and less marked than that seen in CD.

In CD, early inflammation is seen as matted bowel loops and ill-defined mesentery of higher attenuation than normal. Mesenteric stranding, fibrofatty proliferation, lymphadenopathy and fistula or abscess formation are well demonstrated.

Distinguishing active and chronic CD can be difficult; however, features such as the "comb sign" of prominent vasa recta, venous and lymphatic channels suggest actively inflamed bowel.

In chronic UC, low attenuation may be seen paralleling the bowel lumen, which is best seen in the arterial phase. It is

thought to represent a layer of fatty proliferation or submucosal edema between the hypertrophied muscularis mucosa and muscularis propria.

Nonspecific perirectal fat deposition can be seen in any colitis, especially with long-standing inflammation.

Magnetic resonance imaging has only recently been used in the imaging of pediatric IBD. Advantages include the lack of ionizing radiation, multiplanar imaging and excellent soft tissue contrast, and the use of fast breath-hold techniques decreases previous problems with motion artifact. The bowel is distended with non-absorbable oral contrast.

Early superficial CD lesions are not demonstrated well on MRI; however, extramural manifestations and complications and transmural abnormalities are well depicted (Figure 6.31). MRI may also help differentiate active inflammation from fibrosis in a thickened bowel wall segment, with a layered

(A)

(B)

(C)

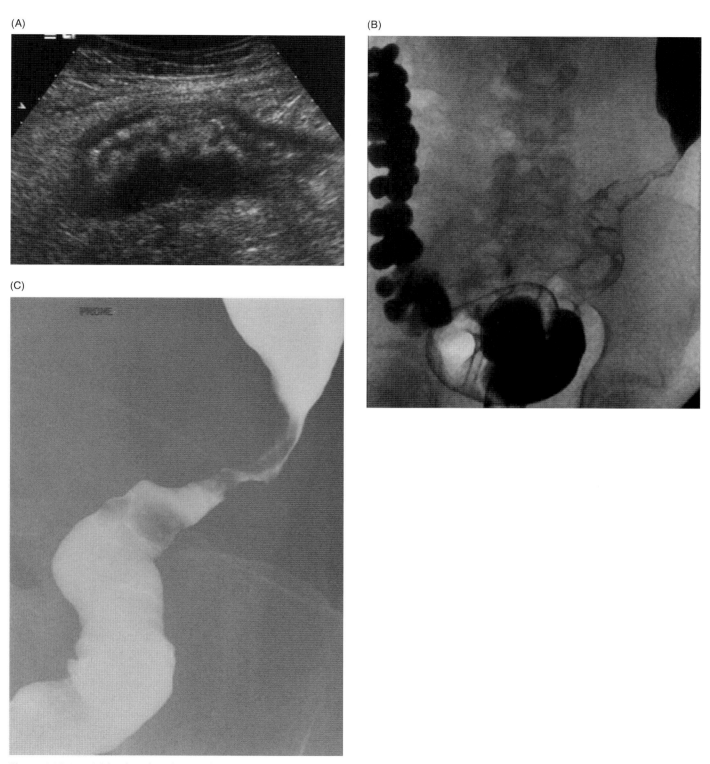

Figure 6.30 In a child with Crohn's disease, ultrasound (A) shows thickening of the colonic wall and echogenicity of the surrounding mesentery. (B), (C) Contrast enema shows a short segment stenosis in the mid-descending colon, with associated ulceration.

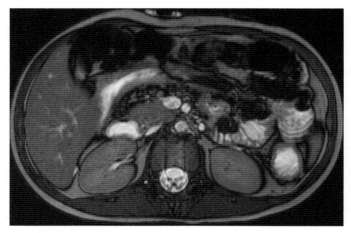

Figure 6.31 Axial fast T2-weighted MR (true FISP – fast imaging with steady state precession) in a child with inflammatory bowel disease shows a thickened and stenosed loop of bowel in the right upper quadrant.

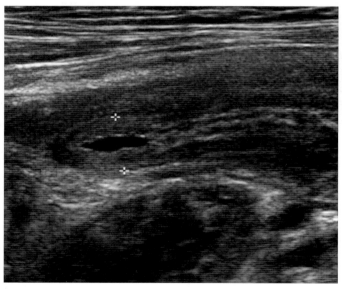

Figure 6.33 Ultrasound in a child with suspected appendicitis shows the fluid-filled, blind-ending appendix of 8 mm in diameter, which was noncompressible.

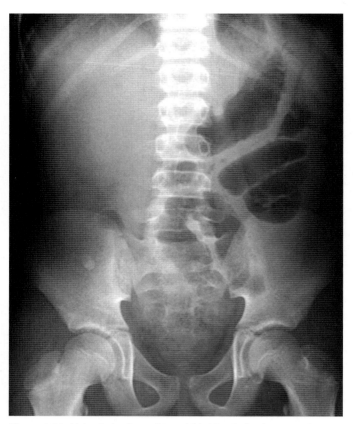

Figure 6.32 Abdominal radiograph in a child with right iliac fossa pain shows an appendicolith, paucity of bowel gas on the right side of the abdomen and prominent loops of bowel on the left, consistent with a diagnosis of appendicitis.

pattern of enhancement on T1 and bright bowel wall due to increased signal of water on T2WSE images suggesting active disease. MRI has also been shown to be superior to CT in assessing perianal complications of CD.

Appendicitis

Acute appendicitis is the most common cause of abdominal pain requiring surgery in children. Appendicitis is typically seen in older children (over two years) and young adults.

The role of imaging in appendicitis is to decrease negative laparotomy rates, decrease time to diagnosis, and identify alternative diagnoses.

"Typical" cases of appendicitis may be taken straight to theatre without any imaging. Abdominal radiographs may be normal (over 50% of cases) or may show an appendicolith (5–10%), air–fluid levels or a focally dilated loop of bowel (sentinel loop) in the

right lower quadrant (Figure 6.32). There may be loss of the right lower psoas margin or scoliosis concave to the right. Small bowel obstruction is common following perforation and a soft tissue mass may be seen in the RIF displacing loops of bowel. Free intraperitoneal gas is uncommon.

Ultrasound has the advantage of being cheap, radiation free and superior to other imaging modalities in the diagnosis of gynecological disease. It is, however, operator dependent and may be difficult in larger or more obese patients. Identification of the site of maximum tenderness by the patient can be of some help.

Using graded compression of the right lower quadrant, the inflamed appendix appears as a fluid-filled, noncompressible, blind-ending structure of 6 mm or more in diameter (Figure 6.33). In the early stages, an inner echogenic submucosal lining may be seen. In the transverse plane, the appendix may have a "target" appearance. Other findings include an appendicolith, pericecal or periappendiceal fluid or periappendiceal hyperechogenicity secondary to infiltration of the surrounding fat. Perforation is more difficult to assess on ultrasound, but focal periappendiceal or pelvic fluid collections or an inflammatory mass are suggestive (Figure 6.34).

CT scanning has become the imaging study of choice in some American centers due to its high sensitivity and specificity, lack of operator dependency, adequacy in obese patients and good performance in the evaluation of perforated appendicitis. It is very rarely used as an initial imaging tool in the

(A)

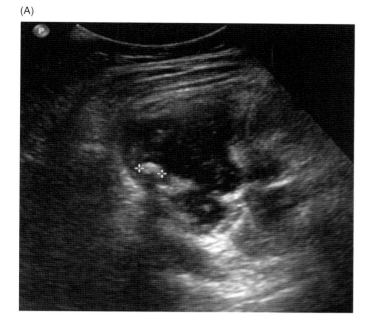

(B)

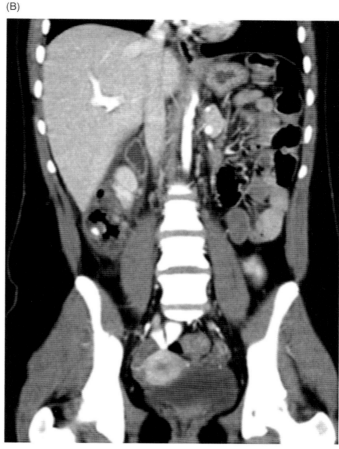

Figure 6.34 (A) Ultrasound and (B) contrast-enhanced coronal CT reformat in a child with suspected appendicitis show an inflammatory mass in the right iliac fossa with an appendicolith within it.

United Kingdom or Europe, due to the high radiation burden. The features seen on CT in acute appendicitis are similar to those described on ultrasound: an appendiceal diameter of 7 mm or greater, wall thickening and enhancement, an appendicolith, circumferential or focal apical cecal thickening, pericecal fat stranding, focal or free peritoneal fluid, mesenteric lymphadenopathy or an intraperitoneal phlegmon or abscess.

Pneumatosis intestinalis

Pneumatosis intestinalis (PI) is a radiological and pathological finding defined as the presence of gas within the bowel wall. Although the cause of PI is not fully understood, the most widely accepted theories are based on bacterial or mechanical causes. Outside the neonatal period, where it is seen in the context of necrotizing enterocolitis, PI is fairly uncommon. It has, however, been associated with a variety of disorders and procedures including transplantation, immunosuppressive medications, ischemia, inflammatory bowel disease, intestinal obstruction and obstructive airway disease. In addition, several concomitant infectious agents have been associated with the development of PI. Pneumatosis intestinalis may present in a variety of ways, ranging from an incidental finding that is clinically benign to an acute and life-threatening illness. It can

be demonstrated on plain film, ultrasound or CT and there may be associated portovenous gas (Figure 6.35).

Genitourinary tract infections

Urinary tract infections (UTIs)

Urinary tract infections are one of the most common childhood bacterial infections and invariably occur secondary to the ascension of periurethral and distal urethral flora. *Escherichia coli* is the commonest cause of first UTIs. Presentation in the neonate and infant is usually with unexplained fever, with or without other systemic symptoms. Older children with pyelonephritis often present with predominantly systemic symptoms, whereas those with cystitis may present with predominantly voiding symptoms.

There is ongoing discussion as to the exact role of imaging in UTI. The diagnosis can usually be made on the basis of clinical and laboratory findings, with the occasional need for imaging in the acute setting to localize infection or detect complications. Imaging is useful in identifying the presence of reflux, detecting renal scarring and identifying any underlying abnormalities of the renal tract, which may predispose to infection. Renal scarring is of concern as it is associated

(A)

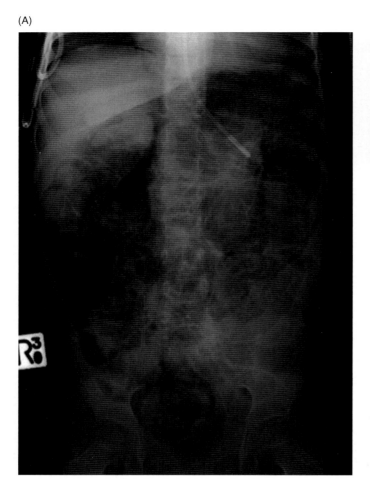

(B)

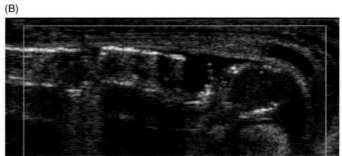

Figure 6.35 (A) Abdominal radiograph in a child with graft-versus-host disease after bone marrow transplant shows widespread pneumatosis intestinalis. (B) Ultrasound in a different child shows echogenicity in both the anterior and superior aspects of the bowel wall consistent with pneumatosis.

with increased risk of hypertension, progressive nephropathy and complications in pregnancies in the future.

Until recently, guidelines advised that imaging be undertaken in all cases of UTI, with ultrasound and either micturating cystourethrography (MCUG) or radionuclide cystography to detect anomalies or the presence of vesicoureteric reflux (VUR) (Figure 6.36).

There is evidence that recurrent renal infections and high-grade VUR are related to renal scarring. However, recent studies have challenged the assumption that prophylactic antibiotics prevent UTI and renal damage; they have also challenged the assumption that there is a relationship between VUR and renal scarring. The available studies are small and generally of poor quality, and a large randomized placebo-controlled trial is currently underway to try and address some of these questions.

Ultrasound is not as sensitive as other imaging modalities in the acute diagnosis of pyelonephritis, and the imaged kidney may appear ultrasonographically normal, or wedge-shaped areas of decreased perfusion may be demonstrated on Doppler ultrasound. Pyelonephritis-induced areas of ischemia and tubular dysfunction can be demonstrated on renal cortical scintigraphy, CT and magnetic resonance imaging.

On CT, signs of acute pyelonephritis include focal or diffuse swelling, loss of definition of the normal corticomedullary differentiation and wedge-shaped poorly enhancing regions. Renal abscesses are seen as rounded areas of parenchyma which fail to enhance.

DMSA studies in the acute phase demonstrate photopenia in the affected areas. The abnormalities may persist for many months following the UTI and therefore DMSA studies looking for scarring should be performed at least six months post-UTI (Figure 6.37).

Gadolinium-enhanced MRI has been shown to be at least as sensitive as DMSA in the diagnosis of pyelonephritis and has the advantage over DMSA of being able to differentiate pyelonephritis from renal scarring. Renal scarring is seen as an area of focal parenchymal loss. More recently, unenhanced sequences have been deemed sufficient for the diagnosis of renal scarring and differentiation from pyelonephritis.

Xanthogranulomatous pyelonephritis

Xanthogranulomatous pyelonephritis (XGP) is a chronic inflammatory kidney disease in which there is destruction and replacement of the renal parenchyma by granulomatous tissue

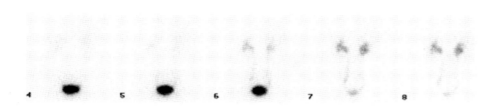

Figure 6.36 Indirect micturating cystourethrogram shows bilateral reflux into the ureters and collecting systems with bladder emptying.

(A)

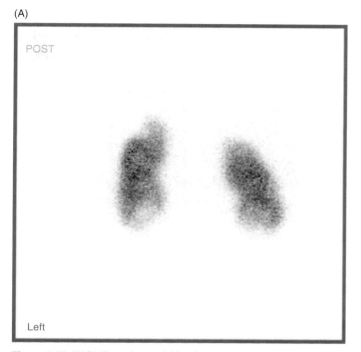

(B)

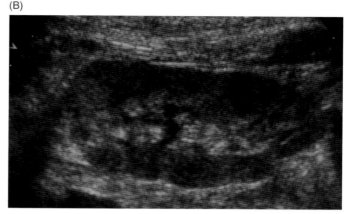

Figure 6.37 (A) DMSA study in a child with previous urinary tract infections and vesicoureteric reflux shows irregularity of the renal outline bilaterally with areas of associated photopenia, consistent with renal scarring. (B) Ultrasound in a different child shows irregularity of the renal contour and focal thinning of the parenchyma, particularly at the lower pole, indicating renal scarring.

containing histiocytes and foamy lipid-laden macrophages. Although rare in children, it is increasingly recognized in the pediatric population, usually in children less than eight years of age. The etiology of XGP is unknown but it is usually associated with urinary tract infections, obstruction and/or renal calculi. Bilateral renal involvement is rare.

Presentation is generally nonspecific with systemic symptoms, and blood tests demonstrate raised inflammatory markers and anemia.

Preoperative diagnosis can be difficult due to clinical and radiological similarities to malignancy, TB or renal abscess.

Plain films may demonstrate an enlarged kidney, renal calculus and renal parenchymal calcification.

Ultrasound findings include increased renal size, renal parenchyma of mixed echogenicity, renal calculus with posterior acoustic shadowing and echoes in a dilated collecting system (Figure 6.38).

Computed tomographic (CT) findings are often strongly suggestive of the diagnosis, with diffuse renal enlargement, a calcific density filling the pelvis and replacement of the renal parenchyma by dilated calyces and abscess cavities. The walls of the cavities may show strong enhancement post-contrast representing the surrounding vascular granulation tissue and compressed parenchyma. Extra-renal spread is common and is well demonstrated on CT. Fistulae have also been described.

MRI may be helpful in demonstrating the accumulated lipid-laden foamy macrophages which should be of high-intensity on T1WSE images due to the fat content.

Pyonephrosis

Pyonephrosis is the presence of infected material in the pelvicalyceal system, usually in association with obstruction. In children, the cause of the obstruction is often congenital, such as ureteropelvic junction (UPJ) obstruction, but can be acquired, for example secondary to renal calculi. Presentation is usually with signs and symptoms of UTI and a positive urine culture.

Plain films may show the presence of renal calculi but are otherwise unhelpful in the diagnosis. IVU is nonspecific with poor visualization of the affected kidney.

(A)

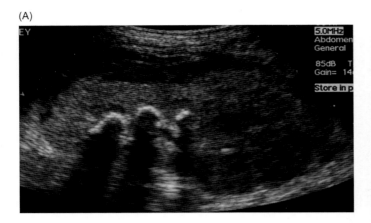

(B)

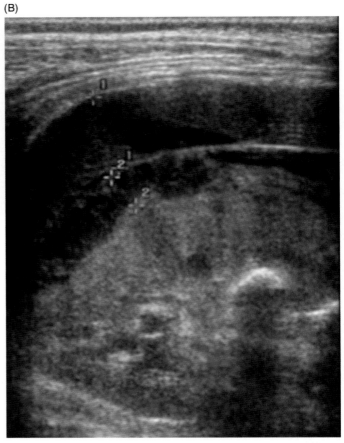

Figure 6.38 (A), (B) Renal ultrasound in a child with fever following multiple urinary tract infections shows a staghorn calculus, a heterogeneous, enlarged lower pole with loss of the normal parenchymal architecture and both subcapsular and extracapsular collections consistent with a diagnosis of xanthogranulomatous pyelonephritis.

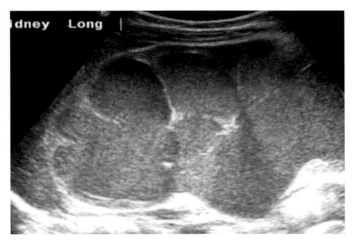

Figure 6.39 Ultrasound in a febrile child with positive urine dipstick and a ureteropelvic junction obstruction shows a dilated pelvicalyceal system containing echogenic fluid consistent with pyonephrosis.

Ultrasound is the imaging technique of choice, classically demonstrating a dilated pelvicalyceal system with coarse intraluminal echoes or a urine–debris level (Figure 6.39). However, the echogenicity of purulent fluid is variable and

ultrasound cannot be used to reliably distinguish sterile from infected fluid.

Fungal infections

Pediatric fungal urinary tract infections are not common but are seen in approximately 0.5% of premature neonates and in older immunocompromised children. *Candida albicans* is the most common pathogen, responsible for 80% of renal fungal infections.

Neonatal *Candida* UTI is thought to occur secondary to hematogenous spread from thrush or colonization of the GI tract, and associated candidemia is found in up to 50% of cases. Presentation varies from mild, nonspecific symptoms to anuric renal failure. "Fungal balls" within the collecting system are more common than parenchymal findings.

In both neonates and older children, ultrasound may be normal or may demonstrate "fungal balls" within the collecting system or, less commonly, parenchymal infiltration. "Fungal balls" are seen as non-shadow casting, echogenic foci within the pelvicalyceal system, and can cause obstruction of the collecting system (Figure 6.40). The differential for this appearance would include blood clot, tumor, necrotic

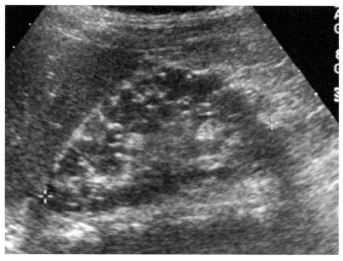

Figure 6.41 Renal ultrasound in a child with previous disseminated fungal infection shows multiple echogenic foci within the kidney consistent with calcification.

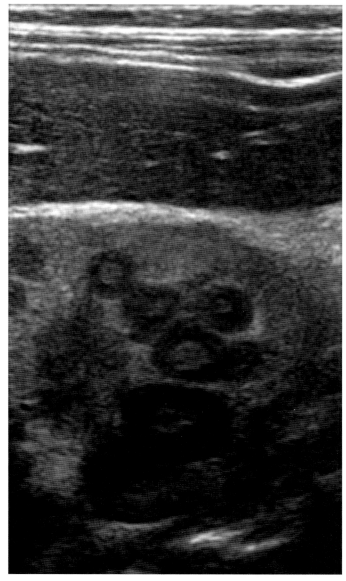

Figure 6.40 Ultrasound in a neutropenic child shows echogenic "fungal balls" within the renal collecting system.

sequestered papillae and nephrocalcinosis. The echogenic foci can persist despite clinical resolution of the fungal infection, leading to suggestions that the findings are sometimes either false positives or sterile aggregates of debris.

Ultrasound findings in renal parenchymal infiltration are nonspecific and are characterized by large, echogenic kidneys. Chronically, calcification may be seen (Figure 6.41).

Tuberculosis of the urinary tract

Genitourinary tract tuberculosis (GUTB) is uncommon in the western pediatric population; however, a rise has been documented in parallel with the spread of HIV-related illness. Presentation is often with vague symptoms and commonly not before 3–10 years after the primary infection. If the diagnosis is made early, cure is almost always possible; however, diagnosis is often delayed.

Radiological abnormalities in GUTB are reported to be as high as 90% and reflect the stage of the disease. Findings are often unilateral. Very acutely, imaging may be normal. With disease progression there is loss of renal parenchyma and the formation of dystrophic calcification, either small, poorly seen nodules or calcification of the whole kidney, which has undergone autonephrectomy. On either IVU or CT there may be delayed renal function and pooling of contrast within the parenchyma at sites of necrotic cavitation. The calyces can appear moth-eaten due to edema, which often precedes papillary necrosis.

Changes in the ureters are rare without visible renal disease. Initial mucosal irregularity progresses to nodularity and notching and there may be narrowing, straightening and a beaded appearance of the affected ureter. Low ureteral strictures can lead to hydroureteronephrosis.

The bladder initially demonstrates mucosal irregularity followed by bladder wall thickening, fibrosis and contraction, which can predispose to vesicoureteric reflux. Bladder wall calcification is rare in children.

Schistosomiasis

Schistosomiasis is a parasitic disease of the tropics which, although not commonly seen as a primary infection in the west, is an important diagnosis to be aware of due to foreign travel, increased immigration and the fact that diagnosis may not be made until a number of years after exposure.

The ova of *Schistosoma haematobium*, one of five described schistosoma fluke species, affect the urinary tract. The parasite's eggs penetrate the bladder and are excreted in the urine. Presentation is usually with urinary symptoms.

Early changes on ultrasound include thickening and nodularity of the bladder and distal ureteric walls, sometimes with resulting lower ureteric distension. The changes progress to nodularity and irregularly dilated lower ureters and then to involve the entire ureter with multiple strictures and dilatations. Involvement is always bilateral, but usually asymmetrical. Fine calcification can be seen in the bladder and ureteric walls (Figure 6.42). The calcification is of the ova in the submucosa and therefore, at least initially, bladder distension is not lost.

If not treated, there is fibrosis of the ureters and bladder wall, often with associated ureteric reflux and hydronephrosis. IVU is not commonly performed but depicts the changes described on ultrasound.

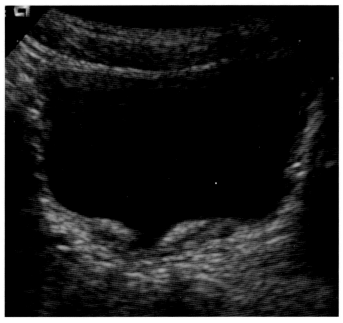

Figure 6.42 Ultrasound of the bladder shows plaques of calcification posteriorly within the bladder wall in a case of schistosomiasis.

Radiological improvement with treatment, particularly in the bladder, can be marked, especially in the early or subacute stages.

Epididymitis

Epididymitis is an inflammatory process, often of unknown cause, most common in boys 9 to 14 years old, but can be seen in younger children with underlying conditions such as Henoch-Schönlein purpura and Kawasaki disease. Although the onset of symptoms in epididymitis is usually more insidious than that of testicular torsion, epididymitis can present with acute scrotal pain and mimic testicular torsion, which must be diagnosed and treated within 6 to 10 hours to avoid loss of the affected testis.

The acutely painful scrotum therefore constitutes an imaging emergency, and ultrasound is the imaging modality of choice for evaluation of the acute scrotum. In testicular torsion, color Doppler demonstrates absence of flow or asymmetrically decreased flow within the affected testis (Figure 6.43). Demonstrating flow within normal testes may be difficult in children less than two years old. Early scanning may show hypoechogenicity of the affected testis when compared to the normal testis, followed later by hyperechogenicity.

Ultrasound findings in epididymitis (or epididymo-orchitis), in contrast to torsion, demonstrate asymmetric and often marked increased flow on Doppler ultrasound, with enlargement and hypoechogenicity of the epididymis (and testis). Reactive hydroceles are common (Figure 6.44).

Musculoskeletal infection and inflammation
Dermatomyositis

Juvenile dermatomyositis is the most common form of idiopathic inflammatory myopathy in childhood. The peak age distribution is between 5 and 14 years old. Presentation is with symptoms of progressive symmetric proximal muscle

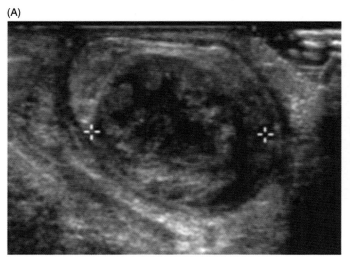

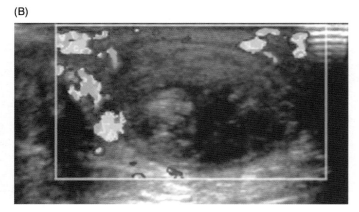

Figure 6.43 (A) Testicular ultrasound shows enlargement and heterogeneity of the testis with a necrotic center and (B) no flow on Doppler, consistent with a testicular torsion of a number of days standing.

(A)

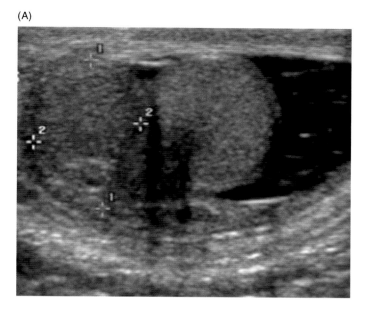

(B)

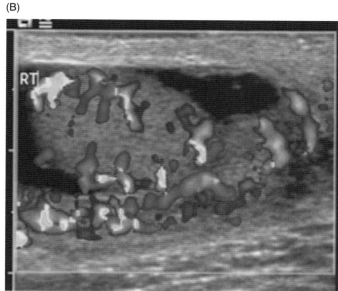

Figure 6.44 Epididymo-orchitis. (A) Testicular ultrasound shows enlargement and hypoechogenicity of the epididymis and a reactive hydrocele. (B) Increased flow is seen on Doppler in both the epididymis and testis.

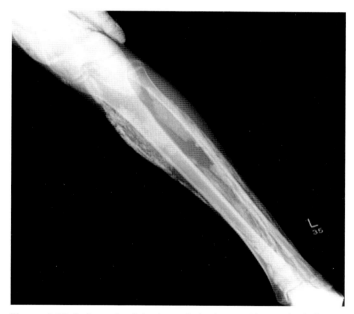

Figure 6.45 Radiograph of the lower limb shows widespread calcification within the visualized soft tissues, in a child with juvenile dermatomyositis.

weakness. Cutaneous findings include a characteristic facial rash and scaly erythematous papules (Gottron's papules) over the small joints on the dorsum of the hands. Muscle enzymes are typically raised.

Soft tissue calcification is seen in 30–70% of patients and may be related to duration of disease. It typically occurs at sites exposed to trauma such as the buttocks, elbows and knees.

The calcification is best demonstrated on plain film or CT (Figure 6.45). On MRI it may be less conspicuous, appearing as areas of signal void on T1- and T2-weighted images, and may enhance on some gradient echo sequences.

Imaging with MR demonstrates abnormal high signal in the affected muscles and fascia on fat-saturated T2-weighted and short tau inversion-recovery (STIR) sequences (Figure 6.46). The findings are nonspecific. In patients with skin involvement, reticulated areas of increased T2 signal may be seen in the subcutaneous fat.

With chronic muscle atrophy, fatty infiltration of the muscles will be apparent on T1W images.

Osteomyelitis

Acute osteomyelitis

The majority of cases of acute osteomyelitis in children are secondary to hematogenous spread from a known focus, or associated with a predisposing condition such as an immune system disorder. It can also be seen secondary to an acute penetrating injury or spread from adjacent tissues.

In children of more than one year old, osteomyelitis initially affects the metaphysis, due to the reduced rate of blood flow in the metaphyseal vessels, from where it spreads. Presentation is with pain, refusal to weight bear and signs of systemic toxicity, and the most common causative organism is *Staphylococcus aureus*.

Under one year of age, nutrient vessels still penetrate the physis, allowing spread of infection into the epiphyses and joints, and osteomyelitis and septic arthritis, therefore, often coexist. Neonates are more prone to multifocal disease than older children, with β-hemolytic streptococcus and *Escherichia coli* the most common causative organisms. Presentation may be very nonspecific.

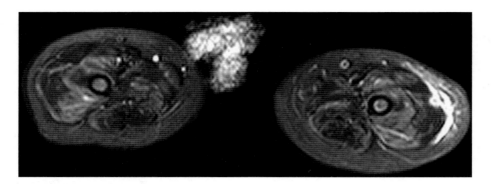

Figure 6.46 Axial T2-weighted MR in a child with proximal muscle weakness shows increased signal in all the muscle groups and involvement of the muscular fascia of the lateral thigh in a child with juvenile dermatomyositis.

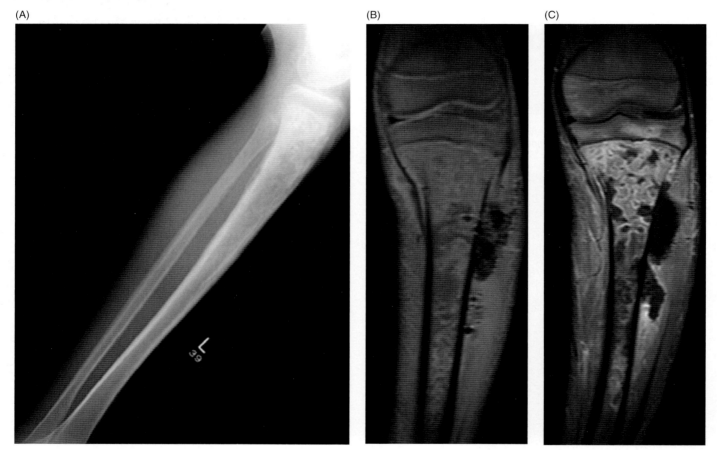

(A)   (B)   (C)

Figure 6.47 Tibial osteomyelitis. (A) Radiograph shows an aggressive lesion in the proximal left tibial metaphysis with a moth-eaten appearance, wide zone of transition and associated periosteal reaction. Coronal (B) pre- and (C) post-contrast T1-weighted MR shows extensive metadiaphyseal inflammation extending into the soft tissues (the low signal area adjacent to the superolateral aspect of the tibia is surgical packing).

Within 48 hours of infection, deep soft tissue swelling may be evident with obliteration of fat planes. In a neonate with associated septic arthritis there may be widening of the joint space with or without subluxation. Bone destruction and periosteal reaction only become evident on plain film by day 10–14. If treated early, radiographic findings may never develop.

In experienced hands, ultrasound may be helpful in making the diagnosis, initially with detection of deep soft tissue swelling, followed by a thin layer of fluid beneath the periosteum, then subperiosteal collections and cortical erosions. Associated joint effusions may also be demonstrated.

On skeletal scintigraphy, a well-defined area of increased uptake is demonstrated within the bone on both early and delayed images, and is often positive as early as 24 hours after onset of symptoms. If the infection is severe enough to cause compromise to the metaphyseal blood flow, an area of photopenia may be seen on scintigraphy. Scintigraphy is also very useful for detecting multiple foci of infection.

On MRI, acute osteomyelitis has low signal intensity on T1 and high signal intensity on T2 and STIR images. The degree of bony involvement may be overestimated as areas of associated reactive inflammation return a similar signal.

Marrow infection enhances following the administration of intravenous gadolinium, and collections can be identified by peripheral enhancement with a low-signal center. MR is helpful in defining the extent of soft tissue and cartilaginous involvement (Figure 6.47).

CT scans may show an increase in density in the marrow cavity caused by the accumulation of purulent material, blood and debris.

Chronic osteomyelitis

Chronic osteomyelitis is a low-grade, recurrent infection characterized by bone sclerosis, Brodie abscess, sequestra and sinus tracts. A Brodie abscess is a focal area of chronic osteomyelitis that may develop *de novo* or in the site of a previous acute osteomyelitis, and contains fluid but not purulent material. Patients may have a history of months or years of recurrent pain, swelling and erythema. The most common causative agent is *Staphylococcus aureus*. A sequestrum is an area of devitalized bone surrounded by the inflammatory process. It appears as a fragment of bone within a region of marrow infection or Brodie abscess. A sinus tract may be seen on imaging as a channel between an area of marrow infection and cortex or subcutaneous tissues.

Imaging demonstrates an area of bone destruction surrounded by reactive bone formation with enhancement of the periphery on post-contrast CT or MRI. CT may be more useful in chronic osteomyelitis than acute, where it is superior to MRI for demonstrating cortical destruction, air and sequestra.

The late sequelae of osteomyelitis include bony bridge formation, producing early physeal fusion and limb deformity, pseudoarthrosis and joint dislocations.

Discitis and vertebral osteomyelitis

Infection of the intervertebral disc (discitis) and vertebral osteomyelitis are both relatively uncommon in children. Discitis generally affects children under the age of five years and is almost always lumbar, presenting with refusal to walk or progressive limp and a normal temperature or low-grade fever. Radiographic changes are seen at two to three weeks, with joint space narrowing and variable degrees of destruction of the adjacent vertebral endplates (Figure 6.48).

Vertebral osteomyelitis typically affects older children who present with back pain, in the lumbar, thoracic or cervical regions, and are usually febrile. Radiographs initially demonstrate osteopenia of one affected vertebral body which progresses to destruction, usually of the anterior portion, and osteophytic bridging.

Bone scintigraphy is more sensitive than radiography in the early stages of disease and may be of use in cases with high clinical suspicion and normal radiographs (Figure 6.49).

MRI is particularly useful in assessing the extent of soft tissue and cartilaginous involvement and to look for complications, such as abscess formation. The degree of bony involvement may be overestimated as active inflammation

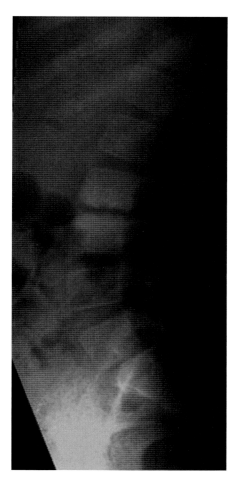

Figure 6.48 Lateral lumbar spine radiograph shows decreased L2–3 joint space with irregularity and sclerosis of the adjacent vertebral bodies consistent with a discitis.

and infection will both be of low signal on T1-weighted images and high signal on T2-weighted and STIR images.

Tuberculous osteomyelitis

Tuberculous osteomyelitis results either from contiguous spread from an adjacent joint or from hematogenous spread, usually from the lungs. It most commonly affects the vertebrae, then large joints and then tubular and flat bones. TB produces a chronic inflammatory reaction in bone more like chronic than acute pyogenic osteomyelitis.

Imaging findings include osteolysis, peripherally located erosions, periarticular osteoporosis and gradual joint space narrowing. Unlike pyogenic osteomyelitis, periosteal new bone formation and subperiosteal involvement are minimal or absent. There may be soft tissue extension with abscess formation.

Congenital infections

Transplacentally acquired infections, which include toxoplasmosis, syphilis, rubella, cytomegalovirus and herpes simplex (TORCH infections) can cause trophic disturbance in the bones, seen in up to 50% of cases. On plain films there is metaphyseal lucency and fraying and longitudinal radiolucent and sclerotic

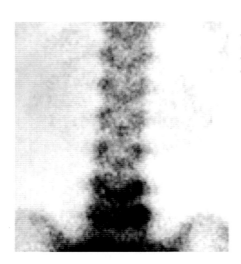

Figure 6.49 Bone scintigraphy shows increased uptake in the L3 and L4 vertebral bodies consistent with discitis.

lines, likened to a "celery stalk." Periosteal reaction is rare and the bones usually return to normal within six months.

Bony changes are seen in up to 95% of cases of congenital syphilis but often do not appear until six to eight weeks after the time of infection. Findings include nonspecific metaphyseal lucent bands and periosteal reaction involving multiple long bones. The Wimberger corner sign is the most specific finding of syphilis and consists of destruction of the medial portion of the proximal metaphysis of the tibia, resulting in an area of triangular lucency (Figure 6.50).

Chronic recurrent multifocal osteomyelitis

Chronic recurrent multifocal osteomyelitis (CRMO) is a multifocal osteomyelitis characterized by bone pain and sometimes fever and swelling. The cause is unknown but it is thought likely to be either due to occult infection or an autoimmune disorder. It has an unpredictable course of exacerbations and remissions and is sometimes associated with other inflammatory conditions such as pustulosis palmoplantaris and psoriasis. The diagnosis is made on the basis of clinical criteria and is often one of exclusion.

The skeletal involvement is multifocal and may be symmetric involving the metaphyses of tubular bones. The commonest sites involved include the distal tibia, distal femur, proximal tibia and clavicle.

Plain films demonstrate an irregular osteolytic lesion and surrounding sclerosis with minimal periostitis and cortical thickening. Nuclear scintigraphy shows increased uptake of tracer and may detect clinically silent lesions.

The lesions are of low signal intensity on T1W MRI images and high intensity on T2W images. More chronic lesions with intense sclerosis may show decreased signal on T2 images (Figure 6.51).

Septic arthritis

As with osteomyelitis, septic arthritis can arise as a result of hematogenous spread, penetrating injury or extension of

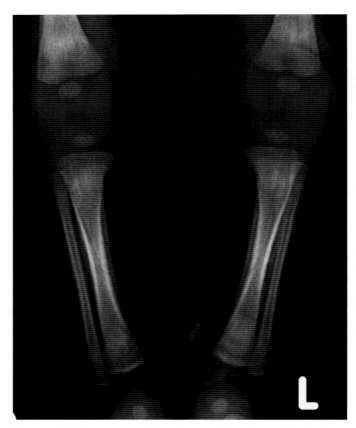

Figure 6.50 Radiograph of the lower limbs in an infant shows periosteal reaction and the "Wimberger" corner sign in the tibiae, and a "celery stalk" appearance of the metaphyses in congenital syphilis. (Kindly donated by Dr. T. Kilborn, Red Cross War Memorial Children's Hospital, Cape Town.)

infection from a focus of osteomyelitis. In neonates, the most common organism is group B *Streptococcus*, and in infants and older children *Staphylococcus aureus*. Presentation in neonates can be very nonspecific but in older children is with fever, pain and lack of movement in the affected extremity.

In early septic arthritis, plain films are often normal, even if there is a small joint effusion, but with increase in effusion size, the joint space widens and may cause displacement of the bone. In the hip, asymmetry of the distance from the medial metaphysis of the femoral neck to the "teardrop" of the acetabulum of 2 mm or more on a nonrotated film suggests joint effusion. In the elbows and knees there may be displacement of the fat pads.

Ultrasound is a sensitive method of detecting joint effusions. In the hip, the normal joint capsule parallels the anterior cortex of the femoral neck and has a concave configuration (Figure 6.52). The distance from the anterior capsule to the bone is normally less than 3 mm. With an effusion, the capsule bulges anteriorly and is convex rather than concave (Figure 6.53). A difference in capsule-to-bone distance of more than 2 mm between the two hips is said to be significant. The echogenicity

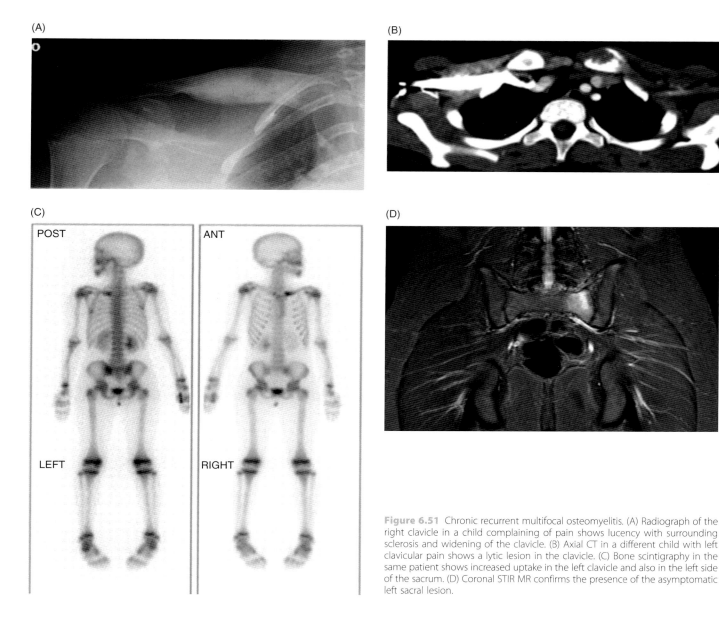

Figure 6.51 Chronic recurrent multifocal osteomyelitis. (A) Radiograph of the right clavicle in a child complaining of pain shows lucency with surrounding sclerosis and widening of the clavicle. (B) Axial CT in a different child with left clavicular pain shows a lytic lesion in the clavicle. (C) Bone scintigraphy in the same patient shows increased uptake in the left clavicle and also in the left side of the sacrum. (D) Coronal STIR MR confirms the presence of the asymptomatic left sacral lesion.

of the fluid is variable and cannot be used to distinguish sterile from infected fluid.

If not treated promptly, complications may ensue, including: osteomyelitis, epiphyseal separation, joint destruction, ankylosis and osteonecrosis of the epiphysis. MRI may be of use in these more complicated cases (Figure 6.54).

Juvenile idiopathic arthritis

Juvenile idiopathic arthritis (JIA), also known as juvenile rheumatoid arthritis (JRA) and juvenile chronic arthritis (JCA), is a chronic inflammatory arthritis of unknown etiology. Pathologically there is chronic inflammation and synovial proliferation. Some 85% of cases are seronegative, and the remainder, seropositive. Classification is complex.

Initial radiographs may be normal or may reflect the acute inflammatory response that accompanies synovial hypertrophy. This can cause soft tissue swelling, periarticular osteopenia and epiphyseal remodeling and widening. Prolonged synovial proliferation will lead to loss of cartilage and bone damage seen as loss of joint space and erosive change along the joint margins on plain films. Progressive damage can eventually lead to bony ankylosis (Figure 6.55). The radiographic changes of chronic JIA are relatively slow to develop and there is significant interobserver variability in their interpretation.

Sonographic evaluation of joint swelling is quick, inexpensive and does not involve radiation. It may be difficult in younger children due to lack of compliance or because of difficulty obtaining a satisfactory acoustic window. Ultrasound can detect effusions, synovial thickening and synovial cysts.

Distinction between fluid and thickened synovium is usually possible (Figure 6.56). Serial US is useful in monitoring disease activity and in evaluating response to therapy. In chronic disease, erosions and thinning of the articular cartilage can be detected. The disadvantage of ultrasound is that, particularly in larger joints, visualization of the whole articular surface may not be possible.

Ongoing advances in MR imaging are allowing increasingly improved assessment of joint disease in JIA, and MRI is superior to both plain films and sonography in the detection of inflammatory changes in the joint and cartilage

damage. Erosions appear as well-circumscribed lesions that are hypointense on T1W and hyperintense on T2W images. They will often show marked enhancement post-contrast.

Normal synovium is of low signal on both T1 and T2W images, less than 2 mm thick, smooth in outline with some

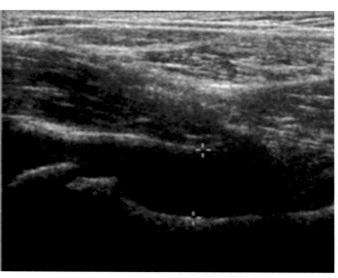

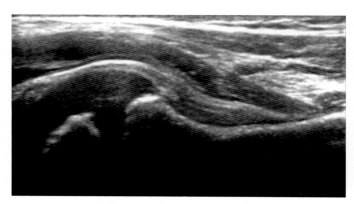

Figure 6.52 Normal ultrasound of the hip with a concave configuration of the joint capsule paralleling the anterior cortex of the femoral neck.

Figure 6.53 Ultrasound shows an anechoic hip effusion with convexity of the bulging joint capsule.

(A)

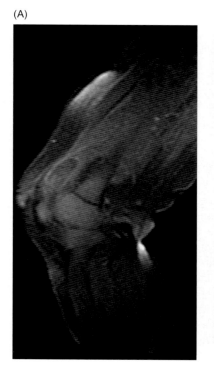

(B)

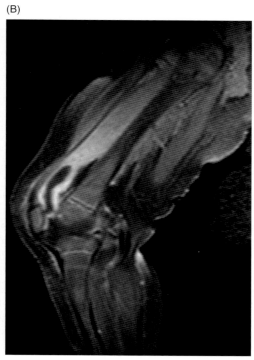

Figure 6.54 (A) Pre- and (B) post-contrast sagittal MR of the knee in a child with septic arthritis shows joint effusion, enhancement of the joint capsule and soft tissue edema involving the quadriceps muscles.

enhancement following contrast administration. Abnormally inflamed synovium is thickened and irregular. It is of low–intermediate signal on T1 and high signal on T2 with a similar intensity to a joint effusion on standard T1 and T2 spin echo (SE) sequences. The best method of differentiating synovial thickening from effusion is the use of gadolinium-enhanced sequences with fat saturation to reduce signal from adjacent fatty marrow. Inflamed synovium enhances rapidly post-contrast, whereas fibrous inactive synovium enhances poorly (Figure 6.57).

The use of T1W spoiled gradient echo volume acquisition sequences allows images to be analyzed using multiplanar reformatting with very thin slices. Cartilage resolution is good and of high signal with defects appearing as low signal change.

Human immunodeficiency virus

Human immunodeficiency virus/acquired immune deficiency syndrome (HIV/AIDS) in the pediatric population is usually acquired through vertical transmission. There is a spectrum of clinical presentation with some children progressing rapidly to AIDS-defining conditions within the first two years of life and others remaining healthy with few or no symptoms of HIV disease by eight years of age. Due to improved anti-retroviral therapy and prevention of opportunistic infections, there has been a marked improvement in overall prognosis and length of survival. The manifestations of AIDS in children are mainly pulmonary and gastrointestinal tract infections. Central nervous system infections are much less common than in adults, and neurological disorders in children are mainly due to HIV itself. Tumors are also less common than in the adult HIV population but can occur and include lymphomas and smooth muscle tumors.

Chest disease

Pulmonary disease is the most common clinical manifestation of AIDS in infants and children and is the primary cause of death in 50% of children with AIDS. Important causes of acute pneumonia in HIV-infected children include pneumococci, gram-negative bacteria and staphylococci, *Pneumocystis carinii* pneumonia (PCP) and cytomegalovirus (CMV), particularly in infants, and pulmonary tuberculosis (TB) in regions endemic

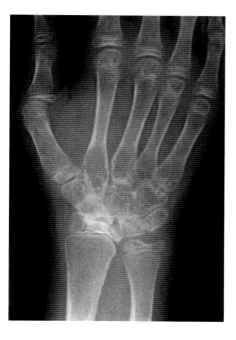

Figure 6.55 Wrist radiograph in a child with chronic juvenile idiopathic arthritis shows loss of joint space, particularly at the carpal bones, erosions and probable bony ankylosis with associated periarticular osteopenia.

(A)

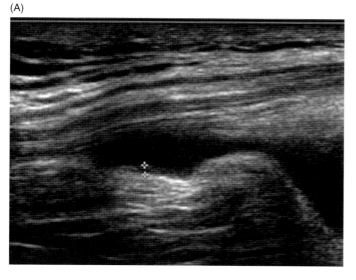

(B)

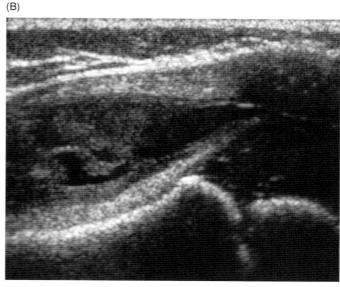

Figure 6.56 Ultrasound of the knee in juvenile idiopathic arthritis shows (A) early changes with mild synovial thickening (between the markers) and a small effusion within the suprapatellar pouch and (B) progression of disease, with significant synovial thickening.

(A)

(B)

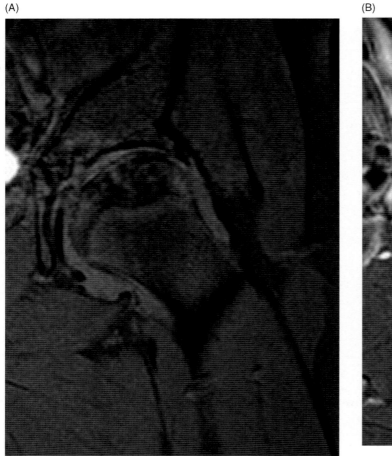 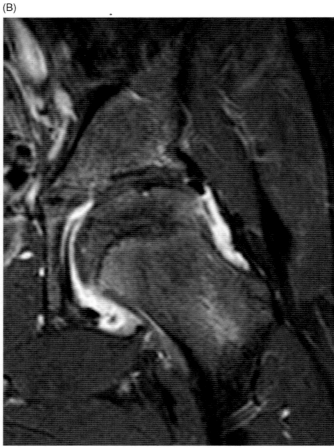

Figure 6.57 (A) Pre- and (B) post-contrast coronal MR of the hip in a child with juvenile idiopathic arthritis shows thickened, irregular synovium with avid enhancement post-contrast.

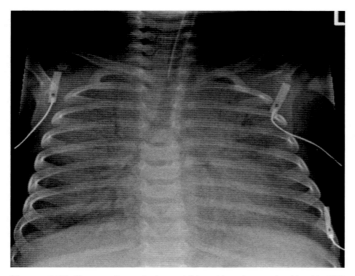

Figure 6.58 Chest radiograph in an HIV-positive six-month-old with PCP shows hyperinflation of the lungs and diffuse bilateral consolidation.

for TB/HIV. With improving survival, chronic pulmonary disease is becoming more common, with important causes including lymphocytic interstitial pneumonia (LIP), chronic infections, immune reconstitution inflammatory syndrome (IRIS), bronchiectasis, malignancies and interstitial pneumonitis. Chronic lung disease may also result from recurrent or persistent pneumonia.

Bacterial pneumonias

Streptococcus pneumoniae and *Haemophilus influenzae* are the most common infecting organisms, although, often, multiple organisms are isolated and infections with unusual bacteria such as *Salmonella* spp. also occur. The chest radiograph usually demonstrates a focal or lobar pneumonia; however, multilobar involvement and diffuse disease are more common than in the normal pediatric population. There is frequently associated adenopathy, effusion or empyema.

PCP is often the initial manifestation of HIV, particularly in infants, and is the leading pulmonary cause of death. Radiographic appearances are variable and include hyperinflation

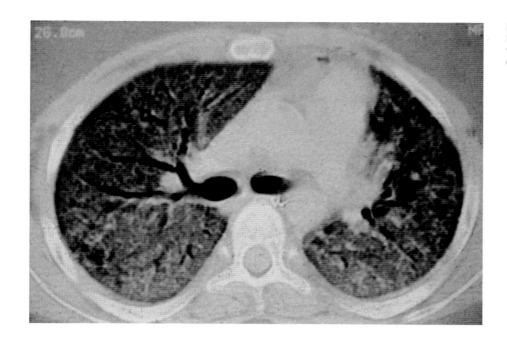

Figure 6.59 HRCT in an HIV-positive child with PCP shows bilateral ground-glass opacification with interlobular septal thickening and cystic change.

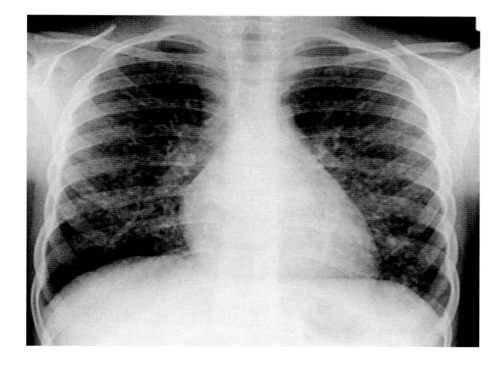

Figure 6.60 Chest radiograph in an HIV-positive child shows bilateral nodular infiltrate consistent with lymphocytic interstitial pneumonitis.

with diffuse bilateral interstitial or nodular infiltrates and widespread alveolar shadowing (Figure 6.58). Asymmetric, focal or patchy infiltrates are also common and cavitatory nodules and cysts are seen in up to a third of patients. Complication with pneumothorax is common. Lymphadenopathy and effusions are uncommon.

HRCT findings include patchy or diffuse ground-glass opacity, consolidation, cysts or cavities, centrilobular opacities, nodules and interlobular septal thickening (Figure 6.59).

Lymphocytic interstitial pneumonitis

Lymphocytic interstitial pneumonitis (LIP) occurs in approximately one-third of infected children and is thought to represent a direct "hyperimmune" lung response to the presence of either HIV or Epstein-Barr virus (EBV).

Radiographic appearances include interstitial reticulo-nodular infiltrates which may progress to patchy airspace opacification (Figure 6.60). Lymphadenopathy is common and often becomes more prominent during episodes of

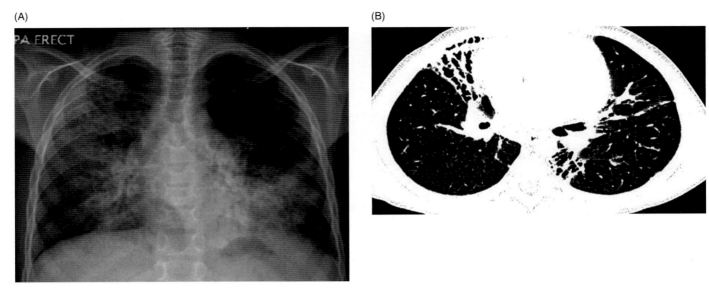

Figure 6.61 (A) Chest radiograph in a child with chronic LIP and intercurrent infection shows reticulonodular shadowing throughout and bilateral consolidation. (B) HRCT in the same patient shows consolidation and bronchiectasis in the right middle lobe and medial segment of the left lower lobe with interstitial nodular infiltrate and some interseptal lobular thickening.

super-added infection. LIP may persist for years and often results in fibrosis and atelectasis with secondary traction bronchiectasis (Figure 6.61). Regression of changes can be seen either as a consequence of treatment or as part of disease progression. HRCT features include poorly defined centrilobular nodules typically of ground-glass density, diffuse ground-glass opacification, interlobular septal thickening and thickening of the bronchovascular interstitium.

Viral infections

Viral infections may result from primary infection or reactivation of a latent virus, and include respiratory syncytial virus (RSV), influenza and parainfluenza viruses, cytomegalovirus (CMV) and occasionally measles and varicella-zoster virus (VZV).

HIV-infected children with VZV often present with a more protracted illness than immunocompetent controls, and the risk of complications increases with increasing immunological impairment. In children with AIDS, the mortality rate is 15%.

The chest radiograph typically shows bilateral diffuse reticulonodular infiltrates which vary in size between 3 and 10 mm and may coalesce, resulting in areas of consolidation. Superimposed bacterial infection is common.

Mycobacterium tuberculosis

TB can occur at any stage of HIV infection and in children usually occurs as a result of primary infection.

Radiological features are similar to those in immunocompetent children and include lobar consolidation, segmental or lobar atelectasis, pleural effusions and lymphadenopathy. Pulmonary cavitation is uncommon. Large-volume lymphadenopathy, most commonly in the paratracheal and hilar regions, is a frequent finding. Occasionally, the chest radiograph may appear normal. Miliary disease is uncommon but, when it does occur, may be indistinguishable from LIP.

Contrast-enhanced CT is invaluable for imaging mediastinal lymphadenopathy, which is typically of large volume and demonstrates peripheral enhancement.

Miliary TB is best imaged on HRCT, which demonstrates the small 1–3 mm nodular infiltrates. Definite distinction between miliary TB, LIP and CMV is not always possible radiologically.

Gastrointestinal tract disease

Gastrointestinal symptoms, caused primarily by opportunistic enteric infections and lymphoproliferative and neoplastic disease, occur in approximately 50% of European and North American children with AIDS.

Esophagus

Esophageal disease in HIV-infected children usually presents as odynophagia and dysphagia. *Candida albicans* is the most common causative organism, followed by CMV and HSV.

Imaging is ideally with a double-contrast esophagogram to detect the fine mucosal lesions seen in *Candida* esophagitis; however, this is not always practical in children. Barium studies demonstrate mucosal edema, plaque formation and eventually deep ulceration. A shaggy, or cobblestone, appearance is seen as barium fills the spaces between the irregular plaques. Pseudodiverticulae may also be seen. *Candida* tends to involve the entire esophagus, whereas CMV is usually focal, commonly affecting the distal esophagus. CMV may cause large ulcers in an otherwise normal esophagus or may cause linear ulcers, nodular thickening, a cobblestone appearance, pseudodiverticulae or strictures.

Either infection may be seen as thickening of the esophageal wall on CT.

HSV usually causes focal esophageal involvement with shallow ulceration. The ulcers are often diamond shaped or stellate.

TB may affect the esophagus via transmural inflammation or sinus/fistula formation from infected mediastinal lymph nodes.

Stomach

Opportunistic infections rarely affect the stomach in HIV-infected children; however, CMV may do so, most commonly at the gastroesophageal junction or in the antropyloric region. Features include deep or aphthous ulceration, submucosal masses secondary to edema, abscesses and perforation.

Thickened gastric folds are a common finding in the stomachs of HIV-infected children and may be secondary to cryptosporidiosis, *Helicobacter pylori* infection or a lymphoproliferative disorder known as gut-associated lymphoid tissue (GALT) which may be part of the disseminated infiltrative lymphocytosis syndrome (like LIP in the chest).

Duodenum and small intestine

Chronic or recurrent diarrhea affects 40–60% of children with AIDS. Stool cultures are often negative for microorganisms, but positive results are often due to common bacterial GI tract pathogens such as *Salmonella, Shigella* and *Campylobacter. Mycobacterium avium intracellulare* (MAI) and TB rarely cause enteritis, being more likely to affect the liver, spleen and mesenteric nodes in the abdomen. Other diarrheal-causing pathogens include *Clostridium difficile, Giardia, Cryptosporidium* and *Isospora belli.*

Features of *Cryptosporidium* on barium study include thickened folds, fragmentation of barium, intestinal spasm and dilatation and mucosal atrophy with the proximal bowel most commonly involved. Nodes are rarely involved. These features are not specific, and *Giardia, Strongyloides, Candida* and gut-associated lymphoid tissue should also be considered.

CMV enteritis can be very severe and lead to ischemic necrosis and perforation seen as pneumatosis intestinalis or free intraperitoneal air.

Although rare, when MAI affects the small bowel it causes a pseudo-Whipple-like condition, with fine nodularity and fold thickening demonstrated on CT and barium follow-through. The mid- and distal small intestine are most commonly involved, whereas *Cryptosporidium* usually involves the more proximal small bowel. MAI will often have associated liver and spleen and mesenteric and retroperitoneal lymph node involvement. Nodes may demonstrate a central area of low attenuation representing necrosis.

Colon and rectum

Shigella and *Salmonella* frequently affect the colon in HIV-infected children but often without severe consequence. CMV, however, can be a devastating colonic infection and is blamed for most of the colonic complications described in children with AIDS, such as typhlitis, pneumatosis, strictures, toxic megacolon and perforation. CMV involves the colon much more commonly than the small bowel.

Radiological features of mild infection include thickened folds, mucosal granularity, spasm (especially cecal) and ulceration. In severe infections, findings include large ulcers, strictures, nodular filling defects and submucosal hemorrhage. CT scan shows thickened bowel wall or a target sign representing a transverse segment of bowel with mucosal edema. The typhlitis-like picture of cecal and ileal inflammation can mimic MAI or TB infection; however, the latter two more commonly demonstrate clusters of associated pericecal nodes.

Pseudomembranous colitis secondary to *Clostridium difficile* results in ulceration and sloughing of mucosal pseudomembranes. CT findings can be identical to those of CMV, but pseudomembranous colitis usually involves the whole colon, whereas CMV is more commonly segmental with less pronounced colonic wall thickening.

Lymph nodes and abdominal cavity

In children, the most common malignant tumor of the gastrointestinal tract is lymphoma, usually of the B-cell non-Hodgkin's type. Other sites of involvement include the liver, adrenal glands, lower genitourinary tract, spleen, peritoneum, omentum and pancreas.

Imaging studies demonstrate enlarged lymph nodes with central low attenuation suggestive of necrosis. The liver and spleen may contain hypoechoic focal lesions, usually of more than 2 cm in diameter, and a variable degree of hepatosplenomegaly (Figure 6.62). CT of the bowel involvement shows diffuse or focal bowel wall thickening or eccentric masses. Ascites is occasionally seen.

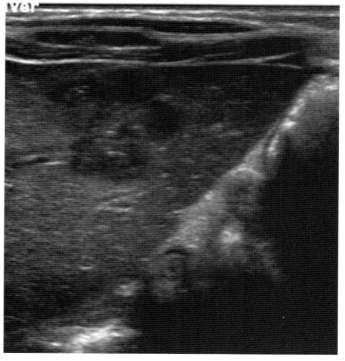

Figure 6.62 Hypoechoic foci in the liver of an HIV-positive child with B-cell non-Hodgkin's lymphoma.

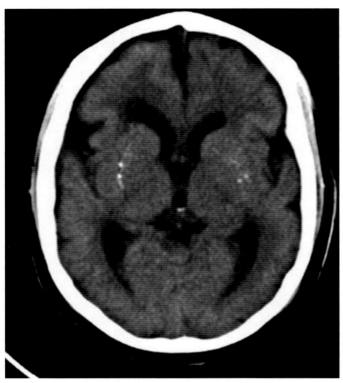

Figure 6.63 Axial CT in a nine-year-old with congenital HIV shows microcephaly, bilateral putaminal calcification, a coarse gyral pattern in the frontal lobes in keeping with cortical malformation, and periventricular white matter low density in keeping with HIV encephalopathy.

Central nervous system disease
HIV encephalopathy

HIV encephalopathy is divided into two major neurological syndromes: progressive encephalopathy, which manifests as a stepwise deterioration of mental status and higher functioning, and static encephalopathy, where the child has better higher functions but does not keep up with age-appropriate milestones. On CT, there is prominence of the subarachnoid spaces and ventricles (secondary to atrophy) and calcification of the basal ganglia and subcortical white matter (Figure 6.63). Subcortical calcification is most common in the frontal lobes.

On MRI, there is diffuse atrophy and commonly bifrontal white matter abnormalities (Figure 6.64). Mild atrophy is associated with static encephalopathy, and severe atrophy with progressive encephalopathy. Antiretroviral therapy may reverse some of the atrophic changes. The white matter lesions have no mass effect and are of low signal on T1-weighted MRI and high signal on T2. They do not enhance post-contrast. The differential diagnosis includes progressive multifocal leukoencephalopathy (PML), lymphoma and toxoplasmosis.

Cranial calcifications

Up to a third of HIV-infected children have basal ganglia calcification on imaging, with 90% showing a calcific vasculitis at autopsy. The calcification is usually bilateral and symmetrical involving the globus pallidus and putamen. The subcortical frontal white matter and cerebellum may also calcify.

(A)

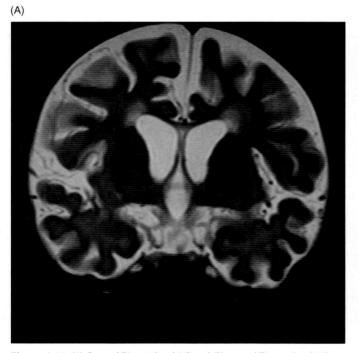

(B)

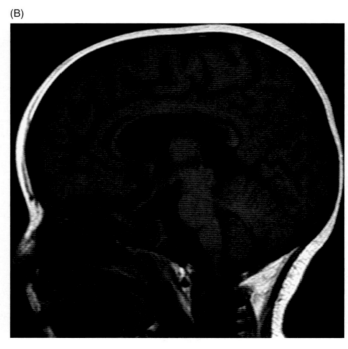

Figure 6.64 (A) Coronal T2-weighted MR and (B) sagittal T1-weighted MR images in an HIV-positive child show marked cerebral atrophy with loss of white matter bulk consistent with HIV encephalopathy.

(A)

(B)

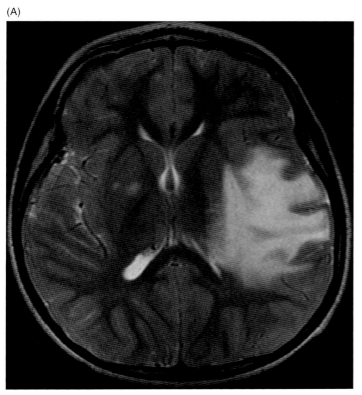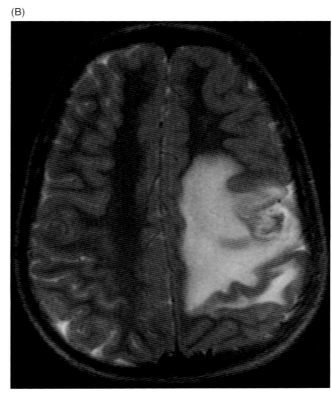

Figure 6.65 Axial T2-weighted MR images in an HIV-positive child show (A) high signal lesions in the right lentiform nucleus and (B) an irregular frontal corticomedullary lesion with marked surrounding vasogenic edema and central hypointensity consistent with toxoplasmosis.

Calcification related to HIV is not usually seen before 10 months of age.

Malignancies

HIV-associated malignancies are less common in children than in adults. The most common is a high-grade B-cell lymphoma associated with EBV and can be primary or metastatic. It usually arises in the periventricular white matter, basal ganglia or corpus callosum and can be multifocal or involve cranial nerves. It may also be associated with LIP and GALT.

Primary lymphoma is commonly hypodense on unenhanced CT, with uniform enhancement post-contrast. A peripheral location, associated hemorrhage and ring enhancement are also common. Mass effect may be less than expected for the size of the lesion. Lymphomatous meningitis is less common and is associated with extracranial lymphoma. Differentiation from toxoplasmosis can be difficult. Lesions in the corpus callosum suggest lymphoma.

Cerebrovascular disease

Pediatric HIV patients have a 1% annual risk of developing cerebrovascular disease ranging from arterial stenoses to aneurysmal dilatation and which may be due to the primary effects of HIV or secondary to opportunistic infections. In the acute stages, diffusion-weighted MR images are the best sequences for detecting infarction.

Infections

Progressive multifocal leukoencephalopathy

Progressive multifocal leukoencephalopathy (PML) is caused by the JC virus, a type of polyomavirus named after the initials of the patient from whose tissue the virus was first successfully cultured. Clinical symptoms are rare. Differentiating white matter disease related to HIV from PML can be difficult. PML is less common than the former, and tends to be more focal and asymmetric. It more commonly affects the posterior parietal lobe. Neither demonstrates mass effect and both are of low attenuation on CT, low signal on T1-weighted MR images and high signal on T2 with no contrast enhancement.

Toxoplasmosis

Reactivated toxoplasmosis is primarily a disease of older children, while congenital toxoplasmosis in the HIV-infected infant is little different from that seen in immunocompetent patients. *Toxoplasma* infection most commonly affects the basal ganglia and corticomedullary junction of the periventricular white matter.

On contrast-enhanced CT, inhomogeneous or ring-like foci of enhancement are seen with both associated mass effect and surrounding edema. MR demonstrates decreased signal on T1–weighted images and increased signal on T2 with enhancement post-contrast (Figure 6.65). The differential diagnosis on imaging includes tuberculosis, abscess or lymphoma.

Meningitis

In addition to the usual causes of meningitis in children, HIV-infected children are at increased risk of fungal, mycobacterial and nocardial meningitis.

Both contrast-enhanced CT and MRI are often normal but may show meningeal enhancement. Fungi and TB may cause noncommunicating or communicating hydrocephalus. Unlike other fungi, *Cryptococcus neoformans* shows perivascular pseudocyst formation, cryptococcomas and no other meningeal enhancement on post-contrast imaging studies.

Further reading

Congenital CNS infections

Barkovich AJ *Pediatric Neuroimaging*, 4th edn. (Philadelphia: Lippincott Williams and Wilkins, 2005).

Martin S (2001) Congenital toxoplasmosis. *Neonatal Netw* **20**(4), 23–30.

Noorbehesht B, Enzmann DR, Sullender W, Bradley JS, Arvin AM (1987) Neonatal herpes simplex encephalitis: correlation of clinical and CT findings. *Radiology* **162**(3), 813–9.

Patel DV, Holfels EM, Vogel NP *et al.* (1996) Resolution of intracranial calcifications in infants with treated congenital toxoplasmosis. *Radiology* **199**(2), 433–40.

Yoshimura M, Tohyama J, Maegaki Y *et al.* (1996) [Computed tomography and magnetic resonance imaging of the brain in congenital rubella syndrome]. *No To Hattatsu* **28**(5), 385–90.

Other CNS infections

Baganz MD, Dross PE, Reinhardt JA (1995) Rocky Mountain spotted fever encephalitis: MR findings. *AJNR Am J Neuroradiol* **16**(Suppl. 4), 919–22.

Barkovich AJ *Pediatric Neuroimaging*, 4th edn. (Philadelphia: Lippincott Williams and Wilkins, 2005).

Chen CY, Chang YC, Huang CC *et al.* (2001) Acute flaccid paralysis in infants and young children with enterovirus 71 infection: MR imaging findings and clinical correlates. *AJNR Am J Neuroradiol* **22**(1), 200–5.

Kim TK, Chang KH, Kim CJ *et al.* (1995) Intracranial tuberculoma: comparison of MR with pathologic findings. *AJNR Am J Neuroradiol* **16**(9), 1903–8.

Kuker W, Nagele T, Schmidt F, Heckl S, Herrlinger U (2004) Diffusion-weighted MRI in herpes simplex encephalitis: a report of three cases. *Neuroradiology* **46**(2), 122–5.

Lee KY, Cho WH, Kim SH, Kim HD, Kim IO (2003) Acute encephalitis associated with measles: MRI features. *Neuroradiology* **45**(2), 100–6.

Silverstein FS, Brunberg JA (1995) Postvaricella basal ganglia infarction in children. *AJNR Am J Neuroradiol* **16**(3), 449–52.

Tuncay R, Akman-Demir G, Gokyigit A *et al.* (1996) MRI in subacute sclerosing panencephalitis. *Neuroradiology* **38**(7), 636–40.

Wallace RC, Burton EM, Barrett FF *et al.* (1991) Intracranial tuberculosis in children: CT appearance and clinical outcome. *Pediatr Radiol* **21**(4), 241–6.

Wilke M, Eiffert H, Christen HJ, Hanefeld F (2000) Primarily chronic and cerebrovascular course of Lyme neuroborreliosis: case reports and literature review. *Arch Dis Child* **83**(1), 67–71.

Upper respiratory tract infections

Buckley AR, Moss EH, Blokmanis A (1994) Diagnosis of peritonsillar abscess: value of intraoral sonography. *AJR Am J Roentgenol* **162**(4), 961–4.

Derkay CS, Wiatrak B (2008) Recurrent respiratory papillomatosis: a review. *Laryngoscope* **118**(7), 1236–47.

Donnelly LF *Pediatric Imaging: The Fundamentals* (Philadelphia: Saunders, 2009).

Marom EM, Goodman PC, McAdams HP (2001) Diffuse abnormalities of the trachea and main bronchi. *AJR Am J Roentgenol* **176**(3), 713–7.

Marra S, Hotaling AJ (1996) Deep neck infections. *Am J Otolaryngol* **17**(5), 287–98.

Miziara ID, Koishi HU, Zonato AI *et al.* (2001) The use of ultrasound evaluation in the diagnosis of peritonsillar abscess. *Rev Laryngol Otol Rhinol (Bord)* **122**(3), 201–3.

Prince JS, Duhamel DR, Levin DL, Harrell JH, Friedman PJ (2002) Nonneoplastic lesions of the tracheobronchial wall: radiologic findings with bronchoscopic correlation. *Radiographics* **22**(Spec. No.), S215–30.

Scott PM, Loftus WK, Kew J *et al.* (1999) Diagnosis of peritonsillar infections: a prospective study of ultrasound, computerized tomography and clinical diagnosis. *J Laryngol Otol* **113**(3), 229–32.

Slovis TL *Caffey's Pediatric Diagnostic Imaging*, 11th edn. (St. Louis: Mosby, 2007).

Stroud RH, Friedman NR (2001) An update on inflammatory disorders of the pediatric airway: epiglottitis, croup, and tracheitis. *Am J Otolaryngol* **22**(4), 268–75.

Bronchiolitis and pneumonia

Andronikou S, Wieselthaler N (2004) Modern imaging of tuberculosis in children: thoracic, central nervous system and abdominal tuberculosis. *Pediatr Radiol* **34**(11), 861–75.

Aquino SL, Kee ST, Warnock ML, Gamsu G (1994) Pulmonary aspergillosis: imaging findings with pathologic correlation. *AJR Am J Roentgenol* **163**(4), 811–5.

Donnelly LF (1999) Maximizing the usefulness of imaging in children with community-acquired pneumonia. *AJR Am J Roentgenol* **172**(2), 505–12.

Donnelly LF *Pediatric Imaging: The Fundamentals* (Philadelphia: Saunders, 2009).

Fjaerli HO, Farstad T, Rod G *et al.* (2005) Acute bronchiolitis in infancy as risk factor for wheezing and reduced pulmonary function by seven years in Akershus County, Norway. *BMC Pediatr* **5**, 31.

Glezen WP, Paredes A, Allison JE, Taber LH, Frank AL (1981) Risk of respiratory syncytial virus infection for infants from low-income families in relationship to age, sex, ethnic group, and maternal antibody level. *J Pediatr* **98**(5), 708–15.

Gopinath A, Strigun D, Banyopadhyay T (2005) Swyer-James syndrome. *Conn Med* **69**(6), 325–7.

Jaffe A, Calder AD, Owens CM, Stanojevic S, Sonnappa S (2008) Role of routine computed tomography in paediatric pleural empyema. *Thorax* **63**(10), 897–902.

Ostapchuk M, Roberts DM, Haddy R (2004) Community-acquired pneumonia in infants and children. *Am Fam Physician* **70**(5), 899–908.

Riccabona M (2008) Ultrasound of the chest in children (mediastinum excluded). *Eur Radiol* **18**(2), 390–9.

Siegel M, Coley B *Pediatric Imaging*, 1st edn. (Philadelphia: Lippincott Williams and Wilkins, 2006).

Slovis TL *Caffey's Pediatric Diagnostic Imaging*, 11th edn. (St. Louis: Mosby, 2007).

Wang EE, Law BJ, Stephens D (1995) Pediatric Investigators Collaborative Network on Infections in Canada (PICNIC) prospective study of risk factors and outcomes in patients hospitalized with respiratory syncytial viral lower respiratory tract infection. *J Pediatr* **126**(2), 212–9.

GIT infections

Alison M, Kheniche A, Azoulay R *et al.* (2007) Ultrasonography of Crohn disease in children. *Pediatr Radiol* **37**(11), 1071–82.

Antao B, Bishop J, Shawis R, Thomson M (2007) Clinical application and diagnostic yield of wireless capsule endoscopy in children. *J Laparoendosc Adv Surg Tech A* **17**(3), 364–70.

Charron M (2000) Pediatric inflammatory bowel disease imaged with Tc-99m white blood cells. *Clin Nucl Med* **25**(9), 708–15.

Darbari A, Sena L, Argani P *et al.* (2004) Gadolinium-enhanced magnetic resonance imaging: a useful radiological tool in diagnosing pediatric IBD. *Inflamm Bowel Dis* **10**(2), 67–72.

Dubinsky M (2008) Special issues in pediatric inflammatory bowel disease. *World J Gastroenterol* **14**(3), 413–20.

Fine JD, Johnson LB, Weiner M, Suchindran C (2008) Gastrointestinal complications of inherited epidermolysis bullosa: cumulative experience of the National Epidermolysis Bullosa Registry. *J Pediatr Gastroenterol Nutr* **46**(2), 147–58.

Fleenor JT, Hoffman TM, Bush DM *et al.* (2002) Pneumatosis intestinalis after pediatric thoracic organ transplantation. *Pediatrics* **109**(5), E78.

Grahnquist L, Chapman SC, Hvidsten S, Murphy MS (2003) Evaluation of 99mTc-HMPAO leukocyte scintigraphy in the investigation of pediatric inflammatory bowel disease. *J Pediatr* **143**(1), 48–53.

Kato S, Sherman PM (2005) What is new related to *Helicobacter pylori* infection in children and teenagers? *Arch Pediatr Adolesc Med* **159**(5), 415–21.

Mann EH (2008) Inflammatory bowel disease: imaging of the pediatric patient. *Semin Roentgenol* **43**(1), 29–38.

Narla LD, Hingsbergen EA, Jones JE (1999) Adult diseases in children. *Pediatr Radiol* **29**(4), 244–54.

Pena BM, Taylor GA, Fishman SJ, Mandl KD (2000) Costs and effectiveness of ultrasonography and limited computed tomography for diagnosing appendicitis in children. *Pediatrics* **106**(4), 672–6.

Rosendahl K, Aukland SM, Fosse K (2004) Imaging strategies in children with suspected appendicitis. *Eur Radiol* **14**(Suppl. 4), L138–45.

Sivit CJ (2004) Imaging the child with right lower quadrant pain and suspected appendicitis: current concepts. *Pediatr Radiol* **34**(6), 447–53.

Slovis TL *Caffey's Pediatric Diagnostic Imaging*, 11th edn. (St. Louis: Mosby, 2007).

Thomson M, Fritscher-Ravens A, Mylonaki M *et al.* (2007) Wireless capsule endoscopy in children: a study to assess diagnostic yield in small bowel disease in paediatric patients. *J Pediatr Gastroenterol Nutr* **44**(2), 192–7.

Tishler JM, Han SY, Helman CA (1983) Esophageal involvement in epidermolysis bullosa dystrophica. *AJR Am J Roentgenol* **141**(6), 1283–6.

Toma P, Granata C, Magnano G, Barabino A (2007) CT and MRI of paediatric Crohn disease. *Pediatr Radiol* **37**(11), 1083–92.

Genitourinary infections

Chang JW, Chen SJ, Chin TW *et al.* (2004) Xanthogranulomatous pyelonephritis treated by partial nephrectomy. *Pediatr Nephrol* **19**(10), 1164–7.

Dacher JN, Pfister C, Monroc M, Eurin D, LeDosseur P (1996) Power Doppler sonographic pattern of acute pyelonephritis in children: comparison with CT. *AJR Am J Roentgenol* **166**(6), 1451–5.

DeMuri GP, Wald ER (2008) Imaging and antimicrobial prophylaxis following the diagnosis of urinary tract infection in children. *Pediatr Infect Dis J* **27**(6), 553–4.

Doehring E (1988) Schistosomiasis in childhood. *Eur J Pediatr* **147**(1), 2–9.

Donnelly LF *Pediatric Imaging: The Fundamentals* (Philadelphia: Saunders, 2009).

Greenfield SP, Chesney RW, Carpenter M *et al.* (2008) Vesicoureteral reflux: the RIVUR study and the way forward. *J Urol* **179**(2), 405–7.

Hoberman A, Charron M, Hickey RW *et al.* (2003) Imaging studies after a first febrile urinary tract infection in young children. *N Engl J Med* **348**(3), 195–202.

Jeffrey RB, Laing FC, Wing VW, Hoddick W (1985) Sensitivity of sonography in pyonephrosis: a reevaluation. *AJR Am J Roentgenol* **144**(1), 71–3.

Karlowicz MG (2003) Candidal renal and urinary tract infection in neonates. *Semin Perinatol* **27**(5), 393–400.

Kirsch AJ, Grattan-Smith JD, Molitierno JA Jr (2006) The role of magnetic resonance imaging in pediatric urology. *Curr Opin Urol* **16**(4), 283–90.

Loffroy R, Guiu B, Watfa J *et al.* (2007) Xanthogranulomatous pyelonephritis in adults: clinical and radiological findings in diffuse and focal forms. *Clin Radiol* **62**(9), 884–90.

Lonergan GJ, Pennington DJ, Morrison JC *et al.* (1998) Childhood pyelonephritis: comparison of gadolinium-enhanced MR imaging and renal cortical scintigraphy for diagnosis. *Radiology* **207**(2), 377–84.

Moorthy I, Easty M, McHugh K *et al.* (2005) The presence of vesicoureteric reflux does not identify a population at risk for renal scarring following a first urinary tract infection. *Arch Dis Child* **90**(7), 733–6.

Munden MM, Trautwein LM (2000) Scrotal pathology in pediatrics with sonographic imaging. *Curr Probl Diagn Radiol* **29**(6), 185–205.

Nerli RB, Kamat GV, Alur SB *et al.* (2008) Genitourinary tuberculosis in pediatric urological practice. *J Pediatr Urol* **4**(4), 299–303.

Pennington DJ, Lonergan GJ, Flack CE, Waguespack RL, Jackson CB (1996) Experimental pyelonephritis in piglets: diagnosis with MR imaging. *Radiology* **201**(1), 199–205.

Samuel M, Duffy P, Capps S et al. (2001) Xanthogranulomatous pyelonephritis in childhood. *J Pediatr Surg* **36**(4), 598–601.

Schneider K, Helmig FJ, Eife R et al. (1989) Pyonephrosis in childhood–is ultrasound sufficient for diagnosis? *Pediatr Radiol* **19**(5), 302–7.

Shah G, Upadhyay J (2005) Controversies in the diagnosis and management of urinary tract infections in children. *Paediatr Drugs* **7**(6), 339–46.

Slovis TL *Caffey's Pediatric Diagnostic Imaging*, 11th edn. (St. Louis: Mosby, 2007).

Musculoskeletal infections

Donnelly LF *Fundamentals of Pediatric Radiology*, 1st edn. (Philadelphia: Saunders, 2001).

El-Shanti HI, Ferguson PJ (2007) Chronic recurrent multifocal osteomyelitis: a concise review and genetic update. *Clin Orthop Relat Res* **462**, 11–9.

Fernandez M, Carrol CL, Baker CJ (2000) Discitis and vertebral osteomyelitis in children: an 18-year review. *Pediatrics* **105**(6), 1299–304.

Johnson K (2006) Imaging of juvenile idiopathic arthritis. *Pediatr Radiol* **36**(8), 743–58.

Offiah AC (2006) Acute osteomyelitis, septic arthritis and discitis: differences between neonates and older children. *Eur J Radiol* **60**(2), 221–32.

Siegel M, Coley B *Pediatric Imaging*, 1st edn. (Philadelphia: Lippincott Williams and Wilkins, 2006).

Slovis TL *Caffey's Pediatric Diagnostic Imaging*, 11th edn. (St. Louis: Mosby, 2007).

Human immunodeficiency virus

Geoffray A, Spehl M, Chami M et al. (1997) [Imaging of AIDS in children]. *J Radiol* **78**(12), 1233–43.

Graham SM (2007) HIV-related pulmonary disorders: practice issues. *Ann Trop Paediatr* **27**(4), 243–52.

Haller JO, Cohen HL (1994) Gastrointestinal manifestations of AIDS in children. *AJR Am J Roentgenol* **162**(2), 387–93.

Jeanes AC, Owens CM (2002) Chest imaging in the immunocompromised child. *Paediatr Respir Rev* **3**(1), 59–69.

Jura E, Chadwick EG, Josephs SH et al. (1989) Varicella-zoster virus infections in children infected with human immunodeficiency virus. *Pediatr Infect Dis J* **8**(9), 586–90.

Kauffman WM, Sivit CJ, Fitz CR et al. (1992) CT and MR evaluation of intracranial involvement in pediatric HIV infection: a clinical-imaging correlation. *AJNR Am J Neuroradiol* **13**(3), 949–57.

Safriel YI, Haller JO, Lefton DR, Obedian R (2000) Imaging of the brain in the HIV-positive child. *Pediatr Radiol* **30**(11), 725–32.

Zar HJ (2008) Chronic lung disease in human immunodeficiency virus (HIV) infected children. *Pediatr Pulmonol* **43**(1), 1–10.

Pediatric tumors

Jane Kim, Soonmee Cha, Heike E. Daldrup-Link and Robert Goldsby

Although cancer is, overall, rare in childhood, it is the most common natural, nontraumatic cause of death in infants, teenagers and adolescents. Approximately 12 000 children and adolescents are diagnosed with cancer annually in the United States. The most common childhood cancers comprise leukemia (30%), brain tumors (22%), lymphoma (11%), neuroblastoma (8%), soft tissue sarcomas (7%), Wilms tumor (6%), bone tumors (5%) and other (11%). Diagnostic imaging plays a critical role in differentiating benign from malignant lesions as well as staging and re-staging tumor extent in order to plan and monitor the most appropriate stage-adapted therapy.

7A PEDIATRIC BRAIN TUMORS

Jane Kim and Soonme Cha

Introduction

Tumors of the central nervous system comprise the second most common type of pediatric malignancy, accounting for about 20% of all childhood tumors and second only to leukemia in incidence.

The basic approach to evaluating pediatric brain tumors on CT or MRI requires consideration first and foremost of the patient's age and tumor location. Additionally, specific imaging features (such as enhancement pattern, solid vs. cystic components, or hemorrhage and calcification) may help to steer the differential diagnosis.

By location, tumors occur with roughly equal frequency in the supratentorial and infratentorial compartment. Table 7.1 is an overview of the frequency of various types of brain tumors in children, grouped by supra- or infratentorial location. The following discussion will emphasize the most common tumors.

Infratentorial tumors

Medulloblastoma, cerebellar astrocytoma, brainstem glioma and ependymoma are the four most common posterior fossa tumors, and account for approximately half of all pediatric brain tumors.

Table 7.1 Brain tumor frequency in children (under 15 years)

Tumor type by location	Percentage of all brain tumors (%)
Infratentorial	50–55
Medulloblastoma	15–20
Cerebellar astrocytoma	10–15
Brainstem glioma	10–15
Ependymoma	5
Other	2–5
Supratentorial	45–50
Astrocytoma (low grade)	10–20
Astrocytoma (high grade)	5–10
Ependymoma	5
Craniopharyngioma	5
Primitive neuroectodermal tumor	1–2
Ganglioglioma/gangliocytoma	1–2
Oligodendroglioma	1–2
Atypical teratoid/rhabdoid tumor	1–2
Choroid plexus papilloma	1–2
Germ cell tumor	1–2
Pineal parenchymal tumor	1–2
Meningioma	1–2
Dysembryoplastic neuroepithelial tumor	<1
Desmoplastic infantile ganglioglioma	<1
Hemangioblastoma	<1
Pituitary adenoma	<1
Metastases	<1

Percentages are based on several large epidemiological studies, with some variability in tumor frequency among the studies (Gjerris *et al.*, 1998; Rickert and Paulus, 2001; Duffner *et al.*, 1986; Pollack, 1999).

Less common tumors include atypical teratoid/rhabdoid tumor, hemangioblastoma, teratoma and dermoid/epidermoid.

Medulloblastoma

Medulloblastomas are the most common posterior fossa tumors in children, and are highly malignant with a propensity for leptomeningeal dissemination. Medulloblastomas most commonly arise from the vermis in children, while assuming

Essentials of Pediatric Radiology, ed. Heike E. Daldrup-Link and Charles A. Gooding. Published by Cambridge University Press.
© Cambridge University Press 2010.

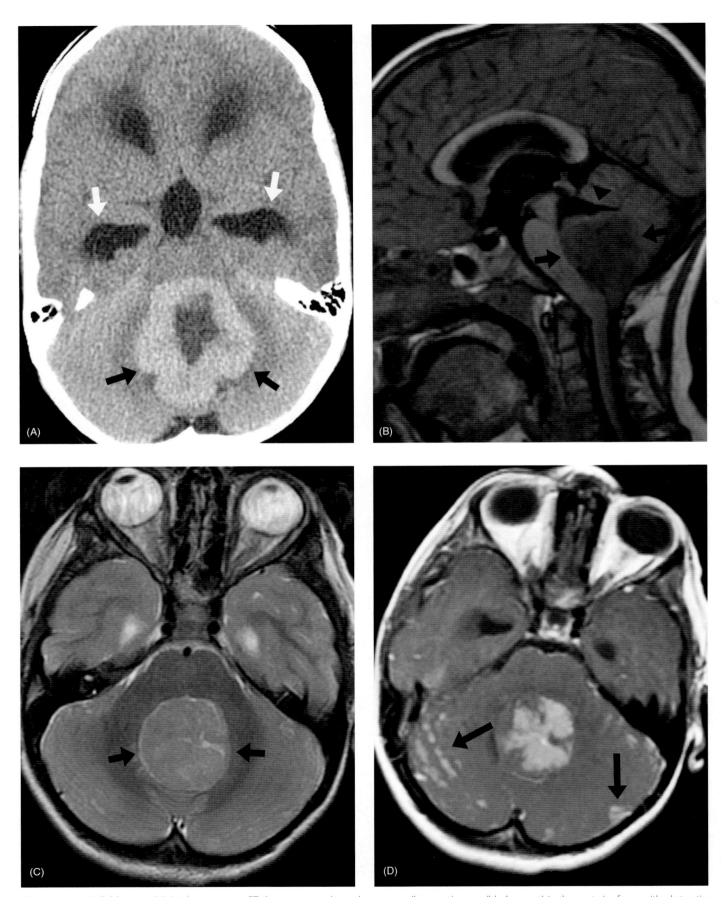

Figure 7.1 Medulloblastoma. (A) Axial noncontrast CT demonstrates a hyperdense, centrally necrotic mass (black arrows) in the posterior fossa, with obstructive hydrocephalus and dilation of the temporal horns (white arrows). (B–E) MR images in a different patient with the same disease. (B) Sagittal T1-weighted image (T1WI) shows a mass centered within and expanding the fourth ventricle (arrowhead). (C) The mass is not particularly bright on T2WI, and appears isointense to gray matter. (D) Axial post-contrast T1WI shows enhancement of the tumor as well as multiple enhancing nodules along the cerebellar folia, consistent with leptomeningeal metastases (long arrows). (E) Sagittal post-contrast T1WI with fat saturation shows further leptomeningeal metastasis (long arrow) along the dorsal aspect of the lower thoracic cord.

a more lateral location in the cerebellar hemispheres in adolescents and adults.

In a child, medulloblastoma classically appears on noncontrast CT as a well-defined, hyperdense mass in the cerebellar

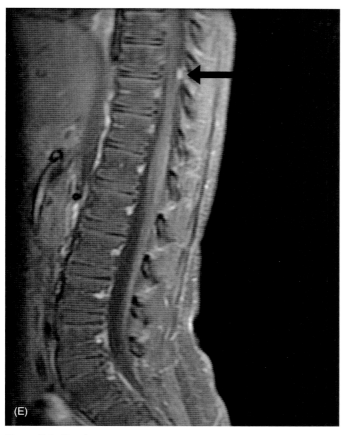

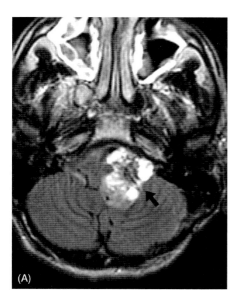

Figure 7.1 (Cont.)

Figure 7.1 (Cont.)

vermis, compressing the fourth ventricle and causing hydrocephalus (Figure 7.1). The small round cells with high nuclear/cytoplasmic ratio that comprise medulloblastoma account for its hyperdense appearance on noncontrast CT and iso/hypointensity to gray matter on T2-weighted MR sequences; this is one of the most useful features for distinguishing medulloblastoma from other posterior fossa tumors such as astrocytoma. However, medulloblastomas can have cystic or necrotic change (approximately 50%) and calcification (approximately 15–20%) that make appearance heterogeneous on both CT and MR.

Medulloblastomas have a propensity for leptomeningeal spread, both in the brain and spine. As one-third of patients may have drop metastases to the spine at presentation, it is critical to image the spine if medulloblastoma is suspected.

Ependymoma

Ependymomas arise from the ependymal cell layer lining the ventricles and central canal in the spinal cord. In children, ependymomas are more commonly intracranial than spinal, and when they are within the brain, more commonly infratentorial (two-thirds) than supratentorial (one-third). While most tumors are of low histological grade, prognosis remains generally poor with five-year overall survival around 50%.

The typical appearance on CT is that of an isodense fourth ventricular mass with heterogeneous areas of calcification and cystic change, and associated obstructive hydrocephalus. Tumor crawling out of the fourth ventricular foramina (of Luschka into the cerebellopontine angle or Magendie into the cisterna magna) is very suggestive of ependymoma (Figure 7.2). Calcification, hemorrhage and/or cystic change will create focal areas of signal heterogeneity on MR. Table 7.2 compares important features of ependymomas and medulloblastomas, which can be difficult to distinguish on imaging when presented with a midline mass in the region of the fourth ventricle.

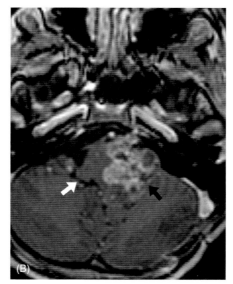
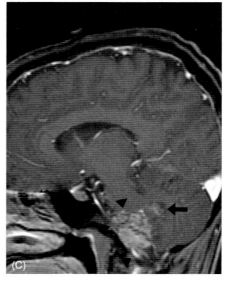

Figure 7.2 Ependymoma. (A) Axial FLAIR MR image shows a heterogeneous fourth ventricular mass. (B) Axial post-contrast T1WI shows the mass extends through the foramen of Luschka on the left (black arrow). Position of the normal, right foramen of Luschka is designated by the white arrow. (C) Sagittal post-contrast T1WI again shows the mass in the fourth ventricle (arrow) extending through Luschka into the lateral cerebellomedullary cistern and cerebellopontine angle (arrowheads). Note the heterogeneous appearance of this mass, which has multiple cystic, nonenhancing areas.

Table 7.2 Medulloblastoma vs. ependymoma in children

	Medulloblastoma	Ependymoma (infratentorial)
Peak age group	Older (5–10 years)	Younger (1–5 years)
Frequency	More common (30–40% of posterior fossa tumors in children)	Less common (8–15% of posterior fossa tumors in children)
Location	Vermis in children Cerebellar hemispheres in adolescents/adults	Fourth ventricle
Imaging hallmarks	Hyperdense on noncontrast CT[a] Solid portions of tumor are iso/hypointense to gray matter on T2[a]	Extension through fourth ventricular foramina (Luschka, Magendie)[b] Heterogeneous with calcifications, cysts, hemorrhage[b]
Leptomeningeal dissemination	Common (30% at presentation)	Less common, unless higher grade (5–10% at presentation)
Remember	Neurosurgical consultation for hydrocephalus Image the spine for drop metastases	Neurosurgical consultation for hydrocephalus Image the spine for drop metastases

[a] Presumably due to high cellularity and increased nuclear/cytoplasmic ratio of small, round tumor cells.
[b] Medulloblastomas may also have this appearance but less commonly than ependymomas. Hemorrhage within medulloblastomas is very rare.

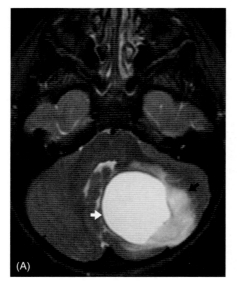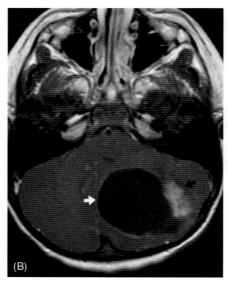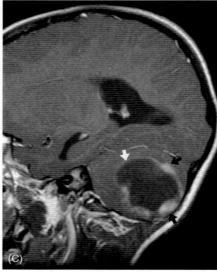

Figure 7.3 Juvenile pilocytic astrocytoma. (A) Axial T2WI shows a predominantly cystic mass (white arrow) with a solid, hyperintense component (black arrows) in the left cerebellar hemisphere, and mass effect on the fourth ventricle. (B), (C) Axial and sagittal post-contrast T1WIs again demonstrate the cystic mass (white arrows) with a solid enhancing nodule (black arrows). Note the high signal of the solid component on T2WI and its intense enhancement after contrast, both of which are characteristic features of this tumor.

Ependymomas may have leptomeningeal dissemination, though this is less common compared to medulloblastomas and occurs in approximately 5–10% overall of cases at diagnosis (with higher frequency for high-grade tumors such as anaplastic ependymoma, and lower frequency for low-grade tumors).

Cerebellar astrocytoma

Most cerebellar astrocytomas in children are low-grade juvenile pilocytic astrocytomas (JPA), as seen in 70% of cases.

High-grade astrocytomas such as anaplastic astrocytomas or glioblastomas are uncommon.

Astrocytomas may arise from the cerebellar hemisphere or vermis, with extension to the brainstem in a subset of cases. They may appear on imaging as (1) a cystic mass with enhancing mural nodule (most common), (2) a solid mass with central necrosis, or (3) a solid mass without necrosis (least common).

JPA classically presents as a cystic mass with an intensely enhancing, mural nodule (Figure 7.3). The solid component of this low-grade tumor is also very bright on T2-weighted

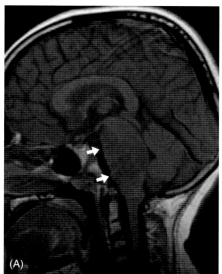

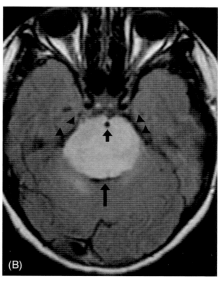

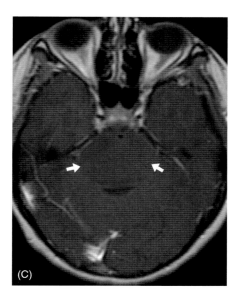

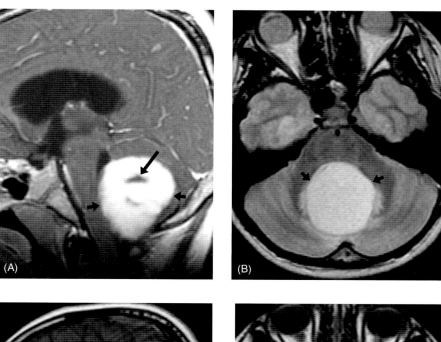

Figure 7.4 Juvenile pilocytic astrocytoma. (A) Sagittal post-contrast T1WI shows an avidly enhancing mass (short arrows) in the inferior cerebellar vermis, with central areas of necrosis (long arrow). (B) Axial T2WI shows a round, midline mass in the region of the fourth ventricle. This could easily be confused with medulloblastoma by location, but note that the mass is very hyperintense on T2WI, which would be atypical for medulloblastoma (compare with Figure 7.1).

Figure 7.5 Diffuse pontine glioma. (A) Sagittal T1WI shows hypointense mass (white arrows) in the pons. (B) Axial FLAIR sequence demonstrates the mass to be hyperintense and expansile, extending into the prepontine cistern (arrowheads), compressing the fourth ventricle (long arrow) and engulfing the basilar artery (short arrow). Engulfment of the basilar artery is characteristic. (C) Post-contrast T1WI shows absence of enhancement, which is typical (though tumors can also show focal or nodular enhancement).

images, which is a useful distinguishing feature from medulloblastoma (Figure 7.4).

Prognosis is generally excellent for children with low-grade cerebellar astrocytomas due to the slow growth rate and indolent behavior of these tumors.

Brainstem glioma

Brainstem gliomas constitute a heterogeneous group of tumors in terms of histology, prognosis and management. They can be divided into two general groups, diffuse and focal, based on their appearance on MR. Diffuse tumors have poorly circumscribed borders and usually correlate with high-grade tumors with poor prognosis. In contrast, focal tumors have circumscribed margins and usually correlate with low-grade tumors with good prognosis, such as pilocytic astrocytoma.

Most diffuse tumors are found in the pons. Diffuse pontine gliomas are infiltrative, expansile masses that are hypointense on T1-weighted sequences and hyperintense on T2, with typically little contrast enhancement (Figure 7.5). The pons often appears expanded, with narrowing of the prepontine cistern, engulfment of the basilar artery and compression of the fourth ventricle. This characteristic MR appearance precludes the need for biopsy, unless there is some question of the diagnosis and entities such as encephalitis need to be excluded. Despite radiation and/or chemotherapy (surgery is avoided because of high morbidity and mortality), the prognosis is very poor.

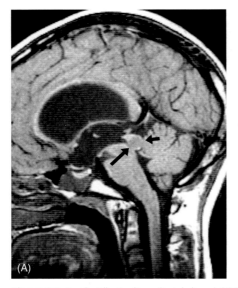
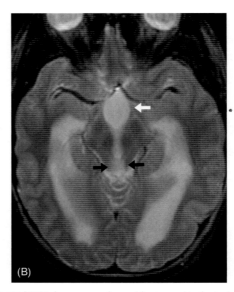
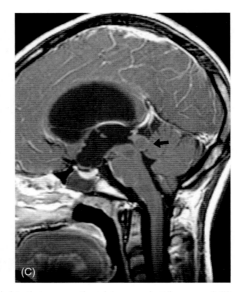

Figure 7.6 Focal midbrain glioma (tectal glioma). (A) Sagittal T1WI shows a round mass (short arrow) in the tectal plate that narrows the sylvian aqueduct (long arrow). (B) Axial T2WI demonstrates focal hyperintensity in the tectum and hydrocephalus (white arrow) caused by aqueductal compression. (C) Sagittal post-contrast T1WI shows absence of enhancement of the mass, which is typical. These tumors, which tend to be low-grade astrocytomas, are usually followed without biopsy because of their precarious location within the brain. Intervention is typically limited to shunting for hydrocephalus unless there is evidence of disease progression.

Focal tumors of the brainstem have distinct margins and are typically hypointense on T1-weighted sequences and hyperintense on T2 with variable enhancement. Specific types of focal tumors include tectal gliomas, which arise from the quadrigeminal plate of the midbrain (Figure 7.6).

Supratentorial tumors

Supratentorial tumors can be divided into two groups on the basis of location: hemispheric and midline. Hemispheric tumors arise from the brain parenchyma or lateral ventricles, while midline tumors arise from the sella, optic chiasm, hypothalamus and pineal gland.

Hemispheric supratentorial tumors

Astrocytoma

Astrocytomas are the most common supratentorial brain tumor in children. Most are of low histological grade (pilocytic or fibrillary), though high-grade tumors (anaplastic astrocytoma and glioblastoma) can occur in children. While astrocytomas can occur in any pediatric age group, older children are more frequently affected.

As with infratentorial astrocytomas, supratentorial tumors have a variety of appearances and can appear as (1) cystic with an enhancing mural nodule, (2) solid, or (3) solid with central necrosis. In general, high-grade tumors are irregular and heterogeneous (due to necrosis and hemorrhage), eliciting more vasogenic edema than low-grade tumors. Pilocytic astrocytomas are very vascular and have portions that enhance very avidly after contrast. However, nonpilocytic low-grade astrocytomas generally do not enhance (Figure 7.7).

Ependymoma

Approximately one-third of ependymomas occur in the supratentorial compartment. Unlike their infratentorial counterparts, supratentorial ependymomas are not necessarily intraventricular. In fact, most are *extraventricular* and located in the white matter adjacent to a ventricular surface, most commonly near the frontal horn or atrium of the lateral ventricle (though they can also arise from within the third or lateral ventricles). It is thought that ependymomas occur outside the ventricular system because of the presence of ependymal cell rests in white matter – streaks or bands of subependymal neural glia that extend into white matter at locations where the ventricles are sharply angled and posterior to the occipital horns. Because of their frequent location outside the ventricles, leptomeningeal dissemination is uncommon. Like their infratentorial counterparts, supratentorial ependymomas are typically heterogeneous on imaging, with approximately half of cases demonstrating areas of calcification and cystic change (Figure 7.8).

Less common hemispheric brain tumors

There are many other types of hemispheric supratentorial brain tumors that are less common. These remaining tumors will be grouped and discussed in terms of differential diagnoses.

Large, heterogeneous supratentorial mass in an infant or young child

A large, heterogeneous supratentorial mass in a younger patient (infant or child less than five years) should bring to mind several types of tumors (see Table 7.3 and Figure 7.9). **Astrocytomas** and **ependymomas** are in the differential diagnosis, as discussed above. **Primitive neuroectodermal tumors**

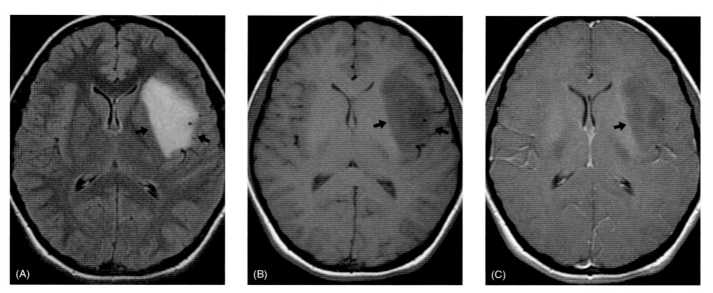

Figure 7.7 Low-grade glioma. (A) Axial FLAIR MR image shows a hyperintense, expansile mass centered in the left insula. (B), (C) Axial pre- and post-contrast T1WIs show that the mass does not enhance with gadolinium. This was presumed to be a low-grade glioma and was followed with serial imaging over several years (biopsy or surgery not initially undertaken given the location of the mass near Broca's area). Eventually, tumor growth and the development of enhancing areas necessitated surgical resection; pathology from this mass (not pictured) showed anaplastic oligoastrocytoma, presumably from de-differentiation of the low-grade glioma depicted above.

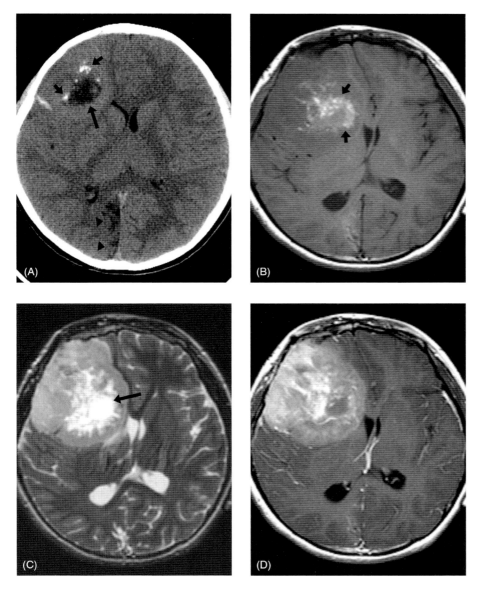

Figure 7.8 Supratentorial ependymoma. (A) Axial noncontrast CT shows a very heterogeneous right frontal mass with calcification (short arrow) and internal presumed cystic change (long arrow). Incidentally, right occipital low attenuation (arrowheads) reflects remote ischemic injury. (B) Axial T1WI shows central areas of intrinsic T1 shortening (short arrows) likely reflecting calcification and/or hemorrhage within the mass. (C) Axial T2WI shows heterogeneous T2 signal with central cystic change (long arrow). (D) Axial post-contrast T1WI demonstrates enhancement of the very large mass. The heterogeneity of the mass with calcification and cystic change is typical of ependymoma, though other tumors such as primitive neuroectodermal tumor (PNET) may have an identical appearance.

Table 7.3 Large, heterogeneous, supratentorial mass in an infant or young child (0–5 years)

Tumor	Imaging hallmarks
Astrocytoma	Most common supratentorial tumor Variable appearance depending on histological grade
Ependymoma	Calcification and cystic areas common Usually extraventricular (next to frontal horn or atrium of lateral ventricle)
Primitive neuroectodermal tumor (PNET)	Calcification and necrosis common Variable enhancement
Atypical teratoid/rhabdoid tumor (ATRT)	Calcification and necrosis common
Desmoplastic infantile ganglioglioma (DIG)	Very large cysts Peripheral solid component involving leptomeninges No calcification (unlike ependymoma, PNET, ATRT) Very young patient (<1 year old)

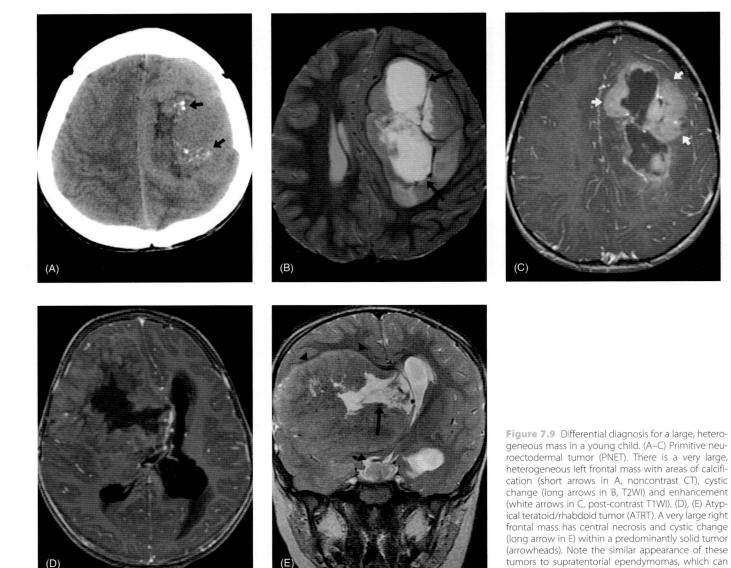

Figure 7.9 Differential diagnosis for a large, heterogeneous mass in a young child. (A–C) Primitive neuroectodermal tumor (PNET). There is a very large, heterogeneous left frontal mass with areas of calcification (short arrows in A, noncontrast CT), cystic change (long arrows in B, T2WI) and enhancement (white arrows in C, post-contrast T1WI). (D), (E) Atypical teratoid/rhabdoid tumor (ATRT). A very large right frontal mass has central necrosis and cystic change (long arrow in E) within a predominantly solid tumor (arrowheads). Note the similar appearance of these tumors to supratentorial ependymomas, which can be indistinguishable on imaging.

Table 7.4 Peripherally located tumor (involving cortex) in an older child or adolescent

Tumor	Imaging hallmarks
Pleomorphic xanthoastrocytoma (PXA)	Classically "cyst with solid nodule" (though appearance can be variable) Temporal lobe most common
Ganglioglioma	Classically "cyst with solid nodule" (though appearance can be variable) Calcification common (30% of cases) Temporal lobe most common
Dysembryoplastic neuroepithelial tumor (DNET)	Microcystic "bubbly" appearance Very bright on T2-weighted sequences Temporal lobe most common
Oligodendroglioma	Calcification common (40% of cases) Frontal lobe most common

(PNET) are tumors that are almost entirely (90–95%) comprised of undifferentiated cells, appearing histologically similar to medulloblastomas, pineoblastomas, neuroblastomas and atypical teratoid/rhabdoid tumors. PNETs are often very large at the time of presentation, and calcification and necrotic areas are common (seen in about half of cases). PNETs characteristically have sharp, well-defined margins and relatively minimal, if any, surrounding edema. **Atypical teratoid/rhabdoid tumors (ATRT)** are indistinguishable from PNETs on imaging. They are typically large at the time of diagnosis and often present as solid, strongly enhancing masses with areas of necrosis. The histological hallmark of ATRT is the rhabdoid cell, but this finding is not always predominant, and the majority of ATRTs contain fields indistinguishable from PNETs, complicating histological diagnosis. Finally, **desmoplastic infantile gangliogliomas (DIG)** are very large tumors in infants who typically present with macrocephaly. These tumors usually affect more than one lobe of the brain and have two components: (1) a dominant cystic portion and (2) a peripheral, avidly enhancing solid component that attaches to the leptomeninges and reflects an intense desmoplastic reaction at the dura.

Peripherally located mass in an older child or adolescent

A peripherally located tumor involving the cerebral cortex in an older child or adolescent should recall several types of tumors (see Table 7.4 and Figure 7.10). Because of their peripheral location and slow growth, all of these tumors can cause erosion of the inner table of the skull. **Pleomorphic xanthoastrocytomas (PXA)** often appear as a well-circumscribed mass in the cerebral cortex and are classically described as a cystic mass with solid enhancing mural nodule, though they may assume any appearance from completely solid to mixed cystic and solid. Half of these tumors arise solely from the temporal lobe, and an additional 10–20% of tumors involve the temporal lobe in addition to another lobe. Not surprisingly, seizure is a common presenting symptom. **Gangliogliomas** are neoplasms comprised of both neuronal and glial cells. Like PXAs, they are characteristically described as cystic masses with solid enhancing mural nodules, though they may also adopt a wide range of appearances. Calcification can be seen in approximately one-third of cases. Similar to PXAs, gangliogliomas most commonly arise from the temporal lobes and are a common cause of long-standing epilepsy. **Dysembryoplastic neuroepithelial tumors (DNET)** are benign tumors of the cerebral cortex that most commonly occur in the temporal lobe (>60% of cases) and present with seizure. These are solid tumors that actually appear cystic on imaging, with very low signal on T1-weighted sequences and extremely bright signal on T2-weighted imaging. They appear to have multiple "cysts" or a microcystic appearance that can be described as bubbly. Focal or nodular contrast enhancement may be seen. Cortical dysplasias can be seen in association with DNETs, raising the question of whether they represent developmental malformations rather than true neoplasms. Finally, **oligodendrogliomas** frequently involve the cortex and periphery of the brain, most commonly arising in the frontal lobes. They commonly calcify (40% of cases) and have variable enhancement, with limited/no enhancement generally correlating with lower histological grade. Recently, it has been discovered that oligodendrogliomas with chromosomal deletions of 1p and 19q respond more favorably to chemotherapy.

Supratentorial intraventricular mass in a child

Subependymal giant cell astrocytomas (SEGA) typically arise from the lateral ventricle near the foramen of Monro and are associated with tuberous sclerosis (Figure 7.11). They are believed to originate from the subependymal nodules that are seen along the ventricular margins in tuberous sclerosis, and are diagnosed when growth of a subependymal nodule is noted on serial MR exams. SEGAs may cause hydrocephalus because of their location, and can rarely degenerate into a higher-grade tumor. **Choroid plexus papillomas and carcinomas** are usually seen in very young children (less than five years) and typically occur in the atrium of the lateral ventricles.

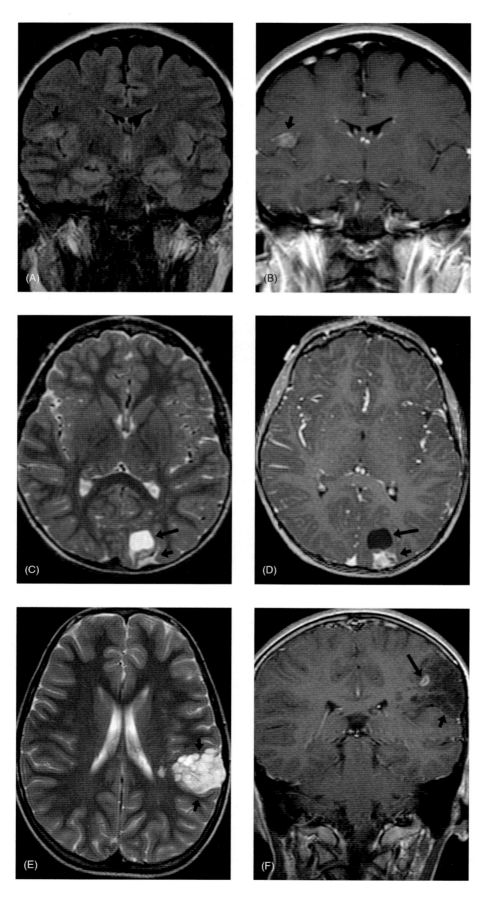

Figure 7.10 Differential diagnosis for a peripherally located tumor in an older child or adolescent. (A), (B) Pleomorphic xanthoastrocytoma (PXA). Right frontal tumor is slightly hyperintense on FLAIR (A) and solidly enhances (B, post-contrast T1WI). (C), (D) Ganglioglioma. Left occipital mass is both solid (short arrows) and cystic (long arrows), involving the cortex. (E), (F) Dysembryoplastic neuroepithelial tumor (DNET). Left parietal mass has multiple small cysts (short arrows in E, axial T2WI) with a "bubbly" appearance. A small enhancing component can be seen (long arrow in F, coronal post-contrast T1WI). (G), (H) Oligodendroglioma. Right frontoparietal mass (short arrows) extends to the cortex and has a solid enhancing component (long arrow in H, axial post-contrast T1WI).

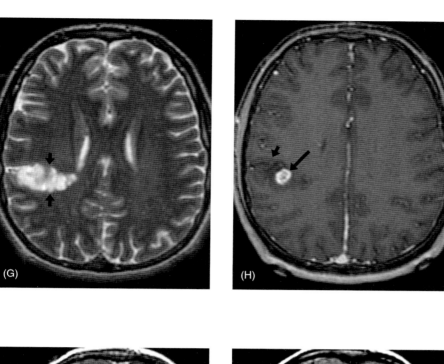

Figure 7.10 (Cont.)

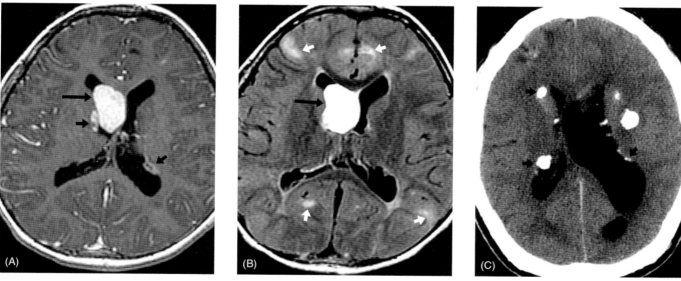

Figure 7.11 Subependymal giant cell tumor (SEGA). (A) Axial post-contrast T1WI shows a large enhancing mass near the right foramen of Monro (long arrow), consistent with a SEGA. Other smaller enhancing subependymal nodules (short arrows) along the ventricular margin are consistent with hamartomas. The presence or absence of enhancement does not help to distinguish SEGA from hamartomas; rather, progressive growth in size seems to be the best indicator. (B) Axial FLAIR shows subcortical and cortical hyperintensities (white arrows) consistent with tubers. (C) Axial noncontrast CT nicely demonstrates calcification of the subependymal nodules, which progresses with the age of the patient.

They have a frond-like appearance with occasional foci of calcification, hemorrhage and/or cystic change, and avid enhancement after contrast (Figure 7.12). While the distinction between papilloma and carcinoma is a histological one, marked heterogeneity of appearance and invasion of adjacent brain parenchyma with vasogenic edema on imaging should raise concern for carcinoma rather than papilloma. Hydrocephalus is common due to marked cerebrospinal fluid (CSF) production by the tumor.

Midline supratentorial tumors
Optic pathway/hypothalamic gliomas

Most of the gliomas affecting the optic pathway and hypothalamus are juvenile pilocytic astrocytomas. Because tumors arising from the optic chiasm and hypothalamus may be difficult to distinguish from each other when large, they are often grouped and discussed together. A significant number of patients with optic pathway/hypothalamic gliomas have neurofibromatosis type 1 (NF1)

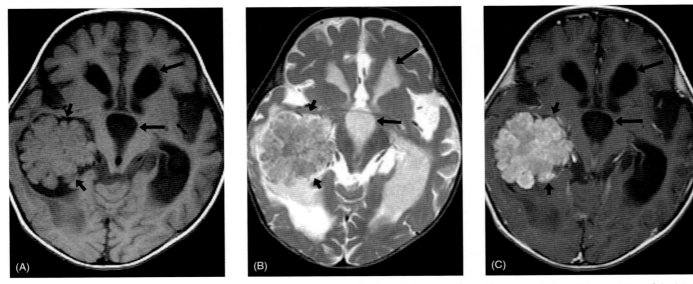

Figure 7.12 Choroid plexus papilloma. (A) This is a characteristic appearance of a choroid plexus papilloma (short arrows), situated in the atrium of the lateral ventricle, which is the most common location in the pediatric age group. It is a lobulated, frond-like tumor with iso/hypointensity to gray matter on T2WI (B) and homogeneous enhancement following contrast (C). There is marked hydrocephalus (long arrows) due to overproduction of CSF by the tumor. Note the absence of parenchymal invasion, which if seen would favor choroid plexus carcinoma.

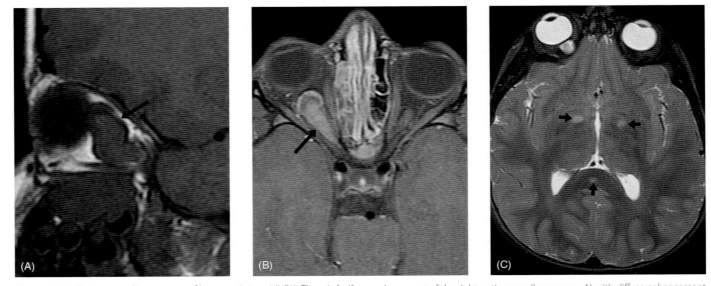

Figure 7.13 Optic nerve glioma in neurofibromatosis type I (NF1). There is fusiform enlargement of the right optic nerve (long arrow, A) with diffuse enhancement following gadolinium (long arrow, B), consistent with optic nerve glioma. Evaluation of the remainder of the brain shows T2-hyperintense foci in the bilateral globus pallidi and splenium of the corpus callosum (short arrows, C) without mass effect. These lesions are seen in the majority of NF1 patients and reflect areas of myelin vacuolization.

(Figure 7.13). Bilateral optic pathway tumors are virtually pathognomonic for NF1.

Interestingly, there appear to be differences in optic pathway tumors between patients with NF1 and those without. In patients with NF1, most tumors involve the optic nerve or chiasm, and extension beyond the optic pathway is rare (2% of cases). However, in patients without NF1, the optic chiasm is much more frequently involved than the optic nerve, and tumor extension beyond the optic pathway is seen in more than two-thirds of cases. Tumors in patients without NF1 more commonly increase in size, compared to patients with NF1 (95% versus 50%). There have been case reports of optic pathway gliomas undergoing spontaneous regression, in patients both with and without NF1. While the frequency of this phenomenon is not known, it raises important questions for treatment planning.

Craniopharyngioma

Craniopharyngiomas are considered histologically benign, though their invasion of critical parasellar structures and risk of recurrence following surgery results in significant morbidity/mortality. They arise from the path of the craniopharyngeal duct and commonly involve the suprasellar compartment or both the sella and suprasellar region; location entirely within the sella is uncommon. There are two histological types: adamantinomatous and papillary; the adamantinomatous variety usually affects the pediatric population.

Table 7.5 The 90% rule (or rule of Cs) for pediatric (adamantinomatous) craniopharyngiomas

90% have a **cystic** component

90% have **calcification**

90% will **contrast-enhance**

On imaging, adamantinomatous craniopharyngiomas have a characteristic appearance: 90% have cystic components, 90% have at least partial calcification, and 90% enhance following contrast (Table 7.5 and Figure 7.14). The cystic components of craniopharyngiomas are characteristically hyperintense on T1-weighted sequences, indicative of a "motor oil" like substance rich in cholesterol, protein and blood products. However, there can be variability of signal intensity of the cysts on both T1- and T2-weighted imaging.

Less common supratentorial midline tumors

Pineal region mass (Figure 7.15): **germ cell tumors** (GCTs) comprise over two-thirds of pineal region masses. The germinoma is the most common tumor of the pineal gland and typically appears as hyperdense on CT and iso/hypointense to gray

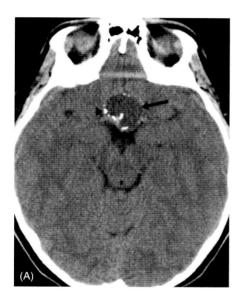
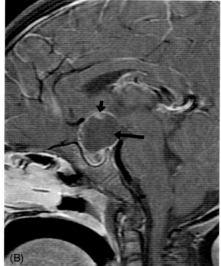
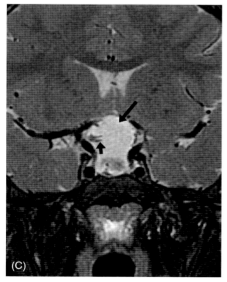
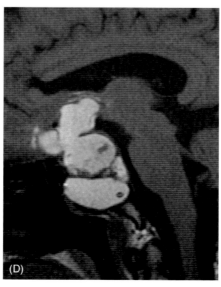

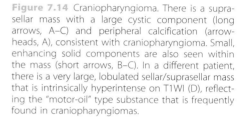

Figure 7.14 Craniopharyngioma. There is a suprasellar mass with a large cystic component (long arrows, A–C) and peripheral calcification (arrowheads, A), consistent with craniopharyngioma. Small, enhancing solid components are also seen within the mass (short arrows, B–C). In a different patient, there is a very large, lobulated sellar/suprasellar mass that is intrinsically hyperintense on T1WI (D), reflecting the "motor-oil" type substance that is frequently found in craniopharyngiomas.

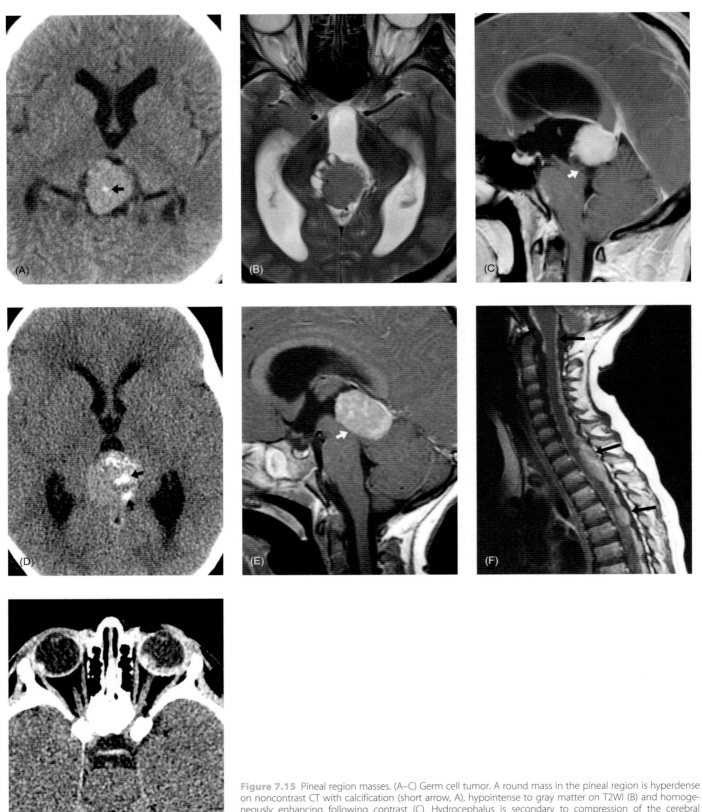

Figure 7.15 Pineal region masses. (A–C) Germ cell tumor. A round mass in the pineal region is hyperdense on noncontrast CT with calcification (short arrow, A), hypointense to gray matter on T2WI (B) and homogeneously enhancing following contrast (C). Hydrocephalus is secondary to compression of the cerebral aqueduct (white arrow, C). (D–G) Pineoblastoma with leptomeningeal metastases and retinoblastoma. A round mass in the pineal gland demonstrates coarse calcification on noncontrast CT (short arrows, D) and avid enhancement with aqueductal compression (white arrow, E) resulting in hydrocephalus. There is also diffuse metastatic coating of the leptomeninges in the spinal cord (long arrows, F). This patient also had bilateral ocular calcifications (G), consistent with retinoblastoma ("trilateral retinoblastoma").

matter on T1- and T2-weighted sequences, presumably due to the lower free water content of the tumor. They are malignant tumors that are not encapsulated and have a propensity for CSF dissemination. Teratomas, another type of germ cell tumor, are the second most common pineal region mass and appear as heterogeneous lesions with mixed fat, calcification, soft tissue and cystic change. Other germ cell tumors like choriocarcinoma, endodermal sinus tumor and embryonal cell carcinoma are less common. **Pineal parenchymal tumors** are much less common than germ cell tumors. There are two types of tumors arising from the pineal cell: pineocytoma and pineoblastoma. Pineocytomas are benign, well-differentiated tumors with mature cells, while pineoblastomas are highly malignant neoplasms with immature, small round cells similar

to medulloblastoma and a similar propensity for CSF dissemination. Pineoblastomas can develop in a small percentage of patients with bilateral and/or familial retinoblastoma ("trilateral retinoblastoma"). Intermediate-grade neoplasms with histological features between pineocytoma and pineoblastoma have also been identified. On imaging, pineoblastomas tend to be larger, more heterogeneously enhancing and more lobular or irregular in shape than pineocytomas, though distinction can be difficult. In distinguishing between germinoma and pineal parenchymal tumors, the gender of the patient can be very helpful: as germinomas have a greater than 10:1 male to female predominance, a pineal tumor in a female patient should raise suspicion for a pineal parenchymal tumor.

Further reading

Akyuz C, Varan A, Kupeli S et al. (2008) Medulloblastoma in children: a 32-year experience from a single institution. *J Neurooncol* **90**, 99–103.

Albright AL, Packer RJ, Zimmerman R et al. (1993) Magnetic resonance scans should replace biopsies for the diagnosis of diffuse brain stem gliomas: a report from the Children's Cancer Group. *Neurosurgery* **33**, 1026–9; discussion 1029–30.

Ashwal S, Hinshaw DB Jr, Bedros A (1984) CNS primitive neuroectodermal tumors of childhood. *Med Pediatr Oncol* **12**, 180–8.

Barkovich AJ *Pediatric Neuroimaging*, 4th edn. (Philadelphia: Lippincott Williams and Wilkins, 2005).

Bernhardtsen T, Laursen H, Bojsen-Moller M, Gjerris F (2003) Sub-classification of low-grade cerebellar astrocytoma: is it clinically meaningful? *Childs Nerv Syst* **19**, 729–35.

Castillo M, Davis PC, Takei Y, Hoffman JC Jr (1990) Intracranial ganglioglioma: MR, CT, and clinical findings in 18 patients. *AJR Am J Roentgenol* **154**, 607–12.

Chang T, Teng MM, Guo WY, Sheng WC (1989) CT of pineal tumors and intracranial germ-cell tumors. *AJR Am J Roentgenol* **153**, 1269–74.

Daumas-Duport C, Varlet P, Tucker ML et al. (1997) Oligodendrogliomas. Part I: Patterns of growth, histological diagnosis, clinical and imaging correlations: a study of 153 cases. *J Neurooncol* **34**, 37–59.

Desai KI, Nadkarni TD, Muzumdar DP, Goel A (2001) Prognostic factors for cerebellar astrocytomas in children: a study of 102 cases. *Pediatr Neurosurg* **35**, 311–17.

Duffner PK, Cohen ME, Myers MH, Heise HW (1986) Survival of children with brain tumors: SEER Program, 1973–1980. *Neurology* **36**, 597–601.

Ernestus RI, Wilcke O, Schroder R (1991) Supratentorial ependymomas in childhood: clinicopathological findings and prognosis. *Acta Neurochir (Wien)* **111**, 96–102.

Farmer JP, Montes JL, Freeman CR et al. (2001) Brainstem gliomas. A 10-year institutional review. *Pediatr Neurosurg* **34**, 206–14.

Finizio FS (1995) CT and MRI aspects of supratentorial hemispheric tumors of childhood and adolescence. *Childs Nerv Syst* **11**, 559–67.

Giannini C, Scheithauer BW, Burger PC et al. (1999) Pleomorphic xanthoastrocytoma: what do we really know about it? *Cancer* **85**, 2033–45.

Gjerris F, Agerlin N, Borgesen SE et al. (1998) Epidemiology and prognosis in children treated for intracranial tumours in Denmark 1960–1984. *Childs Nerv Syst* **14**, 302–11.

Hinshaw DB Jr, Ashwal S, Thompson JR, Hasso AN (1983) Neuroradiology of primitive neuroectodermal tumors. *Neuroradiology* **25**, 87–92.

Jallo GI, Biser-Rohrbaugh A, Freed D (2004) Brainstem gliomas. *Childs Nerv Sys* **20**, 143–53.

Koeller KK, Rushing EJ (2003) From the archives of the AFIP: medulloblastoma: a comprehensive review with radiologic-pathologic correlation. *Radiographics* **23**, 1613–37.

Koeller KK, Rushing EJ (2004) From the archives of the AFIP: pilocytic astrocytoma: radiologic-pathologic correlation. *Radiographics* **24**, 1693–1708.

Koeller KK, Rushing EJ (2005) From the archives of the AFIP: Oligodendroglioma and its variants: radiologic-pathologic correlation. *Radiographics* **25**, 1669–88.

Kornreich L, Blaser S, Schwarz M et al. (2001) Optic pathway glioma: correlation of imaging findings with the presence of neurofibromatosis. *AJNR Am J Neuroradiol* **22**, 1963–9.

Kuroiwa T, Bergey GK, Rothman MI et al. (1995) Radiologic appearance of the dysembryoplastic neuroepithelial tumor. *Radiology* **197**, 233–8.

Meyers SP, Kemp SS, Tarr RW (1992) MR imaging features of medulloblastomas. *AJR Am J Roentgenol* **158**, 859–65.

Ostertun B, Wolf HK, Campos MG et al. (1996) Dysembryoplastic neuroepithelial tumors: MR and CT evaluation. *AJNR Am J Neuroradiol* **17**, 419–30.

Parsa CF, Hoyt CS, Lesser RL et al. (2001) Spontaneous regression of optic gliomas: thirteen cases documented by serial neuroimaging. *Arch Ophthalmol* **119**, 516–29.

Pizzo PA, Poplack DG (eds.) *Principles and Practice of Pediatric Oncology* (Philadelphia: Lippincott Williams and Wilkins, 2005).

Pollack IF (1999) Pediatric brain tumors. *Semin Surg Oncol* **16**, 73–90.

Reni M, Gatta G, Mazza E, Vecht C (2007) Ependymoma. *Crit Rev Oncol Hematol* **63**, 81–9.

Rickert CH, Paulus W (2001) Epidemiology of central nervous system tumors in childhood and adolescence based on the new WHO classification. *Childs Nerv Syst* **17**, 503–11.

Sandhu A, Kendall B (1987) Computed tomography in management of medulloblastomas. *Neuroradiology* **29**, 444–52.

Schild SE, Nisi K, Scheithauer BW *et al.*(1998) The results of radiotherapy for ependymomas: the Mayo Clinic experience. *Int J Radiat Oncol Biol Phys* **42**, 953–8.

Shu HK, Sall WF, Maity A *et al.* (2007) Childhood intracranial ependymoma: twenty-year experience from a single institution. *Cancer* **110**, 432–41.

Smyth MD, Horn BN, Russo C, Berger MS (2000) Intracranial ependymomas of childhood: current management strategies. *Pediatr Neurosurg* **33**, 138–50.

Swartz JD, Zimmerman RA, Bilaniuk LT (1982) Computed tomography of intracranial ependymomas. *Radiology* **143**, 97–101.

Tenreiro-Picon OR, Kamath SV, Knorr JR *et al.* (1995) Desmoplastic infantile

ganglioglioma: CT and MRI features. *Pediatr Radiol* **25**, 540–3.

Tomita T, McLone DG, Yasue M (1988) Cerebral primitive neuroectodermal tumors in childhood. *J Neurooncol* **6**, 233–43.

Viano JC, Herrera EJ, Suarez JC (2001) Cerebellar astrocytomas: a 24-year experience. *Childs Nerv Syst* **17**, 607–10; discussion 611.

7B SOLID TUMORS OUTSIDE OF THE CNS

Heike E. Daldrup-Link and Robert Goldsby

Solid primary tumors account for 30% of all pediatric malignancies. The most common pediatric solid neoplasms are non-Hodgkin's lymphoma (NHL), Hodgkin's lymphoma (HL), neuroblastoma, rhabdomyosarcoma, Wilms tumor, osteosarcoma, Ewing's sarcoma, germ cell tumor and liver tumors, in decreasing order of prevalence. Typical imaging and staging criteria for these tumors will be discussed in this chapter. RECIST criteria for evaluation of response of solid tumors outside of the CNS are shown in Table 7.6

Lymphoma

There are two main forms of pediatric lymphomas. HL represents approximately 45% of pediatric lymphomas and the remainder are included in the category of NHL. Pediatric NHL lymphomas are almost exclusively high-grade lymphomas and usually defined as one of three main categories: lymphoblastic lymphoma, Burkitt's lymphoma and anaplastic large cell lymphoma. Lymphomas are very unusual in infants and more commonly seen in teenagers, with an increasing incidence with age. Boys are more frequently affected than girls. The patients typically present with a rapidly growing, symptomatic mass at a nodal or extranodal site anywhere in the body. Patients with HL can exhibit "B" symptoms such as weight loss, night sweats and fever. They can also have intense pruritis. Patients with lymphoblastic lymphoma often present with respiratory symptoms, such as cough or shortness of breath, due to mediastinal disease. Patients with Burkitt's lymphoma more often present with abdominal complaints due to abdominal disease. Burkitt's lymphoma should be considered in older children that present with intussusception. Radiographically, HL is often localized to a single axial group of nodes (cervical, mediastinal, para-aortic) with continuous spread, while NHL frequently involves multiple peripheral nodes with non-contiguous spread. Mesenteric nodes, the Waldeyer ring and other extranodal sites are rarely involved in HL, but commonly involved in NHL.

A typical presentation of a lymphoma on imaging studies is that of multiple enlarged lymph nodes or a bulky confluent soft tissue mass in the neck or middle mediastinum (Figure 7.16).

Table 7.6 Response evaluation criteria (RECIST) for patients with solid tumors (except neuroblastoma patients with 123I-MIBG positive lesions and patients with Hodgkin's disease)

Criteria	Definition
Measurable disease	The presence of at least one lesion that can be accurately measured in at least one dimension, with the longest diameter at least 10 mm (spiral CT) or 20 mm (other techniques). Up to ten measurable lesions should be followed for response evaluation
Technique	Serial measurements of lesions are to be done with CT or MRI. The same method of assessment is to be used to characterize each identified and reported lesion at baseline and during follow-up
Quantification of disease burden	The sum of the longest diameter (LD) for all target lesions will be calculated and reported as the disease measurement
Complete response (CR)	Disappearance of all target lesions. If immunocytology is available, no disease must be detected by that methodology
Partial response (PR)	At least a 30% decrease in the disease measurement, taking as reference the disease measurement made to confirm measurable disease at study enrollment
Progressive disease (PD)	At least a 20% increase in the disease measurement, taking as reference the smallest disease measurement recorded since the start of treatment, or the appearance of one or more new lesions
Stable disease (SD)	Neither sufficient shrinkage to qualify for PR nor sufficient increase to qualify for PD, taking as reference the smallest disease measurement since the treatment started
Response assessment	Each patient will be classified according to their "best response" for the purposes of analysis of treatment effect. Best response is determined from the sequence of the objective statuses described above

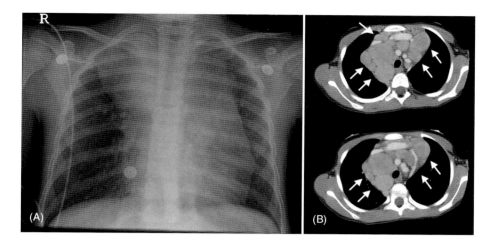

Figure 7.16 Hodgkin's lymphoma. (A) Chest radiograph shows marked widening of the superior mediastinum with mild narrowing of the trachea and unusual low position of the carina (usually projecting at the level of T4). (B) Corresponding axial CT scans through the upper chest show numerous enlarged lymph nodes, predominantly in the middle mediastinum and extending into the anterior and posterior mediastinum (arrows) with displacement and compression of the mediastinal vessels.

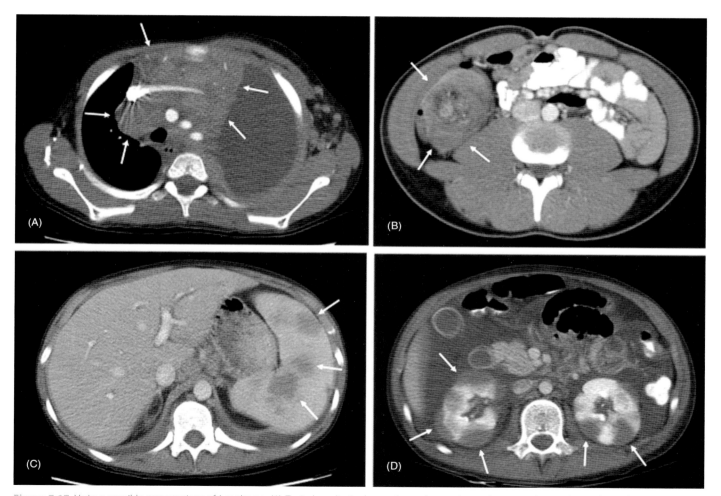

Figure 7.17 Various possible presentations of lymphoma. (A) Typical mediastinal mass (arrows), encasing and compressing mediastinal vessels, with associated large left-sided pleural effusion. (B) Thickened bowel walls (arrows) due to biopsy-proven involvement of the jejunum; (C) multiple focal hypodense lesions in the spleen (arrows) and (D) multiple focal hypodense lesions in both kidneys (arrows) as well as extensive ascites.

Table 7.7 Modified Ann Arbor staging for Hodgkin's lymphoma

Stage	Tumor extent
1	Involvement of single lymph node region (I) or localized involvement of a single extralymphatic organ or site (IE)
2	Involvement of two or more lymph node regions on the same side of the diaphragm (II)
3	Involvement of lymph node regions on both sides of the diaphragm (III), which may also be accompanied by localized contiguous involvement of an extralymphatic organ or site (IIIE), by involvement of the spleen (IIIS), or both (IIIE+S)
4	Disseminated (multifocal) involvement of one or more extralymphatic organs or tissues, with or without associated lymph node involvement, or isolated extralymphatic organ involvement with distant (non-regional) nodal involvement

"B" symptoms: at least one of the following:

Unexplained weight loss >10%, unexplained recurrent fever >38 °C, drenching night sweats

Bulk disease

- Large mediastinal mass: tumor diameter > one-third of the thoracic diameter (measured transversely at the level of the dome of the diaphragm on an upright PA CXR)
- Large extra-mediastinal nodal aggregate: A continuous aggregate of nodal tissue that measures >6 cm in the longest transverse diameter in any nodal area

Table 7.8 Staging of Non-Hodgkin's lymphoma

Stage	Tumor extent
1	A single tumor (extranodal) or a single anatomical site (nodal) with exclusion of the mediastinum or abdomen
2	A single tumor (extranodal) with regional involvement. Two or more nodal areas on the same side of the diaphragm. Two single (extranodal) tumors with or without regional node involvement on the same side of the diaphragm. A primary gastrointestinal tract tumor, usually in the ileocecal area, with or without involvement of associated mesenteric nodes only, grossly completely resected
3	Two single tumors (extranodal) on opposite sides of the diaphragm. Two or more nodal areas above and below the diaphragm. All primary intrathoracic tumors (mediastinal, pleural, thymic). All extensive primary intra-abdominal disease, unresectable. All paraspinal or epidural tumors, regardless of other tumor sites
4	Any of the above with initial CNS and/or bone marrow involvement (>5%, <25%). >25% malignant cells in the bone marrow is defined as leukemia

An enlarged lymph node is defined by an increased diameter of more than 1 cm in the short axis, and bulky disease is defined by a diameter of 6 cm or more of a confluent soft tissue mass. On CT, these masses typically show a homogeneous soft tissue attenuation. Mediastinal lymphomas are often associated with a pleural effusion (Figure 7.17). Central tumor necrosis, hemorrhage or cyst formation may be sometimes seen, while calcifications are extremely rare before treatment. Lymphomas typically encase vascular structures and the trachea or main stem bronchi, which puts the patient at risk for vascular compression and airway collapse with related complications during anesthesia. Pericardial infiltration may also occur. Lung involvement by lymphoma can have a highly variable appearance, presenting as pulmonary nodules, alveolar consolidations or ground-glass opacities. Various other organs can be involved as well (Figure 7.17). Staging of HL is performed according to the Ann Arbor classification (Table 7.7). Several different systems are available for the staging of NHL in children. One of the most popular systems is the St. Jude Children's Research Hospital model (Table 7.8). Patients with lower stage (stage 1 or 2) lymphomas tend to have an excellent outcome (>90% survival). Advanced stage disease (stage 3 or 4) requires more intensive therapy, but patients also generally have a good prognosis (>70%) depending on other risk factors.

PET or PET-CT imaging offers a high sensitivity for staging and treatment-monitoring of lymphomas (Figure 7.18). Metabolically active, presumed viable tumor sites within the body are delineated by increased focal 2-[^{18}F] Fluoro-2-deoxyglucose (fludeoxyglucose (18F), or FDG) radiotracer uptake. Qualitative image evaluation is based on the calculation of the standardized uptake value (*SUV*), which is defined as the activity concentration within the lesion divided by the amount of injected dose per body weight (*bw*), lean body mass (*lbm*) or body surface area (*bsa*):

$$SUV = \frac{\text{activity concentration of lesion } (\text{MBq ml}^{-1})}{\text{injected dose } (\text{MBq ml}^{-1})/bw, \, lbm, \, bsa}$$

The SUV value is an earlier and more accurate predictor of treatment response than changes in tumor size. In addition, the SUV value may be helpful in differentiating rebound thymus and tumor recurrence: at our institution, an SUV of more than 3.5 has been associated with a high likelihood of tumor recurrence. Of note, SUV values differ between different scanners; thus, thresholds have to be adjusted at each institution. A high FDG uptake in both thymus and bone marrow is frequently

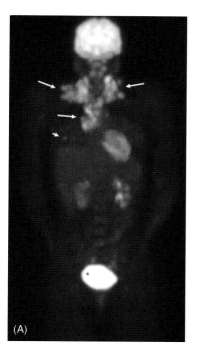

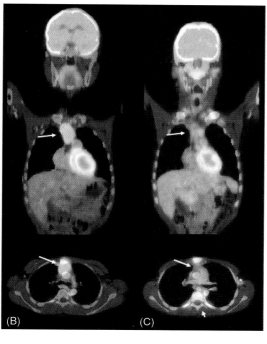

Figure 7.18 PET and PET-CT of patients with lymphoma. (A) Coronal PET scan of a patient with Hodgkin's lymphoma shows numerous FDG-avid lymph nodes in the neck bilaterally, the supraclavicular areas and the mediastinum (arrows). There is also an FDG-positive pulmonary nodule (arrowhead). (B),(C) PET-CT of a patient with Non-Hodgkin's lymphoma. Fusion of PET data with CT data provides improved anatomical detail. This patient shows an FDG-avid mass in the anterior mediastinum (B, arrow). A follow-up scan after six weeks of chemotherapy (C) shows persistent soft tissue in the anterior mediastinum, which showed marked reduction of FDG uptake. Reduced FDG metabolism appears to be a better and earlier predictor of tumor response than change in tumor size. The patient also shows markedly increased FDG-metabolism in the bone marrow (arrowhead), which is due to a therapy-induced red marrow conversion.

Table 7.9 Differential diagnosis of mediastinal masses in children

Anterior mediastinum	Middle mediastinum	Posterior mediastinum
Normal thymus: Homogeneous, does not compress vessels, moves with respiration on US	>> Thymus may extend into middle mediastinum	**Neuroblastoma:** Young child (peak 2–3 years), encases vessels, grows behind aorta, neuroforamina invasion, restricted diffusion on MRI, elevated catecholamine metabolites in urine in >90%, positive MIBG scan
Teratoma: Inhomogeneous, fat, calcifications (Ca^{2+})	**(1) Bronchogenic, (2) pericardial or (3) esophageal cyst:** Well defined, benign mass which may contain simple or complex fluid. Typical location, in particular (1), below carina. (1 and 3): may contain air–fluid levels	
Seminoma: Bulky, lobulated homogeneous mass, no Ca^{2+}, pleural and pericardial effusion		
Malignant nonseminoma: Inhomogeneous and invasive mass, possible gynecomasty, elevated β-HCG and AFP		**Ganglioneuroma:** Older child (peak 6 years), may encase vessels, may invade neuroforamina, increased diffusion on MRI, elevated catecholamines in urine in about 37%, positive MIBG scan in 50%
<< Lymphoma may extend into anterior mediastinum	<< **Lymphoma:** Large mass which encases vessels and airways, adenopathy, possible associated pulmonary consolidation and pleural effusion	
(Thymo)Lipoma: Fat density, very rare in children	**Metastatic nodes:** Round, no identifiable fatty hilum, primary tumor	**Neurofibroma:** Café-au-lait spots, Lisch nodules, neuroforamina involvement, "target sign" (hypointense center in relatively hyperintense lesion) on T2-weighted MRI
Thymic cyst: Fluid density, very rare in children	**Inflammatory nodes:** May show preserved fatty hilum, may be associated with pulmonary consolidation	
Thymoma: Soft tissue density, homogeneous, myasthenia gravis, very rare in children		**Extramedullary hematopoiesis:** Hemolytic anemia, paravertebral soft tissue lesions, positive bone scan
Thyroid: Palpable goiter, positive thyroid scan	>> May extend between trachea and esophagus	**Intrathoracic mengingocele:** Continuity with spinal canal

MIBG = iodine-131-metaiodobenzylguanidine (iobenguane (131I)).
β-HCG = human chorionic gonadotropin.

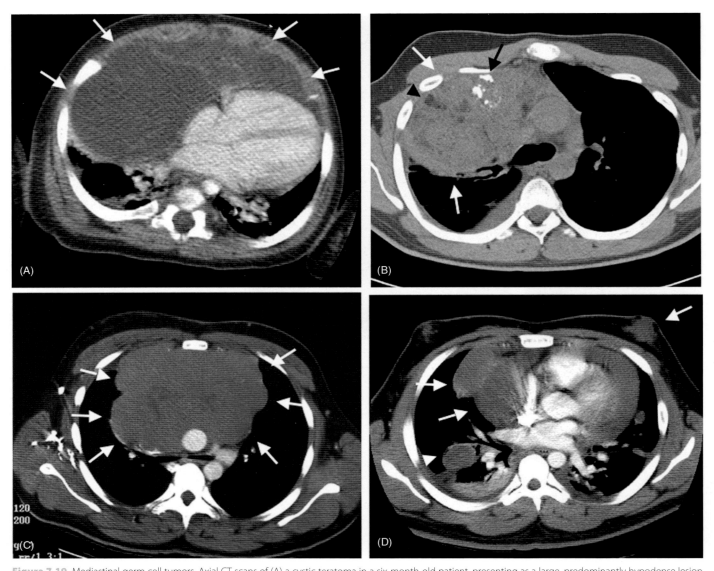

Figure 7.19 Mediastinal germ cell tumors. Axial CT scans of (A) a cystic teratoma in a six-month-old patient, presenting as a large, predominantly hypodense lesion in the anterior mediastinum (arrows) with enhancement of a thin peripheral rim and some internal septae. (B) Mixed mature and immature teratoma in a patient with Klinefelter syndrome (who has increased risk of developing this GCT). The anterior mediastinal mass (white arrows) shows areas of enhancing soft tissue with some areas of calcifications (black arrow) and fat (negative Hounsfield units (HU), arrowhead). (C) Seminoma in a young adolescent, presenting as a relatively homogeneous and relatively well-defined anterior mediastinal mass (arrows). (D) Nonseminomatous germ cell tumor (NSGCT) in an adolescent young man, presenting as an aggressive soft tissue mass in the anterior mediastinum (arrows), infiltrating the pericardium and causing a pericardial and pleural effusion. There are also several lung nodules (arrowhead). Although only seen in a subgroup of patients, the presence of gynecomasty can lead to the diagnosis of a NSGCT.

associated with rebound, while a differential high FDG uptake in the thymus with low FDG uptake in the bone marrow is more frequently seen with tumor recurrence.

Differential diagnosis of mediastinal masses in children

Mediastinal masses in children can be differentiated based on their location, the age of the child and clinical information (Table 7.9). Care has to be taken to not confuse a normal thymus with a mediastinal mass (compare information about

normal thymus in Chapter 1). The most frequent masses in the anterior mediastinum are germ cell tumors (Figure 7.19). These include seminomas and nonseminomatous germ cell tumors (see details below). The latter include teratomas, which may be cystic or present as inhomogeneous lesions with areas of enhancing soft tissue, calcifications and fat (Figure 7.19). The most frequent masses in the middle mediastinum besides lymphoma are infectious causes of lymphadenopathy and mediastinal cysts (Figure 7.20). The most frequent masses in the posterior mediastinum are neurogenic tumors (Table 7.9).

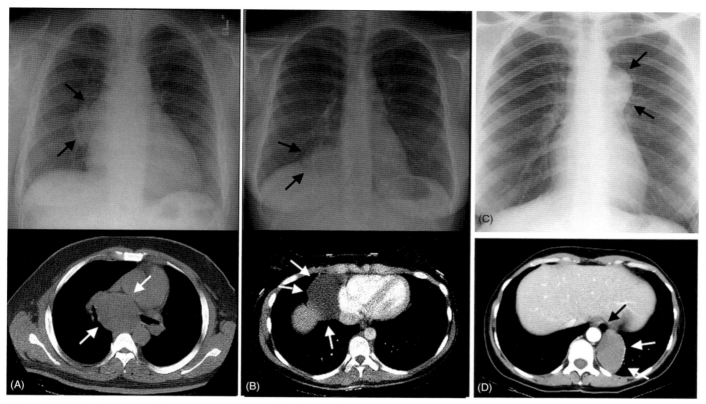

Figure 7.20 Mediastinal cysts. (A) Bronchogenic cyst in typical subcarinal location (arrows): the mass causes a widening of the middle mediastinum along with splaying of the carina and compression of the right main stem bronchus. (B) Pericardial cyst in typical location in the lower mediastinum with contact to the pericardium (arrows). (C), (D) Duplication cyst in the mid- or posterior mediastinum on X-rays and (in a different patient) CT. All mediastinal cysts appear relatively homogeneous on cross-sectional studies with variable density on plain CT images and absent or minimal peripheral enhancement on contrast-enhanced studies.

Neuroblastoma

Neuroblastomas are malignant neoplasms, arising from neural crest cells of the adrenal gland or sympathetic chain in the neck, chest, abdomen or pelvis. Neuroblastomas typically present in young children with a peak age of 2–3 years. They are rare in children over 10 years of age. They are usually sporadic, but fewer than 2% will have other affected family members. The clinical manifestations vary with age, stage, location and metabolic disturbances from excessive catecholamine production. More than 90% of patients show elevated catecholamine metabolites in the urine. Neuroblastomas have a variable biology, but *N-MYC* amplification is associated with aggressive behavior.

Radiographic imaging studies of neuroblastoma usually demonstrate an aggressive, often large, mostly solid, enhancing, inhomogeneous tumor with variable degrees of non-enhancing necrotic areas. Neuroblastomas typically encase vessels and grow behind the aorta (Figure 7.21). Calcifications are found in 40–60% of tumors and often increase in extent during therapy. The tumors may invade adjacent organs and extend into the spinal canal via the neuroforamina. Staging is done based on cross-sectional imaging studies and

MIBG scans (Table 7.10, Figure 7.22). A new staging system was recently proposed that incorporates sites of disease, histological features, tumor biology and age to determine risk groups for treatment. Metastases are found in 75% of patients at the time of diagnosis and may involve the bone marrow, lymph nodes, liver and skin. Bone marrow involvement is rarely solitary. Intracranial or skull base tumors usually originate from the bone marrow and may cause extra-axial soft tissue masses (Figure 7.22). Liver metastases are often multiple and hypervascular compared to liver parenchyma, with early enhancement after contrast media injection, and rapid washout (Figure 7.23). Following successful chemotherapy, on imaging studies the liver can show a "pseudocirrhotic" appearance which does not pathologically resemble a true cirrhosis (Figure 7.23). In addition, focal nodular hyperplasias may develop as late sequelae of aggressive chemotherapy. Lung metastases are rare and are usually only found in patients with extensive or recurrent disease. The abdominal aorta and its major branches may show impaired growth due to irradiation therapy, which may cause significant stenoses many years after successful therapy. Thus, the abdominal vessels have to be carefully examined on follow-up imaging studies.

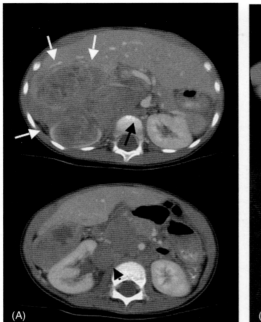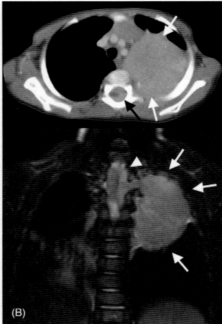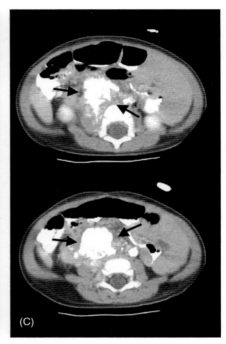

Figure 7.21 Various possible presentations of neuroblastomas. (A) Axial contrast-enhanced CT scans show a typical presentation of an inhomogeneous and aggressive mass in the area of the right adrenal gland. Numerous lymph node metastases are also seen (arrowhead). The mass infiltrates the kidney. However, in contrast to a Wilms tumor, the tumor center is not located in the kidney and grows characteristically behind the aorta (black arrow). (B) A CT scan (upper image) and coronal T2-weighted MR scan (lower image) of another patient with a neuroblastoma in the left upper posterior mediastinum (arrows) show an infiltration of multiple neuroforaminas (CT: black arrow, MR: arrowhead), which is characteristic for neurogenic tumors. (C) Axial CT scans of a mass in the infrarenal retroperitoneum, likely originating from the sympathetic chain. The mass contains large areas of amorphous calcifications (arrows).

Table 7.10 Staging of neuroblastoma

Stage	Definition
1	Limited to organ of origin
2	Regional spread, not crossing the midline (= vertebral body)
3	Extension across the midline (= contralateral margin of vertebral body)
4	Metastatic disease to distant lymph nodes, liver, bone, brain, lung
4S	Stage 1 and 2 with metastatic disease confined to liver, skin, bone marrow; no radiological evidence of bone metastases/osteolysis

Differential diagnosis of adrenal masses in children

Ganglioneuromas are benign neurogenic tumors with imaging features that are very similar to neuroblastomas. Several features can suggest the diagnosis of a ganglioneuroma: (1) a slightly older age than the typical "neuroblastoma age" with a peak presentation at about six years of age. (2) About 50% of ganglioneuromas are not positive on MIBG scans. (3) About 63% show no evidence of elevated catecholamines

in the urine. (4) Follow-up studies often show relatively slow tumor growth; and (5) it has been suggested that neuroblastomas and ganglioneuromas may be distinguishable based on their signal on diffusion-weighted MR scans, with neuroblastomas showing restricted diffusion but ganglioneuromas showing increased diffusion.

Pheochromocytomas are very rare in children and, if they occur, are often associated with multiple endocrine neoplasia (MEN) syndromes. Pheochromocytomas that occur outside of the adrenal gland are called paragangliomas. Patients with pheochromocytomas or paragangliomas present early with signs of hypertensive crises, and the tumors are in general relatively small at diagnosis. In adults, a high T2 signal on MR scans has been found to be diagnostic of pheochromocytomas. This feature is not as helpful in children, as neuroblastomas are also well vascularized and T2 hyperintense. Both pheochromocytomas and neuroblastomas are positive on MIBG scans and, thus, MIBG scans are used for staging. Patients with unresectable disease and MIBG-avid tumors may benefit from high-dose I131-MIBG therapy.

Likewise, the imaging features of an **adrenocortical neoplasm** are not significantly different compared to other adrenal masses. However, a typical combination of clinical and imaging findings should lead to the correct diagnosis: adrenocortical neoplasms present typically in young children (girls more often than boys) with signs of precocious puberty

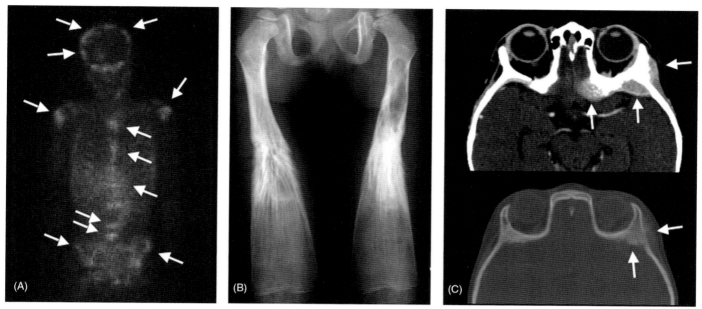

Figure 7.22 Typical neuroblastoma metastases. (A) MIBG scan shows multiple bone metastases in the skull, proximal humeri, numerous vertebrae and pelvis (arrows). (B) Aggressive mixed lytic and sclerotic lesions in both femora with Erlenmeyer flask-like bone expansion, destruction of the cortex and periosteal reaction. (C) Typical metastases to the orbit on CT. These metastases originate in the bone marrow, as evidenced by bone destruction on bone windows (lower image), and then extend to paraosseous soft tissues, causing intraorbital or extra-axial intracranial soft tissue masses, seen on soft tissue windows (upper image, arrows).

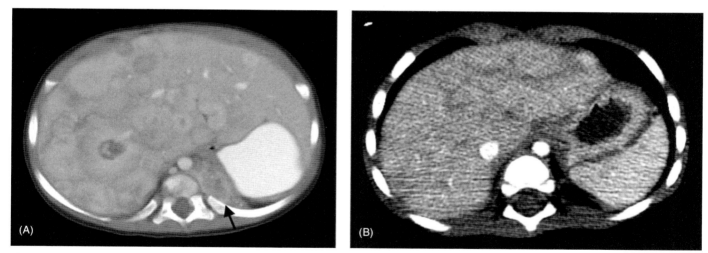

Figure 7.23 Liver metastases from neuroblastoma. (A) Axial contrast-enhanced CT scan shows multiple peripherally enhancing lesions throughout the liver, consistent with metastases. The primary tumor is a neuroblastoma in the area of the left adrenal gland (arrow). (B) Following successful chemotherapy, the liver may show an inhomogeneous parenchyma on imaging studies, which may mimic cirrhosis.

in combination with an adrenal mass and markedly accelerated skeletal maturation on bone radiographs. These lesions are termed "neoplasms" as it is often difficult to determine if they are benign or malignant.

Wilms tumor (nephroblastoma)

Wilms tumors present in young children with a mean age of three years. These malignant tumors arise from the kidney and

may occur bilaterally in 5% of patients. Many patients present with an asymptomatic abdominal mass. Others may present with abdominal pain, hematuria and/or hypertension at diagnosis. The tumor is associated with the *WT1* (11p13) and *WT2* (11p15.5) genes. Patients with Beckwith-Wiedemann syndrome, hemihypertrophy, aniridia and trisomy 18, among others, have an increased risk of developing Wilms tumors and are screened with regular ultrasounds until approximately school age.

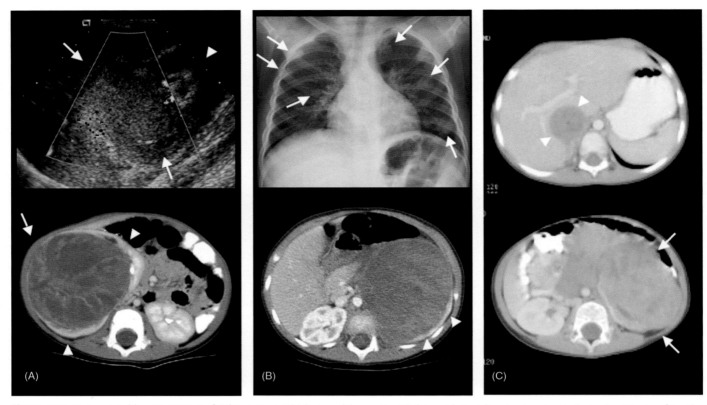

Figure 7.24 Various possible presentations of Wilms tumors. (A) Ultrasound (upper image) shows a large inhomogeneous mass (arrows), originating from the kidney (arrowhead). CT scan (lower image) shows enhancing kidney parenchyma "grabbing" around an inhomogeneous central mass (arrowheads, claw sign). (B) CT scan of a Wilms tumor of the left kidney (lower image). Sometimes, the kidney parenchyma can only form a very thin stripe of enhancing tissue around the mass (arrowheads). The mass pushes vessels to the contralateral side rather than growing around them. A chest X-ray (upper image) shows typical pulmonary metastases, presenting as large bilateral pulmonary nodules. (C) CT scan of an inhomogeneous mass in the left kidney, which extends into the left renal vein and forms a tumor thrombus in the IVC (arrowheads).

The typical imaging feature of a Wilms tumor is an inhomogeneous renal mass with enhancing solid and cystic or necrotic elements. As the tumor grows, the normal kidney may be splayed open around the tumor, called the "claw" sign. This classic appearance indicates a renal origin of the mass (Figure 7.24), as opposed to a neuroblastoma which can sometimes infiltrate a kidney but has its center outside of the kidney (compare Figure 7.21). Wilms tumors can rarely have calcifications. Wilms tumors typically are relatively well defined with a surrounding "pseudocapsule." Any disintegrity of this pseudocapsule and/or large amounts of peritumoral free fluid need to be reported as they may indicate tumor rupture and require a change in therapy with postsurgical irradiation of the whole abdomen. Wilms tumors often infiltrate the renal vein, and a tumor thrombus can extend from the renal vein into the IVC and the right atrium. Careful description of the extent of the tumor thrombus, including extensions into venous branches, is very important for surgery planning. Staging of Wilms tumors is done based on the surgery result and the presence of metastases (Table 7.11). The tumor may

metastasize into lungs, liver or (rarely) brain. Metastases in the liver are more frequently due to venous thrombi than actual parenchymal tumor seeds. Metastases to the bone are

Table 7.11 Staging of Wilms tumor

Stage	Definition
1	Cancer is found only in the kidney and can be completely removed by surgery
2	Cancer has spread to areas near the kidney, fat or soft tissue, blood vessels or renal sinus, and can be completely removed by surgery
3	Cancer has spread to areas near the kidney, and cannot be completely removed by surgery
4	Metastases to lungs, liver, bone and brain
5	Bilateral tumors

Table 7.12 Differential diagnosis of kidney masses in children

Tumor	Patient population	Imaging features	Metastases
Wilms tumor	Young patients, mean age 3 years	Claw sign, inhomogeneous mass, contrast medium enhancement, tumor thrombus in renal vein and IVC, bilateral in 5%	Lungs, lymph nodes, liver, brain
Nephroblastomatosis	Young patients, mean age 3 years	Homogeneous mass, often multiple, often bilateral, no or minimal homogeneous contrast medium enhancement	None, *may regress, or develop into Wilms tumor, follow-up needed*
Mesoblastic nephroma	<1 year of age (*age leads to the diagnosis*)	Homogeneous, well-defined, unilateral enhancing renal mass with claw sign	Very rare
Rhabdoid tumor	Young children, neonates and infants	Ill-defined, aggressive, inhomogeneous unilateral renal mass with claw sign, *concurrent or metastatic CNS tumor*	Lymph nodes, lung, CNS
Clear cell sarcoma	Young children	Very aggressive inhomogeneous unilateral renal mass with claw sign, often metastases at diagnosis	Lymph nodes, lung, *bone metastases in 10–40%*, CNS
Renal medullary carcinoma	Teenage or young adult men with sickle cell trait	Very aggressive inhomogeneous unilateral renal mass with claw sign, often metastases at diagnosis	Lymph nodes, lung, *bone*, CNS
Renal cell carcinoma	Teenagers or adults, increased incidence in *van Hippel Lindau (VHL)* patients	Well- or ill-defined, homogeneous or inhomogeneous unilateral renal mass, often metastases at diagnosis (VHL patients also have multiple cysts)	Lymph nodes, lung, *bone*, CNS
Multilocular cystic renal tumor	1. Cystic partially differentiated nephroma = baby boys 2. Cystic nephroma = young women	Homogeneous, well-defined multicystic mass, some septae may enhance, cysts do not enhance, may rarely have small foci of enhancing soft tissue	None
Angiomyolipoma	Tuberous sclerosis	Usually multiple homogeneous, small, well-defined lesions with fat attenuation, often bilateral, some areas of the lesions may enhance	None

extremely rare and should lead to considerations of other differential diagnoses.

Differential diagnosis of kidney masses in children

A variety of possible other renal masses have to be considered in children. The differential diagnosis can be narrowed based on the age of the child, the morphology of the renal mass and the pattern of metastatic disease (Table 7.12). It is important to recognize **nephroblastomatosis**, primarily benign rests of embryonic renal tissue, which present focal or confluent, often multiple and bilateral homogeneous soft tissue masses within the peripheral or – more rarely – central renal parenchyma

(Figure 7.25). The lesions are homogeneous and show no or only minimal enhancement. They may sometimes be associated with intralesional cysts. Nephroblastomatosis lesions may regress spontaneously. However, they can also progress to a Wilms tumor (nephroblastoma) and, thus, have to be followed with imaging techniques. Rapid growth, tumor inhomogeneities and marked contrast enhancement are not definite, but highly suspicious signs for possible malignant transformation, and may warrant biopsy or resection. Other differential diagnoses are listed in Table 7.12 and shown in Figure 7.26. Typical kidney tumors in children less than one year of age are mesoblastic nephromas and rhabdoid tumors. Rhabdoid tumors are particularly aggressive cancers that occur in the kidney and/or brain.

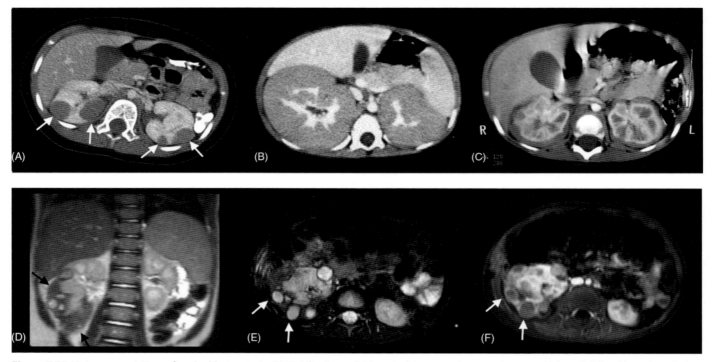

Figure 7.25 Various presentations of nephroblastomatosis. (A) Multifocal superficial nephroblastomatosis, presenting as multiple well-defined hypodense lesions on the periphery of the kidney on a CT scan. (B) Diffuse pancortical nephroblastomatosis on CT: the kidneys are greatly enlarged; there is no normal renal tissue. The whole kidney parenchyma consists of hypodense metanephric blastema. A pelvicalyceal system is present and shows accumulation and excretion of intravenously administered contrast agent. (C) Superficial diffuse nephroblastomatosis (late infantile type) on CT: diffuse subcapsular distribution of hypodense metanephric blastema which may extend into the interlobular areas. The kidneys are symmetrically enlarged. (D–F) Cysts of various types may accompany nephroblastomatosis. Coronal (D) and axial (E) T2-weighted scans demonstrate nephroblastomatosis as hypointense tissue in the periphery of the right kidney (black arrows). Within this tissue, there are several well-defined round T2-hyperintense lesions, consistent with accompanying cysts (white arrows). On contrast-enhanced T1-weighted scans (F), nephroblastomatosis shows minimal enhancement, and the intralesional cysts show no enhancement (arrows).

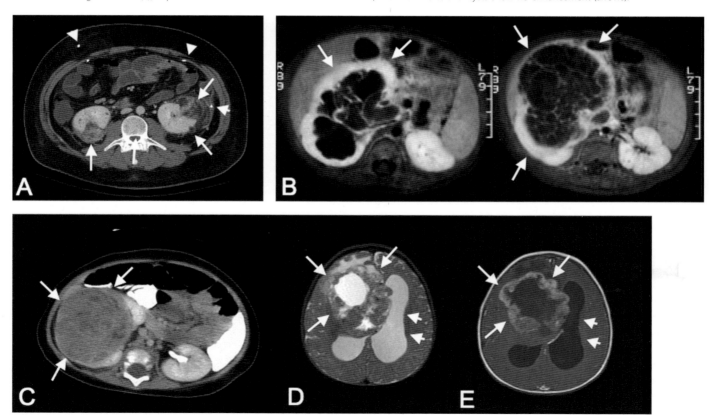

Figure 7.26 Other kidney tumors in children. (A) Axial CT scan in a patient with tuberous sclerosis shows innumerable hypodense lesions in both kidneys (arrow), with areas that contain fat (negative Hounsfield units) and variable proportions of enhancing soft tissue. These are typical angiomyolipomas. A ventriculoperitoneal (VP) shunt is also seen (arrowhead). (B) Axial contrast-enhanced T1-weighted MR scans show a large, multiseptated mass in the right kidney. The majority of the mass shows a signal equivalent to fluid (compare CSF as internal standard) and does not enhance. Only the periphery and internal septae show contrast enhancement. This is characteristic for a cystic nephroma. (C–E) Axial CT scan shows an inhomogeneous, enhancing mass in the right kidney (C). Axial T2-weighted (D) and contrast enhanced T1-weighted (E) MR scans of the brain show a very large, peripherally enhancing and centrally necrotic mass in the right brain hemisphere, causing marked hydrocephalus. The combination of a kidney mass and brain tumor in an infant is highly suspicious for a rhabdoid tumor.

Hepatoblastoma

The majority of liver tumors in children are malignant. Hepatoblastomas are the most common primary liver tumors in young children, with a peak presentation at one to two years of age and a male : female ratio of 2 : 1. Predisposing conditions include Beckwith-Wiedemann syndrome, hemihypertrophy, familial polyposis coli, Gardner's syndrome, fetal alcohol syndrome and prematurity. The alpha fetoprotein (AFP) is typically markedly elevated. Hepatoblastomas typically present as a well-defined, solitary, inhomogeneous hepatic mass, with similar attenuation or signal compared to liver tissue, with or without calcifications. Hepatoblastomas show a heterogeneous enhancement after contrast media administration. The tumor may invade the portal vein or liver veins (Figure 7.27). Metastases may be seen in lymph nodes and lung parenchyma, rarely in the bones and brain. Imaging is essential to determine if the tumor is resectable.

Differential diagnosis of liver masses in children

A differential diagnosis of liver tumors in children can be obtained based on the age of the child, clinical information (in particular AFP) and imaging characteristics.

Hepatocellular carcinoma (HCC) typically affects children over 10 years of age with no specific sex predilection. Predisposing conditions include cirrhosis due to biliary atresia, other causes of infantile cholestasis, hemochromatosis and glycogen storage disorders. Imaging features are similar to adult HCCs, with early arterial contrast enhancement and a rapid washout, although imaging signs of cirrhosis may be minimal or non-appreciable (Figure 7.28).

Infantile hepatic hemangiomas and hemangioendotheliomas are the most common vascular hepatic tumors. They typically present in neonates and infants, may be rapidly growing in the perinatal period and may involute in the natural course. Infantile hepatic hemangiomas are benign vascular lesions. Epitheloid hemangioendotheliomas are also primarily benign, but may show a malignant potential. Imaging characteristics are similar to hemangiomas in adults, with high T2 signal on MR images (similar to CSF as an internal standard, Figure 7.29) and characteristic persistent enhancement on delayed post-contrast CT or MR images. Extensive arteriovenous shunting can lead to high-output congestive heart failure.

Adenomas and focal nodular hyperplasia (FNH) show similar imaging features as those described for adults, with a characteristic early arterial enhancement and rapid washout of contrast material on CT or MR images. The T1 and T2 signal on MR images is usually very similar to liver tissue, except for central necroses or hemorrhages in adenomas or central, vascularized scars in FNH. Of note, FNHs were previously thought to occur preferentially in young women. However, these tumors are also increasingly seen in young children. Children at higher risk for FNH include those who have been previously treated with chemotherapy and those who have undergone a Kasai procedure. FNH and adenomas may be seen in patients with glycogen storage disorder.

Focal hepatic lesions with fluid-equivalent contents on imaging studies comprise simple cysts, cysts associated with polycystic kidney diseases, biliary cysts, cysts in Caroli's syndrome, liver abscesses, mesenchymal hamartoma and centrally necrotic malignant tumors (Figure 7.29).

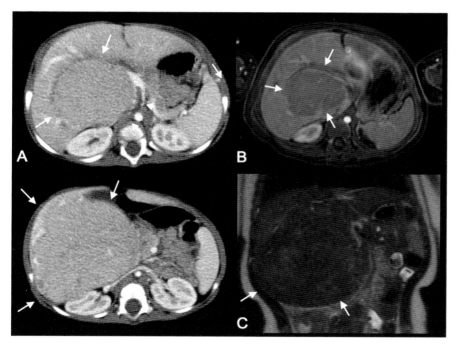
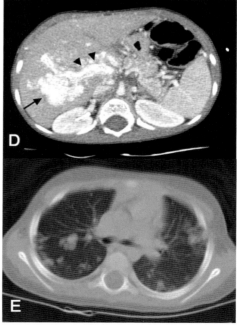

Figure 7.27 Hepatoblastoma. (A) Contrast-enhanced CT scan of a nine-month-old infant shows a large inhomogeneous mass in the right liver lobe with exophytic extension inferiorly (arrows). The lesion appears hypointense on contrast-enhanced T1-weighted MR scans (B), and nearly isointense to liver tissue on T2-weighted scans (C). (D) CT scan of a hepatoblastoma, which contains extensive calcifications (arrows) and extends with a tumor thrombus into the portal vein (arrowheads). (E) Typical pulmonary metastases.

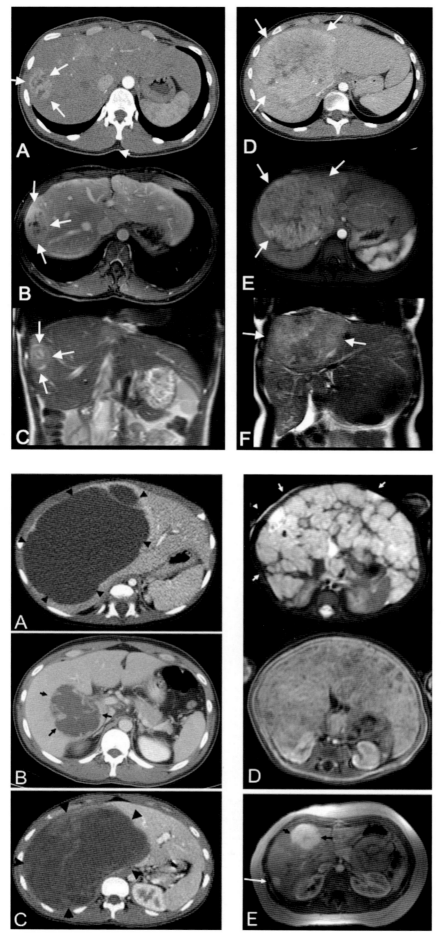

Figure 7.28 Typical imaging features of hepatocellular carcinoma (HCC). Relatively small (A–C) or large (D–F) inhomogeneous, ill-defined lesion in the right liver lobe (arrows). The lesions show an early arterial enhancement on contrast-enhanced CT (A, D) and contrast-enhanced T1-weighted MR images (B, E). The lesions show a similar enhancement compared to liver parenchyma on T2-weighted MR scans (C, F).

Figure 7.29 Differential diagnosis of liver tumors in children. (A) Mesenchymal hamartoma, a benign lesion in infants, which appears largely cystic and homogeneously hypodense on CT scans. The lesion shows some peripheral or septal enhancement (arrowheads). (B) Liver abscess: may occur in various age groups, and appears largely hypodense with relatively thick enhancing rim on contrast-enhanced CT scans (arrowheads). (C) Embryonal sarcoma, a malignant liver tumor, typically occurring in teenagers, with extensive central necroses, which may be mistaken as cysts or abscesses (arrowheads). The mass shows areas of inhomogeneous internal enhancement on delayed contrast-enhanced CT and MR scans. (D) Hemangioendothelioma, a vascular lesion, typically occurring in infants. The lesion may be solitary or multiple, and can involve the whole liver parenchyma. On T2-weighted MR images (upper image), these lesions show a very high signal, similar to CSF. On contrast-enhanced MR scans (lower image) or CTs (not shown), the lesions show similar enhancement compared to liver tissue. Some of these lesions may show a persistent enhancement on delayed scans, similar to hemangiomas. (E) Typical FNHs, which may be seen in young children or teenage girls and which typically show an early arterial enhancement on contrast-enhanced CT scans (arrows). Larger lesions may show a central scar (arrowheads), which appears hypodense/hypointense on early post-contrast scans, and hyperdense/hyperintense on delayed scans.

Germ cell tumors

Germ cell tumors are based on primordial germ cells, which originate in the yolk sac and migrate to the genital ridge on the posterior abdominal wall. Aberrant migration accounts for the occurrence of germ cell tumors in midline sites. Germ cell tumors may occur at many different sites, such as – in decreasing frequency – the ovaries (mostly adolescents, 70% benign), sacrococcygeal area (newborns, 80% girls, benign or malignant), testes (80% malignant), retroperitoneum (usually newborns, 90% benign), the anterior mediastinum (various ages, 90% boys, 20% malignant) and head and neck (usually newborns and usually benign), among other sites. The various histopathological subtypes of ovarian and testicular masses are listed in Table 7.13. Teratomas and yolk sac tumors comprise the majority of germ cell tumors in children. Teratomas typically present as primarily cystic masses (dermoid cyst) or, classically, as masses with elements of all three germ cell layers, i.e. soft tissue, fat and calcifications. These lead to characteristic, inhomogeneous features on ultrasound, CT and MR imaging studies. Malignant germ cell tumors, which include yolk sac tumors, or tumors with other malignant elements in primarily benign tumors are rare, but increase with increasing age. Malignant germ cell tumors may metastasize to the lungs, peritoneal cavity, pleura, liver, CNS and bone.

Sacrococcygeal teratomas represent the most common tumors in newborns. They are often diagnosed on prenatal ultrasound exams (Figure 7.30). More detailed information may be obtained by pre- and postnatal MR imaging studies (Figure 7.30). Imaging studies have to determine the extrapelvic and intrapelvic extension of these masses, as this information affects the delivery mode of the child and the prognosis of the disease. Completely extrapelvic tumors have a very low risk of malignant elements, while partially or completely intrapelvic masses have an increasing incidence of malignant elements. Differential diagnoses include a myelomeningocele, which shows continuity with the spinal canal. Evaluations of postoperative scans must include confirmation of removal of the coccyx. If the coccyx is not removed, there is a higher risk of local tumor recurrence and development of metastases.

Ovarian germ cell tumors are most frequently teratomas. Other histopathologies are much less common (Table 7.13). Of note, the ovaries in young girls are located in the lower abdomen or upper pelvis, higher than in adults. Thus, germ cell tumors should be considered in the differential diagnosis of abdominal masses in girls (Figure 7.30). Mature cystic teratomas or dermoid cysts represent the most common cause for an ovarian mass in premenarchal girls. On imaging studies, dermoid cysts are visualized as fluid-filled, well-delineated, often large cystic masses. The cystic component can have an increased density on CT, or increased signal on T1-weighted MR images due to protein contents. Teratomas composed of all germ cell layers present as inhomogeneous masses with areas of fat, hemorrhage or calcification. Ill-defined margins, infiltration of adjacent anatomical structures, free abdominal/pelvic fluid and enlarged lymph nodes may indicate malignancy. Ovarian masses may be accompanied by a torsion of the ovary, which may be diagnosed by an absence of intralesional vascularization on Doppler ultrasound or cross-sectional imaging studies, associated fallopian tube thickening or T1-/T2-hypointense hemorrhagic content on MR images due to hemorrhagic infarction. Of note, contralateral teratomas occur in about 10–20% of patients. Thus, the contralateral ovary has to be carefully evaluated as well.

Table 7.13 Differential diagnosis of gonadal masses in children and adolescents

1. Ovarian masses in girls

70% germ cell	Dermoid cyst, mature and immature teratoma Dysgerminoma = germinoma, choriocarcinoma (extremely rare, HCG+)
15% epithelial	Cystadenoma/cystadenocarcinoma
10% stroma	Granulosa cell tumor (estrogen production)/arrhenoblastoma (testosterone production), gynandroblastoma
5% others	Gonadoblastoma (mixed germ cell and stroma, occurs in dysgenetic gonads, in patients with true or pseudohermaphroditism, estrogen production, 30% of patients have an additional germinoma elsewhere)

2. Testicular masses in boys

70% germ cell	Seminoma = germinoma (AFP−), teratoma (AFP−) Yolk sac tumor = endodermal sinus tumor (AFP+) Choriocarcinoma (extremely rare, HCG+), embryonal carcinoma (adults)
20% stroma	Leydig cell tumor, Sertoli cell tumor, granulosa cell tumor (hormone production)
5% gonadoblastoma	Mixed germ cell and stroma, occurs in dysgenetic gonads, in patients with chromosome abnormality, estrogen production, 30% of patients have an additional germinoma elsewhere
5% others	Metastases from leukemia/lymphoma, neuroblastoma Paratesticular: rhabdomyosarcoma

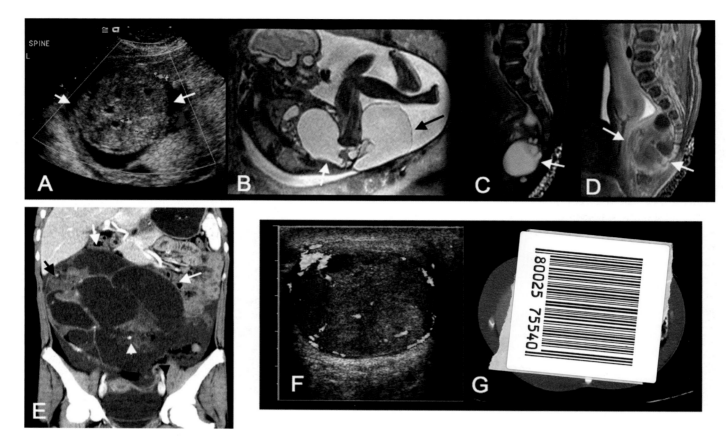

Figure 7.30 Different presentations of germ cell tumors. (A–D) Sacrococcygeal teratoma. (A) Prenatal ultrasound shows an inhomogeneous, predominantly solid and partly cystic mass posterior to the sacrum. (B) Prenatal T2-weighted MR scan in a different patient shows a predominantly cystic sacrococcygeal mass with large intrapelvic (white arrow) and extrapelvic (black arrow) components, which show a high T2 signal, indicating predominately cystic content. (C) Postnatal sagittal T2-weighted and (D) contrast-enhanced T1-weighted MR scans of the lumbar spine and sacrum show an inhomogeneous, predominantly intrapelvic mass with enhancing solid and T2-hyperintense cystic components. Of note, the location of the conus medullaris should be determined with all presented diagnostic techniques to evaluate for a possible associated tethered cord. (E) Coronal CT scan of a young woman with a mature teratoma of the left ovary. The lesion is very inhomogeneous and contains nonenhancing cysts (white arrow), enhancing soft tissue (black arrow) and small calcifications (white arrowhead). The lesion shows close contact to the left adnexa (black arrowhead). (F, G) Nonseminomatous germ cell tumor, presenting as a relatively homogeneous mass in the right testicle on ultrasound (F) and showing typical nodal metastases at the level of the hila of the kidneys, where testicular veins drain (G, arrows).

Testicular germ cell tumors usually occur between 15 and 30 years of age and are differentiated into seminomas and nonseminomas. Patients with a history of cryptorchidism have a 10- to 40-times increased risk of testicular cancer. Seminomas are typically homogeneous hypoechoic intratesticular masses on ultrasound. Larger lesions may be more inhomogeneous. The AFP is not elevated and metastases at the time of diagnosis are rare. Nonseminomatous germ cell tumors (NSGCTs) contain embryonic stem cells and comprise yolk sac tumors, teratomas, choriocarcinomas and embryonal carcinomas. An elevated AFP, found in about 60–70% of patients with NSGCTs, excludes a seminoma. NSGCTs often appear inhomogeneous on ultrasound studies, with intralesional cysts, hemorrhage or calcifications, and metastases are more frequent than in semi-nomas (Figure 7.30). An abdominal and pelvic CT has to be obtained for staging of both seminomas and nonseminomas in order to detect lymph node metastases. The left testicular vein drains into the left renal vein, and the right testicular vein drains into the IVC at the level of the right renal vein. Thus, nodal metastases are typically found in the para-caval and para-aortic region inferior to the renal vessels (Figure 7.30).

Previous studies suggested that testicular microcalcifica-tions noted on scrotal sonograms were associated with the development of testicular carcinomas. However, it has been recently found that over 98% of patients with asymptomatic microcalcifications do not develop a malignancy. Therefore, no imaging follow-up exams are needed and self-examination is recommended as the only method to evaluate for the devel-opment of a mass.

Rhabdomyosarcoma

Rhabdomyosarcoma (RMS), a malignant neoplasm of skeletal muscle origin, is the most common soft tissue sarcoma in childhood. It can occur at any age (peak around one to five years of age) and anywhere in the body, involving the head and neck (40%), retroperitoneum and genitourinary tract (20%), extremities (20%) or other areas of the trunk (20%). Histolo-gically, there are two subtypes in children: embryonal RMS (60–70% of cases) with a relatively better prognosis, and alveo-lar RMS (about 20% of cases) with a relatively worse prognosis. A third subtype, pleomorphic RMS (10%), occurs primarily in

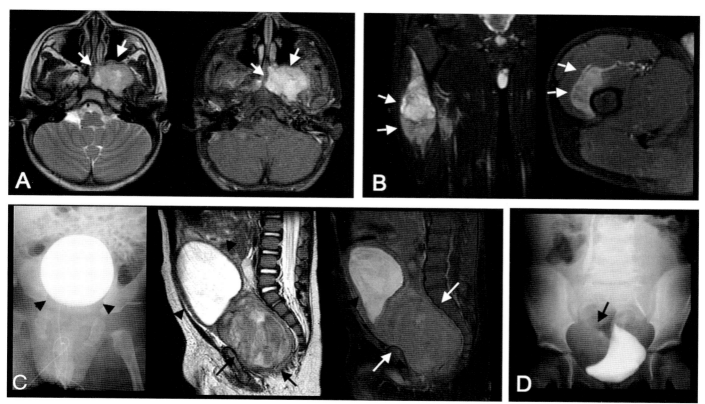

Figure 7.31 Different presentations of rhabdomyosarcomas. (A) Six-year-old boy with mass in the left nasopharynx extending down the left parapharyngeal space to involve the medial left pterygoid plate (arrows). The lesion shows relatively low signal on T2-weighted scans (left) and moderate enhancement on contrast-enhanced T1-weighted scans (right). (B) Thirteen-year-old boy with RMS within muscles of the right thigh. The lesion appears inhomogeneous and hyperintense on coronal STIR images (left, arrows) and shows inhomogeneous contrast enhancement (right, arrows). (C) Five-month-old boy with inhomogeneous soft tissue mass in the region of the prostate gland (arrows). A VCUG shows a markedly elevated bladder (left image, arrowheads). MR scans delineate a pelvic mass which shows relatively low signal on T2-weighted scans (middle) and moderate enhancement on contrast-enhanced T1-weighted scans (right). The bladder is displaced superiorly (arrowheads). (D) Intravenous pyelogram (IVP) of a three-year-old girl with a botryoid RMS, which causes a filling defect within the bladder. Any large pelvic mass could cause this appearance. The sharply defined margin of the impression on the right side of the bladder is, however, slightly more suggestive of an intramural, submucosal mass than an intraluminal or extrinsic lesion.

adults. The principal sites of distant metastases are lymph nodes, lung, liver, bone marrow and brain.

Head and neck RMS may arise in the sinuses, nasopharynx, orbit or skull base (among other locations) and may be associated with bone destructions, intracranial extension or dural involvement. Genitourinary RMS typically arises from the prostate, paratesticular region or bladder base in boys or from the anterior vaginal wall or bladder base in girls, and presents as a bulky, heterogeneous mass which invades the periurethral and perivesical tissues or may extend into the ischiorectal fossa. Tumors that arise in the bladder or vagina show a typical grape-like growth pattern and morphology, called "botryoid" RMS. Rhabdomyosarcomas of the extremities are most commonly of alveolar histology and have a worse prognosis than head and neck or genitourinary RMS. Extremity RMS may infiltrate the bone directly or may be distant from bone. All RMS can be associated with extensive bone marrow metastases.

The imaging appearance of RMS is nonspecific. The tumors present as aggressive, homogeneous or inhomogeneous soft tissue masses with a variable degree of contrast enhancement and invasion of adjacent structures (Figure 7.31). Calcifications are extremely rare and should lead to consideration of

other diagnoses. Cross-sectional imaging studies for staging of RMS should determine the local tumor extent along with associated local or distant lymph node metastases, pulmonary metastases, bone marrow infiltrations and other organ metastases. RMS can metastasize to the pancreas, and thus careful attention to the pancreas is warranted on imaging studies. Staging of RMS is complex and involves assigning a surgico-pathological stage and a risk group. Details can be found under: www.cancer.gov/cancertopics/pdq/treatment/childrhabdo myosarcoma/HealthProfessional/page4.

Differential diagnosis of soft tissue masses in children

Soft tissue tumors in children comprise a large variety of different histopathologies, ranging from relatively common vascular malformations to rare tumors (Figures 7.32, 7.33). Benign tumors outnumber malignant tumors. Ultrasound is usually used as the initial diagnostic tool. MR imaging is the technique of choice for determining tumor extent prior to surgery. An overview of characteristics of soft tissue tumors in children other than RMS is provided in Table 7.14.

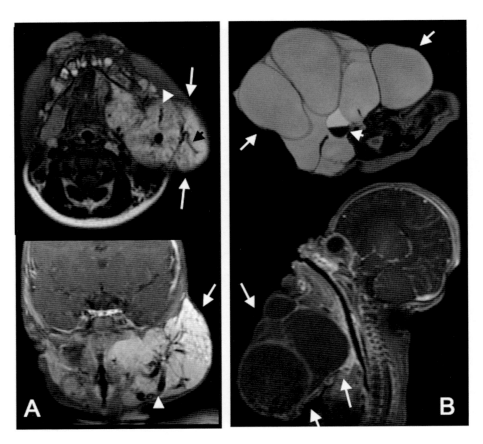

Figure 7.32 Vascular masses. (A) Twelve-month-old girl with large, multilobulated, left facial hemangioma (arrows), centered in the left parotid space, and extending into the carotid/masticator and parapharyngeal spaces. The mass shows a very high signal on T2-weighted MR scans (upper image) and marked enhancement on contrast-enhanced T1-weighted scans (lower image). There is typically no perilesional edema. Fast-flow vessels are identified by voids in and around the mass. Additional smaller hemangioma in the chin. (B) Newborn baby with huge macrocystic lymphatic malformation of the neck (arrows), diagnosed based on prenatal ultrasound (not shown). The lesion demonstrates multiple large cysts with very high signal on T2-weighted MR scans (upper image) and some focal areas of intralesional hemorrhage, which causes a fluid–fluid level (arrowhead). The lesion shows only peripheral and septal enhancement on contrast-enhanced T1-weighted scans (lower image).

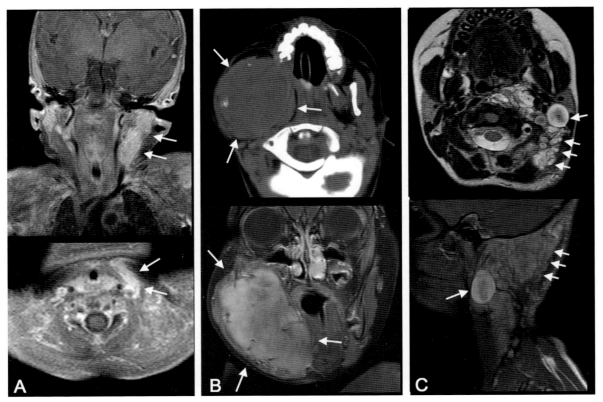

Figure 7.33 Other soft tissue masses in children. (A) Congenital torticollis in a six-month-old due to shortening and contraction of one sternocleidomastoid muscle with resulting rotation and lateral bending of the neck. The clinical presentation is usually characteristic and self limited and does not warrant imaging studies. In some equivocal cases, ultrasound or even cross-sectional imaging is done and care has to be taken to not confuse this benign condition with a mass. MR images show enhancement of the sternocleidomastoid muscle on contrast-enhanced T1-weighted scans without any mass effect. (B) Conversely, an infantile myofibromatosis, a benign but locally aggressive and infiltrative soft tissue mass, may cause a marked mass effect (arrows). On CT scans, these lesions have a similar attenuation compared to muscle (upper image). In contrast to adult-type fibromatoses, infantile fibromatoses can be highly vascularized and may appear hyperintense on T2-weighted scans (not shown) and may demonstrate marked enhancement on contrast-enhanced MR scans (lower image). (C) Multiple neurofibromas in a patient with neurofibromatosis I. There are multiple oval and sausage-shaped lesions noted in the left neck and hypopharynx (arrows). The lesions show a characteristic "target sign" on T2-weighted MR scans (upper image), with a relatively hypointense center in a hyperintense lesion. The neurofibromas show a marked enhancement on contrast-enhanced MR scans (lower image); larger lesions may also show the target sign on contrast-enhanced scans.

Table 7.14 Differential diagnosis of soft tissue tumors other than rhabdomyosarcoma in children

Soft tissue mass	Characteristics
Lipoma/lipoblastoma	Fat-equivalent density on CT (negative HU) or MR (T1 and T2 hyperintense, decreasing signal on fat-suppressed images)
Cyst	Fluid-equivalent signal (<30 HU on CT, CSF-equivalent on MR), no or only peripheral rim enhancement
Lymphangioma	Contains CSF-equivalent fluid (<30 HU on CT, CSF-equivalent on MR), or fat-containing fluid (negative HU on CT, brighter than muscle on plain T1 MR images), no or only peripheral and septal enhancement
Hemangiomas and vascular malformations	Fluid equivalent signal on T2w MR or area of hemorrhage. Hemangiomas: well defined mass, serpiginous "fast flow" vessels, marked enhancement. Low flow vascular malformations: phleboliths, absence of flow voids, variable enhancement. High flow vascular malformations: little tissue matrix, flow voids, poorly defined mass, may infiltrate adjacent structures (bone).
Fibromatosis colli (infants)	Fusiform expansion of the sternocleidoid muscle, usually diagnosed with ultrasound. If MR is performed, the lesion appears T1 isointense, T2 isointense or slightly hyperintense to muscle. May grow during first weeks of life, followed by spontaneous regression
Infantile myofibromatosis (infants)	Aggressive hypodense (CT), T1-hypointense and T2-variable (MR) lesions with variable degree of enhancement. Three types: 1. Solitary (most often in deep soft tissues of neck or leg) 2. Multiple lesions without visceral involvement 3. Multiple lesions with visceral involvement (2) and (3) nearly always associated with lesions in bone
Aggressive fibromatosis, desmoid (usually >3 years)	>90% solitary lesions, very rarely multifocal, any location, relatively homogeneous, CT-hypodense, T1-hypointense and T2-variable lesions with poorly defined margins and infiltration of adjacent bones and organs. Mild to moderate contrast enhancement
Neurofibromas	NF1 patients, usually benign and multiple lesions; characteristic dumbbell shape of partly intradural and partly extradural paraspinal tumors; characteristic "target" signal on T2-weighted MR images: hypointense center, hyperintense periphery
Plexiform neurofibromas	Aggressive, large neurogenic tumors, close association to nerve roots or peripheral nerves
Malignant peripheral nerve sheath tumor (MPNST)	NF1 patients, same imaging features for benign schwannomas and MPNSTs; thickened nerve proximal and distal to the tumor due to tumor spread along the perineurium; local recurrence and pulmonary metastases are common, lymph node metastases are rare
Synovial sarcoma	Relatively well-defined but inhomogeneous lesion near a joint and bone with intralesional hemorrhage, fluid–fluid levels and hyper-, hypo- and isointense areas relative to fat (triple signal) on T2-weighted sequences
Clear cell sarcoma	Adolescents and young adults; malignant, apparently well-circumscribed soft tissue mass developing in tendons and aponeuroses, >90% in the extremities, most frequently in the foot and ankle; no calcifications or fluid–fluid levels. High frequency of lymph node metastases, dismal prognosis if positive

Bone tumors

Benign bone tumors are much more common than malignant ones and include true neoplasms and tumor-like lesions (Tables 7.15, 7.16). The most common benign tumors are osteochondroma, nonossifying fibroma, and enchondroma (Figure 7.34). Among primary malignant bone tumors, osteosarcoma, Ewing's sarcoma and lymphoma are most common. Benign bone tumors are generally well circumscribed, with (less aggressive) or without (more aggressive) a sclerotic margin and possible associated cortical thickening or cortical scalloping and thinning. Malignant lesions are ill defined, difficult to delineate, have a "wide zone of transition" to apparently normal bone and show onion-skin, Codman triangle (elevated periost with sharp triangular end) or spiculated periosteal reactions.

Osteosarcoma is the most common malignant bone tumor in children, typically presenting in teenagers. Osteosarcomas typically develop in the metaphyses of long bones, but can arise in other locations. The most frequent sites of primary disease are distal femur, proximal tibia, proximal humerus or proximal femur, in that order. Most osteosarcomas are sporadic. Etiological and predisposing factors have been described for patients with bilateral retinoblastomas, Li-Fraumeni syndrome, Rothmund-Thomson syndrome, osteogenesis imperfecta, benign cartilage bone tumors and status post-radiation therapy.

On radiographic imaging studies, osteosarcomas present as aggressive, destructive, ill-defined metaphyseal lesions with poorly defined margins and cloud-like amorphous dense areas of osteoid formation. About 10% of osteosarcomas present as purely lytic lesions and may show only minimal cortical erosions and periosteal reactions. Few osteosarcomas may present as diaphyseal rather than metaphyseal lesions. Typical periosteal reactions include the "Codman triangle" and "sunburst" spiculae (Figure 7.35). The tumors almost always extend into the paraosseous soft tissues (Figure 7.36). There are several histological subtypes with specific imaging characteristics: telangiectatic osteosarcomas present as expansile medullary lesions that rarely show osteoid formation but contain multiple fluid-filled cysts, which show fluid–fluid levels on MR images (Figures 7.35, 7.36). These lesions can look very similar to an aneurysmal bone cyst. Periosteal osteosarcomas typically involve the bone diaphysis with sessile growth on the bone surface, a thickened cortex and a broad, cortex-based soft tissue component. A paraosteal osteosarcoma is a well-differentiated low-grade tumor of the bone surface with a large, osteoid-producing extraosseous component, attached to the bone by a small-based "pedicle," minor or absent marrow component and usually absent periosteal reaction (Figures 7.35, 7.36).

A biopsy of a suspected osteosarcoma has to be planned carefully and should only be performed by oncological surgeons since the biopsy canal needs to be later resected with the primary tumor. Staging should include imaging of the whole affected bone, including adjacent joints, in order to facilitate planning of surgery and to detect skip lesions. Skip lesions are tumor deposits in the bone marrow, which are distinctly separate from the primary tumor. These lesions are iso- or hypointense to bone marrow on plain T1-weighted spin echo MR images, in contrast to hematopoietic marrow which is hyperintense to muscle on these images. MR imaging is also very useful in determining joint invasion of the primary tumor and vascular invasion of the soft tissue component. Of note, the tumor usually displaces and rarely infiltrates adjacent vessels. The latter would necessitate amputation, and thus this diagnosis should be carefully considered. A tumor that surrounds adjacent vessels by more than 180° can be considered to infiltrate the neurovascular bundle.

Metastases in osteosarcoma patients can occur at any site, with the most common being the lungs and bone. These metastases may produce osteoid and may contain calcifications and should not be mistaken for granulomas.

The **Ewing's sarcoma** family of tumors (ESFT) comprises Ewing's sarcoma of the bone, extraosseous Ewing's sarcoma, peripheral primitive neuroectodermal tumor (PPNET) and Askin tumor (a chest wall tumor). ESFTs have a common genetic lesion, with over 90% exhibiting a translocation between the *EWS* gene on chromosome 22 and the *FLI1* gene on chromosome 11. Histologically, these tumors have been found to originate from the neural crest and represent "small round blue cell tumors." Ewing's sarcomas typically present in teenagers and are very rare in children of Asian or African descent. The Ewing's sarcoma of the bone is classically located in the diaphyseal region of the distal long bones (52%) or flat bones, such as the femur, pelvic bones, rib and tibia. On conventional radiographs and CT scans, a Ewing's sarcoma of bone presents as an aggressive permeative osteolysis with a wide zone of transition, classically "onion-skin," lamellated periosteal reactions and a paraosteal soft tissue mass (Figure 7.37). There are many variations to this typical appearance. Typical locations of metastases are the lungs (20% of patients at diagnosis), bone, bone marrow and more rarely, lymph nodes.

Langerhans' cell histiocytosis (LCH) is a histiocytic disorder due to a clonal proliferation of Langerhans' cells (histiocytes) in bones, various organs and/or skin. There is a highly variable clinical manifestation.

A solitary LCH (i.e. eosinophilic granuloma) represents a lytic bone lesion, a solitary lesion in an internal organ, or involvement isolated to the skin. The most frequently involved bones are, in decreasing order, the skull, ribs, femur, pelvis, vertebrae, mandible and humerus. In the skull, the lesion develops as a well-defined, "punched-out" osteolysis in the diploic space with beveled, scalloped or confluent edges (Figure 7.38). Some lesions show a characteristic central sequestrum, representing residual bone. Vertebral body involvement can cause collapse, resulting in vertebra plana. In long bones, LCH presents as well- or ill-defined, lytic lesions, with or without a sclerotic margin, periosteal reaction or soft tissue component (Figure 7.38).

Polyostotic unisystem LCH is characterized by multiple lytic bone lesions. Hand-Schüller-Christian disease belongs

Table 7.15 Differential diagnosis of bone tumors in children

Tumor type	Clinical characteristics	Imaging characteristics
Osteoma	Sporadic or with polyposis and Gardner's syndromes	Small focal bony lesion in another bone
Osteoid osteoma	Teenagers and young adults; night pain, aspirin-responsive	Mainly cortical lesion with vascularized, enhancing lucent center (nidus) and sclerotic rim
>2 cm diameter = osteoblastoma	Lack of intense pain	Larger nidus, smaller or absent sclerotic rim
Osteosarcoma 1. Conventional 2. Telangiectatic 3. Paraosteal 4. Periosteal	Teenagers; typical location: metaphysis of long bones	Variable proportions of aggressive osteolyses and new bone formation, Codman triangle, "sunburst" spiculae, intramedullary and extraosseous component

Cartilage-forming tumors: lucent lesions with punctate "popcorn" calcifications, high signal on T2-weighted MR images, "rings and arcs" on contrast-enhanced MR images

Enchondroma Multiple = Ollier's disease + hemangiomas = Maffucci's syndrome	Metaphyses, mostly in bones of hands and feet	Well-circumscribed metaphyseal intramedullary lytic lesion with fine sclerotic rim
Osteochondroma Multiple = hereditary or acquired (e.g. post-radiation) multiple exostoses	Any age; cartilage cap >3 cm in children (>1 cm in adults) indicates malignant transformation, metaphysis	"Cartilage-capped bone exostosis," continuity of cortex of lesion with cortex of associated bone; cartilage cap not seen on radiographs
Chondroblastoma	Age 10–30, boys > girls; epiphysis	Well-delineated, lucent, expansile epiphyseal lesion
Chondromyxoid fibroma	Age 10–30; metaphyses of long bones, femur and tibia	Large, eccentric, ovoid, expansile, bubbly, metadiaphyseal lesion
Chondrosarcoma	Extremely rare in children, may occur years after irradiation; pain in the absence of fracture is indicative of sarcoma	Lobulated, ill-defined mass with endosteal erosions and bone destruction. Greater than two-thirds cortical destruction, size >5 cm and extraosseous extent indicate sarcoma

Giant cell tumors of bone: usually affect young adults after closure of growth plates, rare in teenagers. Lytic, eccentric epiphyseal lesion without sclerotic rim on radiographs and CT, "fluid–fluid levels" and areas of hemorrhage on T2-weighted MR images, positive on bone scans

Small round blue cell tumors of bone: ill-defined lucencies on radiographs and CT, iso- or hypointense compared to muscle on plain T1-weighted spin echo sequences (normal hematopoietic marrow appears hyperintense to muscle on plain T1SE)

Ewing's sarcoma (and other PNETs)	Teenagers, boys > girls; typical location: diaphyses of long bones or pelvis	Ill-defined, "moth-eaten" bone destruction, "onion-skin" periosteal reaction, usually extraosseous soft tissue component
Lymphoma, leukemia	Malignant cells in the bone marrow: <25% lymphoma >25% leukemia	Patchy lytic bone marrow lesions: multifocal in lymphoma/AML, typically diffuse in ALL; may develop reactive sclerosis under therapy

Vascular tumors of bone: bone destruction on radiographs and CT, very high signal (similar to CSF) on T2-weighted MR images with serpiginous flow voids and possible areas of fat or hemorrhage

Hemangiomas and vascular malformations	Most common in newborns/infants; solitary or multiple (multiple = hemangio/lymphangiomatosis)	Little or no extraosseous component; hemangiomas enhance, lymphangiomas do not enhance after contrast injection
Gorham disease ("vanishing bone disease")	Underlying lymphatic malformation that destructs bone	Very aggressive, extensive osteolysis, T2-hyperintense mass in the area of bone destruction on MR

Fibrous/fibrohistiocytic tumors: lytic lesions on radiographs and CT, hyperintense on T2-weighted MR images

1. Fibrous cortical defect	Most frequent benign bone lesion in children	

Table 7.15 (cont.)

Tumor type	Clinical characteristics	Imaging characteristics
2. >2 cm lesion = nonossifying fibroma (NOF) = fibroxanthoma		Grape-like, well-delineated lytic lesion in cortex of bone metaphyses, "migrates" towards diaphysis with growth, FDG+
Ossifying fibroma	Rare, arising most commonly in molar regions	Expansile, well-circumscribed lytic lesion of mandible or maxilla, with or without calcification
Fibrosarcoma	Extremely rare in children	Expansile, ill-defined lytic lesion
Other primary bone tumors:		
Chordoma	Rare, arise from notochord, most commonly clivus or presacral, rarely associated with tuberous sclerosis	Ill-defined lytic lesions, with or without calcification, high signal on T2-weighted MR scans, mild to moderate contrast enhancement
Differentiated adamantinoma	Rare, age 10–20 years; 90% in tibia, typically in the diaphysis and classically involving anterior tibial cortex	Eccentric, lobulated, well delineated, expansile lytic lesion with "soap bubble" appearance, intense contrast enhancement

AML = acute myeloid leukemia; ALL = acute lymphocytic leukemia.

Table 7.16 Tumor-like lesions of bone in children

Type of lesion	Clinical characteristics	Imaging characteristics
Unicameral bone cyst (simple bone cyst)	Typically located in proximal metaphysis of humerus or femur; may give rise to pathological fracture	Well-delineated, fluid-filled lytic lesion with sharp borders and sclerotic margin, "fallen fragment sign" with fractures
Aneurysmal bone cyst	Age 10–30 years, located in long bones or vertebrae, one-third arise in or are a component of another bone tumor	Eccentric metaphyseal multicameral lytic lesion with enhancing rim and septae; "fluid–fluid" levels on MR
Fibrous dysplasia	Diaphysis of tubular bones, + skin pigmentation + precocious puberty = McCune-Albright syndrome	Monostotic or polystotic, well-defined, expansile, intramedullary "ground-glass" lesion in craniofacial or long bones; may lead to bowing of long bones
Langerhans' cell histiocytosis (histiocytosis X; eosinophilic granuloma, Hand-Schüller-Christian disease, Letterer-Siwe disease)	Possible association with pituitary stalk or hypothalamic lesions, hepatosplenomegaly, fatty liver, thymus mass with calcifications, interstitial lung changes, bowel thickening	Solitary or multiple "punched-out" lytic lesions of the skull and tubular bones, well delineated or ill defined, vertebra plana, "floating teeth"
Myositis ossificans	Post-trauma, 80% proximal arm or leg, usually in soft tissues, may involve adjacent bone	Relatively well-circumscribed lesion with peripheral, circular calcification and central "lucency," perilesional edema on STIR and T2-weighted MR

in this category and is defined as multiple bone lesions associated with diabetes insipidus and exophthalmus. Polyostotic and multisystem involvement of LCH is a very rapidly progressing disease of bones and multiple organs in young children (usually less than two years of age). This includes Letterer-Siwe disease, which is characterized by lytic bone lesions, lymphadenopathy, skin rash, hepatosplenomegaly, fever, anemia and thrombocytopenia. Lung involvement can present as interstitial disease with honeycomb appearance.

Differential diagnosis of bone tumors in children

The age of the child is extremely helpful for the differential diagnosis: in young children, 0–10 years of age, simple bone cysts, Langerhans' cell histiocytosis, leukemia, Ewing's sarcoma and bone marrow metastases from neuroblastoma or rhabdomyosarcoma are most common. Differential diagnoses for bone tumors in children 10–20 years of age are listed in Tables 7.15 and 7.16. The location of a bone lesion can also help in the differential diagnosis: in the epiphyses,

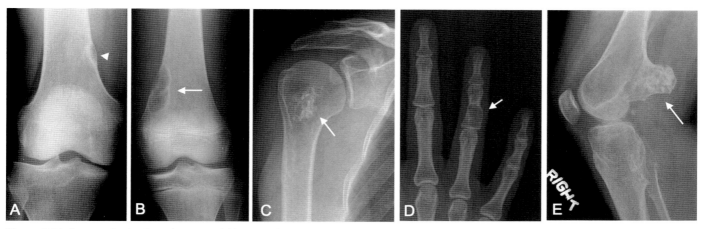

Figure 7.34 Common benign bone lesions in children. (A) Fibrous cortical defect: small, lytic, well-defined lesion in the cortex of the distal femur metaphysis (arrowhead). (B) Nonossifying fibroma (NOF): grape-like, well-delineated lytic lesion in cortex of the distal femur metaphysis (arrow). (C) Enchondroma: well-circumscribed metaphyseal intramedullary lytic lesion with fine sclerotic rim and popcorn-like calcifications (arrow). (D) Enchondroma: the lesion can be purely lytic, especially in distal small bones (arrow). (E) Multiple osteochondromas in a patient with multiple hereditary exostoses. The largest lesion arises from the posterior right femur (arrow).

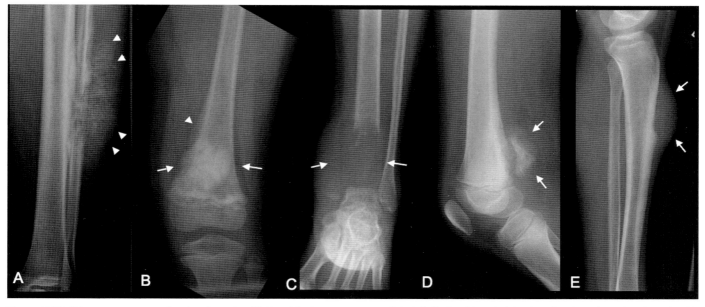

Figure 7.35 Osteosarcoma, conventional radiography. (A) Osteoblastic osteosarcoma of the left fibula with typical "sunburst" periosteal reaction (arrowheads). (B) Osteoblastic osteosarcoma in the distal femur metaphysis with extensive new bone formation and typical "Codman triangle" periosteal reaction (arrowhead). (C) Telangiectatic osteosarcoma of the left distal tibia, presenting with extensive aggressive osteolysis. (D) Paraosteal osteosarcoma with erosions along the distal posterior right femur and associated lesion extending from these erosions into the posterior soft tissues and showing extensive new bone formation. There is a characteristic lucent zone between the lesion and the femur cortex. (E) Periosteal osteosarcoma presenting as focal cortical thickening in the anterior proximal tibial diaphysis, with associated sessile soft tissue mass.

chondroblastomas (typically with open growth plate), giant cell tumors (closed growth plate) and (rarely) Langerhans' cell histiocytosis may be seen. In the metaphyses, lesions centered in the cortex include NOF or osteoid osteoma. Lesions centered in the medullary canal comprise a larger group of differential diagnosis, as listed in Tables 7.15 and 7.16. In the diaphyses, lesions centered in the cortex include osteoid osteoma or (very rarely) adamantinoma. Lesions centered in the medullary canal include enchondroma, fibrous dysplasia, Ewing's sarcoma and lymphoma.

Most bone tumors present as solitary lesions. The differential diagnosis of multiple bone lesions in children includes: Langerhans' cell histiocytosis, enchondromatosis, fibrous dysplasia, multiple nonossifying fibromas, hemangiomatosis, leukemia/lymphoma, metastases, infantile myofibromatosis, multifocal osteomyelitis and hyperparathyroidism. Possible primary tumors that cause bone metastases in children are neuroblastoma, rhabdomyosarcoma, clear cell sarcoma or renal cell carcinoma of the kidney, retinoblastoma, Ewing's sarcoma, osteosarcoma, lymphoma and medulloblastoma.

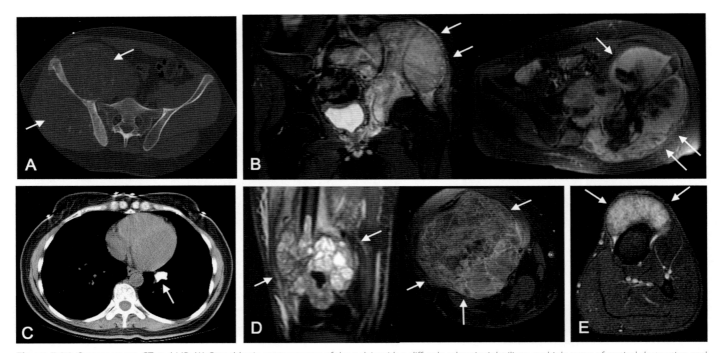

Figure 7.36 Osteosarcoma, CT and MR. (A) Osteoblastic osteosarcoma of the pelvis with a diffusely sclerotic right ilium, multiple areas of cortical destruction and large soft tissue mass (arrows) with small internal areas of new bone formation. (B) Osteoblastic osteosarcoma (arrows) with extensive bone marrow involvement of the whole left hemipelvis and sacrum and a large intra- and extrapelvic soft tissue mass. The lesion is hyperintense on fat-saturated T2-weighted scans (left), and shows areas of enhancement and central nonenhancing necrosis on contrast-enhanced T1-weighted scans (right). (C) Calcified pulmonary metastasis in a patient with osteosarcoma (arrow). (D) Telangiectatic osteosarcoma of the distal femur shows multiple focal hyperintense, fluid-equivalent areas on T2-weighted scans (left) and peripheral enhancement of these areas on contrast-enhanced scans (right). (E) Periosteal osteosarcoma: sessile soft tissue mass along the anterior cortex of the proximal tibia; no bone marrow involvement.

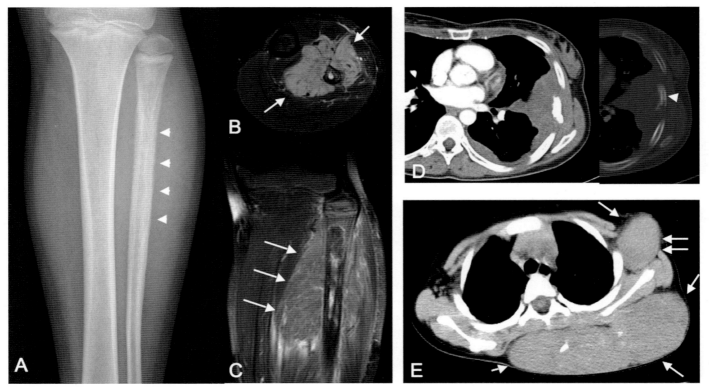

Figure 7.37 Ewing's sarcoma. (A–C) Ten-year-old boy with Ewing's sarcoma of the left fibula, which shows a permeative/moth-eaten destruction of the cortex of the proximal and mid-diaphysis (A, arrowheads). T2-weighted MR scans demonstrate abnormal bone marrow signal and a large associated soft tissue mass (B, arrows). The mass shows marked enhancement on contrast-enhanced scans (C, arrows). (D) CT scan of a young woman with an Askin tumor, arising from the eighth left lateral rib (arrowhead on bone window) and extending into the chest; (E) CT scan of a two-year-old boy with rapidly growing back mass (arrows) without evidence of associated bone destruction; biopsy revealed extraosseous Ewing's sarcoma.

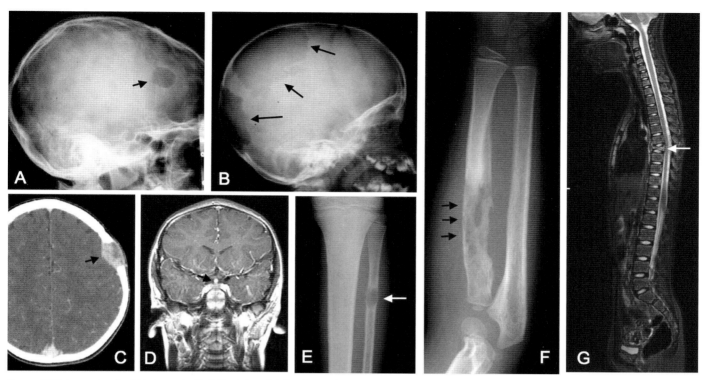

Figure 7.38 Langerhans' cell histiocytosis. (A–C) Typical, well-defined, "punched-out" lesions of the skull may be relatively small (A, arrow), or large (B, arrows) and show enhancing soft tissue in the defect on contrast-enhanced CT scans (C, arrow). (D) Coronal contrast-enhanced MR scan shows an enhancing lesion in the pituitary stalk (arrow) in a patient with Langerhans' cell histiocytosis and diabetes insipidus. (E, F) Focal osteolysis in long bones may be well defined and small (E, arrow) or large with aggressive cortical destruction (F, arrows). (G) Whole-body MRI is a new technique that allows whole-body scanning of Langerhans' cell histiocytosis patients without radiation exposure. This sagittal T2-weighted scan through the whole spine shows a vertebra plana (arrow).

Further reading

Abramson SJ, Price AP (2008) Imaging of pediatric lymphomas. *Radiol Clin North Am* **46**(2), 313–38.

Barksdale EM Jr, Obokhare I (2009) Teratomas in infants and children. *Curr Opin Pediatr* **21**(3), 344–9.

Benz MR, Tchekmedyian N, Eilber FC *et al.* (2009) Utilization of positron emission tomography in the management of patients with sarcoma. *Curr Opin Oncol* **21**(4), 345–51.

Cohn SL, Pearson ADJ, London WB *et al.* (2009) The International Neuroblastoma Risk Group (INRG) Classification System: an INRG Task Force report. *J Clin Oncol* **27**(2), 289–97.

Darge K, Jaramillo D, Siegel MJ (2008) Whole-body MRI in children: current status and future applications. *Eur J Radiol* **68**(2), 289–98.

Fayad LM, Bluemke DA, Weber KL, Fishman EK (2006) Characterization of pediatric skeletal tumors and tumor-like conditions: specific cross-sectional imaging signs. *Skeletal Radiol* **35**(5), 259–68.

Fitzgerald PA, Goldsby RE, Huberty JP *et al.* (2006) Malignant pheochromocytomas and paragangliomas: a phase II study of therapy with high-dose 131I-metaidobenzylguanidine (131I-MIBG). *Ann N Y Acad Sci* **1073**, 465–90.

Jadvar H, Connolly LP, Fahey FH, Shulkin BL (2007) PET and PET/CT in pediatric oncology. *Semin Nucl Med* **37**(5), 316–31.

Jha P, Chawla SC, Tavri S *et al.* (2009) Pediatric liver tumors – a pictorial review. *Eur Radiol* **19**(1), 209–19.

Laffan EE, Ngan BY, Navarro OM (2009) Pediatric soft-tissue tumors and pseudotumors: MR imaging features with pathologic correlation: Part 2. Tumors of fibroblastic/myofibroblastic, so-called fibrohistiocytic, muscular, lymphomatous, neurogenic, hair matrix, and uncertain origin. *Radiographics* **29**(4), e36.

Marabelle A, Campagne D, Déchelotte P *et al.* (2008) Focal nodular hyperplasia of the liver in patients previously treated for pediatric neoplastic diseases. *J Pediatr Hematol Oncol* **30**(7), 546–9.

Monclair T, Brodeur GM, Ambros PF *et al.* (2009) The International Neuroblastoma Risk Group (INRG) staging system: an INRG Task Force report. *Journal of Clinical Oncology* **27**(2), 298–303.

Reaman GH (2009) What, why, and when we image: considerations for diagnostic imaging and clinical research in the Children's Oncology Group. *Pediatr Radiol* **39**(Suppl. 1), S42–5.

Stehr M (2009) Pediatric urologic rhabdomyosarcoma. *Curr Opin Urol* **19**(4), 402–6.

Wootton-Gorges SL (2009) MR imaging of primary bone tumors and tumor-like conditions in children. *Magn Reson Imaging Clin N Am* **17**(3), 469–87.

Wright CD (2009) Mediastinal tumors and cysts in the pediatric population. *Thorac Surg Clin* **19**(1), 47–61.

Kevin M. Baskin, Charles R. Fitz, Max Wintermark and John J. Crowley

Ischemia is a pathophysiological state of hypoperfusion with cellular, local and systemic consequences that can be severe and threatening to tissue and organ function and consequently to the life of the patient. Brief ischemia may result in reversible injury with preservation of cellular integrity, and may even be protective against the harmful effects of subsequent and more prolonged ischemia. If the underlying abnormality has been corrected and perfusion restored after prolonged ischemia, reperfusion injury may occur. Reperfusion injury is caused by an imbalance between increased production of reactive oxygen and nitrogen species and decreased availability of such free-radical scavengers as nitric oxide. This results in a cascade of effects characteristic of an acute inflammatory reaction and most profoundly affecting the endothelial cells lining microscopic blood vessels. The intensity of this inflammatory reaction may extend to involvement of remote tissues and organs, leading to multiple organ dysfunction with a high degree of morbidity and mortality. When uncorrected, prolonged ischemia leads to irreversible injury: necrosis or cell death.

The final common pathway of disorganized and contiguous cell death after prolonged ischemia is indistinguishable from that evoked by other nonphysiological disturbances such as metabolic poisoning, hypoxia, trauma, lytic viruses, hypothermia and complement attack. This stands in opposition to the highly organized and tightly regulated process of programmed cell death, or apoptosis. Interestingly, damage to the cell related to ischemia or ischemia-reperfusion injury may *induce* cell death from apoptosis. The imaging findings and related approaches to imaging management of ischemia and its consequences in the broader sense of unregulated cell death from nonphysiological disturbances will be the primary focus of this chapter.

Clinicians seldom consider consulting radiologists to diagnose and treat ischemia *per se*. The imaging findings related to ischemia are often subtle and nonspecific, related to hypoperfusion, visualized as absence of contrast where it might be expected, and to increased extravascular and extracellular edema, visualized as free fluid where it might not be expected. These findings are often interpreted in the more familiar context of organ-based

pathologies such as stroke, necrotizing enterocolitis, coronary artery disease, avascular necrosis, frostbite, etc. In turn, radiologists should anticipate the prior probability of these subtle findings in the face of relevant history, and similarly should seek a relevant history in the face of these subtle findings!

Sickle cell disease: a prototype for pediatric ischemia

While there are many potential examples of medical conditions that predispose to ischemia, a few serve well to illustrate the principles. For example, the child with sickle cell anemia accompanied by factors that potentiate decreased end-organ oxygen tension (e.g., dehydration) may develop microvascular occlusions due to sickled erythrocytes that manifests most characteristically as recurrent painful vaso-occlusive crises which present variously as stroke, acute chest syndrome, splenic infarction, aseptic necrosis of bone, low-flow priapism, and leg ulcers. The sickle cell acts as a procoagulant with exposed phosphatidylserine, and as an irritant that provokes an inflammatory response and impairs perfusion. Secondary effects of sickling may relate to increased degradation of erythrocytes as well as local and distant effects of hypoxia, inflammatory mediators, and activated cells that result in reperfusion injury and organ dysfunction manifesting as stroke, pulmonary embolic disease, acute splenic sequestration crisis, renal failure, cholelithiasis and pain.

Because the combined effects of the decreased immunocompetence and local tissue ischemia or necrosis that commonly accompany sickle cell disease predispose both to localized infection and to overwhelming sepsis, abnormal imaging findings in children with sickle cell disease must be interpreted with a high degree of suspicion for both ischemic changes and infection (Figure 8.1). So-called "acute chest syndrome" is emblematic of this concept, as a new pulmonary infiltrate on the chest radiograph of a child with sickle cell disease, usually accompanied (or preceded) by pain in the chest or extremities, fever, respiratory distress and decreased oxygen saturation, may develop because of infection, infarction or both (Figure 8.2).

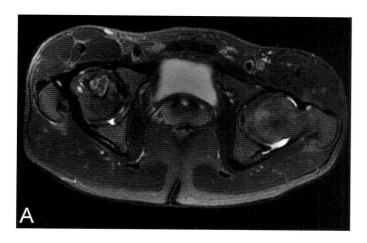

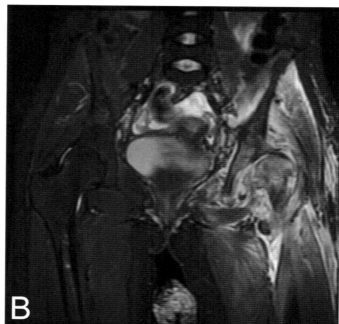

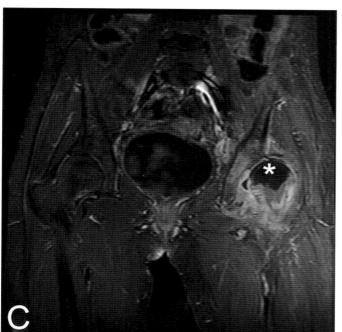

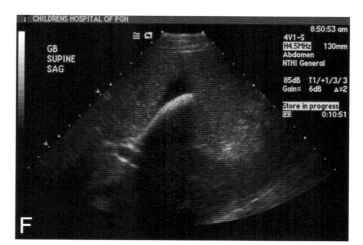

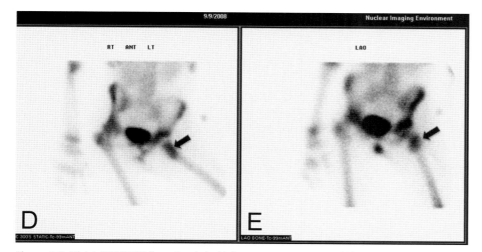

Figure 8.1 (A) Axial T2 MR FSE (fast spin echo) with fat saturation in a 12-year-old female with hemoglobin SS disease, left hip pain and fever shows osteonecrosis without inflammation in the right femoral head, and abnormal marrow signal and joint effusion in the left hip consistent with acute inflammation or infection. (B) Coronal inversion recovery MR imaging of the pelvis shows abnormal signal in the left femoral head and neck, with profound inflammatory changes in the surrounding tissues and hip effusion. Note lateral and superior subluxation of the left femoral head with preservation of its contour. (C) Coronal T1SE MR with contrast demonstrates both osteonecrosis, with lack of enhancement of the left femoral head (asterisk), and superimposed infection, with inflammation of surrounding tissues, marrow edema of the femoral neck and acetabulum, and joint effusion. (D) Blood pool and (E) delayed images (arterial phase not shown) from a positive ^{99m}Tc MDP (technetium 99m methylene diphosphonate) bone scan show coexisting osteonecrosis of the left femoral head (decreased uptake in all three phases) and intertrochanteric osteomyelitis (arrows) of the left femoral neck (increased uptake in all three phases). Biopsy proved a *Salmonella* infection. (F) Grayscale right upper quadrant US shows a large shadowing stone in the gallbladder. Pigment gallstones are common in sickle cell patients and related to the increased enterohepatic cycling of heme pigments from increased erythrocyte destruction.

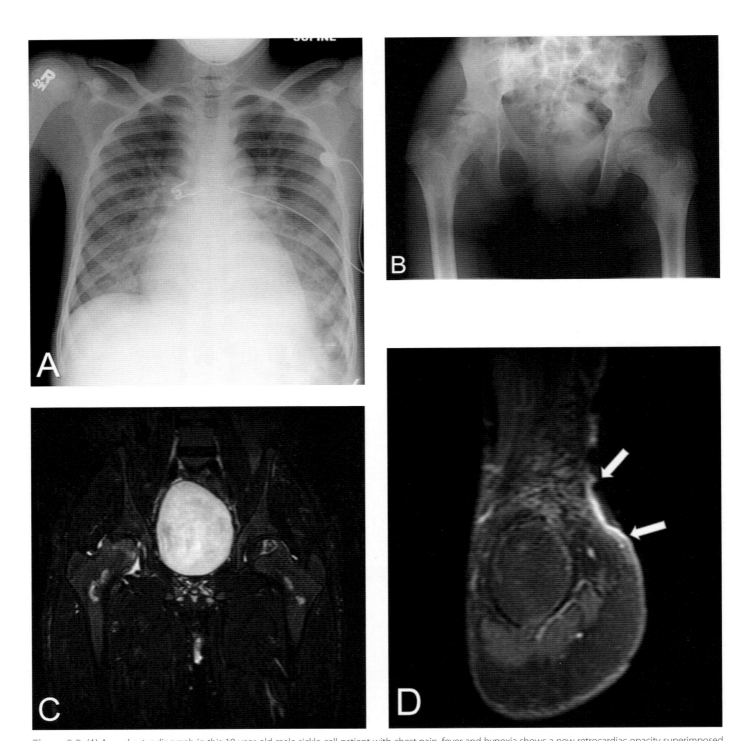

Figure 8.2 (A) A pa chest radiograph in this 19-year-old male sickle cell patient with chest pain, fever and hypoxia shows a new retrocardiac opacity superimposed on chronic cardiomegaly. He was admitted to the intensive care unit and treated with supportive therapy and antibiotics. His symptoms and radiographic findings resolved within three days. (B) An ap radiograph of the hips shows chronic deformity of the right femoral head after avascular necrosis. (C) Coronal inversion recovery MR of the hips shows multiple areas of increased signal from bone infarctions, with irregularity of the right femoral head and a small right hip effusion, but without evidence of osteomyelitis. (D) Coronal T1SE MR and (E) coronal T1 3D spoiled-gradient recalled (SPGR) MR of the left ankle show contrast enhancement of the tissues at the base of the known left medial malleolar skin ulcer (arrows), without extension to the underlying bone. (F) A temporary central venous access device was placed in the right groin. The patient's right leg became acutely swollen and painful. Grayscale US shows a noncompressible thrombus (arrows) in the common femoral vein.

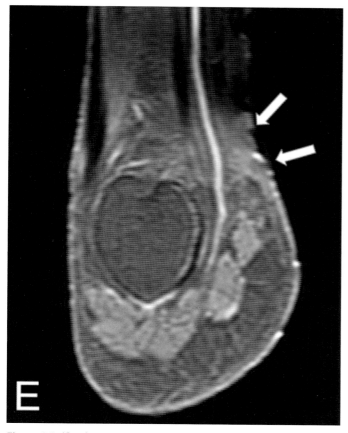

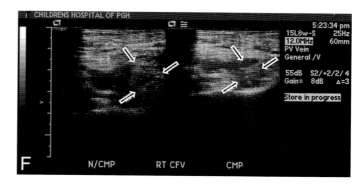

Figure 8.2 (Cont.)

Acute chest syndrome commonly leads to sudden clinical deterioration, so the imaging findings should provoke a rapid response including admission to a pediatric intensive care unit, initiation of oxygen and antibiotic therapy, and consideration of simple or exchange transfusions as necessary.

Ischemia in musculoskeletal tissues

Bone infarcts are most often encountered in the setting of sickle cell disease (Figure 8.2B, C). In this disease, various processes result in endothelial adherence and microvascular occlusion by sickled nondeformable erythrocytes that are sequestered in the bone marrow spaces. This microvascular occlusion promotes local hypoxia and results in increased erythrocyte sickling and sequestration with resultant marrow infarction. Clinically, the presentation of a child with sickle cell disease, fever, and a swollen and painful limb raises suspicion of either bone infarction, which will resolve with supportive therapy, or osteomyelitis, which will require antibiotic therapy.

Clinical and laboratory analysis alone may not differentiate these processes. A radionuclide bone scan (Figure 8.1D, E; Figure 8.3B, C) in conjunction with a bone marrow scan may be both the most accurate and most cost effective approach to distinguish these two entities. It has recently been claimed that an unenhanced T1 fat-saturated sequence alone is diagnostic for

acute bone infarcts, with contrast enhancement aiding in the differentiation of osteomyelitis from simple infarct (Figure 8.2C).

Bone infarcts result directly from the sickling of red blood cells in the bone marrow, which causes stasis of blood and sequestration of cells. Bone infarcts typically occur in the medullary cavities and epiphyses (Figure 8.3E, F) and are often the source of painful bone crises, although they may be clinically silent and discovered incidentally at radiography. Osteonecrosis of bone can occur in relation to many other predisposing factors or may be idiopathic. In certain select populations, such as older children undergoing intensive therapy for leukemia (Figure 8.4), the prevalence may be as high as 20%. The precise pathophysiological process leading to osteonecrosis or avascular necrosis is as yet undetermined, but the consequences can be severe, with joint derangement, chronic pain and gait dysfunction often leading to joint fusion or replacement.

In infants and young children, infarction often occurs in the diaphyses of small tubular bones in the hands and feet. Infarction of these sites is termed sickle cell dactylitis or hand foot syndrome, and results from the presence and persistence of red marrow in these regions. Sickle cell dactylitis is common between six months and two years but is rare after the age of six years, because of regression of red marrow in these areas with increasing age. This syndrome will occur in approximately half of children with sickle cell disease. Plain radiography shows

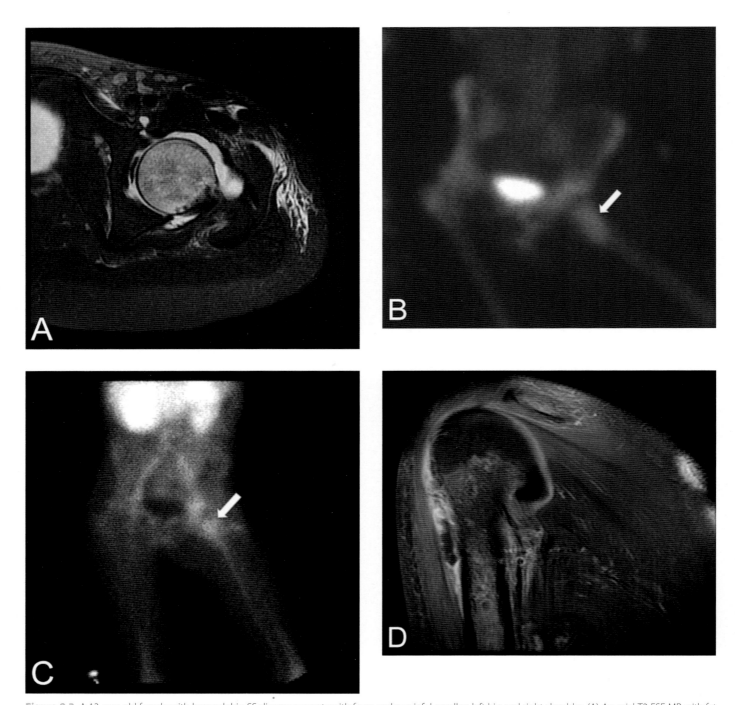

Figure 8.3 A 13-year-old female with hemoglobin SS disease presents with fever and a painful, swollen left hip and right shoulder. (A) An axial T2 FSE MR with fat saturation shows abnormal signal in the left femoral head and a left hip effusion, without significant inflammation in the surrounding tissues. A three-phase bone scan showed (B) increased uptake of radiotracer in the venous or blood pool phase in the left femoral neck and head (arrow) and (C) increased uptake in the delayed images in the same region (arrow), suggesting osteomyelitis rather than osteonecrosis. (D) A T1SE MR with fat saturation shows contrast enhancement of the tissues around the humeral head and neck, and abnormal increased signal in the bone. Blood cultures confirmed *Salmonella* sepsis and osteomyelitis. (E) Coronal T1-weighted MR image and (F) an axial T2 MR with fat saturation shows infarction in the medial femoral condyle. Note diffusely abnormal marrow signal in the femoral shaft due to marrow replacement.

patchy areas of lucency with periosteal reaction. In more severe cases, bone destruction and resultant deformity may be seen.

Epiphyseal ischemic necrosis in sickle cell disease is common, frequently seen in the femoral and humeral heads and more often bilateral than avascular necrosis in other diseases. About 50% of patients develop avascular necrosis by the age of 35 years. The contribution of synovial fluid to epiphyseal nutrition may offer some protection against infarction in children, among whom there is a lower prevalence of that complication. The earliest radiographic signs of avascular

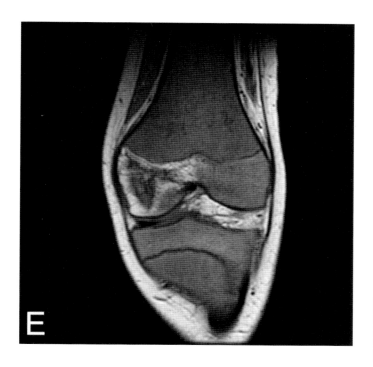

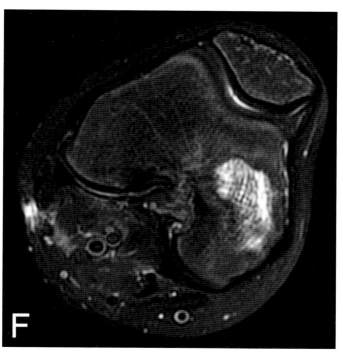

Figure 8.3 (Cont.)

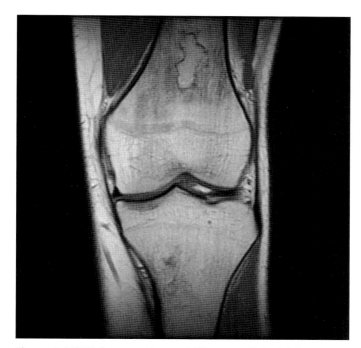

Figure 8.4 SPGR fat-saturated coronal MR image of the left knee shows infarction in the distal left femur in this 17-year-old male with high-risk leukemia on high-dose steroids and chemotherapy.

necrosis are shown on T2-weighted inversion recovery MR images, which show high signal intensity indicative of bone marrow edema. Early plain film signs include lucency and sclerosis within the epiphysis. Subsequently, crescent-shaped subchondral lucencies develop and eventually lead to depression of the articular surface, collapse and fragmentation. In weight-bearing joints such as the hip, secondary degenerative changes are produced by altered mechanical factors following collapse; these changes are less prominent features of osteonecrosis in non-weight-bearing joints such as the humeral head.

The soft tissues are also susceptible to ischemic injury from a variety of mechanisms, including trauma (Figure 8.5), hypothermia, metabolic disturbances, autoimmune diseases and infection. Examples include: trauma- or infection-induced rhabdomyolysis and compartment syndromes; microvascular thrombosis and vasculopathy from frostbite (Figure 8.6); myositis and pyomyositis related to connective tissue disorders; viral infections and metabolic disturbances such as diabetes mellitus, vasculitis and Raynaud's phenomenon related to such autoimmune disorders as systemic sclerosis; recurrent thrombosis in such autoimmune disorders as the catastrophic antiphospholipid antibody syndrome (Figure 8.7); and microvascular thrombosis and aneurysm formation in small arteries related to viral infections such as HIV and varicella-zoster.

Pulmonary infarct

Lung infarction is relatively rare due to the dual blood supply to the lung from the pulmonary and bronchial arteries. Hence, pulmonary infarction occurs with pulmonary artery obstruction only if the bronchial artery circulation is compromised. Pulmonary infarction is more commonly seen with occluded pulmonary artery branches ≤3 mm in diameter, perhaps because rapid bronchial flow into an isolated segment of the arterial circulation may cause extravasation of red blood cells into the alveoli,

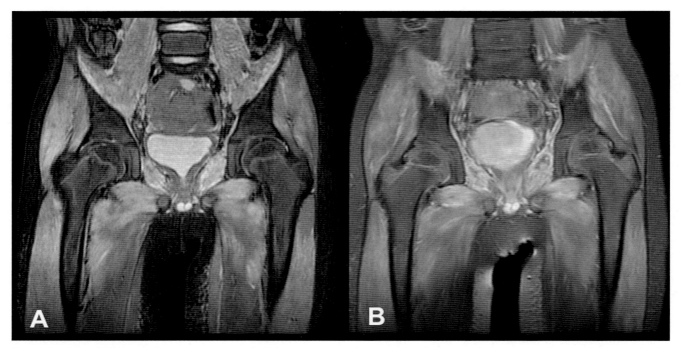

Figure 8.5 Coronal MR images show symmetric muscular T2 hyperintensity (A – STIR image) and contrast enhancement (B – fat-saturated, T1-weighted scan after Gd injection) around the pelvic girdle and proximal thighs consistent with myositis. The myositis in systemic autoimmune diseases is the result of tissue *ischemia* from the underlying vasculopathy.

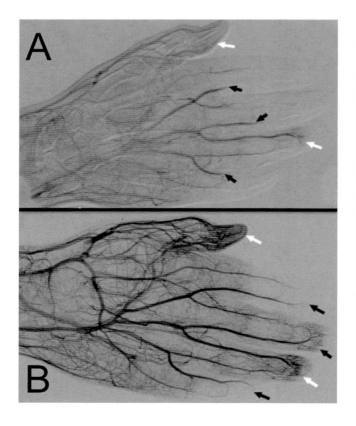

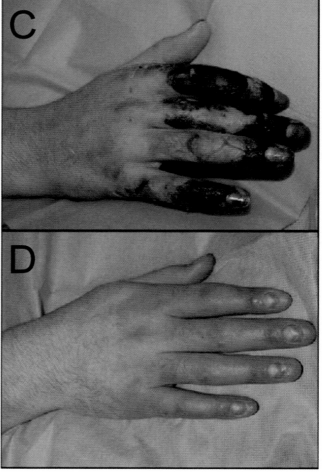

Figure 8.6 A 16-year-old male was unconscious in the snow due to inebriation, with his right hand exposed for approximately 10 hours. These angiographic images demonstrate (A) hypoperfusion of the entire right hand, with some perfusion to the tips of the first and fourth digits (white arrows) and abrupt loss of perfusion beyond the bases of the remaining digits (black arrows). (B) After 24 hours of transcatheter infusion of tissue plasminogen activator (tPA), there has been significant improvement in perfusion of all digits, although the second and fifth digits show persistently poor flow. Photographs show the right hand (C) immediately after tPA and (D) six months later, showing complete recovery. (Courtesy of T. Gregory Walker, MD, Massachusetts General Hospital, Boston, MA.)

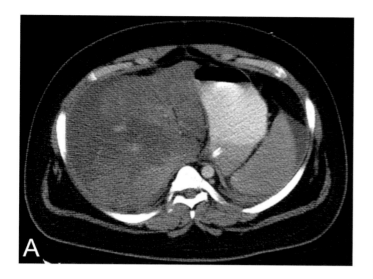

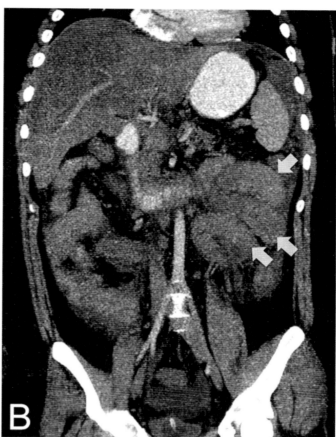

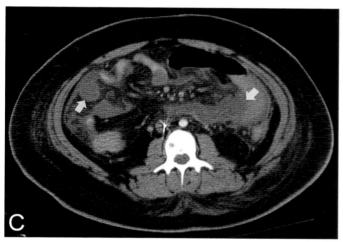

Figure 8.7 A 21-year-old male with Down syndrome and antiphospholipid antibodies presented with a two-month history of intermittent abdominal pain, and was found to have extensive portomesenteric thrombosis. (A) Contrast-enhanced axial CT of the abdomen shows a persistent irregular pattern of hepatic hypoperfusion and edema, consistent with chronic mild ischemia. (B) Coronal images from the same acquisition also show loops of proximal jejunum that are edematous and variably enhancing (arrows). (C) Three weeks after admission, a contrast-enhanced axial CT image demonstrates multiple loops of grossly edematous and hypoperfused bowel. Incidental note is made of a retrievable IVC filter, implanted to protect the patient from thromboembolic disease related to a pelvic venous thrombosis. A necrotic segment of proximal jejunum was removed at surgery the following day.

which may lead to pulmonary infarction. Congestion of a pulmonary vein is a contributing factor in the development of pulmonary infarcts, and congestive left heart failure is also a risk factor.

Splenic ischemia and infarction

Splenic infarction is seen in a wide variety of diseases including sickle cell disease, thalassemia embolic disease, hematological malignancies, aortic dissection, splenic torsion and vasculitis. On ultrasound, the infarct tends to be isoechoic in the acute phase, becoming increasingly hypoechoic after a few days. There is currently interest in the use of ultrasound contrast agents which are said to increase sensitivity; however, these are not yet universally available. With sulfur colloid technetium 99m, splenic infarction presents as a cold lesion (Figure 8.8).

On CT scans, in the acute phase, a wedge-shaped core of decreased enhancement is seen on contrast-enhanced scans. In a review of 59 patients with splenic infarction, one study found that 17% developed splenic abscess and 3.4% splenic rupture. Transcatheter splenic artery embolization is frequently carried out in trauma patients to treat acute hemorrhage or traumatic pseudoaneurysm. In one study, post-embolization splenic infarctions occurred in 63% of patients following proximal splenic artery embolization, and 100% after distal embolization. Partial splenic embolization may also be used to treat hypersplenism or to reduce portomesenteric overperfusion (Figure 8.9). Post-embolization syndrome may occur, with increasing severity associated with infarction of a larger volume of the organ. This is itself a manifestation of the systemic effects of local ischemia, and commonly includes pain, fever, nausea and ascites.

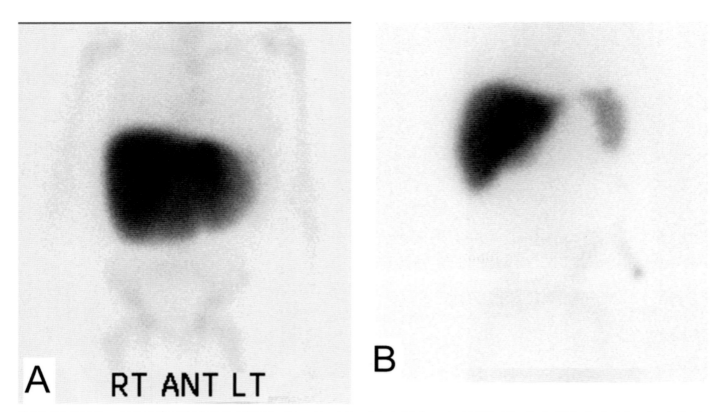

RT ANT LT

Figure 8.8 (A) A liver–spleen sulfur colloid scintigraphic scan shows no splenic uptake in this five-year-old sickle cell patient with "autosplenectomy" secondary to splenic infarction. (B) A repeat scan two years after bone marrow transplant demonstrates the unexpected return of splenic function.

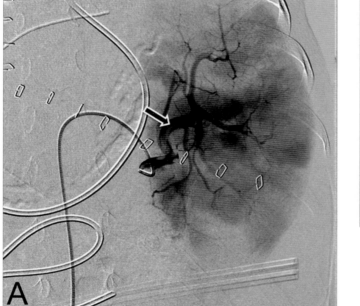

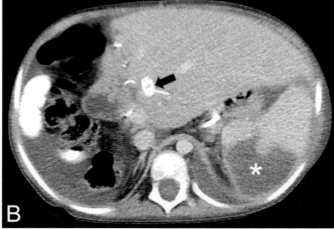

Figure 8.9 (A) A seven-year-old recipient of a living related left lobe liver transplant developed "small for size" syndrome from overperfusion of the transplant graft with over 12 l of ascites per day. He was referred to interventional radiology for a therapeutic reduction of splenic venous return to the liver. (A) Partial splenic embolization with PVA (polyvinyl alcohol) particles delivered through a catheter (arrow) via the splenic artery results in acute occlusion of microvessels in approximately 60% of the spleen, which shows a patchy pattern of hypoperfusion at angiography. (B) Contrast-enhanced CT six weeks later shows patchy areas of liquefactive necrosis (asterisk) with preservation of approximately 40% of viable splenic tissue. This resulted in temporary relief, but permanent resolution of symptoms required a transjugular intrahepatic portosystemic shunt (TIPS; arrow) insertion.

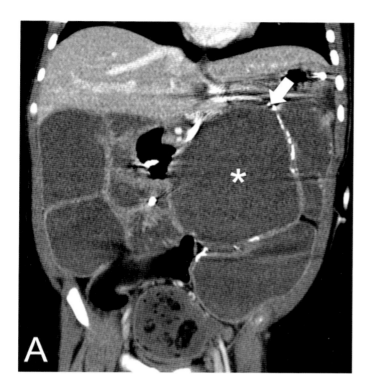
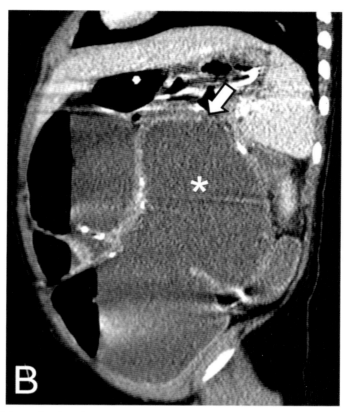

Figure 8.10 A two-year-old boy with short gut syndrome developed increased abdominal girth and pain. A stricture was suspected. (A) Coronal and (B) sagittal images from CT enterography performed with enteric administration of VoLumen (0.1% barium suspension) low density contrast shows the transition point from dilated loops (asterisk) to normal-caliber bowel (arrow). Although a high-quality 3D image could not be constructed, the ability to "fly through" the bowel with volumetric software permitted the stricture to be located with precision, enabling a more efficient surgical procedure at resection.

Mesenteric ischemia

Mesenteric ischemia is defined as impaired arterial or venous flow to or from the intestines. One percent of patients present-ing with an acute abdomen have ischemic intestinal disease. Morbidity and mortality have remained high over the past 30 years, with mortality rates in patients with acute ischemia exceeding 60%; an aggressive approach to the diagnosis and intervention is therefore warranted. Angiography has been considered the gold standard, although it is time consuming, invasive and costly. Considerable interest has therefore been focused on the use of CT and CT enterography (Figure 8.10).

In cases of acute ischemia, the most common finding is circumferential bowel wall thickening. The bowel may be of high or low attenuation; the low attenuation reflecting sub-mucosal edema and inflammation; the high attenuation due to submucosal hemorrhage. Sometimes the affected loops may show decreased contrast enhancement due to compromised blood flow (Figure 8.11).

CT and MR imaging findings include bowel wall thickening with or without the target sign, intramural pneumatosis, mesen-teric or portal gas and mesenteric arterial or venous thromboem-bolism. Other CT findings include engorgement of mesenteric veins and mesenteric edema, lack of bowel wall enhancement

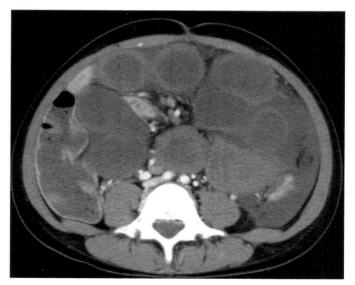

Figure 8.11 This 15-year-old female with Crohn's disease developed acute right epigastric pain, fever and diarrhea. Contrast-enhanced CT of the abdomen shows multiple loops of grossly edematous small bowel, although some perfu-sion of the bowel wall is still visualized. At surgery, the bowel appeared viable, and a short region of stricture was resected. The patient recovered without further loss of bowel.

(Figure 8.7B, C), increased enhancement of the thickened bowel wall, bowel obstruction and infarction of other abdominal organs.

Radiographic findings of bowel ischemia on plain film and barium studies are well described and include bowel wall thickening, submucosal focal mural thickening or thumb-printing, dilated bowel loops, intramural pneumatosis and mesenteric or portal venous gas. Bowel dilatation reflects the interruption of peristaltic activity in ischemic segments; it is a common but nonspecific finding in bowel ischemia. Owing to the edema that accompanies bowel ischemia, the mesenteric fat may be abnormally increased in attenuation.

Intramural gas is a less common but more specific CT sign of ischemic bowel disease. The intramural gas is caused by dissection of luminal gas into the bowel wall and across the compromised mucosa. Mesenteric or portal venous gas is an even less common manifestation of ischemic bowel disease, and represents the propagation of intramural gas into the mesenteric venous system. Free intraperitoneal air is an ominous sign in ischemic bowel disease because it indicates perforation of an infarcted bowel segment. While transcatheter thrombolysis may be indicated for treatment of ischemic bowel related to arterial or venous thrombosis, it is contraindicated in the face of evidence of bowel necrosis or perforation.

Absent or poor enhancement of the bowel wall appears to be the most specific finding for bowel ischemia. In some cases, the ischemic segment shows prolonged enhancement. An abnormal enhancement pattern in ischemic segments is attributable mainly to perfusion problems, i.e. delayed return of venous blood with subsequent slowing of the arterial supply or arteriospasm. Chronic intestinal ischemia frequently presents with a history of recurrent abdominal pain after meals. Such cases may result from congenital cardiovascular malformations (e.g. aortic coarctation, hypoplastic left heart syndrome), atherosclerosis or radiation treatment (e.g. as a long-term complication after abdominal irradiation for neuroblastoma) with stenosis and/or decreased perfusion of the mesenteric arteries and typically large collateral pathways are present.

Torsion, volvulus and herniation

Any organ suspended from a vascular pedicle is at risk for ischemia and necrosis due to torsion or volvulus. While this most commonly affects the testis and appendix testis, the ovary and adnexa, and the bowel, it may also affect the fallopian tube, omentum, spleen, and under unusual circumstances even gallbladder, lung and transplant kidney. Similar vascular compromise occurs when an organ partially herniates through a rigid bony, fibrous or muscular ring, whether mesentery or bowel herniating through the inguinal ring, bowel herniating through a diaphragmatic hernia, or diencephalon herniating through the tentorium cerebelli. The result is tissue ischemia, and the outcome is determined, as in all other cases of ischemia, by the intrinsic vulnerability of the tissue, the duration of ischemia, and the extent of either necrosis or reperfusion injury.

Torsion is characterized by twisting of the vascular pedicle. The resulting hypoperfusion of the testis or ovary may lead over time to irreversible necrosis (Figure 8.12). If this is unrecognized, such as in the antenatal period, the gonadal tissue may be resorbed and become unapparent on subsequent imaging. Presence of vascular flow, for example on color Doppler imaging, is predictive of reversible injury and sustained function (Figure 8.13), while absence of vascular flow in a twisted pedicle is usually associated with irreversible necrosis. Although similar findings may be made with CT and MR imaging of adnexal torsion, these modalities tend to be less sensitive than US in this application. However, CT evaluation for abdominal pain may reflect findings suggestive of ovarian torsion, including a twisted vascular pedicle, pelvic fluid, an enlarged ovary, uterine deviation, fallopian tube thickening and adnexal cystic structures. Perhaps due to the intermittent

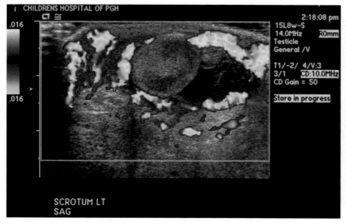

Figure 8.12 A three-year-old male presented with scrotal swelling and pain of approximately 12 hours duration. The testis shows no flow on color Doppler evaluation, and shows alternating strands of hyper- and hypoechoic tissue. There is profound hyperemia and swelling of the scrotum and hydrocele. At surgery, the torsed testis was not viable.

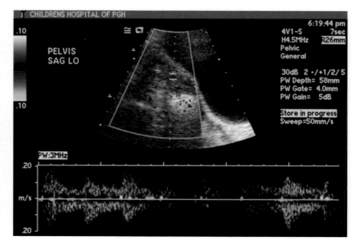

Figure 8.13 Pulse-wave Doppler imaging of the left adnexa shows abnormally poor perfusion of an edematous left ovary in this 18-year-old female with intermittent pelvic pain radiating to the flank. At surgery, the viable ovary was detorsed and orchidopexy performed to prevent future torsion.

nature of gonadal torsion and potentially to the protective effects of brief ischemic episodes, salvage by detorsion is often possible despite prolonged symptoms and even despite subjective intraoperative evidence of severe ischemia.

As volvulus represents progression of malrotation to complete intestinal obstruction with significant compromise of the SMA territory, affected bowel may include anything from proximal duodenum to mid-transverse colon. Intermittent volvulus may in addition lead to mesenteric cyst formation and chylous ascites (from lymphatic congestion), as well as chronic malabsorption, vomiting, and alternating constipation and diarrhea. Arterial compromise may lead to mucosal necrosis, pneumatosis, sepsis, perforation, peritonitis and death. The imaging modality of choice to diagnose a midgut volvulus is dynamic contrast fluoroscopy. Ultrasound may show an inversion of the position of the superior mesenteric vein and artery with a "whirlpool" appearance of these vessels. Pneumatosis coli on plain film may represent necrosis and gangrene and is especially ominous (Figures 8.14, 8.15). While these findings should

provoke an immediate referral for laparotomy, absence of conclusive imaging findings in the face of strong clinical suspicion of volvulus warrants prompt contrast studies for confirmation. Incidental note of bowel wall thickening due to edema and venous congestion may also support the diagnosis. An upper GI contrast series remains the gold standard for diagnosis of volvulus. It should demonstrate partial or complete duodenal obstruction. A "birdbeak" obstruction of the proximal duodenum with a "corkscrew" appearance of the lower duodenum with abnormal positioning and adhesive obstruction is characteristic of volvulus. Continuation of the small bowel series to show abnormally positioned proximal jejunal loops leading into the right lower quadrant can be very helpful confirmation. Although abnormal position of the cecum is suggestive, lower GI studies are not particularly helpful and may obscure findings on a subsequent upper GI study. The role of ultrasound in volvulus is limited primarily to evaluation of the vascular relationships, and demonstration of the SMV to the left of the SMA is highly suggestive of the diagnosis. Vascular-contrast-enhanced CT may also demonstrate the same abnormal mesenteric vascular relationships, with a "hurricane" appearance of the SMA, and may show the extent of mural edema and hypoperfusion.

Cerebrovascular disease and ischemic injury

Stroke in the pediatric population is rare, but actually occurs approximately as often as pediatric brain tumors, with an estimated incidence of about 1 to 13 per 100 000 per year, and may be even higher in the perinatal period. Risk factors differ: in the perinatal period, fetal distress and post-term delivery are predictors of stroke, whereas in neonates and older children cyanotic congenital heart disease, hemoglobinopathies like sickle cell disease, trauma and infections are the leading causes of stroke. However, numerous other entities may contribute to risk of stroke in children, including but not limited to hyperviscosity syndromes, hypercoagulable states, inborn errors of metabolism, autoimmune disorders, vasculitis, radiation injury, both prescribed and illicit drugs, and many syndromes. In at least one-third of cases, no specific etiology can be identified (Figure 8.16). The symptoms of stroke in children are similar to those in adults, with weakness, numbness, etc., but because children have frequent minor trauma and illnesses the symptoms are often attributed to these. Symptoms may be absent, fleeting or transient, may be delayed by developmental capability, or may be profound, including acute hemiplegia, flaccidity, seizures, lethargy or coma. First-line radiological studies may include CT, MR, MR arteriography (and MR venography), which should be accomplished immediately in the case of suspected acute stroke, at the minimum within the first 48 hours of presentation. Transcranial Doppler US is a second-line examination that may be helpful within the first week for non-acute presentations.

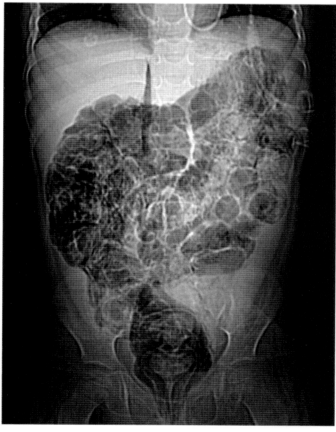

Figure 8.14 A plain radiograph of the abdomen and pelvis in this 13-year-old female with acute lymphocytic leukemia on high-dose steroid therapy shows a "bubbly" pattern of intramural air in the bowel as well as free air to the right of the spine and adjacent to the sigmoid colon. While in a patient with infection this pattern would indicate a very poor prognosis, this patient was nearly asymptomatic and had no long-term sequelae.

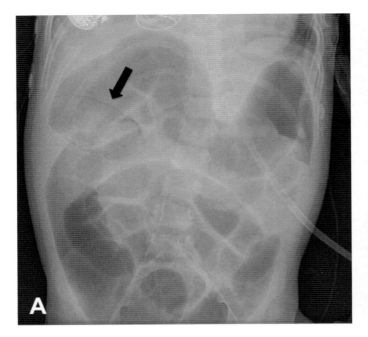

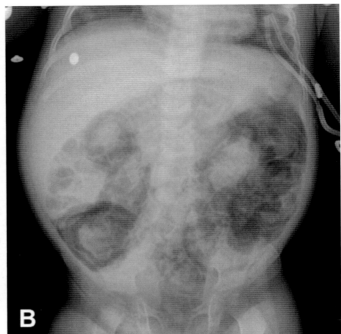

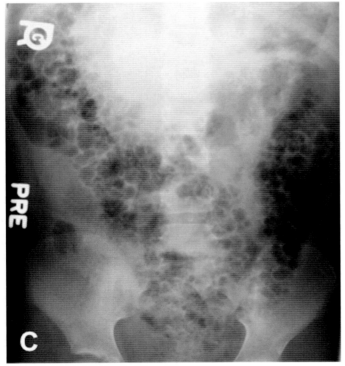

Figure 8.15 Various forms of pneumatosis intestinalis. (A) Infant with Marfan syndrome after heart surgery, developing abdominal pain and distension. A radiograph of the abdomen showed pneumatosis intestinalis (arrow), which proved to be due to bowel infarction at laparotomy. Echocardiography demonstrated a thrombus in the left ventricle as the probable cause. (B) Twenty-seven-month-old with leukemia and benign pneumatosis after chemotherapy. (C) Nine-year-old girl with systic fibrosis and benign pneumatosis cystoides intestinalis, dissection of gas from ruptured alveoli along vessels and bronchi into the mediastinum and then along major vessels into the retroperitoneum, from which it moves via the mesentery to the subserosa of bowel loops.

In general, cerebral angiography or venous sinus venography is reserved to answer specific clinical questions or to evaluate candidacy for therapeutic interventions on an elective basis as indicated. Many, if not most, pediatric strokes are first imaged beyond the time window of treatment established for adults. There is currently no consensus on how and when to treat pediatric stroke patients, although multicenter trials of thrombolytic therapy are ongoing.

Neonates

Cerebral palsy is a group of disorders involving movement, learning, hearing, seeing and thinking that occur in premature

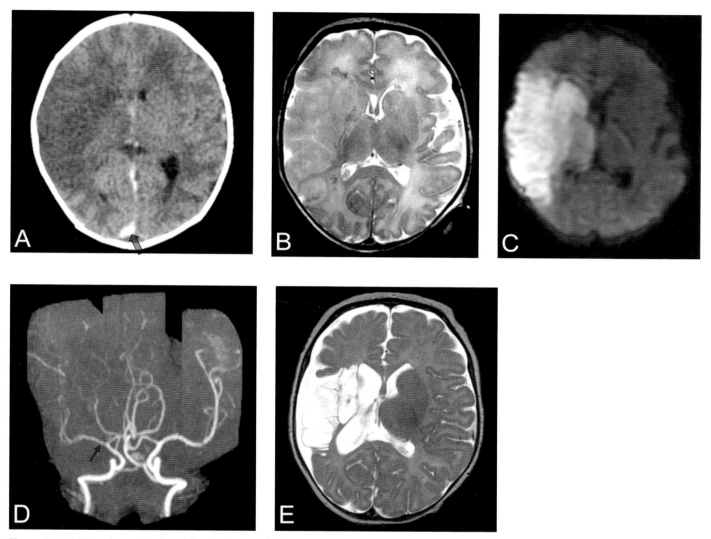

Figure 8.16 A 39-week-gestational-age infant had a normal delivery with Apgar scores at one and five minutes of 9 and 9. He developed seizures on the second day of life. (A) CT on the third day of life shows edema in right middle cerebral artery; distribution consistent with neonatal arterial occlusion. The right basal ganglia and thalamus are also involved. High density in the superior sagittal sinus (arrow) is due to the high hemoglobin concentration of the neonate and is not thrombosis. (B) On axial T2-weighted imaging, note the swelling of the right operculum and basal ganglia with compression of the frontal horn. (C) Axial diffusion-weighted imaging confirms restricted diffusion in the middle cerebral artery territory including the basal ganglia and the thalamus. (D) Time-of-flight MRA shows stenosis of the right middle cerebral artery (arrow) and a marked decrease in peripheral perfusion. (E) On follow-up axial T2-weighted MR, most of the middle cerebral territory has undergone cystic encephalomalacia with dilation of the lateral ventricle and subarachnoid space.

infants as a result of hypoxia, sometimes with periventricular hemorrhagic infarction, in the periventricular white matter, causing a typical injury pattern referred to as "periventricular white matter injury of the premature infant." This injury pattern reflects the arterial supply of the brain and metabolism approximately in week 26–34 of gestation. At this period of development, the arterial supply in the premature infant is primarily from the cortex. As a result, deep vascular "border zones," especially at the depth of the sulci in parasagittal regions (the end zones of long penetrating arteries) and distal vascular fields such as the posterior occipital regions, are most vulnerable to hypoxic injury. The veins of the germinal matrix are also large and fragile, accounting for the frequency of subependymal hemorrhage. It is also thought that the deep white matter at this stage, until around 32 weeks, has a high population of late oligodendrocyte precursors, which are quite susceptible to hypoxic injury. Maternal infections of any type are associated with a higher risk of cerebral palsy. Experimental work in fetal sheep suggests that preexisting circulatory instability may play a role. The final pattern of periventricular leukomalacia (PVL) with white matter loss and ventricular enlargement is usually not clearly

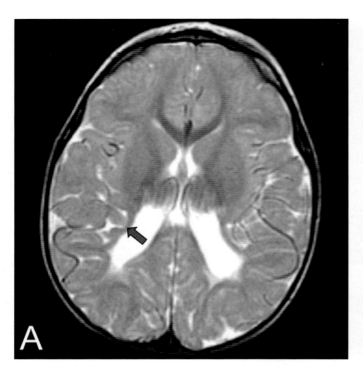 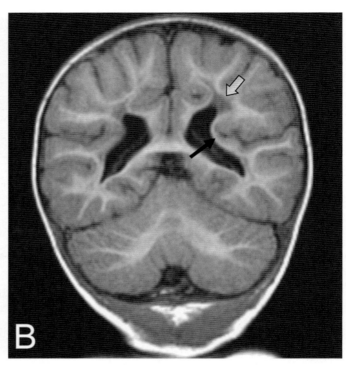

Figure 8.17 A 13-month-old former premature infant with PVL. (A) Axial T2-weighted MR shows sulci down close to the ventricular surface (arrow) because of loss of white matter. There is also mild focal ex vacuo enlargement of the ventricles from the white matter loss. (B) A coronal MR image shows unmyelinated periventricular white matter (white arrow) and the loss of white matter (black arrow).

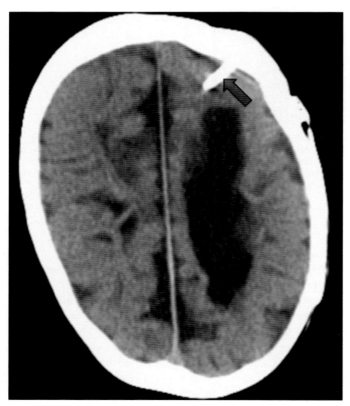

Figure 8.18 CT in a former 34-week-gestation infant with previous grade 4 intraventricular and cerebral hemorrhage shows severe loss of white matter and superimposed ex vacuo hydrocephalus characteristic of severe PVL. Note shunt in left frontal region (arrow).

visible until most of the white matter is well myelinated around 18–24 months. At this time, the imaging findings may be moderate (Figure 8.17) or severe with volume loss of the periventricular white matter and ex vacuo hydrocephalus (Figure 8.18).

In the newborn, one may see only periventricular cysts or small hemorrhages on US (Figure 8.19). This in part reflects the inability of cranial US to resolve subtle findings of white matter gliosis and glial scarring. Term infants may occasionally have PVL from an earlier in utero insult. They are more likely to have a variety of abnormalities secondary to acute hypoxia, infection, venous or venous sinus occlusion, or less commonly arterial occlusion. Severe total hypoxic-ischemic encephalopathy typically involves the central gray matter and possibly the cortex (Figures 8.20, 8.21), depending on the severity. These areas are most involved because of higher metabolic activity, and they are also the most myelinated. Clinical signs are variable, ranging from hypotonia and apnea to seizures. In milder prolonged hypoxia, blood is shunted to the central structures for preservation, and the more peripheral watershed regions suffer the hypoxic changes. Chronic hypoxia may be milder and usually less severe and is quite variable in appearance. Since there is considerable variability as to the severity and duration of hypoxia, the imaging findings vary.

MRI is more sensitive than CT to early signs of cerebral ischemia, though the ease of CT imaging still makes it useful.

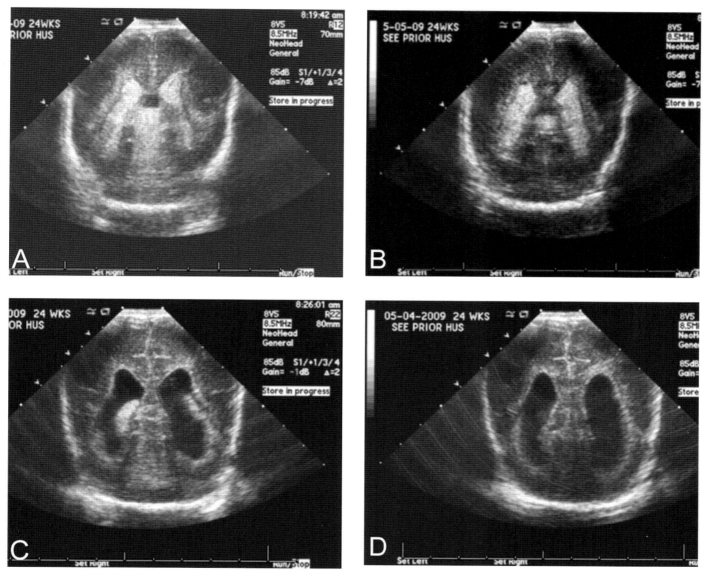

Figure 8.19 Coronal transcranial Doppler ultrasound images at the mid- (A) and posterior (B) ventricles from a head ultrasound examination in a 24-week-gestational-age infant shows echogenic blood within dilated lateral ventricles. Increased echogenicity is also visible around the ventricles. Five days later, on a repeat examination at the same levels (C, D) the ventricular hemorrhage has almost completely cleared, but there is further enlargement of the lateral ventricles.

CT findings may lag in visibility for the first 24 hours. They include patchy or generalized edema with blurring of gray–white matter borders, sometimes with a "bright" cerebellum because of sparing, and the "reversal sign" with the central gray matter remaining normal but appearing higher in attenuation compared to the surrounding low-attenuation edema. Diffusion imaging may demonstrate abnormalities of perinatal ischemic insult much earlier than conventional MR imaging. While generally positive after 6–8 hours, it has also been reported to be falsely negative up to 24 hours in both full-term and preterm infants. Even when positive, it may underestimate the severity of injury, and exhibits an evolving pattern that changes significantly over time. The combination of diffusion-weighted imaging (DWI),

perfusion imaging and spectroscopy (MRS) can be very useful in the neonate (Figures 8.22–8.24), though it requires infant head coils and high-level software. Assuming no new injuries, diffusion returns to "normal" within seven days. The lack of abnormal diffusion after seven days does not mean the injury has reversed.

Metabolic disorders are also commonly related to cerebral injury. Hypoglycemia in the newborn and in older children typically causes occipital lobe edema followed by atrophy or infarction, though involvement may be more diffuse with the occipital lobes being most severely involved (Figure 8.25). Extracorporeal membrane oxygenation (ECMO), used for severe respiratory and cardiac problems, occasionally leads to

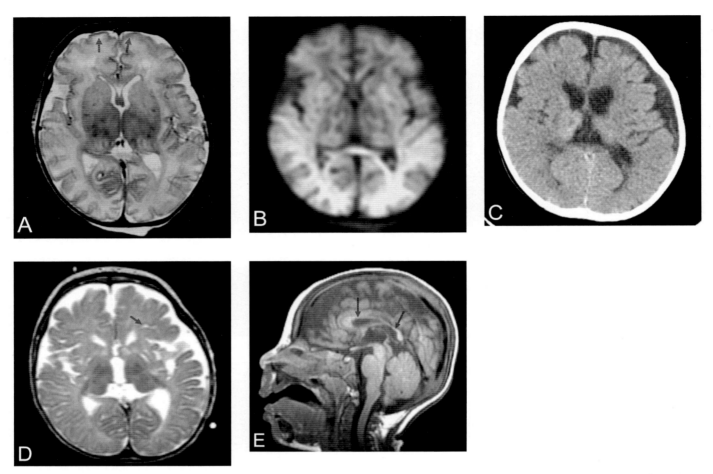

Figure 8.20 (A) T2 axial MR image in a term infant with placental abruption shows abnormally increased, somewhat heterogeneous signal in the basal ganglia and thalami. The white matter is also somewhat increased in signal. Multiple areas of cortex, particularly the frontal lobes (arrows), are swollen. (B) Diffusion-weighted MR (DWI) demonstrates increased signal (decreased diffusion) throughout the white matter, and somewhat heterogeneously in the central gray matter, especially the putamina. (C) Axial noncontrast CT at five months of age shows mild enlargement of the ventricles. There is increased density in the thalami secondary to microcalcification, and loss of volume of thalami and basal ganglia. The subarachnoid space is enlarged from atrophy, worse on the left side. (D) At six months of age, a T2-weighted axial image shows diffuse white matter volume loss, enlargement of the lateral and third ventricles, and atrophy of the basal ganglia. The cortex is thin. Some widening of the base of the sulci (arrow) indicates mild ulegyria, which is typical of severe term hypoxic-ischemic encephalopathy. (E) A sagittal T1 image obtained at six months shows extreme thinning of the corpus callosum (arrows) from severe white matter loss. The head is microcephalic.

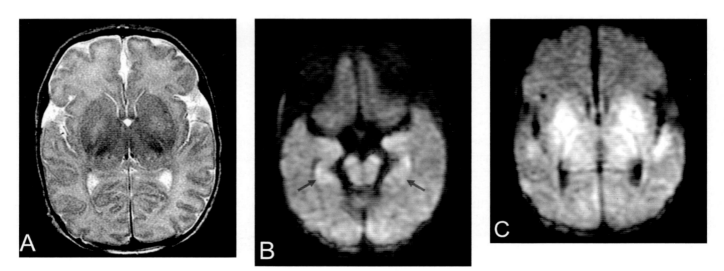

Figure 8.21 (A) A 39-week-gestational-age infant had one and five minute Apgar scores of 2 and 4, and subsequently died. Axial T2-weighted MR imaging shows some mildly increased signal in the basal ganglia, posterior thalami, and to a lesser degree within the white matter. (B) Diffusion-weighted image shows restricted diffusion in the mesial temporal lobes and central midbrain, typical for severe term hypoxia. (C) Diffusion-weighted image through the central gray matter shows restricted diffusion particularly in the basal ganglia, but also in the thalami, the mesial temporal lobes, and minimally in the occipital gray matter and subcortical white matter consistent with severe hypoxic-ischemic encephalopathy.

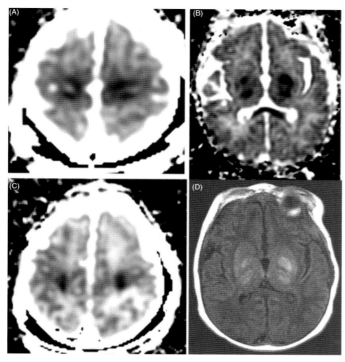

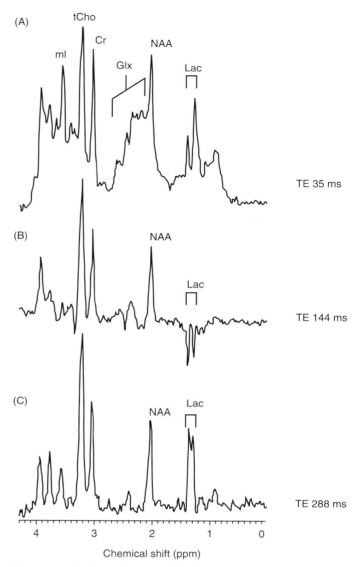

Figure 8.22 (A–C) Average diffusion coefficient (ADC) mapping of a term infant on the first day of life with acute hypoxic-ischemic injury shows abnormal restricted diffusion in the perirolandic cortex, cortical spinal tract at the level of the corona radiata, basal ganglia, and thalamus, representing the "central" pattern of acute perinatal hypoxic-ischemic injury. Of note, the corresponding conventional T1-weighted MR images (D) showed abnormal signal intensity on follow-up imaging at day five. (Courtesy of Ashok Panigrahy, MD, University of Pittsburgh. Used with permission.)

Figure 8.23 Single-voxel proton MR spectroscopy (MRS) at three different echo times in the basal ganglia of a hypoxic-ischemic term infant. Note the character-istic modulation of lactate. (A) A spectrum acquired using short echo time (35 ms) shows an mI peak (left side of the spectrum), elevated glutamine/glutamine peak next to a reduced NAA peak (middle spectrum), and an elevated lactate doublet next to a lipid peak (right side of spectrum). (B) A spectrum acquired using long echo time (144 ms) shows a lactate doublet peak, inverted, and reduced NAA, but nonvisualization of mI, glutamate and lipids. (C) A spectrum acquired using longer echo time (288 ms) is similar to 144 ms, except that the lactate doublet reverts to the other side of the spectrum. (Courtesy of Ashok Panigrahy, MD, University of Pittsburgh. Used with permission.)

intracerebral hemorrhage, which can be severe (Figure 8.26). Newborns and older infants are especially prone to venous sinus and cerebral venous thrombosis from dehydration. Cerebral injury from cerebral venous thrombosis can be benign (Figure 8.27) or devastating, depending on the extent of the thrombosis and the severity of venous involvement (Figure 8.28).

Newborns are also prone to a variety of infections. TORCH infection in utero causes classical findings of calcifications and volume loss (Figure 8.29) with or without ex vacuo hydro-cephalus. Herpes (HSV) encephalitis is a relatively common newborn infection although it occurs in only 1 in 3000 births. Transmission is usually direct from the infected birth canal and is most commonly type 2 virus. Unlike the classical type 1 herpes infection in older children and adults, the effects are usually more diffuse. If treated early, the infection may be mild and leave no residual damage (Figure 8.30); if left untreated, the infection can be devastating and cause brain infarction (Figure 8.31). Bacterial infections, especially from *E. coli* and group B *Streptococcus*, can cause severe damage to the new-born brain (Figure 8.32). Again, the topology is usually diffuse, may include hemorrhage, and cannot be easily separated from HSV by imaging.

Older children

Cerebral ischemic damage from trauma is often devastating. Direct trauma, other than birth trauma, rarely occurs in the newborn infant. On the contrary, child abuse, or non-accidental trauma, most often occurs before the age of three years, but is uncommon before the age of three months. Early edema may be very subtle. Lesions are frequently multiple and

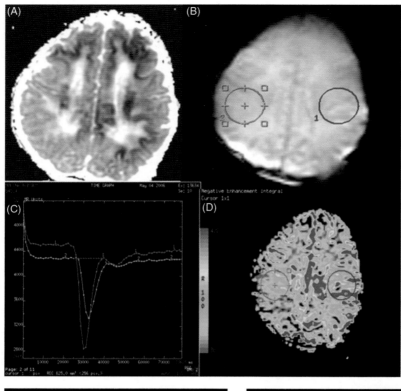

Figure 8.24 Dynamic contrast susceptibility perfusion MRI of hypoxic-ischemic injury in the neonatal brain. (A) Diffusion map shows abnormal restricted diffusion in the bilateral cerebral cortex, left greater than right, with a "peripheral" pattern of injury. (B) A GRE-planar perfusion-weighted MR raw image obtained at the same level with placement of two regions of interest (ROIs). (C) Time–activity curve showing the signal change over time of the contrast bolus through the ROI. (D) A generated cerebral blood volume map shows increased cerebral blood volume in the regions of acute infarction likely representing compensatory luxury perfusion. (Courtesy of Ashok Panigrahy, MD, University of Pittsburgh. Used with permission.)

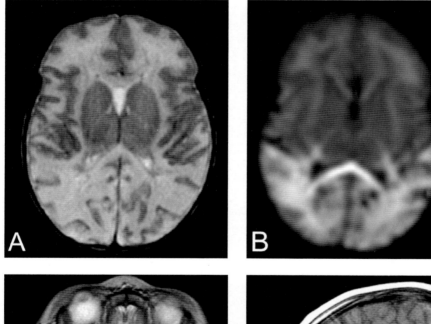

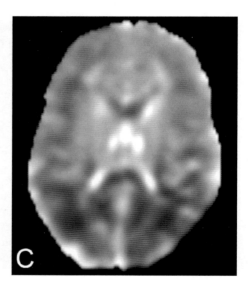

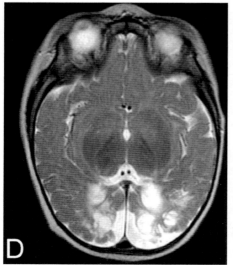

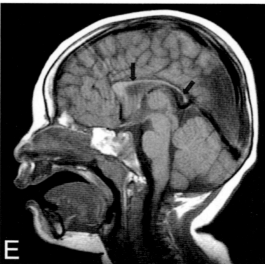

Figure 8.25 Term infant with severe hypoglycemia. (A) Initial T2-weighted MR image shows diffuse cerebral edema, which is worst in the occipital lobes where the outline of the cortex is more difficult to see. (B) On diffusion-weighted MR imaging there is marked restriction of diffusion in the occipital and posterior temporal regions along with the posterior corpus callosum. (C) ADC map at a slightly higher level than (B) shows severely restricted diffusion in the occipital lobes (darker signal), and some involvement of more anterior white matter and corpus callosum. (D) Follow-up axial T2-weighted imaging at 11 months of age demonstrates severe atrophy/encephalomalacia of the occipital lobes. (E) Sagittal T1 imaging obtained at the same time as (D) shows marked thinning of the corpus callosum (arrows) in addition to the severe atrophy of the occipital lobes.

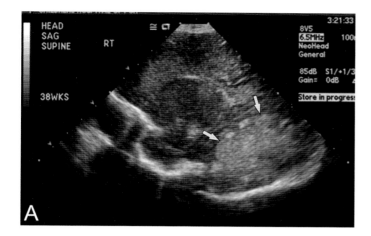

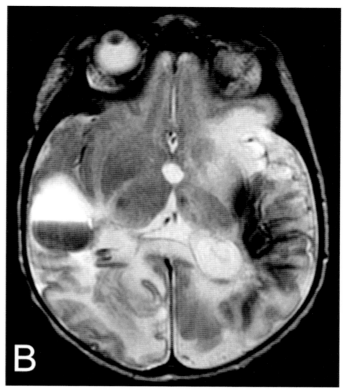

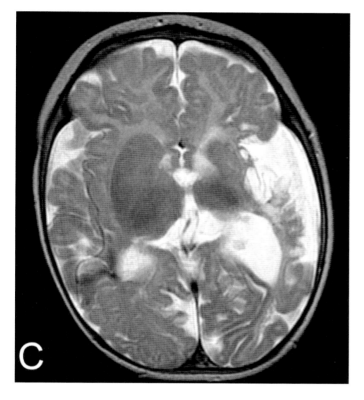

Figure 8.26 (A) A parasagittal image from a head ultrasound in a 38-week-gestation infant on ECMO for sepsis reveals a large cerebral hematoma (arrows). (B) On axial T2-weighted images 10 days later, there is a right temporal hemorrhage with fluid levels. There is cortical and subcortical hemorrhage on the left in the temporal and occipital lobes. Increased signal from edema is noted in the occipital lobes, left temporal lobe and left basal ganglia. (C) At two months post-hemorrhage, axial T2 MR imaging shows extensive left-sided atrophy including the left basal ganglia and thalamus.

sometimes of multiple ages, including subdural and intracerebral hemorrhage and more diffuse lesions such as diffuse axonal injury (Figure 8.33). Gunshot wounds are uncommon in children, with damage usually resulting from the shock wave and dispersion of debris as the projectile fragments (Figure 8.34). Blunt trauma varying from blows to the head to severe ATV and other vehicular accidents are common in children, especially those with ADHD. Injury may be minor and localized without permanent sequelae (Figure 8.35), or severe in the case of high-energy trauma from high-speed collisions (Figure 8.36). Changes of acute edema, contusional hemorrhage, secondary complications,

and severe local malacia are often present. "Growing fractures" (leptomeningeal cysts) are more likely to occur in children than in adults due to continuing head growth. They result from dural tears that allow CSF to leak through the fracture, with CSF pulsations progressively enlarging these fractures (Figure 8.37).

Moyamoya vasculitis is another identifiable cause of pediatric stroke, albeit a rare disease, affecting approximately 1 person per 100 000 population. The etiology of moyamoya itself is usually unclear. It can be primary or be found in children with neurofibromatosis type 1, tuberous sclerosis, Down syndrome, sickle cell disease, and like

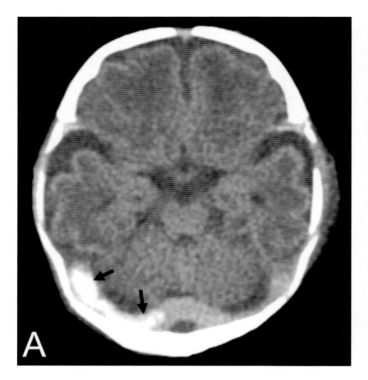

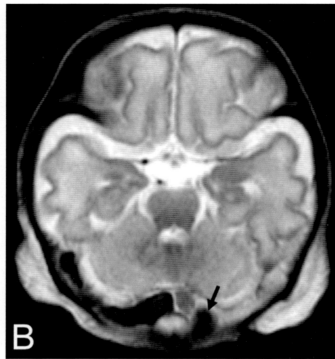

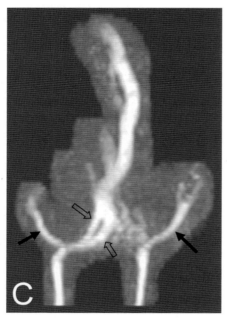

Figure 8.27 (A) CT of the head was performed in a 35-week-gestation infant with congenital diaphragmatic hernia and congenital heart disease. There is thrombus in the right transverse sinus (arrows), which is denser than the left transverse sinus. (B) Axial T2-weighted MR image obtained the following day shows extension of clot into the left proximal transverse sinus (arrow). (C) On coronal MR venogram, both transverse sinuses are not visualized due to absent or very slow flow. However, the sagittal sinus is connected to a bifid occipital sinus (open arrows), and there is also good drainage remaining in the sigmoid sinuses (solid arrows). Infants typically have large occipital sinuses that can bypass transverse sinus occlusion.

unrelated infarcts, a variety of syndromes. Moyamoya presents as progressive stenosis and occlusion of cavernous and supraclinoid internal carotid arteries, with development of multiple collaterals through the central gray matter from the external carotid circulation and from the posterior circulation. Because of the collaterals, symptoms usually present late in the disease with infarcts, though there may be warning

transient ischemic attacks, headaches etc. MRI and MRA will define the disease, but catheter angiography remains the gold standard for preoperative planning (Figure 8.38). The most effective treatment currently available is synangiosis, in which a branch of the external circulation, usually the superficial temporal artery, is placed on the pia through a craniotomy. If successful, the artery "grafts" itself to the

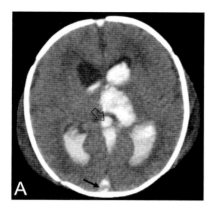
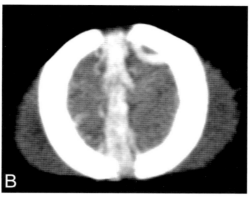

Figure 8.28 A 38-week-old infant presented with tetralogy of Fallot, which was repaired. The patient subsequently developed fungal sepsis. (A) CT at 20 days of age shows clot in the vein of Galen (hollow arrow), the straight sinus immediately behind it and the distal superior sagittal sinus (arrow). In addition, there is significant intraventricular and left thalamic hemorrhage. (B) A superior slice from the CT shows clot filling the superior sagittal sinus and the adjacent veins draining into the sinus. Venous thrombosis extended into the internal jugular veins. The patient died shortly after.

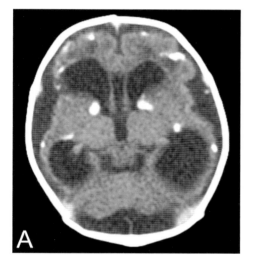
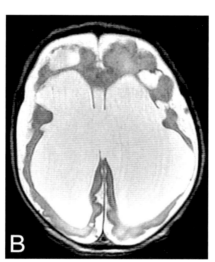

Figure 8.29 (A) Axial noncontrast CT shows multiple calcifications typical for TORCH, most commonly CMV or toxoplasmosis. The ventricles are markedly dilated, and the cortex is poorly formed, suggesting that the ventricular dilation is primarily due to atrophy. Hydrocephalus can occur, usually due to aqueduct occlusion. (B) Axial T2-weighted MR image shows infarcts in the frontal lobes, and severe volume loss of white matter and cortex. There is some suggestion of enlarged gyri in the left front lobe. TORCH infections are commonly associated with cortical dysplasia.

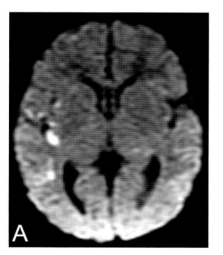
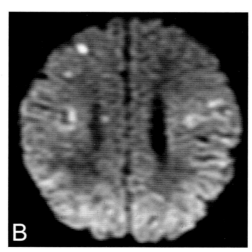
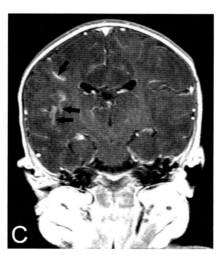

Figure 8.30 This full-term newborn infant began seizing at 17 days of age. (A) Diffusion-weighted imaging shows scattered abnormalities in the right opercular cortex. (B) Diffusion-weighted imaging at a higher level shows scattered abnormal foci in the frontal lobes. (C) A coronal post-contrast T1-weighted image shows scattered foci of abnormal enhancement deep in the sulci (arrows).

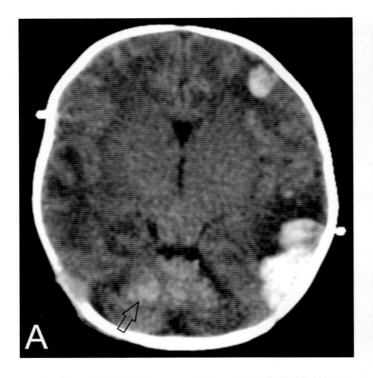

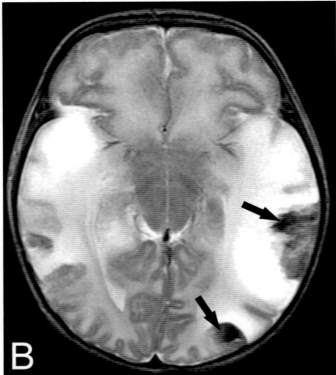

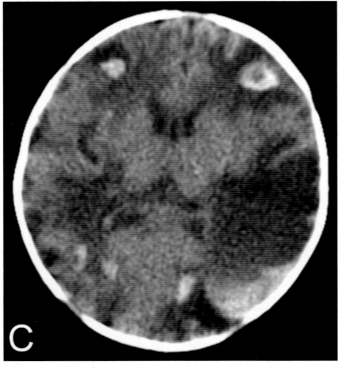

Figure 8.31 A three-week-old infant developed seizures, and HSV type 2 titers were positive. (A) Axial noncontrast CT shows bilateral cerebral edema, multiple hemorrhages in left hemisphere, and subtle hemorrhage in right cerebellum (arrow). (B) Axial T2-weighted MRI shows severe diffuse bilateral edema primarily involving temporal lobes with temporal and occipital hemorrhages (arrows). (C) Follow-up CT obtained two weeks later demonstrates multiple areas of low-density edema. Focal frontal, temporal and occipital foci of hemorrhage remain visible.

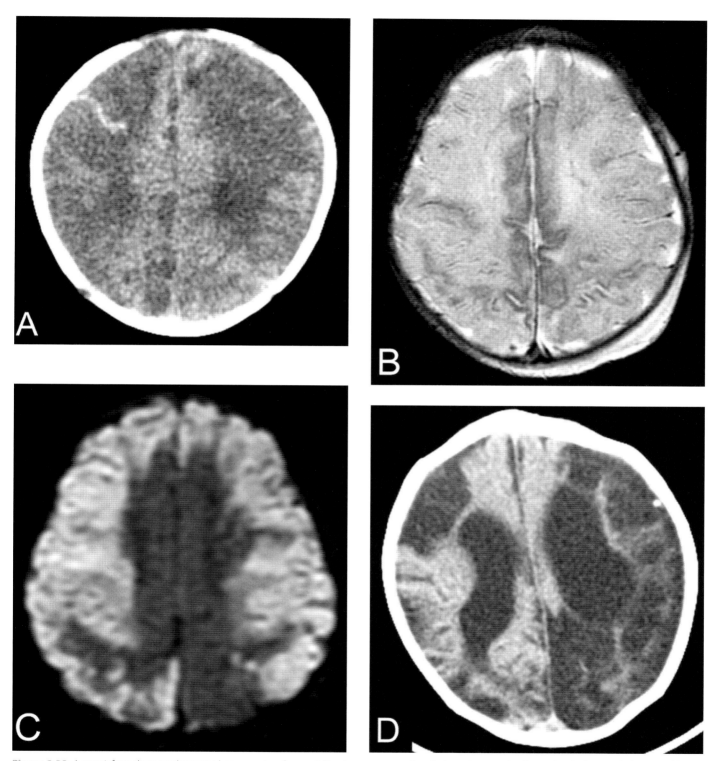

Figure 8.32 A term infant whose mother was a known carrier of group B *Streptococcus* was well until about three weeks of age when he became lethargic and began seizing. (A) A noncontrast CT shows patchy diffuse edema, and focal right subarachnoid hemorrhage. (B) Axial T2-weighted MRI shows severe diffuse edema with some relative sparing along the medial cortical borders. (C) Diffusion-weighted imaging demonstrates markedly restricted diffusion throughout most of the cortex and subcortical white matter. (D) A follow-up CT shows severe atrophy and encephalomalacia, especially on the left side. The ventricles are enlarged due to parenchymal volume loss.

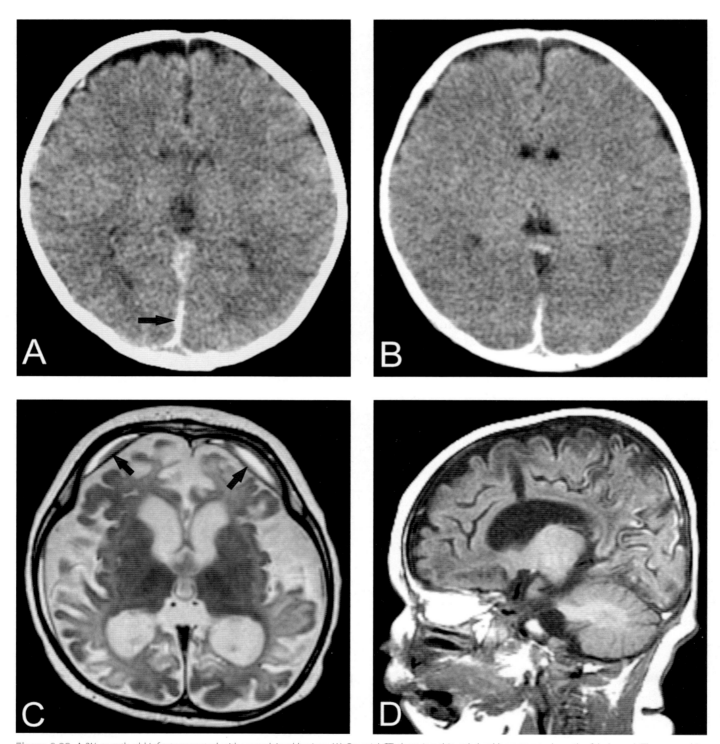

Figure 8.33 A 3½-month-old infant presented with unexplained bruises. (A) On axial CT, there is a thin subdural hematoma along the falx (arrow). The gray–white matter borders are somewhat blurred. There is also an occipital fracture present. (B) Repeat CT 16 hours later shows small ventricles, further blurring of gray–white matter borders, and lack of differentiation of basal ganglia and thalami. Subdural hematoma is now visible behind the occipital lobes. (C) On a follow-up T2-weighted MR three months after non-accidental trauma, there is diffuse severe cerebral atrophy with atrophic dilatation of the ventricles. Bilateral chronic subdural hematomas (arrows) are also present. (D) Sagittal T1-weighted MR imaging in the follow-up examination shows multiple ribbons of bright cortex especially in the parietal and occipital lobes. This is typical for cortical necrosis.

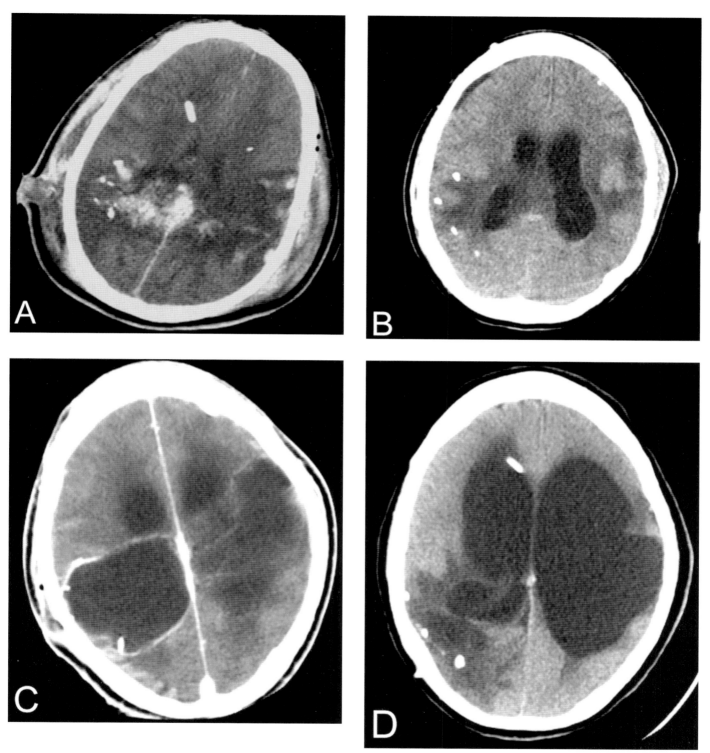

Figure 8.34 A 12-year-old boy received a 9 mm gunshot wound to the head. (A) Axial CT shows multiple bullet fragments in the right periatrial region from the entry site, hemorrhage across occipital lobe and corpus callosum, and a widening fan of edema with small hemorrhages toward the left exit site. (B) A noncontrast CT obtained three days later shows improvement in edema, but there is some increase in left-sided hemorrhages. The ventricles are enlarging from hydrocephalus related to intraventricular blood. (C) Follow-up post-contrast CT at 18 days shows worsening edema across area of primary injury and peripheral enhancement of porencephalic cysts. Infection is secondary to debris through the brain from the initial gunshot wound. (D) Follow-up CT obtained eight months after injury demonstrates severe encephalomalacia across the right posterior hemisphere, hydrocephalus and porencephaly. MRI could not be done because of bullet fragments.

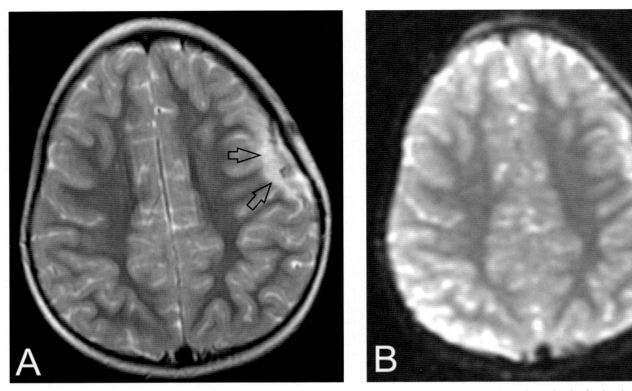

Figure 8.35 A 33-month-old girl was hit in the head with a large stick. (A) Axial T2-weighted MR examination 17 hours later, shortly after headache and lethargy began. There is a small epidural hematoma and underlying cortical edema (arrows). (B) An ADC map shows susceptibility within the hematoma, but no evidence of restricted diffusion in the cortex. The patient recovered without sequelae.

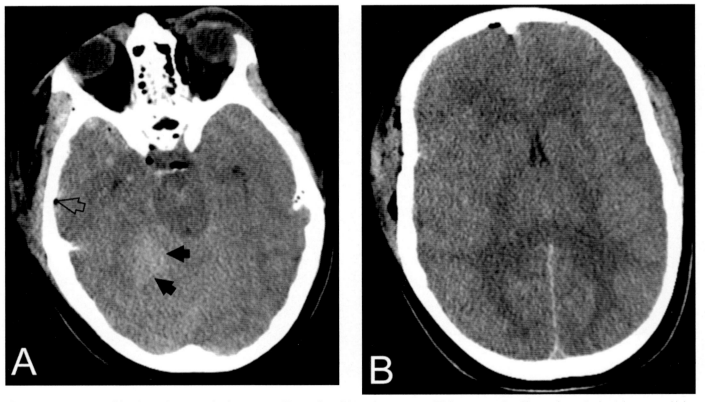

Figure 8.36 A 12-year-old with ADHD was involved in a severe ATV accident. (A) Initial noncontrast CT shows contusional hemorrhages in the right temporal lobe, punctate air (open arrow) from open fracture, and a thin layer of subdural tentorial hematoma (solid arrows). (B) Initial noncontrast CT at the ventricular level shows compression of frontal horns from edema. Gray and white matter are still well defined. Punctate air is present beneath the frontal bone from facial fractures. (C) Axial T2-weighted MRI three days following the trauma shows evidence of the temporal and frontal craniectomy. There is edema in the frontal and temporal lobes. A partial temporal lobe resection has been done. There is also edema in the left global pallidus (arrow). (D) An axial T2-weighted MR image obtained one month later shows a new large right parenchymal hemorrhage with low signal and edema surrounding the hemorrhage. There is also a large right-sided pseudomeningocele. (E) A follow-up noncontrast CT five years after injury shows ventricular dilation due to both atrophy and hydrocephalus, as well as bilateral frontal lobe low densities from atrophy and gliosis.

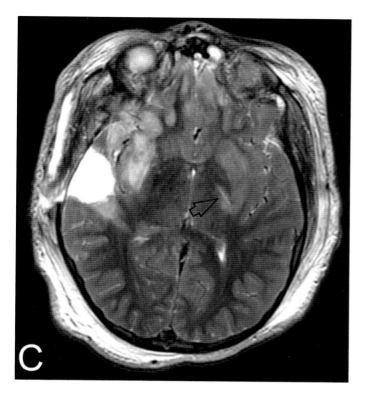

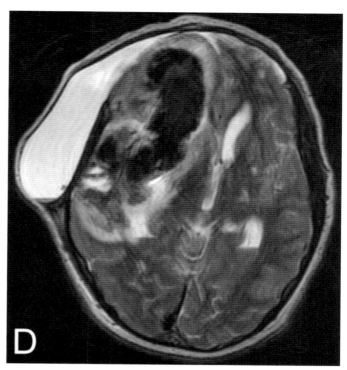

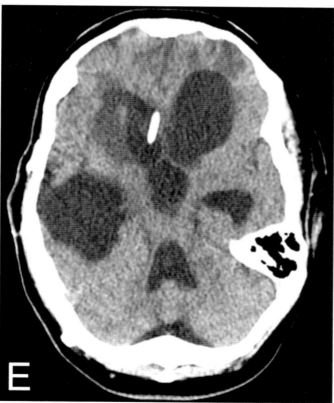

Figure 8.36 (Cont.)

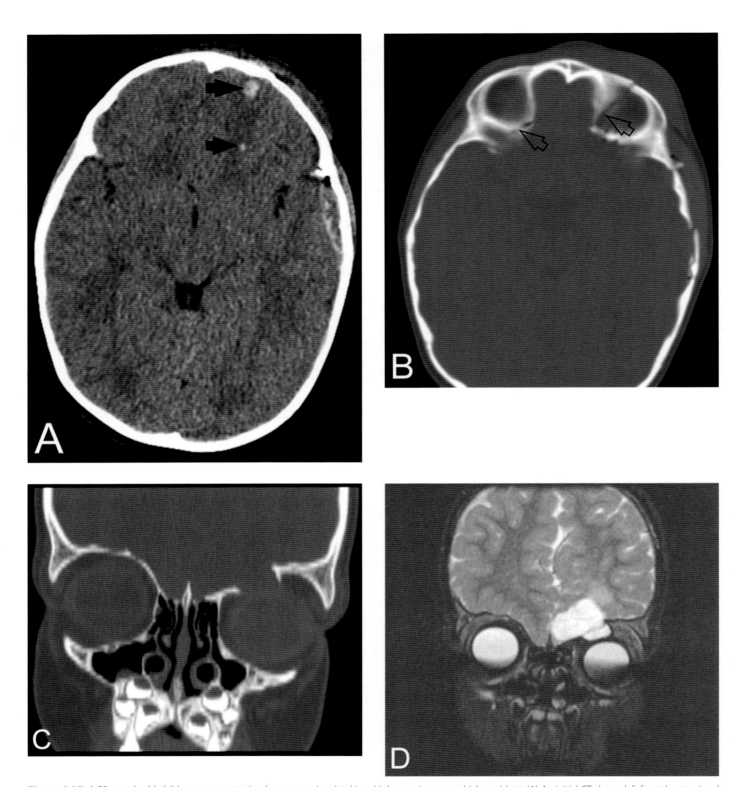

Figure 8.37 A 22-month-old child was an unrestrained passenger involved in a high-speed motor-vehicle accident. (A) An initial CT shows left frontal contusional hemorrhages (arrows), and a small left temporal region epidural hematoma. (B) Bone window of the CT shows a fracture across orbital roofs (arrows). Left temporal fractures are also present. (C) Coronal CT, 21 months after injury, was done for proptosis. A large gap in the orbital roof is visible. (D) A coronal fat-saturated T2-weighted MRI shows focal encephalomalacia with a pseudomeningocele, or leptomeningeal cyst, protruding through the growing fracture into the orbit. Note the downward displacement of the globe.

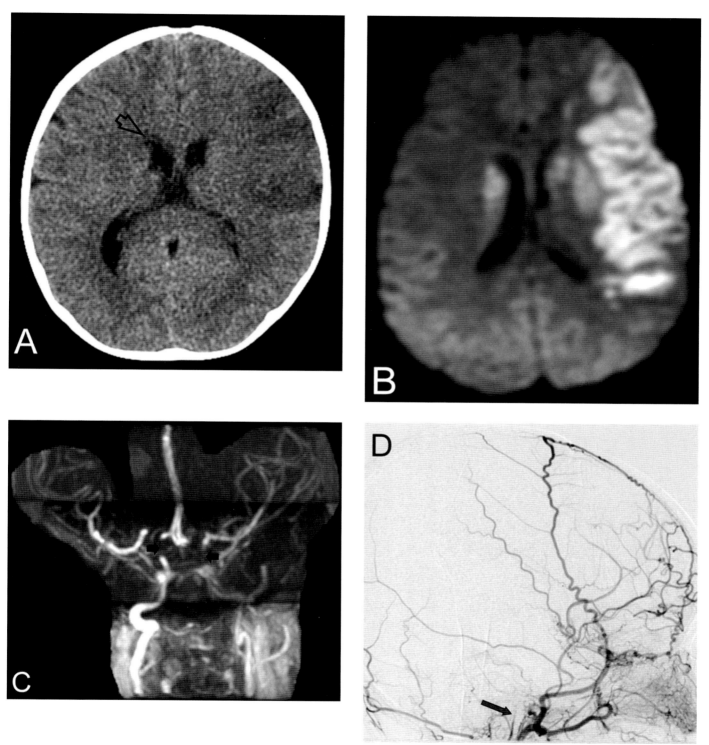

Figure 8.38 A child with both neurofibromatosis type 1 and Down syndrome presented at age 20 months with left-sided weakness. (A) Noncontrast CT shows edema in left middle cerebral artery (MCA) territory and a small hypodense lesion in the right basal ganglia (open arrow). (B) Diffusion-weighted image confirms restricted diffusion in the left MCA territory and in the basal ganglia bilaterally. (C) MRA (somewhat limited quality) shows occlusion or lack of flow in distal internal carotid arteries (horizontal arrows) characteristic of moyamoya disease, with poor flow through proximal anterior cerebral arteries. (D) Lateral projection from a digital subtraction angiography (DSA) of the right common carotid artery shows multiple collaterals from the external carotid circulation. The tiny right internal carotid artery ends blindly (arrow). (E) Lateral projection from DSA of the left internal carotid shows marked narrowing of the distal carotid artery, with a large ophthalmic artery (open arrow) providing collateral flow, and vertically oriented moyamoya collateral vessels through basal ganglia (opposing arrows). (F) Time-of-flight MRA at age three shows no flow through the left internal carotid artery, and nearly a complete occlusion of the distal right internal carotid artery (open arrow). Most of the flow is via the large external carotid branches on the periphery of the image. (G) An anterior projection from a DSA in the external carotid following bilateral synangiosis shows middle cerebral arterial filling via the superficial temporal artery, which has been surgically placed on the pia (arrow). (H) Lateral projection from a left external carotid DSA following synangiosis shows collateral flow through the surgical synangiosis (arrow), and multiple collaterals through the anterior falcine artery (open arrow) which is fed by ethmoid branches.

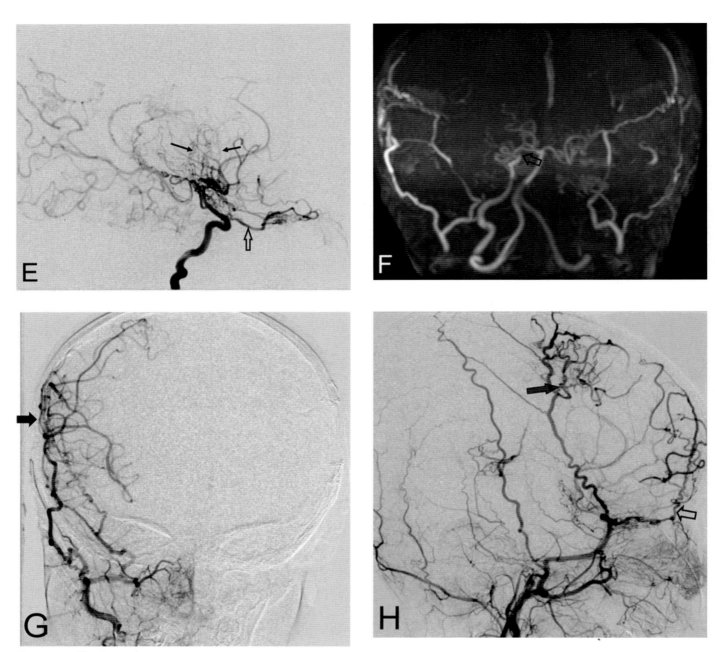

Figure 8.38 (Cont.)

middle cerebral branch on which it is placed, and grows collateral branches.

Future directions

The definitive features of ischemic injury involve impaired perfusion, decreased bioavailability of free-radical scavengers, disruption of microvascular circulation, provocation of acute inflammation, leakage across semipermeable membranes, chemotaxis of activated leukocytes and, ultimately, loss of cellular integrity. Conventional imaging demonstrates predominantly late events in this evolution, such as decreased perfusion, tissue edema, and necrosis, in a largely nonspecific manner at the level of ischemic effects on tissues.

Perfusion imaging has traditionally been accomplished with transvascular angiography, although MR and CT perfusion imaging now offer less-invasive imaging of arterial, capillary and venous blood flow with the added advantage of volumetric analysis (Figures 8.39, 8.40). There are few examples of CT perfusion in children, primarily due to the higher than normal

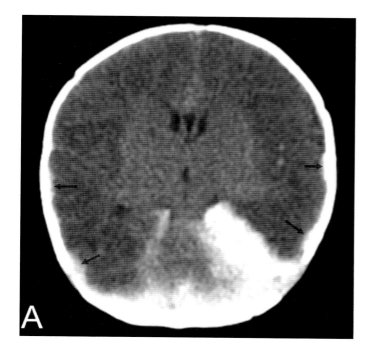

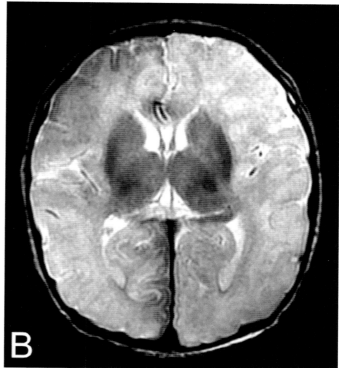

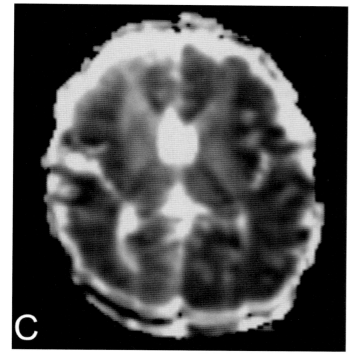

Figure 8.39 A normal term infant with normal cesarian section and good Apgar scores was noted to have a poor suck, and began seizing on day two of life. (A) At nine weeks of age, contrast-enhanced CT shows a large tentorial subdural hematoma, extending along the hemispheres (arrows), and low density throughout the peripheral gray and white matter with central sparing. (B) On axial T2-weighted MR images, there is diffuse peripheral cortical and white matter edema with relative sparing of the central structures. Note also some sparing of the medial right occipital cortex and the right frontal cortex with more normal dark signal. (C) An ADC map shows restricted diffusion in the peripheral cortex. Sparing of the medial right occipital and interior frontal areas is again visible.

radiation doses required. Work is ongoing to develop significantly lower dose algorithms that may make pediatric CT perfusion imaging reasonable in select cases.

However, there are many physiological features at an even finer level of physiological resolution that can potentially be exploited to evaluate ischemic changes. For example, chronically ischemic tissues do not respond effectively to a stressful challenge. Therefore, exposure of ischemic bowel to a caloric challenge will show hypoperfusion on MR after intravenous infusion of paramagnetic contrast material that will not be apparent on non-stress imaging. Long-term viability of ischemic tissues is an issue when under consideration for resection. Leaving nonviable tissue behind risks sepsis and death, while taking too much tissue risks critical organ failure. Both infrared imaging and contrast-enhanced (pulse-inversion) ultrasound have been proposed to differentiate viable from nonviable tissue, and both have shown promise in animal studies.

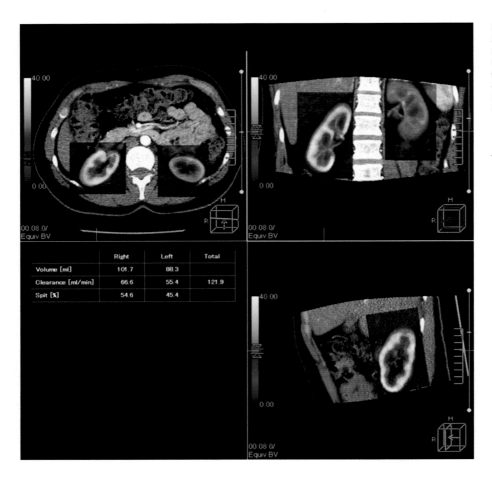

Figure 8.40 Fusion of CT-perfusion imaging on a 320-slice scanner and scintigraphic measurement of renal clearance permits visualization of differential renal function, with decreased perfusion and poor clearance of the left kidney and normal perfusion and function of the right kidney in this 50-year-old renal donor candidate. (Courtesy of Patrik Rogalla, MD, University of Toronto, Canada.)

	Right	Left	Total
Volume [ml]	101.7	88.3	
Clearance [ml/min]	66.6	55.4	121.9
Spit [%]	54.6	45.4	

Cellular processes may also be amenable to imaging. During exposure to an ischemic insult, tissue autofluorescence induced by laser light decreases. Monitoring changes in autofluorescence imaging during warm ischemia at transplantation may permit continuous evaluation of the transplant graft. Ischemic cell injury also results in abnormal ion fluxes. For example, Ca^{2+} may be a major mediator of cell death in ischemia. The ability to image unlabeled target ions, such as with time-of-flight secondary ion mass spectrometry (TOF-SIMS), may reveal very specific pathophysiological events in the progression of ischemic injury, and may potentially allow monitoring of such related therapeutic interventions as calcium chelation.

Apoptosis itself may lead to predictable changes in cytoplasmic binding sites or cell surface markers. Labeled agents that bind to these sites, such as ^{18}F-DFNSH and [124]I-annexin V, accumulate in regions of active apoptosis. In conjunction with agents such as ^{18}F-FDG, which demonstrates marrow edema, and such agents as ^{13}N-NH$_3$ (Figure 8.41) and ^{18}F-fluorine, which show blood flow, strategies can be envisioned for identifying and elucidating the specific temporal evolution of ischemic injury and prognosis for recovery, as for example would be desirable in evaluating the early changes of avascular necrosis not evident on conventional imaging. Precise treatment or excision of injured cells could be contemplated before injury propagates to involve contiguous or distant tissues, or causes irreversible injury, such as fragmentation of the femoral head.

Conclusions

Imaging features of ischemia are better understood and anticipated when the radiologist considers the underlying pathophysiology of disease and the progression from brief, reversible ischemia to ischemia with reperfusion injury or to necrosis with irreversible cell death. While ischemia ultimately affects all cells and tissues, the most profound effects involve the microvasculature. Since early or intermittent ischemia may be reversible, confirmation, recognition and communication of suspected ischemia should proceed without delay. It is certain that the fields of molecular imaging, high-field MR perfusion, diffusion and spectroscopic imaging, CT perfusion imaging, contrast and elastographic US imaging, optical imaging, etc. will in the near term significantly change our approach to imaging and intervention in ischemic disease.

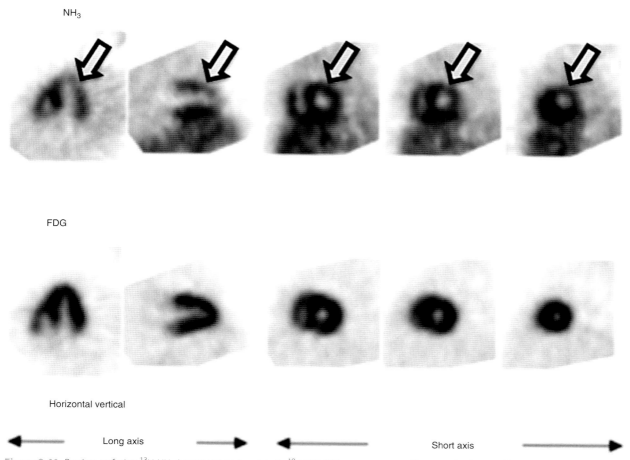

NH₃

FDG

Horizontal vertical

Long axis   Short axis

Figure 8.41 Resting perfusion ¹³N-NH₃ (ammonia) and metabolic ¹⁸F-FDG PET are reconstructed in a standard array of horizontal, vertical, long axis and short axis of the left ventricle of an infant with a history of D-TGA after an arterial switch operation, who developed sudden angina. Perfusion images on top show a reduced perfusion of the anterior and anterolateral walls (arrows). Metabolic FDG images demonstrate preserved uptake consistent with viable but jeopardized myocardium in the territory of the left anterior descending coronary artery. (Courtesy of Miguel Hernandez-Pampaloni, MD, University of California, San Francisco.)

Further reading

Adekile AD, Gupta R, Yacoub F et al. (2001) Avascular necrosis of the hip in children with sickle cell disease and high Hb F: magnetic resonance imaging findings and influence of alpha-thalassemia trait. *Acta Haematol* **105**(1), 27–31.

Aidlen J, Anupindi SA, Jaramillo D, Doody DP (2005) Malrotation with midgut volvulus: CT findings of bowel infarction. *Pediatr Radiol* **35**(5), 529–31.

Anders JF, Powell EC (2005) Urgency of evaluation and outcome of acute ovarian torsion in pediatric patients. *Arch Pediatr Adolesc Med* **159**(6), 532–5.

Armstrong-Wells J, Johnston SC, Wu YW, Sidney S, Fullerton HJ (2009) Prevalence and predictors of perinatal hemorrhagic stroke: results from the kaiser pediatric stroke study. *Pediatrics* **123**(3), 823–8.

Aziz D, Davis V, Allen L, Langer JC (2004) Ovarian torsion in children: is oophorectomy necessary? *J Pediatr Surg* **39**(5), 750–3.

Babhulkar SS, Pande K, Babhulkar S (1995) The hand-foot syndrome in sickle-cell haemoglobinopathy. *J Bone Joint Surg Br* **77**(2), 310–2.

Back SA, Luo NL, Borenstein NS et al. (2001) Late oligodendrocyte progenitors coincide with the developmental window of vulnerability for human perinatal white matter injury. *J Neurosci* **21** (4), 1302–12.

Barkovich AJ, Miller SP, Bartha A et al. (2006) MR imaging, MR spectroscopy, and diffusion tensor imaging of sequential studies in neonates with encephalopathy. *AJNR Am J Neuroradiol* **27**(3), 533–47.

Bartnicke BJ, Balfe DM (1994) CT appearance of intestinal ischemia and intramural hemorrhage. *Radiol Clin North Am* **32**(5), 845–60.

Beltran J, Knight CT, Zuelzer WA et al. (1990) Core decompression for avascular necrosis of the femoral head: correlation between long-term results and preoperative MR staging. *Radiology* **175**(2), 533–6.

Breuer C, Janssen G, Laws HJ et al. (2008) Splenic infarction in a patient hereditary spherocytosis, protein C deficiency and acute infectious mononucleosis. *Eur J Pediatr* **167**(12), 1449–52.

Carden DL, Granger DN (2000) Pathophysiology of ischaemia-reperfusion injury. *J Pathol* **190**(3), 255–66.

Chang HC, Bhatt S, Dogra VS (2008) Pearls and pitfalls in diagnosis of ovarian torsion. *Radiographics* **28**(5), 1355–68.

Chawla S, Boal DK, Dillon PW, Grenko RT (2003) Splenic torsion. *Radiographics* 23(2), 305–8.

Chen Y, Zhang J, Dai J et al. (2009) Angiogenesis of renal cell carcinoma: perfusion CT findings. *Abdom Imaging*, in press. DOI: 10.1007/s00261-009-9565-0.

Chiou SY, Lev-Toaff AS, Masuda E, Feld RI, Bergin D (2007) Adnexal torsion: new clinical and imaging observations by sonography, computed tomography, and magnetic resonance imaging. *J Ultrasound Med* 26(10), 1289–301.

Dalen JE, Haffajee CI, Alpert JS 3rd et al. (1977) Pulmonary embolism, pulmonary hemorrhage and pulmonary infarction. *N Engl J Med* 296(25), 1431–5.

Dokmeci D (2006) Testicular torsion, oxidative stress and the role of antioxidant therapy. *Folia Med (Plovdiv)* 48(3–4), 16–21.

Ejindu VC, Hine AL, Mashayekhi M, Shorvon PJ, Misra RR (2007) Musculoskeletal manifestations of sickle cell disease. *Radiographics* 27(4), 1005–21.

Gorg C (2007) The forgotten organ: contrast enhanced sonography of the spleen. *Eur J Radiol* 64(2), 189–201.

Gross M, Blumstein SL, Chow LC (2005) Isolated fallopian tube torsion: a rare twist on a common theme. *Am J Roentgenol* 185(6), 1590–2.

Han BK, Towbin RB, De Courten-Myers G, McLaurin RL, Ball WS Jr (1989) Reversal sign on CT: effect of anoxic/ischemic cerebral injury in children. *AJNR Am J Neuroradiol* 10(6), 1191–8.

Horton KM, Fishman EK (2001) Multidetector row CT of mesenteric ischemia: can it be done? *Radiographics* 21(6), 1463–73.

Huang BY, Castillo M (2008) Hypoxic-ischemic brain injury: imaging findings from birth to adulthood. *Radiographics* 28(2), 417–39; quiz 617.

Hunter JV (2002) Magnetic resonance imaging in pediatric stroke. *Topics Magn Res Im* 13, 23–38.

Jain R, Sawhney S, Rizvi SG (2008) Acute bone crises in sickle cell disease: the T1 fat-saturated sequence in differentiation of acute bone infarcts from acute osteomyelitis. *Clin Radiol* 63(1), 59–70.

Kaul DK, Hebbel RP (2000) Hypoxia/reoxygenation causes inflammatory response in transgenic sickle mice but not in normal mice. *J Clin Invest* 106(3), 411–20.

KeenHG, Dekker BA, Disley L et al. (2005) Imaging apoptosis in vivo using 124I-annexin V and PET. *Nucl Med Biol* 32(4), 395–402.

Killeen KL, Shanmuganathan K, Boyd-Kranis R, Scalea TM, Mirvis SE (2001) CT findings after embolization for blunt splenic trauma. *J Vasc Interv Radiol* 12(2), 209–14.

Kim JH, Kim JH, Ahn BJ et al. (2008) Label-free calcium imaging in ischemic retinal tissue by TOF-SIMS. *Biophys J* 94(10), 4095–102.

Kimura T, Yonekura T, Yamauchi K et al. (2008) Laparoscopic treatment of gallbladder volvulus: a pediatric case report and literature review. *J Laparoendosc Adv Surg Tech A* 18(2), 330–4.

Lanthier S, Carmant L, David M et al. (2000) Stroke in children: the coexistence of multiple risk factors predicts poor outcome. *Neurology* 54, 371–8.

Lauenstein TC, Ajaj W, Narin B et al. (2005) MR imaging of apparent small-bowel perfusion for diagnosing mesenteric ischemia: feasibility study. *Radiology* 234(2), 569–75.

Lee EJ, Kwon HC, Joo HJ, Suh JH, Fleischer AC (1998) Diagnosis of ovarian torsion with color Doppler sonography: depiction of twisted vascular pedicle. *J Ultrasound Med* 17(2), 83–9.

Lund EC, Han SY, Holley HC, Berland LL (1988) Intestinal ischemia: comparison of plain radiographic and computed tomographic findings. *Radiographics* 8(6), 1083–108.

Malafaia O, Brioschi ML, Aoki SM et al. (2008) Infrared imaging contribution for intestinal ischemia detection in wound healing. *Acta Cir Bras* 23(6), 511–9.

Marumo G, Kozuma S, Ohyu J et al. (2001) Generation of periventricular leukomalacia by repeated umbilical cord occlusion in near-term fetal sheep and its possible pathogenetical mechanisms. *Biol Neonate* 79(1), 39–45.

Mattano LA Jr, Sather HN, Trigg ME, Nachman JB (2000) Osteonecrosis as a complication of treating acute lymphoblastic leukemia in children: a report from the Children's Cancer Group. *J Clin Oncol* 18(18), 3262–72.

McKinsey JF, Gewertz BL (1997) Acute mesenteric ischemia. *Surg Clin North Am* 77(2), 307–18.

Meza MP, Amundson GM, Aquilina JW, Reitelman C (1992) Color flow imaging in children with clinically suspected testicular torsion. *Pediatr Radiol* 22(5), 370–3.

Miller LA, Mirvis SE, Shanmuganathan K, Ohson AS(2004) CT diagnosis of splenic infarction in blunt trauma: imaging features, clinical significance and complications. *Clin Radiol* 59(4), 342–8.

Neary P, Redmond HP Ischaemia-reperfusion injury and the systemic inflammatory response syndrome. In *Ischaemia-Reperfusion Injury*, ed. PA Grace, RT Mathie (London:Blackwell Science,1999) pp. 123–36.

Neufeld MD, Frigon C, Graham AS, Mueller BA (2005) Maternal infection and risk of cerebral palsy in term and preterm infants. *J Perinatol* 25(2), 108–13.

Nores M, Phillips EH, Morgenstern L, Hiatt JR (1998) The clinical spectrum of splenic infarction. *Am Surg* 64(2), 182–8.

Nowak-Göttl U, Sträeter R, Sébire G, Kirkham F (2003) Antithrombotic drug treatment of pediatric patients with ischemic stroke. *Paediatr Drugs* 5(3), 167–75.

Paltiel HJ, Kalish LA, Susaeta RA et al. (2006) Pulse-inversion US imaging of testicular ischemia: quantitative and qualitative analyses in a rabbit model. *Radiology* 239(3), 718–29.

Panigrahy A, Bluml S (2007) Advances in magnetic resonance neuroimaging techniques in the evaluation of neonatal encephalopathy. *Top Magn Reson Imaging* 18(1), 3–29.

Park JH, Sung YK, Bae SC et al. (2009) Ulnar artery vasculopathy in systemic sclerosis. *Rheumatol Int* 29(9), 1081–6.

Patsalides AD, Wood LV, Atac GK et al. (2002) Cerebrovascular disease in HIV-infected pediatric patients: neuroimaging findings. *Am J Roentgenol* 179(4), 999–1003.

Platt OS (2000) Sickle cell anemia as an inflammatory disease. *J Clin Invest* 106(3), 337–8.

Pratl B, Benesch M, Lackner H et al. (2008) Partial splenic embolization in children with hereditary spherocytosis. *Eur J Haematol* 80(1), 76–80.

Ramos C, Whyte CM, Harris BH (2006) Nontraumatic compartment syndrome of the extremities in children. *J Pediatr Surg* 41(12), e5–7.

Resnick D Hemoglobinopathies and other anemias. In *Diagnosis of Bone and Joint*

Disorders, ed. D Resnick (Philadelphia: Saunders, 2002) pp. 2146–87.

Rha SE, Ha HK, Lee SH *et al.* (2000) CT and MR imaging findings of bowel ischemia from various primary causes. *Radiographics* **20**(1), 29–42.

Robertson RL, Ben-Sira L, Barnes PD *et al.* (1999) MR line-scan diffusion-weighted imaging of term neonates with perinatal brain ischemia. *AJNR Am J Neuroradiol* **20**(9), 1658–70.

Rovira A, Alonso J, Cordoba J(2008) MR imaging findings in hepatic encephalopathy. *AJNR Am J Neuroradiol* **29**(9), 1612–21.

Roza AM, Johnson CP, Adams M (1999) Acute torsion of the renal transplant after combined kidney-pancreas transplant. *Transplantation* **67**(3), 486–8.

Saemi AM, Johnson JM, Morris CS (2009) Treatment of bilateral hand frostbite using transcatheter arterial thrombolysis after papaverine infusion. *Cardiovasc Intervent Radiol* **32**(6), 1280–3.

Schoenberg BS, Mellinger JF, Schoenberg DG (1978) Cerebrovascular disease in infants and children: a study of incidence, clinical features, and survival. *Neurology* **28**(8), 763–8.

Scott RM, Smith ER (2009) Moyamoya disease and moyamoya syndrome. *N Engl J Med* **360**(12), 1226–37.

Sharma J, Karthik S, Rao S *et al.* (2005) Catastrophic antiphospholipid antibody syndrome. *Pediatr Nephrol* **20**(7), 998–9.

Smith JL (2009) Understanding and treating moyamoya disease in children. *Neurosurg Focus* **26**(4), E4.

Steinauer-Gebauer AM, Yee J, Lutolf ME (2001) Torsion of the greater omentum with infarction: the vascular pedicle sign. *Clin Radiol* **56**(12), 999–1002.

Stevens MC, Padwick M, Serjeant GR(1981) Observations on the natural history of dactylitis in homozygous sickle cell disease. *Clin Pediatr (Phila)* **20**(5), 311–7.

Takahashi M, Murakami Y, Nitta N *et al.* (2008) Pulmonary infarction associated with bronchogenic carcinoma. *Radiat Med* **26**(2), 76–80.

Taourel PG, Deneuville M, Pradel JA, Régent D, Bruel JM (1996) Acute mesenteric ischemia: diagnosis with contrast-enhanced CT. *Radiology* **199**(3), 632–6.

Telen MJ (2007) Role of adhesion molecules and vascular endothelium in the pathogenesis of sickle cell disease. *Hematology Am Soc Hematol Educ Program* **2007**, 84–90.

Tirapelli LF, Bagnato VS, Tirapelli DP *et al.* (2008) Renal ischemia in rats: mitochondria function and laser autofluorescence. *Transplant Proc* **40**(5), 1679–84.

Traubici J, Daneman A, Navarro O, Mohanta A, Garcia C (2003) Original report. Testicular torsion in neonates and infants: sonographic features in 30 patients. *Am J Roentgenol* **180**(4), 1143–5.

Tsao MS, Schraufnagel D, Wang NS (1982) Pathogenesis of pulmonary infarction. *Am J Med* **72**(4), 599–606.

Volpe JJ *Neurology of the Newborn*, 5th edn. (Philadelphia: Saunders, 2008).

Ware HE, Brooks AP, Toye R, Berney SI (1991) Sickle cell disease and silent avascular necrosis of the hip. *J Bone Joint Surg Br* **73**(6), 947–9.

Wintermark M, Cotting J, Roulet E *et al.* (2005) Acute brain perfusion disorders in children assessed by quantitative perfusion computed tomography in the emergency setting. *Pediatr Emerg Care* **21**(3), 149–60.

Zahuranec DB, Brown DL, Lisabeth LD, Morgenstern LB (2005) Is it time for a large, collaborative study of pediatric stroke? *Stroke* **36**(9), 1825–9.

Zeng W, Yao ML, Townsend D *et al.* (2008) Synthesis, biological evaluation and radiochemical labeling of a dansylhydrazone derivative as a potential imaging agent for apoptosis. *Bioorg Med Chem Lett* **18**(12), 3573–7.

Chapter 9

Metabolic bone disorders

Paul Babyn

Rickets

Rickets is a clinical syndrome that represents a spectrum of metabolic disorders with similar radiological and histopathological abnormalities resulting from inadequate or delayed mineralization of newly synthesized organic matrix (osteoid) in the immature skeleton before physeal fusion. When seen in adults, the same radiological, biochemical and clinical changes are termed as "osteomalacia" as these refer to the mature skeleton. By definition, rickets is found only in children prior to the closure of the growth plates, while osteomalacia occurs in adults.

Pathophysiology

Vitamin D is a steroid hormone that plays a major role in calcium and phosphorus homeostasis and hence bone mineralization. Vitamin D prohormone undergoes two sequential hydroxylations in the body to become biologically active, the first one being in the liver and then the kidney. Vitamin D in its active form is biochemically 1,25-dihydroxyvitamin D, $1,25(OH_2)$ D. The second hydroxylation is closely regulated by parathyroid hormone (PTH), calcium, phosphorus and vitamin D. The main targets of vitamin D action at the organ level are the intestine and bone. Vitamin D has two actions that have diametrically opposite outcomes. In conjunction with PTH, it acts on bone, to promote osteolysis by osteoclasts, which results in release and mobilization of calcium from bone to blood. It also mediates the mineralization of organic matrix by calcium and phosphorus deposition. Understanding this basic mechanism is integral in approaching metabolic bone diseases involving abnormalities of vitamin D or PTH.

The etiological factors for rickets may be congenital or acquired. Any factor that interferes with vitamin D metabolism involving intake, its hydroxylation in the liver or kidney, or end-organ resistance to the action of the hormone can lead to rickets. Malnutrition, decreased sun exposure, malabsorption states involving the pancreas, small intestine and liver, and abnormal hydroxylation states are the usual suspects.

As rickets results from a disturbance in metabolism, the underlying disease should be diagnosed. The causes of rickets can be classified into 11 main categories, as shown in Table 9.1.

Imaging findings

The clinical and radiographic features of rickets depend on the age of the patient at which it occurs, the relative maturation of the affected bones and the severity of vitamin D deficiency. There is delayed or abnormal ossification of bone leading to skeletal retardation and osteopenia. The earliest radiographic finding of rickets consists of widening at the growth plate along the longitudinal axis of the bone followed by a decrease in the density of the bone along the metaphyseal side of the growth plate (Figure 9.1). With progressive disease, the widening of the growth plate increases and the zone of provisional calcification becomes irregular. Fraying and disorganization of spongy bone in the metaphyses follows (Figures 9.2, 9.3).

The radiographic changes are maximally seen in zones of active and rapid growth, including the costochondral junctions of the middle ribs, distal femur, proximal humerus, both ends of the tibia and distal ends of the radius and ulna.

In the skull, incessant accumulation of unossified osteoid in the frontal and parietal regions results in the prominence of the frontal bones, called frontal bossing. Other manifestations include Wormian bones, flattening of the posterior skull, basilar invagination and squaring of the skull (craniotabes).

Other key findings including sequelae of bone weakening include deformities of the long bones, both of the shaft and its junction with the cartilage. Genu varum (bow legs) or genu valgum (knock knees) can be seen in toddlers. Anterior bowing of the tibia (saber shin) is also seen. In the pelvis and hips, one may see a triradiate pelvis due to intrusion of the spine into the soft pelvis, appearing as a triflanged-shaped pelvis, and slipped capital femoral epiphysis may be seen. With increasing age, other deformities like scoliosis and bending of long bones may lead to reduced height. Greenstick fractures in the weakened long bones, delayed eruption of teeth, hypoplasia

Essentials of Pediatric Radiology, ed. Heike E. Daldrup-Link and Charles A. Gooding. Published by Cambridge University Press.
© Cambridge University Press 2010.

Table 9.1 Etiological causes of rickets

- Vitamin D deficiency
  - Dietary deficiency
  - Deficient endogenous synthesis

- Gastrointestinal tract disorders
  - Small intestine diseases with malabsorption
  - Partial or total gastrectomy
  - Hepatobiliary disease
  - Chronic pancreatic insufficiency

- Disorders of vitamin D metabolism
  - Hereditary – pseudovitamin D deficiency or vitamin D dependency (types I and II)
  - Acquired
    - Use of anticonvulsants
    - Chronic renal failure

- Acidosis
  - Distal renal tubular acidosis (classic or type I)
  - Secondary forms of renal acidosis
  - Ureterosigmoidostomy
  - Drug-induced disease
    - Chronic acetazolamide ingestion
    - Chronic ammonium chloride ingestion

- Chronic renal failure

- Phosphate depletion
  - Dietary – low phosphate intake plus ingestion of non-absorbable antacids
    - Hereditary – X-linked hypophosphatemic rickets or adult-onset vitamin D-resistant hypophosphatemic osteomalacia
    - Acquired – sporadic hypophosphatemic osteomalacia (phosphate diabetes), tumor-associated (oncogenous) rickets, osteomalacia, neurofibromatosis and fibrous dysplasia

- Generalized renal tube disorders
  - Primary renal tube disorders
  - Renal tube disorders associated with systemic metabolic abnormality
    - Cystinosis
    - Glycogenosis
    - Lowe syndrome
  - Systemic disorder with associated renal disease
    - Hereditary – inborn errors (Wilson's disease, tyrosinemia) and neurofibromatosis
    - Acquired – multiple myeloma, nephrotic syndrome and kidney transplantation
    - Intoxication-related – cadmium, lead, outdated tetracycline

- Primary mineralization defects
  - Hereditary
  - Acquired
    - Diphosphonate treatment
    - Fluoride treatment

- States of rapid bone formation with or without a relative defect in bone resorption
  - Postoperative hyperparathyroidism with osteitis fibrosa cystica
  - Osteopetrosis

- Defective matrix synthesis – fibrogenesis imperfecta ossium

- Miscellaneous
  - Magnesium-dependent conditions
  - Axial osteomalacia
  - Parenteral alimentation
  - Aluminum intoxication
  - Ifosfamide treatment

of enamel with dental caries, beading of costochondral junctions of ribs due to accumulation of unossified osteoid in the ribs, also called the rachitic rosary, and pectus carinatum of the sternum are other important findings to look for (Table 9.2).

Most of the clinical manifestations become obvious after the first six months of life.

Other imaging modalities may assist in evaluation, diagnosis and follow-up of rickets. Computed tomography (CT) can help in evaluation of fractures and bone density, while magnetic resonance imaging is optimum for detection of Looser's zones and widened physes. Scintigraphy may reveal cortical infractions that later develop into Looser's zones. Bone scans using technetium 99m methylene diphosphonate (MDP) may show areas of bilateral and symmetric increased uptake, which may show an initial flare up after initiating therapy. Sonography helps in evaluating slipped capital femoral epiphysis of femur.

With healing, there is reappearance of the zone of provisional calcification. This recalcified zone casts a transverse linear shadow of increased density in the rachitic metaphyses beyond the visible ends of the shaft. The radiolucent rachitic metaphyses are interposed between the newly calcified zone of calcification and the visible ossified end of the shaft. As the rachitic metaphyses are not mineralized they are of soft tissue density.

As healing continues, the new zone of provisional calcification thickens into a transverse band; at the same time, the metaphyseal spongiosa is gradually recalcified and fills the previously radiolucent intermediate rachitic zone, fusing with that of the zone of provisional calcification. This may produce a false appearance of rapid increase in the length of the shaft. In due course of time, with re-strengthening of the bony osteoid, there is reduction in the cupping, fraying, splaying and deformity of the metaphysis. However, healing of cortical bone is usually slower and less conspicuous radiographically, although periosteal reaction may be noted.

Drug-induced rickets

This is known to be seen in long-term therapy with anticonvulsants, disphosphonates, deferoxamine, anticancer agents like

(A)

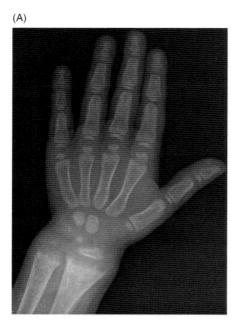

(B)

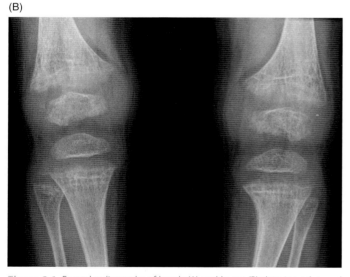

Figure 9.1 Frontal radiographs of hands (A) and knees (B) showing advanced changes of rickets including cupping, fraying and splaying of metaphyses, widening of the provisional zone of calcification and generalized reduction in bone mineral density.

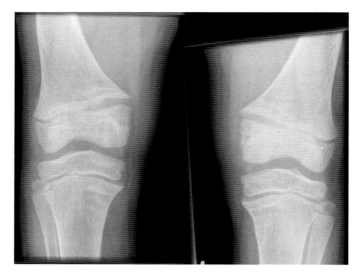

Figure 9.2 Frontal view of knees reveals metaphyseal growth recovery lines and other changes after initiation of therapy.

Table 9.2 Radiographic findings of rickets

Widening of growth plates

Irregularity or loss of sclerotic zone of provisional calcification

Widening or cupping of metaphyses

Skull deformities including frontal bossing, craniotabes

Bowing deformities

Greenstick fractures

Rachitic rosary

Pectus carinatum

Scoliosis

Triradiate pelvis

Slipped capital femoral epiphysis

(A)

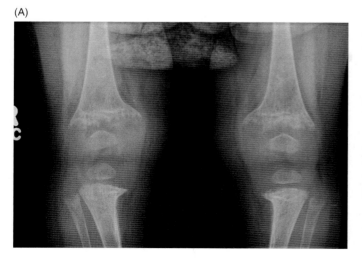

(B)

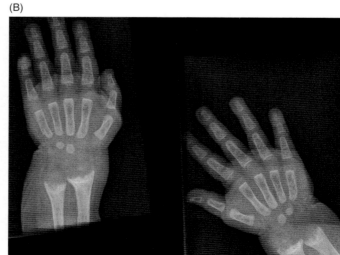

Figure 9.3 Frontal radiographs of knees and wrists reveal advanced changes of rickets.

(A)

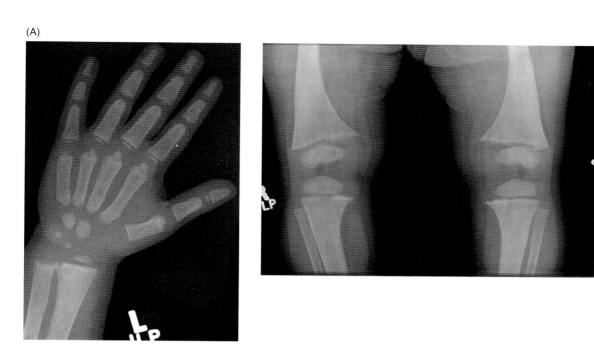

(B)

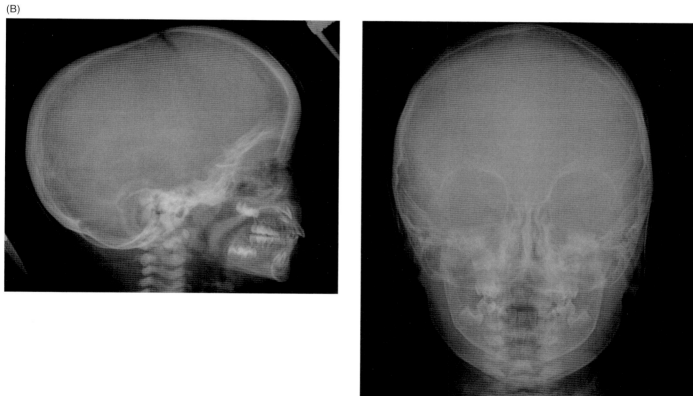

Figure 9.4 Hypophosphatemic rickets. (A) Frontal views of hands and knees reveal trabecular coarsening with cupping and fraying of radial and ulnar metaphyses. (B) Frontal and lateral views of skull show frontal bossing and dolichocephaly.

Table 9.3 Radiographic appearances of X-linked hypophosphatemic rickets

Appears at 12–18 months of age

Clinical and radiographic manifestations are worse at the knees than the wrists

Premature fusion of cranial sutures

Bowing of long bones

Thick cortices with increased bone density

Looser's zones

Enthesopathy with calcified annulus fibrosus, paraspinal ligaments

ifosfamide, aluminum in patients with chronic renal failure, and rifampicin – a first line antitubercular drug.

Hereditary vitamin D-dependent rickets

This is an autosomal recessive disorder and has two types: type I, i.e. pseudovitamin D-dependent rickets, and type II or the hereditary hypocalcemic vitamin D-resistant rickets. Type I is due to a defective renal hydroxylation mechanism. Although radiographic and biochemical changes (low calcium, phosphorus and vitamin D with increased PTH) remain the same, it typically manifests within the first three months of life, becoming florid by one year of age.

Type II disease results from receptor insensitivity to the action of vitamin D and, in contrast to other forms, the amounts of vitamin D are high.

Hypophosphatemic rickets

This form of rickets is caused by an X-linked hypophosphatemic state due to defective phosphorus reabsorption at the level of the renal tubule. Hypophosphatemic rickets is transmitted by an autosomal dominant trait that typically presents between 12 to 18 months of age.

Patients are stocky and short with bowed legs and may develop spontaneous dental abscesses. Skull deformities may occur due to premature fusion of cranial sutures and can lead to increased intracranial pressure.

Bowing of the legs is common in the lower limbs, and radiographs reveal thick cortices and coarse trabeculae. By adulthood, generalized increase in bone density, particularly in the axial skeleton is seen (Figure 9.4). Enthesopathic changes (inflammation at and around attachment sites of ligaments, tendons and joint capsules to bone, with subsequent calcification and ossification) are unique in this form of rickets and occur in the annulus fibrosus, paravertebral ligaments, and capsules of appendicular and apophyseal joints, and may mimic ankylosing spondylitis (Table 9.3).

Mucopolysaccharidosis
Background

One of the lysosomal storage disorders (LSDs), mucopolysaccharidosis encompasses a heterogeneous group of inherited metabolic disorders resulting from defects in the degradation or transport of several distinct by-products of cellular turnover. The resultant clinical problems reflect the pattern of involved cell. There is similarity between the several clinical subtypes, which partly explains the overlap in clinical manifestations seen in this group of diseases. Diagnostic confirmation is established only when an assay is performed to measure the activity of a specific enzyme.

LSDs are divided in two subgroups: sphingolipidoses and mucopolysaccharidoses (MPSs). The commonly encountered sphingolipidoses encompass Gaucher disease (GD, caused by deficiency of acid β-glucosidase) and Niemann-Pick disease (NPD, caused by deficiency of acid sphingomyelinase) types A and B.

On the other hand, the MPSs comprise a group of seven metabolic disorders, known as mucopolysaccharidosis types I–VII: (I) Hurler, Hurler-Scheie, and Scheie syndrome; (II) Hunter syndrome; (III) Sanfilippo syndrome; (IV) Morquio syndrome; (VI) Maroteaux-Lamy syndrome; and (VII) Sly syndrome (mucopolysaccharidosis V is now considered a form of type I and is known as mucopolysaccharidosis IS).

Of the MPSs, mucopolysaccharidosis type I (MPS I) is by far the most common type. MPS I is heterogeneous, and the severity of symptoms widely varies. Generally, the range of most-to-least severe forms is as follows: Hurler syndrome, Hurler-Scheie syndrome, and Scheie syndrome.

Pathophysiology

The MPSs are caused by a deficiency of lysosomal enzymes required for the degradation of mucopolysaccharides or glycosaminoglycans (GAGs). GAGs are oligosaccharide components of proteoglycans (macromolecules that provide structural integrity and function to connective tissues). The chronic progressive course is caused by the accumulation of partially degraded GAGs, with resulting thickening of tissue and compromising of cell and organ function over time. Eleven distinct single lysosomal enzyme deficiencies are known to cause the recognized phenotypes of MPS. All of the MPSs are inherited in an autosomal recessive fashion, except for Hunter syndrome, which is X-linked.

Mucopolysaccharidosis type I (MPS I) is a rare, inherited lysosomal storage disorder caused by a deficiency of the lysosomal enzyme alpha-L-iduronidase. This deficiency leads to accumulation of undegraded mucopolysaccharides, especially dermatan sulfate (DS), in tissues and organs. The buildup of excess dermatan sulfate leads to the gradual development of numerous morphological abnormalities in tissues and organs. The α-L-iduronidase gene has been mapped to chromosome band 4p16.3.

MPS type II (Hunter disease) is an X-linked disorder that results from the deficiency of iduronate sulfatase and subsequent accumulation of heparan and dermatan sulfate.

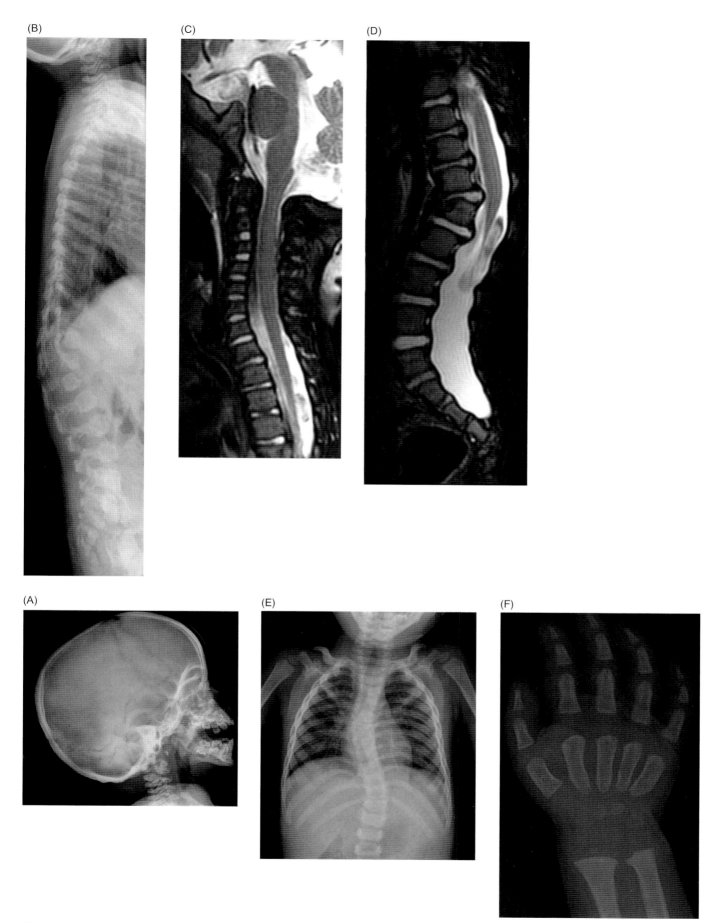

Figure 9.5 A 19-month-old male newly diagnosed with MPS type I (Hurler disease). (A) Skull radiograph showing scaphocephaly. There is abnormal excavated J-shaped sella turcica. (B, C, D) Spine X-ray and MRI demonstrating reversal of the physiological cervical lordosis, kyphosis centered at L2–L3 level and inferior beaking of L2 vertebral body. (E) Anteroposterior chest view showing "oar-shaped" ribs, which are thin anteriorly and wide posteriorly. (F) Proximal metacarpal pointing is seen on hand X-ray, a typical finding in MPS.

(A)

(B)

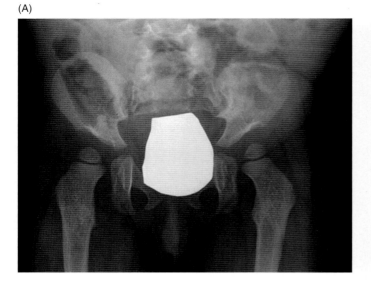
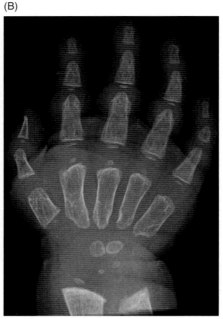

Figure 9.6 (A) Pelvis in a two-year-old female with Hurler disease. There are small iliac wings with inferior tapering and slanted, irregular acetabular roofs. (B) Metacarpal proximal pointing is again noted.

MPS type III or Sanfilippo syndrome results from the deficiency or absence of four different enzymes that are necessary to degrade the GAG heparan sulfate. Each enzyme deficiency defines a different form of Sanfilippo syndrome, as follows: type IIIA (Sanfilippo A), type IIIB (Sanfilippo B), type IIIC (Sanfilippo C), and type IIID (Sanfilippo D).

In MPS type IV or Morquio syndrome, the degradation of the GAG keratan sulfate is defective because of deficiency of either *N*-acetyl-galactosamine-6-sulfate sulfatase (*GALNS* gene) in Morquio syndrome type IVA, or β-galactosidase (*GLB1* gene) in Morquio syndrome type IVB. Defective *GALNS* also affects the catabolism of chondroitin 6-sulfate.

MPS type VI results from the deficiency of *N*-acetylgalactosamine 4-sulfatase (arylsulfatase B) activity and the lysosomal accumulation of dermatan sulfate.

Finally, in MPS type VII the molecular defect on the gene that encodes β-glucuronidase protein (*GUSB*) leads to deficiency of the enzyme β-glucuronidase. This enzyme is required for the breakdown of several GAGs, including dermatan sulfate (DS), heparan sulfate (HS) and chondroitin sulfate (CS). The *GUSB* is located on chromosome 7q11.21–7q11.22, is 21 kb long and contains 12 exons. The defect in *GUSB* is responsible for Sly syndrome.

Imaging findings

The classic and typical common features in mucopolysaccharidoses include short stature, flattened vertebra with anterior beaking (due to anterior hypoplasia of the thoracic and lumbar vertebral bodies), "bullet-shaped" phalanges (tapering of the proximal phalanges), kyphoscoliosis and genu valgum. Large skull with a J-shaped sella, hypoplasia of the pelvis with small

femoral heads and coxa valga, oar-shaped ribs (narrow at the vertebrae and widening anteriorly), diaphyseal and metaphyseal expansion of long bones with cortical thinning are also well known features. All these findings are evident on X-rays and are referred to as dysostosis multiplex. Patients can develop "claw hand," carpal tunnel syndrome and atlantoaxial subluxation due to undevelopment of the odontoid process (Figure 9.5).

MPS type I

The first abnormality detected in these patients is coarsening of the facial features, which often becomes apparent by three to six months of age. The head is large with bulging frontal bones. The skull is often scaphocephalic, secondary to premature closure of the metopic and sagittal sutures. The nasal bridge is depressed with broad nasal tip and anteverted nostrils, and the eyes may be widely spaced. Musculoskeletal findings comprise progressive flattening and beaking of the vertebrae, often leading to spinal deformity. Typically, the pelvis is abnormal, with small femoral heads and coxa valga. Clavicles may be short, thickened, and irregular ("oar shaped") (Figures 9.6, 9.7). Visceral involvement may be present and include corneal clouding, progressive hepatosplenomegaly and valvular disease, specifically aortic valve disease.

MPS type II

This entity has two subtypes: type A disease (severe form) and type B (milder form). Type A usually presents by two to four years of age and is characterized by progressive involvement of the nervous system and somatic effects. Initial suggestive features may include coarse facies, short stature, skeletal deformities, joint stiffness and mental retardation (Figure 9.8).

(A)

(B)

(C)

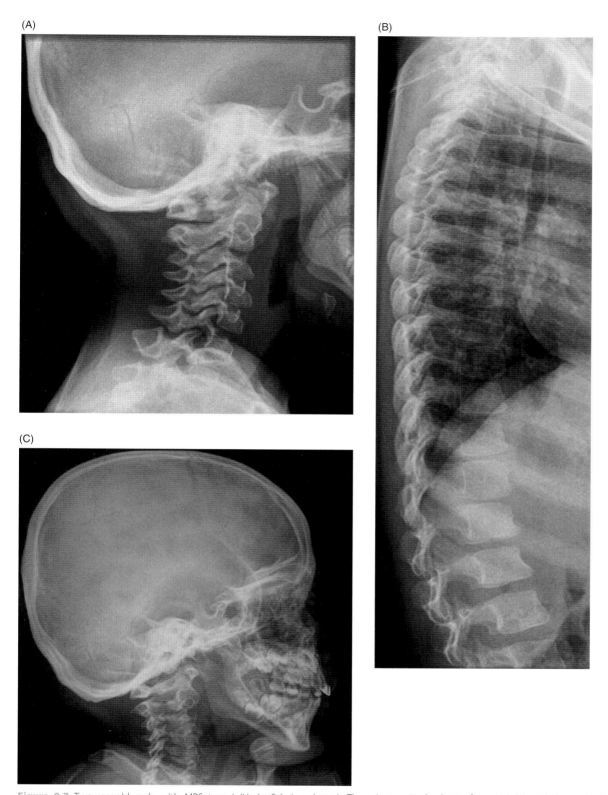

Figure 9.7 Two-year-old male with MPS type I (Hurler-Scheie subtype). There is anterior beaking of cervical (A) and thoracolumbar (B) vertebral bodies. (C) Skull radiograph showing marked excavated sella turcica.

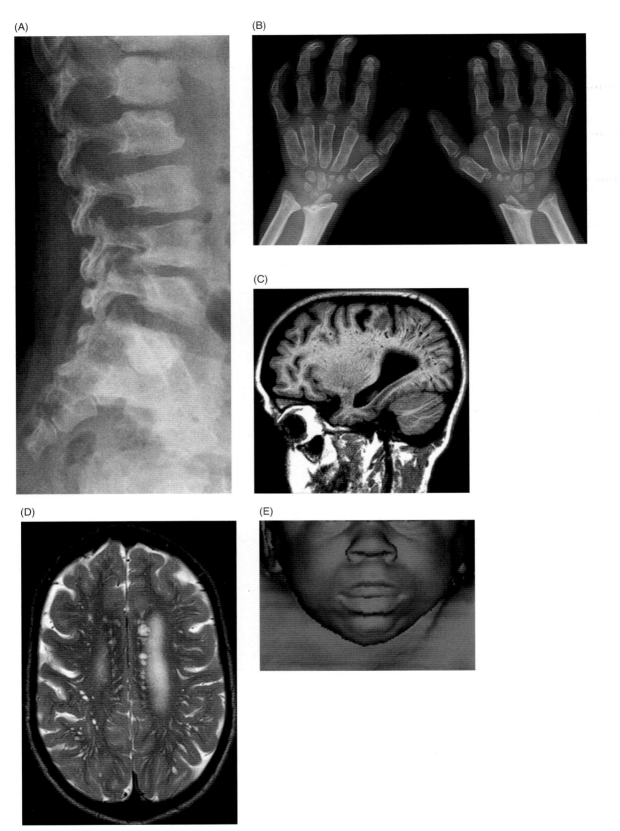

Figure 9.8 An 11-year-old male with MPS type II (Hunter disease). (A) Lateral view of the lumbar spine demonstrates anterior beaking of L2 and posterior scalloping of the lumbar vertebrae. (B) Images of the hands demonstrate osteopenia and broadening of the short tubular bones. In addition, there is irregularity and pointing of the bases of the metacarpals. The carpal bones are small and irregular. The distal radius and ulna have a pseudo-Madelung's appearance with flaring of the metaphysis and a decreased radiocarpal angle. (C, D) Sagittal T1 and axial T2 images of the brain. There is prominence of Virchow-Robin (VR) spaces in the supratentorial white matter, basal ganglia and corpus callosum. (E) A 10-year-old male also with Hunter disease. Soft tissue 3D reconstruction showing coarsening of the facial features with depressed nasal bridge, broad nasal tip and anteverted nostrils.

(A) (B)

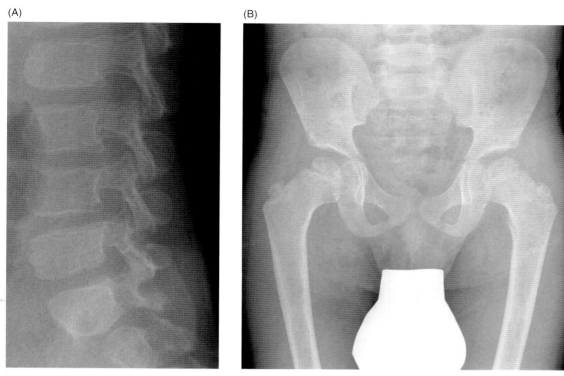

Figure 9.9 Five-year-old male with MPS type III (Sanfilippo syndrome). (A) Subtle anterior beaking is present at L2, L3 and L4. (B) There is moderate bilateral coxa vara, with small, under-formed femoral heads and greater trochanteric apophyses.

Type B usually presents later in adolescence or childhood. Most of these patients have normal intelligence, and features such as hearing impairment, joint stiffness, coarse facial features, upper airway disease and carpal tunnel syndrome remain hallmarks, but only with a more protracted time frame.

MPS type III

Patients with Sanfilippo syndrome are asymptomatic at birth and typically have normal development for the first two years of life. In all types of this syndrome, central nervous system (CNS) disease predominates, with less skeletal and soft tissue involvement compared with the other MPSs. Mild facial coarsening may be present, and the skeletal features are usually subtle (Figure 9.9).

MPS type IV

Compared with other patients who have MPS, those with Morquio syndrome (mucopolysaccharidosis type IV) tend to have greater spine involvement, with scoliosis, kyphosis and severe gibbus, as well as platyspondyly, rib flaring, pectus carinatum and ligamentous laxity. Odontoid hypoplasia is the most critical skeletal feature to recognize in any patient with Morquio syndrome. On the other hand, as lysosomal accumulation of keratan sulfate (KS) continues, mild coarsening of facial features, corneal clouding and hepatomegaly become apparent (Figure 9.10).

MPS type VI

This entity is characterized by somatic features but not by mental retardation. There is progressive connective tissue organ involvement that results from continuous storage of dermatan sulfate in the skeleton, heart valves, spleen, liver, lung, dura and cornea. Facial features include coarse facial features, macrocephaly, enlarged tongue and prominent forehead. Hepatomegaly, splenomegaly and umbilical and inguinal hernias are also often present in patients with MPS VI.

MPS type VII

MPS type VII can present in the fetal period as hydrops fetalis in the severe early form, or with later onset, frequently in patients over four years. Dysmorphic features, such as coarse facies, macrocephaly, frontal prominence, premature closure of sagittal lambdoid sutures, and short neck, may be seen. The abnormal skeletal findings include short stature and dwarfism, dislocated hip, joint contractures, kyphoscoliosis and wide rib cage/shield chest. In addition, dysostosis multiplex is associated with the severe form of Sly syndrome. This syndrome also can present with pectus carinatum or excavatum, oar-shaped ribs, talipes, underdeveloped ilium, aseptic necrosis of femoral head, and shortness of tubular bones (Figure 9.11). Recurrent pulmonary infections, hepatomegaly and splenomegaly can also occur. Finally, these patients have growth and motor skill abnormalities as well as mental retardation.

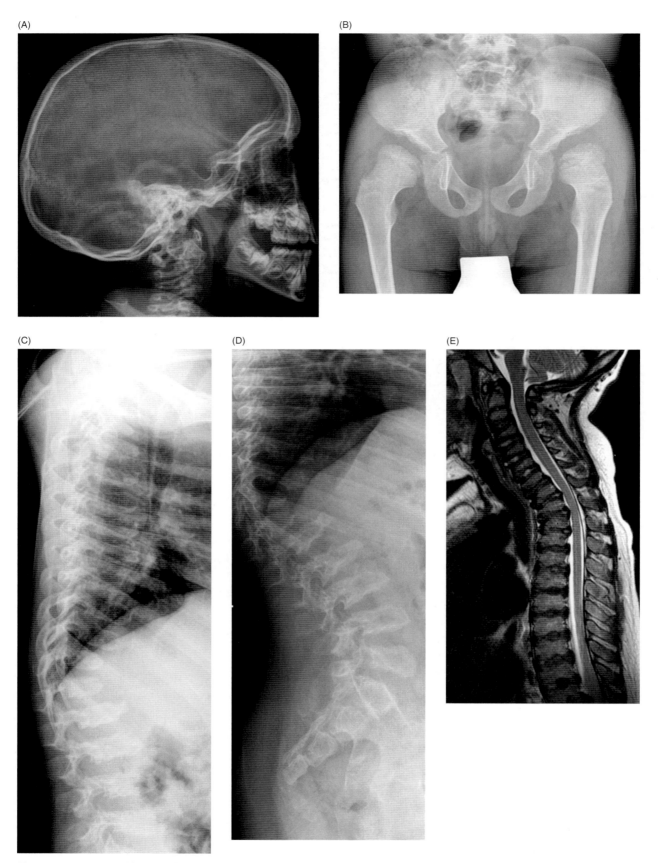

Figure 9.10 Four-year-old male with Morquio syndrome (MPS type IV). (A) Skull radiograph again demonstrates excavated sella turcica. (B) The epiphyses of the femoral head are abnormal with mild fragmentation. In addition the femoral heads are somewhat flattened. (C–F) Spine X-ray and MRI. There is evidence of diffuse platyspondyly involving the vertebral bodies of the cervical, thoracic and lumbar spine with increase of the lumbar lordosis and marked kyphosis centered at T1–T2 and T12–L1. (G) MRI spine of an eight-year-old female with Morquio syndrome. A short clivus, short posterior arch of C1 and hypoplastic dens are noted. There is also diffuse platyspondyly, bullet-shaped vertebrae and enlargement and posterior bulging of lower thoracic and upper lumbar discs with prominent osteochondral bars causing thecal sac compression.

(F)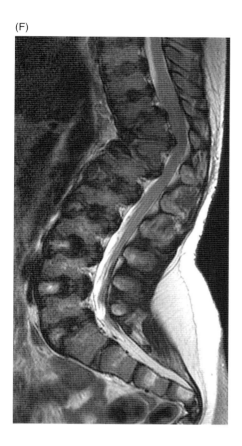

(G)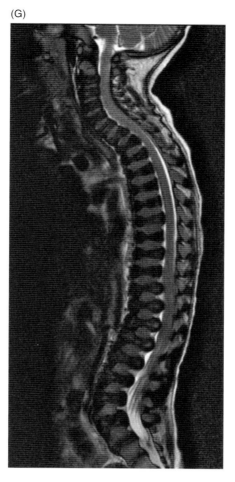

Figure 9.10 (Cont.)

Cushing syndrome and Cushing disease

Background

Cushing disease refers to adrenal cortical hyperfunction secondary to adrenocorticotropic hormone (ACTH)-secreting pituitary adenoma, whereas Cushing syndrome is a term used to describe the manifestations of glucocorticoid excess.

Cushing syndrome (CS) takes its name from Harvey Cushing, who, in 1912, was one of the first physicians to report a patient affected with excessive glucocorticoid. More than 99% of cases of Cushing syndrome are due to administration of excessive amounts of glucocorticoid. CS can be endogenous or exogenous and its differentiation is usually straightforward.

Cushing syndrome can be divided into ACTH-dependent and ACTH-independent forms. The proportion of adrenal and pituitary disease varies in different regions; however, in western countries, 90–95% of cases of Cushing syndrome in children older than five years are ACTH-dependent, and 90–95% of those cases are due to Cushing disease caused by an ACTH-secreting pituitary adenoma. Tumors that ectopically secrete ACTH are rare, and tumors that secrete corticotropin-releasing hormone (CRH) are extremely rare, together accounting for fewer than 5% of cases of Cushing syndrome. Beside this, in children younger than five years, the proportion of ACTH-independent cases of Cushing syndrome approaches 50%. Such cases are due to a combination of congenital disorders of the adrenal cortex and adrenocortical neoplasms that result in autonomous overproduction of cortisol and other adrenal cortical hormones (summarized below). All children in this age group who have been proven to have ACTH-independent Cushing syndrome require adrenalectomy because of the significant incidence of malignancy in this age group (Figures 9.12, 9.13).

Pathophysiology

Glucocorticoid synthesis and release is strictly regulated by the pituitary and hypothalamus by negative feedback and, to a lesser extent, by catecholamines from the adrenal medulla and neural inputs from the autonomic system. The glucocorticoid receptor is an intracellular protein that, in its ligand-bound form, acts as a nuclear transcription factor to regulate the expression of

(A)

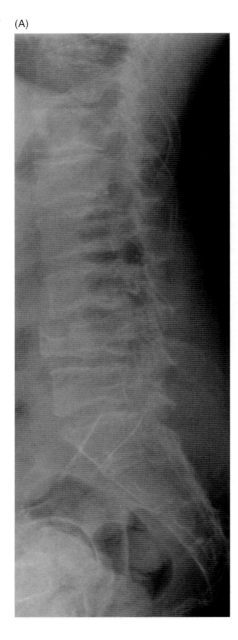

(B)

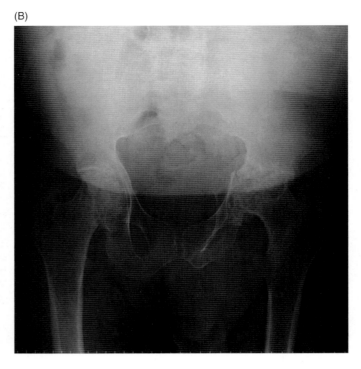

Figure 9.11 (A, B) Forty-year-old male with Sly syndrome (MPS type VII). Lumbar spine demonstrates marked endplate irregularity as well as loss of disc space height at T12/L1; L4 demonstrates significant loss of vertebral body height anteriorly, with extensive superior endplate irregularity. There is a large anterior wedge defect along the superior endplate which could represent anteriorly disc herniation or a large Schmorl's node.

a diverse array of genes in many areas of the body. Factors that influence the spectrum of adverse effects observed in hyper-cortisolemic individuals include duration of treatment, potency of the steroid, dose and route of administration, and the site and rate of metabolism and clearance.

All patients with Cushing syndrome who receive pharmacological glucocorticoid treatment develop cushingoid features if exposed to a high-enough dose for long enough (usually one month or more). With the exception of abnormal growth, the signs of hypercortisolism are frequently subtler in pediatric patients than in adults. In children, the most common features that are observed include an increase in body weight due in part to an increase in appetite and a decrease in linear growth.

The effects of glucocorticoids on the skeleton are multiple and vary from impairment of physeal chondrogenesis (by decreasing growth hormone secretion) to effects on mineralization by both systemic and direct action on bone. The systemic effects imply the impairment of sex hormones and reduction of the absorption of calcium in the gut. Direct effects on bone include decrease of bone formation and increase of reabsorption.

Osteonecrosis is also a well-known complication of endogenous or exogenous glucocorticoid excess. Many hypotheses have been postulated and include fat deposition with resultant increase in intra-osseous pressure and therefore decreased perfusion, fat embolization from a fatty liver and increased blood viscosity.

(A)

(B)

(C)

(D)

(E)

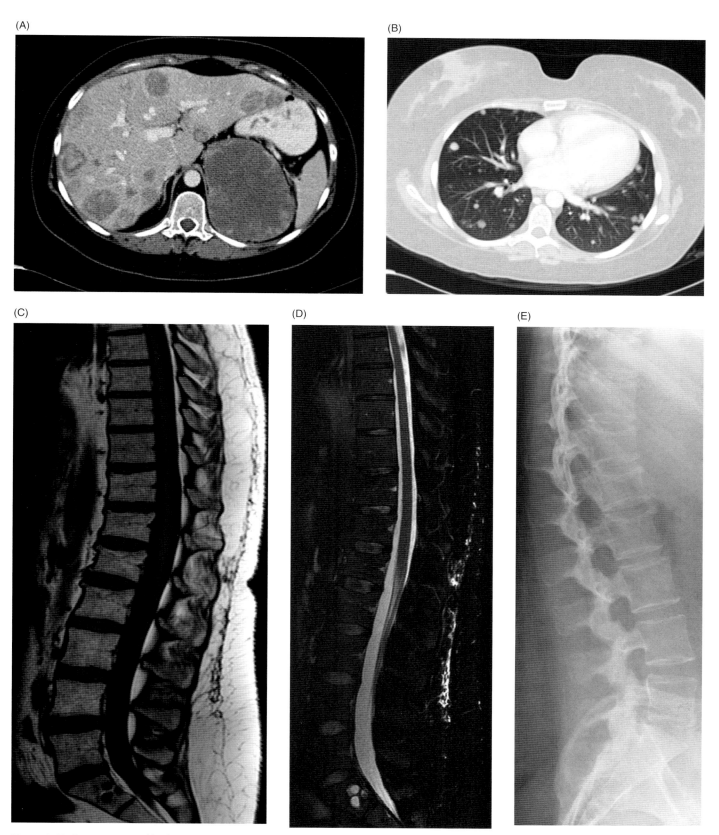

Figure 9.12 Seventeen-year-old girl with acne and cushingoid features. (A) CT demonstrates a large, left adrenal mass, with extensive liver and lung metastatic pattern (B) and prominent subcutaneous fatty tissues. The patient complained of back pain two weeks later and thoracolumbar spine X-ray and MRI were performed (C–E), demonstrating acute compression fractures involving T12, L1 and L2.

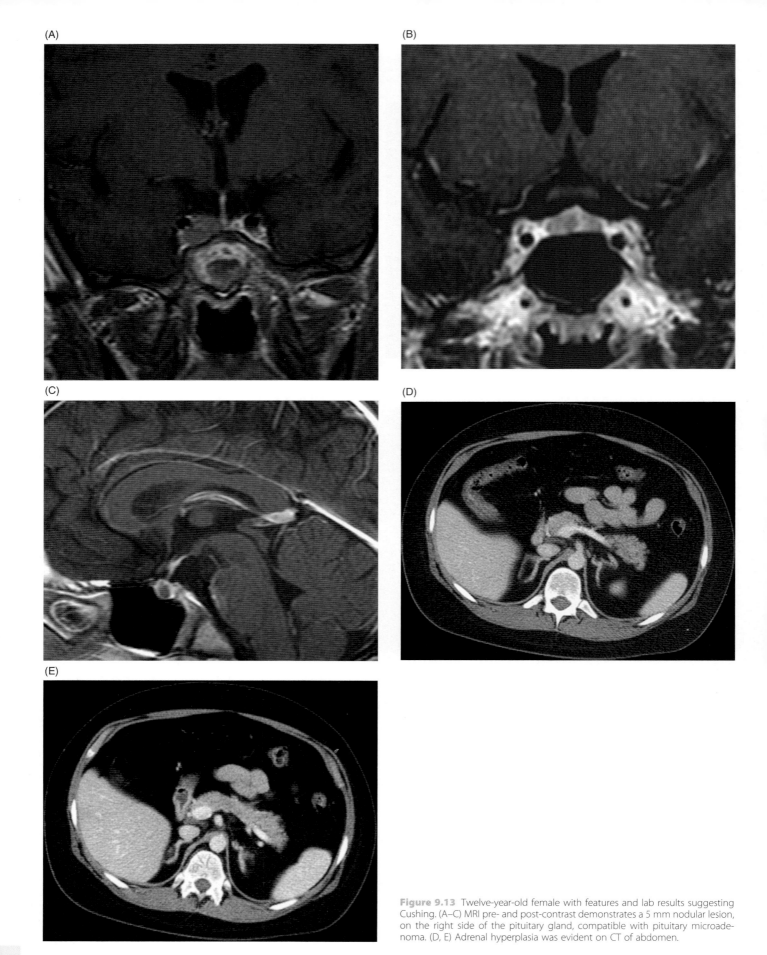

(A)

(B)

(C)

(D)

(E)

Figure 9.13 Twelve-year-old female with features and lab results suggesting Cushing. (A–C) MRI pre- and post-contrast demonstrates a 5 mm nodular lesion, on the right side of the pituitary gland, compatible with pituitary microadenoma. (D, E) Adrenal hyperplasia was evident on CT of abdomen.

Imaging findings

Endocrine and metabolic effects include growth failure in children, hyperinsulinemia/insulin resistance and abnormal glucose tolerance test result/diabetes mellitus. Gastrointestinal effects comprise gastric irritation, peptic ulcer, acute pancreatitis (rare, secondary to insulin resistance and hypertriglyceridemia) and fatty infiltration of liver (hepatomegaly, rare). Hematopoietic manifestations in these patients include leukocytosis, neutrophilia (increased recruitment from bone marrow, decreased migration from blood vessels), lymphopenia (migration from blood vessels to lymphoid tissue), eosinopenia and monocytopenia. Spontaneous fractures, avascular necrosis of femoral and humeral heads and other bones as well as myopathy (particularly of the proximal muscles, e.g., unable to comb hair or climb stairs) are well known musculoskeletal manifestations in these patients. Ophthalmological manifestations include posterior subcapsular cataracts and elevated intraocular pressure/glaucoma. Other cushingoid features include moon facies (broad cheeks with temporal muscle wasting), facial plethora, generalized and truncal obesity (more marked in adults), supraclavicular fat collection, posterior cervical fat deposition (dorsocervical hump), glucocorticoid-induced acne, thin and fragile skin, violaceous striae (more common in adults) and menstrual irregularity.

Radiological findings are usually nonspecific and include osteopenia, cortical thinning, trabecular rarefaction and vertebral compression fractures. However, more specific findings have been described, such as endplate sclerosis, exuberant callus formation at fracture sites and osteonecrosis. The most affected site in osteonecrosis is the femoral head, followed by the humeral head and femoral condyles. Peculiar features of Cushing-related osteonecrosis have also been described and include absence of enhancement following contrast-enhancement in MRI and decreased uptake on scintigraphy.

Gigantism and acromegaly

Background

Gigantism refers to abnormally high linear growth due to excessive action of insulin-like growth factor-I (IGF-I) while the epiphyseal growth plates are still open during childhood. Gigantism is a nonspecific term that refers to any standing height more than two standard deviations above the mean for the person's sex, age and Tanner stage (i.e., height Z-score > +2). On the other hand, acromegaly is the same disorder of IGF-I excess when it occurs after the growth plate cartilage fuses. Therefore acromegaly is seldom seen in children.

Pathophysiology

The growth hormone (GH) hypersecretion originates from a monoclonal benign pituitary tumor (adenoma) in more than 90% of the cases. However, GH hypersecretion does not always have a pituitary origin. Acromegaly can therefore be due to ectopic hypothalamic growth hormone releasing hormone (GHRH) hypersecretion (gangliocytoma, hamartoma, choristoma, glioma, etc.) or, more often, to ectopic, peripheral GHRH hypersecretion from a pancreatic or bronchial carcinoid tumor that stimulates the normal somatropes to become hyperplastic and to hypersecrete. In addition, GH can be secreted by an ectopic pituitary adenoma (sphenoidal sinus, petrous temporal bone or nasopharyngeal cavity) or, in exceptional cases, by a peripheral tumor such as pancreatic islet tumor or lymphoma.

GH stimulates periosteal and endochondral bone formation and produces hypertrophy of the cartilage and soft tissue, with hands, feet and face being the most affected sites. In response to both GH and IGF-I, periosteal new bone formation leads to increase in skeletal growth, especially at the level of the mandible (prognathism); jaw thickening; teeth separation; frontal bossing; malocclusion and nasal bony hypertrophy. Radiographic findings include thickening of the cranial vault and protuberances, frontal internal hyperostosis, condensation of the walls of the sella turcica with clinoid hypertrophy and hypertrophy of the sinuses, especially the frontal sinus. This, along with laryngeal hypertrophy, explains why the voice tends to be deeper in patients with acromegaly (Figure 9.14).

Imaging findings

The changes in the extremities are explained by the soft tissue hypertrophy and excess growth of bone and cartilage and bone deformation. The tubular bones are thickened by periosteal bone formation with excrescences arising from the trochanters and tuberosities through subtendinous and subligamentous bone formation. The phalanges show distal tufting with widening of the bases and osteophyte formation. "Acromegalic rosary" can be seen, and refers to the reactivation of endochondral bone at the costochondral junctions. The prevalence of spinal involvement is about 40–50%. Spinal findings include: ossification of the anterior and lateral surface of the vertebral bodies, contributing to enlarging their anteroposterior diameter; biconcave vertebral appearance; and scalloping of the vertebral bodies by osteophytosis. The mechanism seems to be related to hypertrophy of the intraspinal soft tissues (including ligamentous hypertrophy and epidural lipomatosis) or of the bone.

Peripheral joint symptoms are frequent, with arthralgias and myalgias occurring in up to 30–70% of patients. Joint effusion is rare, and synovial aspirate shows no evidence of inflammation, but may point to the presence of calcium microcrystals related to associated chondrocalcinosis. Radiological studies demonstrate widening of the joint spaces as a result of hypertrophy of the hyaline cartilage, osteophytes, bone proliferation at the attachment sites of tendons and ligaments, periarticular calcium deposit and exostosis of the bone surface. The joint space subsequently diminishes due to destructive arthropathy. Acromegaly also can cause a variety of symptoms such as malodorous sweating (in up to 70%), especially at night; headache; acroparesthesia (carpal tunnel syndrome), which occurs in 20–70% of the cases; Raynaud's disease and joint pain. Hypertension is also

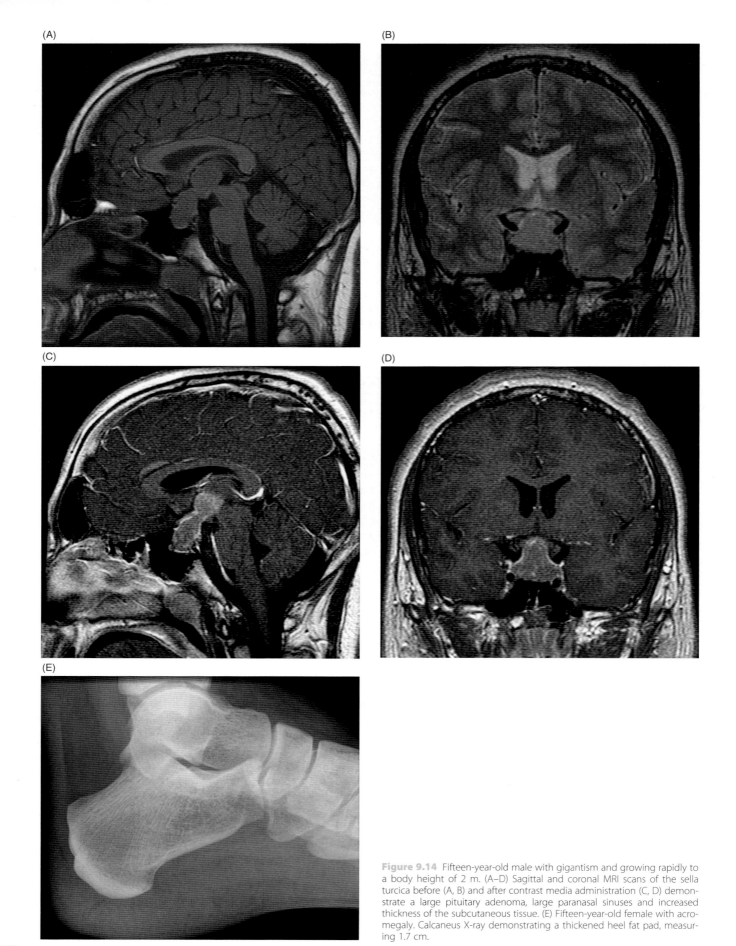

(A)

(B)

(C)

(D)

(E)

Figure 9.14 Fifteen-year-old male with gigantism and growing rapidly to a body height of 2 m. (A–D) Sagittal and coronal MRI scans of the sella turcica before (A, B) and after contrast media administration (C, D) demonstrate a large pituitary adenoma, large paranasal sinuses and increased thickness of the subcutaneous tissue. (E) Fifteen-year-old female with acromegaly. Calcaneus X-ray demonstrating a thickened heel fat pad, measuring 1.7 cm.

seen in 20–50% of patients. Two theories have been postulated; the first one implies chronic hypovolemia, and the second one, endothelial dysfunction. Sixty to eighty percent of patients have sleep apnea, with most of the cases obstructive in nature, and 25–90% of patients have goiter.

Oxaluria and oxalosis
Background
Hyperoxaluria, defined as excessive urinary oxalate, is a common abnormal finding in patients with calcium oxalate kidney stones. Some degree of excessive urinary oxalate is found in 20–30% of all patients with recurrent calcium oxalate stones.

Pathophysiology
Oxalate is absorbed primarily in the colon, but it can be absorbed directly from anywhere in the intestinal tract. In addition, oxalate is created from endogenous sources in the liver as part of glycolate metabolism. In the kidney, oxalate is secreted in the proximal tubule via two separate carriers involving sodium and chloride exchange. Hyperoxaluria is defined as a urinary oxalate excretion that exceeds 40 mg day^{-1}. The four main types of hyperoxaluria include: (1) primary hyperoxaluria (types I and II), (2) enteric hyperoxaluria, (3) dietary hyperoxaluria, and (4) idiopathic or mild hyperoxaluria.

Primary hyperoxaluria type 1 is an inherited disease due to an inborn error of glyoxylate metabolism within the hepatocyte peroxisome. This results in increased urinary excretion of oxalate and glycolate and, eventually, renal failure and end-stage renal disease (ESRD). Insoluble calcium oxalate (CaOx) is deposited in extra-renal tissue, which is known as oxalosis.

Imaging findings
The most consistent findings in oxalosis are condensations on the metaphyseal side of long bone growth plates (dense metaphyseal bands), which correlates with the presence and duration of the ESRD. In addition, ESRD is associated with lucent metaphyseal bands between the physis and the adjacent dense metaphyseal bands in long bones and vertebral condensations involving at first the superior and inferior vertebral endplates, creating a rugger-jersey spine appearance. Bone-within-bone appearance can also be seen.

Other less specific findings are subperiosteal resorption, osteolysis of the distal phalanges, periosteal apposition, spondylolysis and osteopenia. These nonspecific changes are the result of CaOx deposition, renal osteodystrophy and secondary hyperparathyroidism (Figure 9.15).

Galactosemia
Background
This is a rare autosomal recessive disorder, but the second most common cause of chronic severe liver disease in children. Incidence is approximately 1 case per 40 000–60 000 persons.

Pathophysiology
Hypergalactosemia is associated with the following three enzyme deficiencies: galactokinase, which converts galactose to galactose-1-phosphate; uridine diphosphate (UDP)-galactose-4-epimeras (both are not common deficiencies); and galactose-1-phosphate uridyltransferase (GALT; EC 2.7.7.12), which is the most common deficiency. This enzyme catalyzes conversion of galactose-1-phosphate and UDP glucose to UDP galactose and glucose-1-phosphate. The gene encoding GALT is located on chromosome 9p13, and the most common mutation in classical galactosemia is the p.Q188R mutation, changing the glutamine at position 188 into arginine.

Imaging findings
Most patients present in the neonatal period after ingestion of galactose-containing feeds. Symptoms and signs include jaundice, hepatosplenomegaly, hepatocellular insufficiency, food intolerance, hypoglycemia, renal tubular dysfunction, muscle hypotonia, sepsis and cataract. Pseudotumor cerebri may also occur and may cause a bulging fontanelle. The long-term complications include retarded mental development, verbal dyspraxia, motor abnormalities and hypergonadotropic hypogonadism (Figure 9.16). Although some of the damage is believed to occur in utero, it appears that a substantial portion of these long-term complications originate from ongoing toxicity during life. Most recent studies have revealed that, except for a diagnosis after two months of age, neither the age at the time of diagnosis nor the severity of clinical illness at the time of diagnosis correlate with the presence and severity of late complications.

In many patients, growth is delayed in childhood and early adolescence, but the final height is usually normal. On the other hand, diminished bone mineral density due to premature ovarian failure is a well-known complication in women with classical galactosemia.

Alpha-1 antitrypsin deficiency
Background
This is a genetic disorder that manifests clinically as pulmonary emphysema or chronic obstructive pulmonary disease, liver cirrhosis and less frequently as the skin disease panniculitis.

Pathophysiology
The protein alpha-1 antitrypsin is produced primarily in hepatocytes and released into the blood circulation by the liver. A serum concentration below 0.5 g l^{-1} is considered a reason for further analysis. Patients with a gene defect in both alleles of the chromosome are defined as having Z deficiency. Neonatal hepatic syndrome is a condition that occurs in a small percentage of newborns with homozygous Z genotype alpha-1 antitrypsin. These newborns have prolonged jaundice after birth, with conjugated hyperbilirubinemia and abnormal

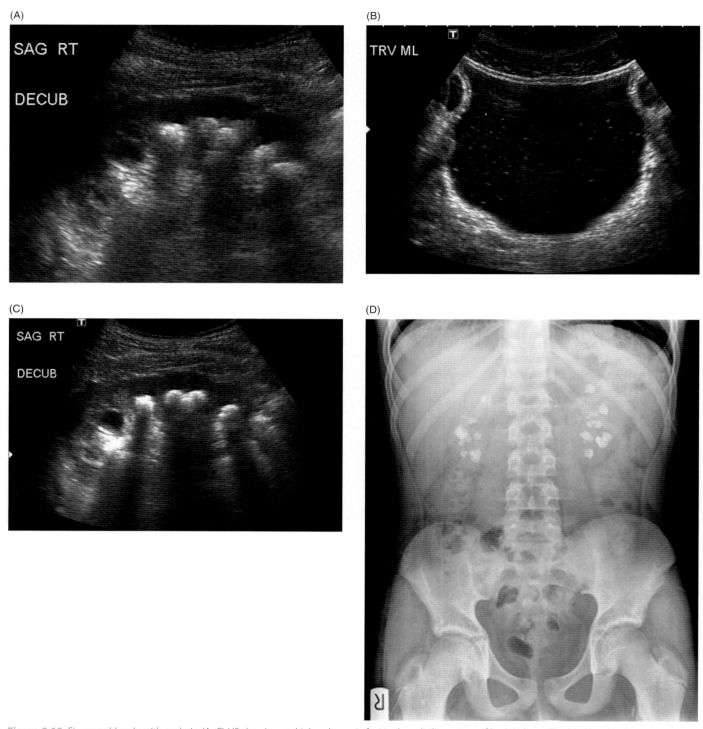

Figure 9.15 Six-year-old male with oxaluria. (A–C) US showing multiple echogenic foci in the caliciliar system of both kidneys. The bladder also demonstrates tiny echogenic debris. (D) Abdomen radiograph confirms bilateral kidney stones.

liver enzymes. Panniculitis is also associated with the Z genotype and manifests as spontaneous necrotic areas of the skin without previous trauma of the skin. These lesions have a predilection for the gluteal region, trunk, limbs and arms.

Two mechanisms have been postulated to contribute to the development of lung disease. The first one is related to the

serum level of alpha-1 antitrypsin. This theory is supported by the fact that individuals with the very rare homozygote null variant (no production of the enzyme in their liver or monocytes) develop emphysema at a younger age than subjects with the homozygous Z allele-related deficiency. The second theory states that the Z mutant of alpha-1 antitrypsin has

(A)

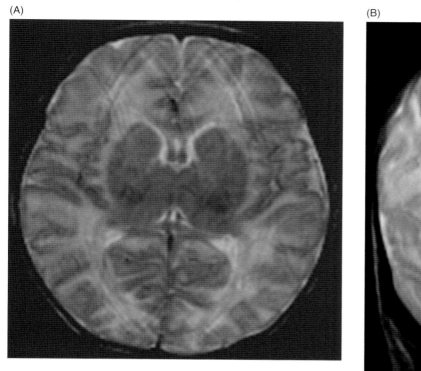

(B)

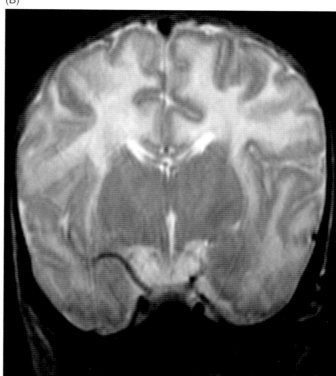

(C)

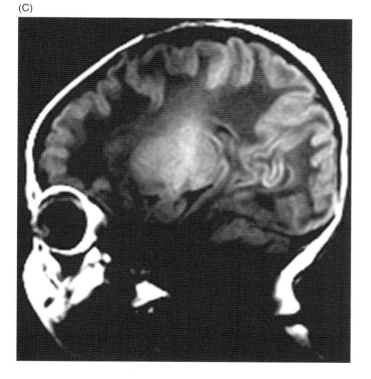

Figure 9.16 Ten-day-old male with hyperbilirubinemia and edema on US of head. (A–C) MRI demonstrates diffuse white mater edema supratentorially and restricted diffusion in deep white matter tracts, periventricular region, internal capsules and corpus callosum. These findings are consistent with galactosemia.

a point mutation, Glu342Lys, in the molecule that renders it prone to polymerization of the protein. The A allele results in hepatic polymerization in hepatocyte inclusions, and decreased serum concentrations.

Imaging findings

Newborns presenting with a bleeding disorder or prolonged neonatal jaundice, individuals with history of asthma or chronic obstructive lung disease (especially before age 40) and individuals with unexpected liver cirrhosis should be tested for alpha-1 antitrypsin deficiency.

The treatment options for patients with this entity are still limited. Only end-stage liver and lung disease can be treated by organ transplantation. For treatment of lung disease, intravenous alpha-1 antitrypsin augmentation therapy is advised in individuals with FEV1 between 35 and 65% of predicted. Also, annual flu vaccination and pneumococcal vaccine every five years are recommended. Once diagnosed, the prognosis of both liver and lung disease is variable.

Hyperparathyroidism

Hyperparathyroidism can be classified into the primary, secondary or tertiary forms. Primary hyperparathyroidism is caused by overproduction of the parathyroid hormone (PTH), due to a primary parathyroid gland abnormality within the gland, leading to an overproduction of PTH, in excess of the amount required by the body. The secondary form of disease is due to an excess of production of the PTH caused by a systemic stimulus. Tertiary hyperparathyroidism results from an autonomous hyperfunction of the parathyroid glands. Parathyroid hormone has a dynamic state of equilibrium, driven by serum calcium levels. It has a direct effect on vitamin D production to increase calcium homeostasis in the gut and kidney, and subsequently modulates bone metabolism.

Pathophysiology

In 75–80% of cases of primary hyperparathyroidism, one or more adenomas account for the overproduction, whereas approximately 20% of cases are due to diffuse hyperplasia of all glands. Carcinoma accounts for less than 2% of all cases. At the cellular level, parathyroid hormone acts on the osteoclasts, causing resorption and demineralization of bone. Thus, the hallmark of osseous disease is resorption of bone, with or without formation of brown tumors, coupled with replacement of bone by fibrous tissue.

Pathology

Historically, the term "osteitis fibrosa cystica" was used to describe the advanced skeletal disease in primary hyperparathyroidism. Bone findings are characterized by osteoclastic resorption of bone, osteoblastic bone formation and fibrous replacement of marrow, with radiographic findings of subperiosteal resorption, brown tumors, bone cysts, and sclerosis.

The affected bones may have microfractures, with subsequent hemorrhage and growth of fibrous tissue followed by an influx of macrophages. The resulting mass is called a brown tumor because of its color, attributable to the vascular elements and blood contained within.

The process of bone resorption and fibrous replacement results in the characteristic radiological features of generalized bone demineralization, resorption, cysts, brown tumors,

erosion of the dental lamina dura, and pathological fractures. Other manifestations include nephrolithiasis, nephrocalcinosis, neurological changes, peptic ulcer disease and pancreatitis. Hence, it is called the disease with "moans, bones, groans and stones."

Symptomatic bone disease may be present in 10–25% of patients. The diagnosis is based on an elevated PTH level in the setting of elevated calcium levels.

Imaging findings

Bone resorption is the hallmark, which may be subdivided into subperiosteal, intracortical, trabecular, endosteal, subchondral, subligamentous, or subtendinous. Subperiosteal bone resorption is "pathognomonic" of hyperparathyroidism and is marked by marginal erosions with adjacent resorption of bone and sclerosis. A lace-like appearance may be seen beneath the periosteum, with an occasional spiculated external cortex, and may progress to complete cortical disappearance. The most common sites include radial aspects of the middle phalanges of the index and middle fingers (Figure 9.17), phalangeal tufts (acro-osteolysis), medial aspect of tibia, humerus, femur and distal clavicle and absent lamina dura around the teeth.

Resorption may extend to the margins of joints, particularly in the hands, wrists, and feet (Figure 9.17). In the skull, areas of decreased radiopacity are intermingled with sclerotic radiopaque areas, resulting in a classic appearance called the "salt-and-pepper skull" (Figure 9.18). In endosteal resorption, the medullary cavity widens with thinning of the inner cortex, usually best seen in the hands, appearing as scalloped lucencies on the inner aspect of the cortex.

Subchondral bone resorption is most common in the joints of the axial skeleton, such as the sacroiliac, acromioclavicular, discovertebral, sternoclavicular and symphysis pubis, but may also occur at other joints. Subchondral bone is resorbed, leading to bone collapse with subsequent new bone formation, and fibrous replacement may result. On radiographs, areas of subchondral lucency are noted with surrounding sclerosis. In the sacroiliac joint, the ilium is affected more than the sacrum and may produce an irregular articular margin with the appearance of a widened joint. At the acromioclavicular joint, erosions affect the clavicle more than the acromion, whereas the sternum and clavicle are equally affected at the sternoclavicular joint. Subligamentous and subtendinous resorption occur at insertion sites on bones, common sites being the plantar aspect of the calcaneus, dorsal aspect of the patella, inferior margin of the distal clavicle, trochanters, and ischial and humeral tuberosities.

Brown tumors are well-circumscribed lytic lesions of bone that represent the osteoclastic resorption of bone with subsequent fibrous replacement. They may be single or multiple, with expansion of overlying bone; common sites include the mandible, clavicle, ribs, pelvis, and femur (Figure 9.19). On radiography, they are geographic, lytic lesions.

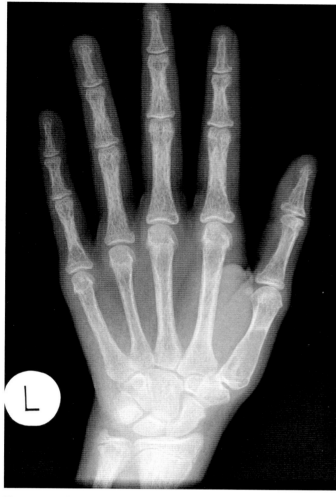

Figure 9.17 Anteroposterior hand radiograph reveals generalized coarsening of trabecular pattern, acro-osteolysis and subperiosteal resorption, more pronounced along the radial aspects of the second to fifth middle phalanges, typical for hyperparathyroidism.

In the presence of subperiosteal resorption these polyostotic, geographic, lytic lesions are pathognomonic for brown tumors. Due to the presence of hemosiderin, there is a classic MR appearance with T1- and T2-hypointense lesions and blooming on gradient echo sequences. Once considered a finding that was characteristic of primary hyperparathyroidism, brown tumors are more common in the secondary form of disease with increasing life expectancy of patients with renal disease.

Other radiological manifestations include varying degrees of sclerosis and vascular calcification. Generalized sclerosis is more common in secondary hyperparathyroidism, as is

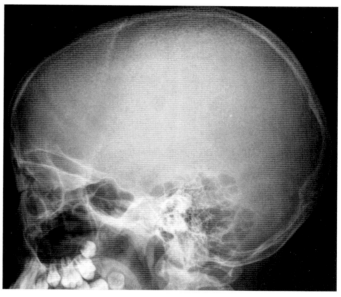

Figure 9.18 Hyperparathyroidism. Lateral radiograph of the skull with classic "salt-and-pepper" appearance.

(A)

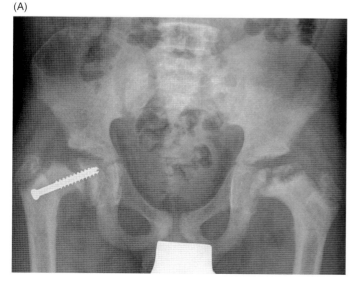

(B)

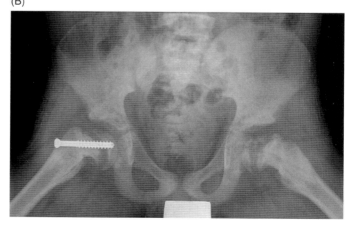

Figure 9.19 (A, B) Frontal neutral and frog-leg abduction views of both hip joints show bilateral slipped femoral capital epiphyses with avascular necrosis and a lucent lesion in the right ilium, a brown tumor.

(A)

(B)

(C)

(D)

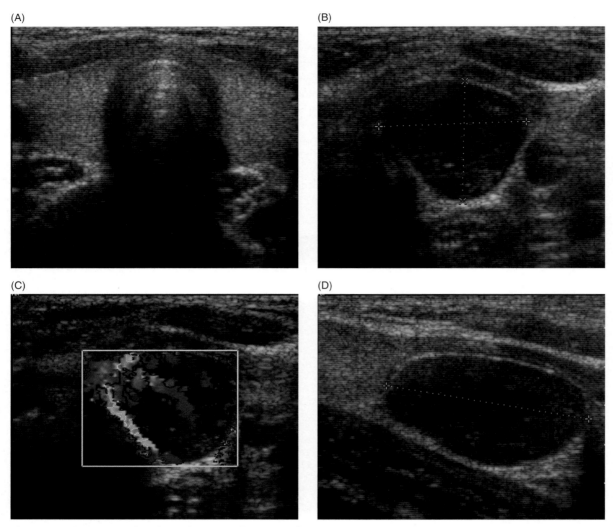

Figure 9.20 (A–D) Gray-scale and Doppler sonographic images of neck reveal a solitary, vascular, solid parathyroid nodule, representing an adenoma.

Table 9.4 Radiological imaging findings in primary hyperparathyroidism

Subperiosteal bone resorption – radial aspects of index and middle fingers, phalangeal tufts, absent lamina dura, medial aspect of the tibia, humerus, femur and distal clavicle

Salt-and-pepper skull

Endosteal bone resorption with widened medullary cavity and thinning of the inner cortex

Subchondral bone resorption around sacroiliac, acromioclavicular, discovertebral, sternoclavicular joints

Subligamentous and subtendinous resorption at plantar aspect of the calcaneus, dorsal aspect of the patella, inferior margin of the distal clavicle, trochanters, and ischial and humeral tuberosities

Brown tumors, common sites include mandible, clavicle, ribs, pelvis and femur

Varying generalized or focal sclerosis

Parathyroid adenoma

soft tissue and vascular calcification in secondary disease. The sclerosis may be in the superior and inferior endplates of the spine, termed as "rugger-jersey spine."

Imaging of parathyroid adenoma

On ultrasound, adenomas are classically well-defined, hypo-echoic nodules, separate from the thyroid glands (Figure 9.20). On contrast CT, they are iso- to hypodense relative to the thyroid, and hyperdense to muscle. On MRI scans, adenomas are typically seen as masses that are isointense on T1W sequences and hyperintense on T2W sequences, with post-gadolinium enhancement. Technetium 99m sestamibi studies reveal areas of increased uptake.

Secondary hyperparathyroidism

Hyperparathyroidism may be secondary to hypocalcemia due to various etiologies, such as chronic renal failure, intestinal malabsorption and vitamin D deficiency. Chronic renal

(A)

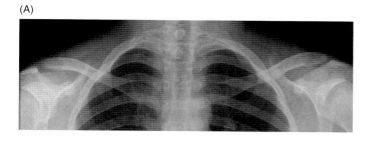

(B)

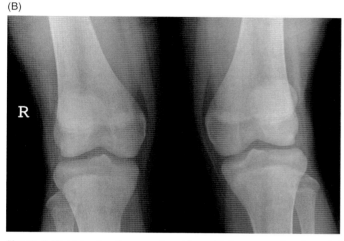

(C)

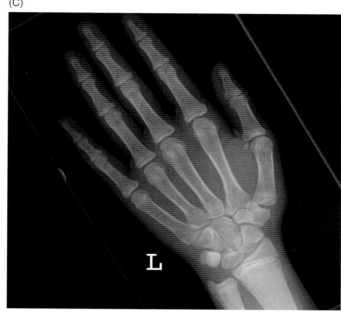

Figure 9.21 Secondary hyperparathyroidism. (A) Posteroanterior view of the chest reveals subperiosteal resorption around distal clavicular ends bilaterally. (B) Anteroposterior views of knees and hands reveal patchy sclerosis around the knee joints and (C) anteroposterior view of the hands demonstrates subperiosteal resorption along the radial aspects of the middle phalanges.

insufficiency with rickets and osteomalacia is a frequent cause of secondary hyperparathyroidism: often referred to as renal osteodystrophy (ROD).

The radiological features of secondary hyperparathyroidism are similar to those of the primary form of the disease. The basic defect is generalized hyperplasia of the parathyroid glands (Figure 9.21). The combination of the two pathological processes of hyperparathyroidism and resultant hypocalcemia is responsible for the osseous abnormalities in renal osteodystrophy.

Pathophysiology

Biochemical abnormalities and skeletal manifestations of ROD are a consequence of two major hormonal changes: deficient 1,25-dihydroxyvitamin D, and excess PTH.

Imaging findings

The common radiological manifestations include widening of the growth plates of the long bones, with irregular metaphyseal margins and disorganization of the growth plate indicative of advanced rickets. These changes have been likened to the "rotting of a wooden post at its stem." Severe osteopenia may be seen with or without pathological fractures. Epiphyseal displacement of metaphyseal fractures is also seen; the most commonly involved sites include distal radius,

proximal humerus, distal femur, and heads of metacarpal and metatarsals.

Secondary hyperparathyroidism also remains a common cause of retarded skeletal maturation. Blount disease may occur as a result of lateral angulation of the proximal tibial epiphysis. Genu valgum and jaw enlargement have also been described.

The secondary form of disease predictably shares some features of the primary form, including subperiosteal bone resorption (Figure 9.22A), intracortical and endosteal, subligamentous and subchondral resorption, which has been described above. An erosive-type arthropathy is reported with secondary hyperparathyroidism.

Brown tumors occur, but are less common with secondary hyperparathyroidism than with primary disease. The skull may show a granular pattern, which may be associated with thickening, particularly in the inner table (Figure 9.23). Osteomalacia may be predominant in patients with renal osteodystrophy (Figures 9.24, 9.25). Associated Looser transformation zones and pathological fractures, possibly symmetric, may be seen. Osteosclerosis may affect the epiphyses, metaphyses, pelvis and ribs (Figure 9.21B, Figure 9.23). Frequently, a classic "rugger-jersey" spine is observed; it is caused by ill-defined bands of increased bone density adjacent to the vertebral endplates. Extraosseous calcification is more common in secondary hyperparathyroidism than in the primary form of the

(A)

(B)

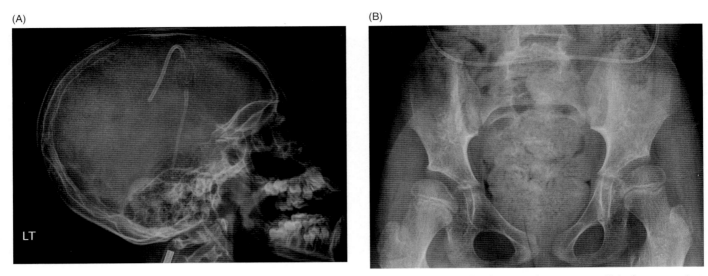

Figure 9.22 Secondary hyperparathyroidism. (A) Lateral radiograph of skull reveals patchy sclerosis with fine, lacy, reticular appearance. (B) In the same patient, frontal radiograph of pelvis including bilateral hips reveals coxa valga deformity of both hips.

(A)

(B)

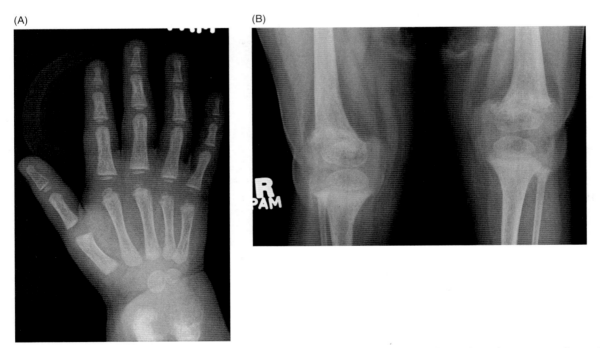

Figure 9.23 (A, B) Frontal views of the wrist and knee joints reveal changes of rickets and renal osteodystrophy are a case of secondary hyperparathyroidism, comprising of a metaphyseal fracture, flaring and cupping of metaphyses, generalized osteopenia, coarsened trabeculae and subperiosteal resorption of middle phalanges.

disease. Abnormal calcification and other abnormalities include the following:

- Tumoral calcification associated with bone erosions
- Chondrocalcinosis
- Vascular calcification
- Calcified pulmonary nodules
- Cerebral subcortical calcification
- Calcification within the eyes
- Layering of soft tissue calcification
- Cardiac calcifications
- Breast calcifications
- Renal calcification
- Hepatic calcification.

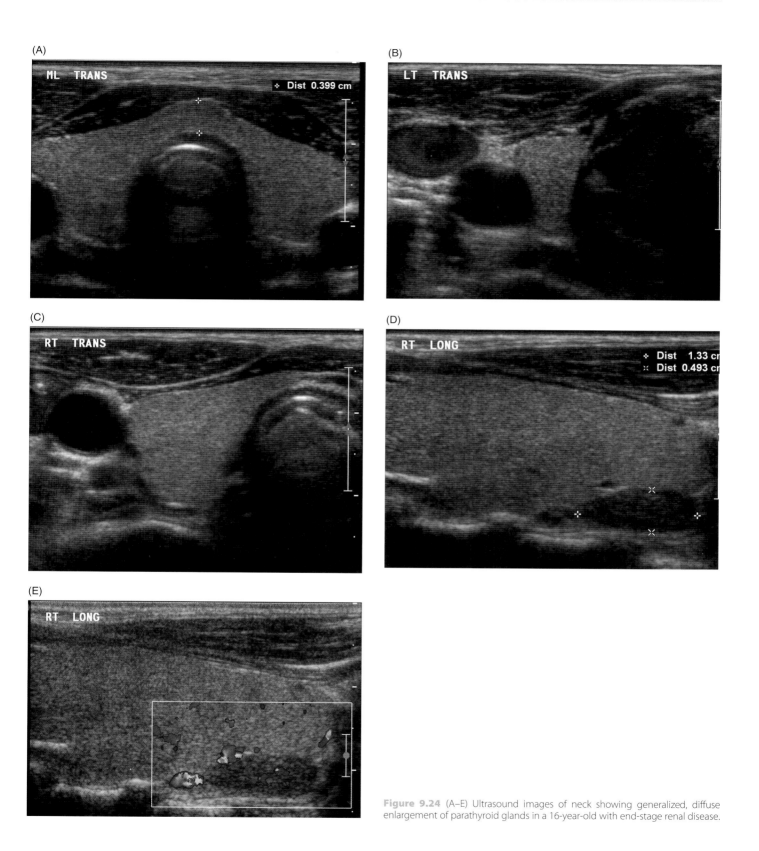

Figure 9.24 (A–E) Ultrasound images of neck showing generalized, diffuse enlargement of parathyroid glands in a 16-year-old with end-stage renal disease.

(A)

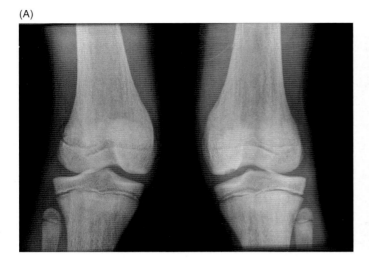

(B)

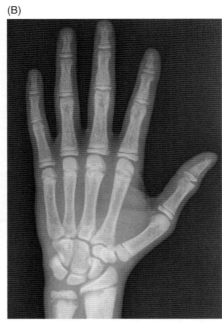

Figure 9.25 Osteomalacia in a patient with renal osteodystrophy. (A) Frontal view of knees reveals undertubulation of proximal tibiae and distal femora accompanied by patchy sclerosis and inhomogeneous bone density. (B) Frontal view of hands reveals acro-osteolysis with subperiosteal resorption.

Tertiary hyperparathyroidism

In some patients with improved renal function following renal transplantation for chronic renal insufficiency, hyperparathyroidism may persist as a result of autonomous hyperfunction of the parathyroid glands. This is called tertiary hyperparathyroidism.

Skeletal findings are similar to those in ROD. In severe cases, parathyroidectomy is the treatment of choice. SPECT (single photon emission computed tomography) imaging, ultrasound and MRI play a significant role in preoperative localization and demonstration of morphological abnormalities of parathyroid glands.

Hypoparathyroidism

Hypoparathyroidism is the clinical syndrome of underproduction of the parathyroid glands, mostly as a result of inadvertent excision or trauma or due to end-organ resistance.

It may also result from congenital absence of the parathyroid glands or from atrophy in infants born to mothers with hyperparathyroidism. An idiopathic, familial form has been observed in some children. It is also seen in various auto-immune disorders, often associated with other endocrine abnormalities, especially of the adrenal gland.

Pathophysiology

Reduced levels of PTH lead to reduced absorption or activation of vitamin D, adversely affecting calcium reabsorption at the level of the renal nephron as well as gastrointestinal tract. Hypoparathyroidism can be inherited when congenital or may be secondary when acquired.

DiGeorge's syndrome is an example of the congenital type, due to a defective embryological development of the third and fourth pharyngeal pouches leading to agenesis of the gland.

Pseudohypoparathyroidism is an inherited disorder resulting from mutations in the end-organ receptors, leading to a state of PTH resistance. But in contrast to hypoparathyroidism, the serum PTH levels are high.

Imaging findings

Common radiographic findings in hypoparathyroidism include localized or diffuse osteosclerosis, with thickening of facial and calvarial bones and increased bone density being the most important findings (Figure 9.26). Sutural diastasis may be present due to increased intracranial pressure. Other intracranial findings include calcification of the basal ganglia, choroid plexus, falx and cerebellum (Figure 9.27). Dental manifestations, e.g. hypoplastic dentition, failure or delay of tooth eruption and thickened lamina dura, may be seen. Subcutaneous calcifications around hips and shoulders are also seen.

It is also a cause of advanced bone age due to premature physeal fusion in contradiction to the retarded skeletal maturation noted in states of excess PTH hormone (Figure 9.28). Spinal ossification resembling diffuse idiopathic skeletal hyperostosis (DISH) or ankylosing spondylitis (occurs due to anterior and posterior longitudinal ligament calcification with osteophytes) is also a feature.

Ancillary findings may include nephrocalcinosis (Figure 9.29), and, as baseline, renal ultrasound is recommended at the commencement of therapy.

(A)

(B)

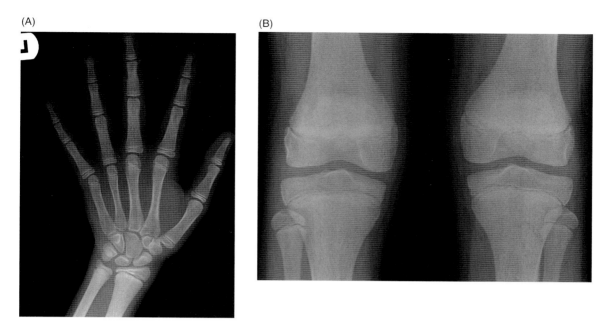

Figure 9.26 Hypoparathyroidism. Frontal radiographs of hands (A) and knees (B) reveal generalized osteosclerosis with coarsened trabeculae. Short fourth metacarpal is also seen.

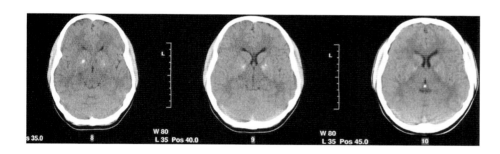

Figure 9.27 Hypoparathyroidism. Axial noncontrast CT of head reveals bilateral basal ganglia calcification.

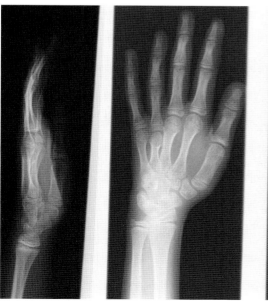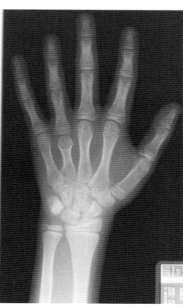

Figure 9.28 Hypoparathyroidism. Frontal, lateral and oblique views of hands reveal short fourth metacarpal and accelerated skeletal maturation.

(A)

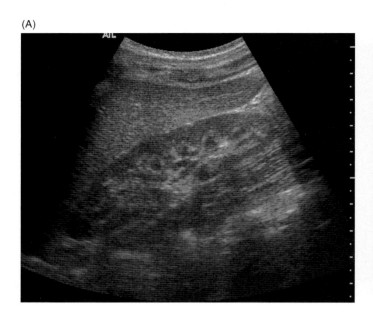

(B)

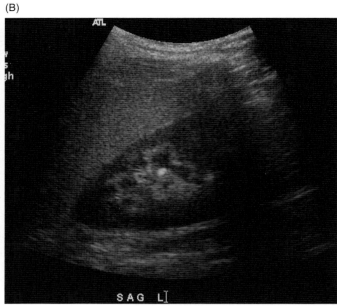

Figure 9.29 Hypoparathyroidism. Ultrasound examination of the abdomen reveals bilateral renal nephrocalcinosis with bilateral nonocclusive renal calculi.

Pseudohypoparathyroidism and pseudopseudohypoparathyroidism

Pseudohypoparathyroidism is a disorder characterized by end-organ resistance to PTH, leading to decreased serum levels of calcium and phosphorus as in idiopathic hypoparathyroidism, but with elevated PTH levels.

Some patients present with somatic features of Albright's hereditary osteodystrophy (AHO), which include short stature, obesity, brachydactyly, subcutaneous calcifications and ossifications and subnormal intelligence.

The radiographic findings in the hands include disproportionate shortening of the fourth and fifth metacarpals and distal phalanges, accompanied by punctate soft tissue and subcutaneous calcifications.

Pathophysiology

End-organ resistance at the renal tubule site of action of PTH is clinically confirmed by renal excretion of cyclic AMP and phosphorus following intravenous administration of PTH.

In contrast, pseudopseudohypoparathyroidism is characterized by somatic features of AHO but without clinical or biochemical evidence of hypoparathyroidism. Serum calcium, phosphorus and PTH levels are all normal. The radiographic findings in pseudohypoparathyroidism (PHP) or pseudopseudohypoparathyroidism (PPHP) may include soft tissue calcification and ossification, basal ganglion calcification, premature physeal fusion, metacarpal and metatarsal shortening, calvarial thickening and exostoses. Abnormalities of bone density may be seen, whether increased or decreased, along with bowing deformities of the extremities (Figures 9.30).

Hypophosphatasia (HP)

Hypophosphatasia refers to an inborn error of metabolism characterized by reduced alkaline phosphatase (which is an important catalyst of normal mineralization) in serum and tissue, leading to overall demineralization of the skeleton.

Pathophysiology

Marked clinical radiographic variability of perinatal (lethal) HP exists. Clinical manifestations include marked calvarial softening, large fontanelle, wide cranial sutures, low-set ears, depressed nasal bridge, funnel chest and short and bowed distal limbs.

Pathology

One of the biochemical hallmarks of this disease is an abnormal amount of phosphoethanolamine in urine and blood.

Imaging findings

Various manifestations include generalized absent or deficient mineralization with coarsening of trabeculae, fractures with deformities and shortening with or without metaphyseal cupping and irregularities (Figure 9.31). Subsequently, modeling defects in the long bones and spurs in the mid-portion of the ulna and fibula can also be seen.

Survivors may show bone changes similar to rickets, but characteristically demonstrate irregular, prominent lucent extensions into the metaphyses. Other radiographic findings include widened sutures and Wormian bones.

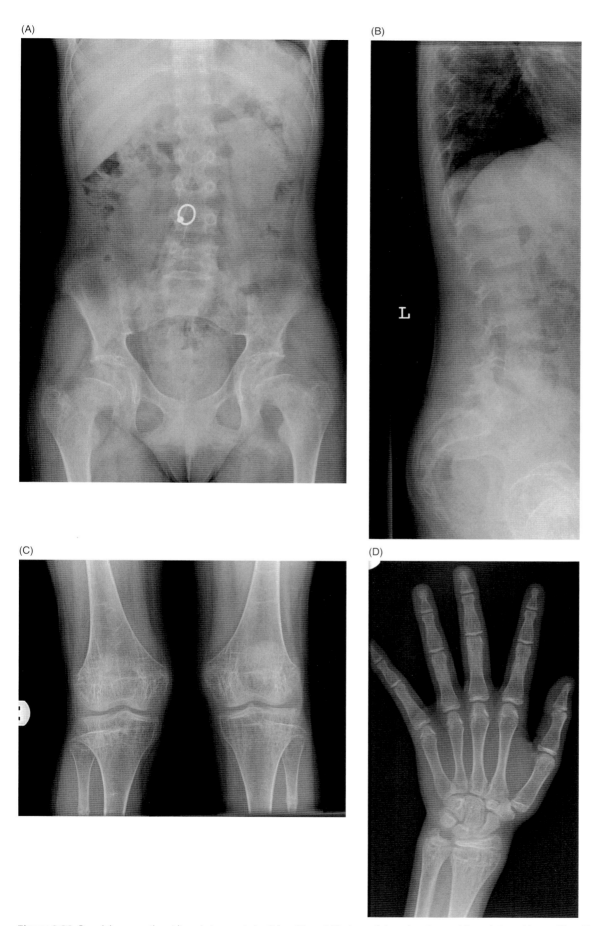

Figure 9.30 Pseudohypoparathyroidism. Anteroposterior (A) and lateral (B) views of thoracic spine, and frontal view of knees (C) and hands (D) reveal generalized osteopenia accompanied by changes of renal osteodystrophy, focal sclerosis of phalangeal epiphyses and delayed bone age.

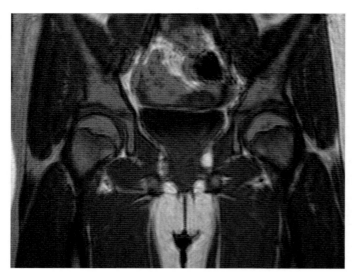

Figure 9.31 Hypophosphatasia. Coronal T2-weighted image of proximal femora and hip joints reveals decreased height of left femoral head along with inhomogeneity suggestive of avascular necrosis.

Gaucher disease

Gaucher disease is a familial storage disorder of cerebroside metabolism, leading to abnormal lipid accumulation in reticulo-endothelial cells of the body. The underlying enzymatic defect is transmitted in an autosomal recessive fashion. Clinically it is categorized into three types. Type 1 is the chronic non-neuropathic or adult type, type 2 the acute neuronopathic type, while type 3 is the subacute neuronopathic/juvenile Gaucher disease.

Pathophysiology

Gaucher disease is due to a defective enzyme, i.e. beta glucosi-dase, leading to an abnormal accumulation of a cell membrane metabolite, glucosylceramide, in lysosomes of monocyte/macrophage lineage. This is referred to as a reticulum cell, also called the "Gaucher cell" in various tissues, predominantly involving the spleen, bone marrow and lymph nodes. It is mostly seen in older infants, children and adults who suffer from the more chronic forms.

Pathology

At the cellular level, accumulation of these abnormal cells may lead to marrow infiltration, cause osteopenia, cortical thinning and subsequent fractures, modeling deformities and may also predispose to secondary superinfections.

These cells also have a tendency to accumulate in the reticuloendothelial system and affect organs like the liver, spleen and lymph nodes.

Diagnosis of Gaucher disease is made by enzyme assay, DNA analysis, bone marrow biopsy, spleen or liver biopsy or some combination of these methods. The most reliable assay is for glucocerebrosidase activity in peripheral blood leukocytes.

Imaging findings

Various radiological findings can be seen, pertaining to diffuse replacement or focal deposits within the bone marrow, fractures, avascular necrosis, remodeling deformities and superimposed infections.

Bone marrow replacement

In Gaucher disease, normal bone marrow is infiltrated by cellular elements containing foam cells. Due to diffuse bone marrow infiltration, Gaucher disease may present as increased bone lucency, cortical scalloping and thinning. These findings are typically seen in the axial skeleton and then proceed to the proximal and finally distal long bones. There is relative epiphyseal sparing. It may also have a more permeative geographic or moth-eaten appearance of osteolysis. On MRI, marrow affected by Gaucher disease demonstrates patchy or homogeneous low signal intensity on both T1- and T2-weighted sequences.

Other presentations include spinal osteopenia, compression fractures and secondary sequelae of generalized osteopenia.

Focal Gaucher deposits

Focal accumulation of Gaucher cells may result in osteolytic lesions. These are typically asymptomatic until fracture or infection supervenes. Extraosseous Gaucher disease may occur when focal marrow deposits grow large enough to violate the cortex and then they may simulate malignancies and are called "gaucheromas."

Fractures are most commonly vertebral and may lead to vertebral collapse or "vertebra plana." It may also present in the ribs and appendicular tubular bones, leading to long-standing deformities, e.g. coxa vara in the femur. Remodeling abnormalities are the most characteristic, and commonly seen features include expansion of the contour of the long tubular bones leading to a straightened or convex osseous appearance called the "Erlenmeyer flask" deformity, which is not pathognomonic, but very suggestive, of Gaucher disease.

Gaucher disease may also cause epiphyseal and diaphyseal osteonecrosis, simulating bone-within-bone or "endobone" appearance. Osteonecrosis may affect the ends of bones, and leads to collapse of the articular cortex and destruction of the adjacent joint space. It may also cause medullary necrosis that affects the shafts and metaphyses of the bones. Following an episode of infarction due to small vessel disease, the bone marrow may appear diffusely sclerotic. If larger areas are affected, it may appear as a focal lucency or partially calcified margin. During an episode of pain, CT and radiographs may remain normal, but MRI shows bright signal within the affected marrow on T2-weighted sequences.

The altered metabolic milieu predisposes to various secondary superinfections of both bone and soft tissue.

Extraskeletal imaging findings

Accumulation of glucocerebrosides in the lysosomes of visceral macrophages may cause hepatosplenomegaly (Figure 9.32),

(A)

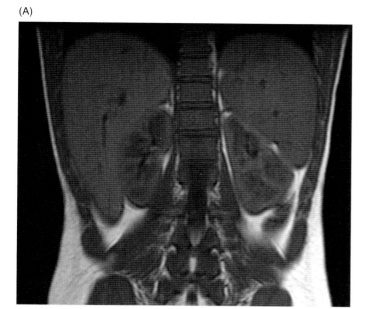

(B)

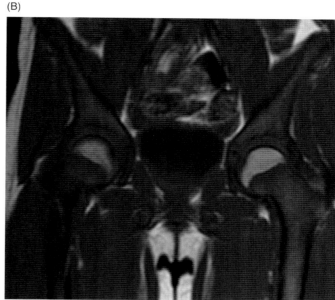

(C)

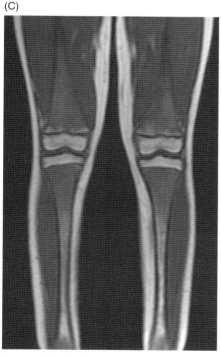

Figure 9.32 (A–C) Gaucher disease. Coronal images from MRI of abdomen and lower limbs reveal hepatosplenomegaly, and inhomogeneous reduced T1 signal of bone marrow of lower limb long bones and "Erlenmeyer flask" deformity.

anemia, thrombocytopenia, growth retardation and skeletal disease.

Soft tissue manifestations include pulmonary infiltrates and thoracic lymph node enlargement. On chest radiography, one may find reticular lung disease, while CT shows interlobular and intralobular septal thickening, pleural reaction and ground-glass opacities. Liver and spleen enlargement is almost universal (Figure 9.32), while 5% of children may have focal hepatic or splenic lesions, which may be hypo- or hyperechoic on sonography. Though cardiac involvement is rare in Gaucher disease, a few cases with pericardial involvement and mitral regurgitation due to immobile aortic and mitral valves have been reported. Brain involvement includes severe neuronopathic forms, multifocal hypoperfusion of the brain and progressive cerebral atrophy in the frontal and temporal lobes.

Hemochromatosis and hemosiderosis

Hemochromatosis is characterized by abnormal iron deposition in various tissues, and is caused by a genetic defect in metabolism leading to abnormally high gastrointestinal absorption of iron, from a variety of causes.

Hemosiderosis is a state of abnormal iron deposition in various reticuloendothelial organs of the body, secondary to causes like liver cirrhosis, multiple blood transfusions and chronic anemias.

Musculoskeletal manifestations seen in this disease spectrum include symmetric and progressive noninflammatory arthropathy, initially involving small joints of the hands followed by larger joints. Articular abnormalities are due to abnormal hemosiderin deposition and calcium pyrophosphate dehydrate (CPPD) crystal deposition.

Pathophysiology

Hemochromatosis is an autosomal recessive condition and leads to abnormal deposition of iron in the parenchyma of liver, spleen, pancreas, heart and other organs. Pancreatic involvement and subsequent insufficiency has been historically referred to as "bronze diabetes." The classic triad of hemochromatosis consists of cirrhosis, diabetes and bronze skin.

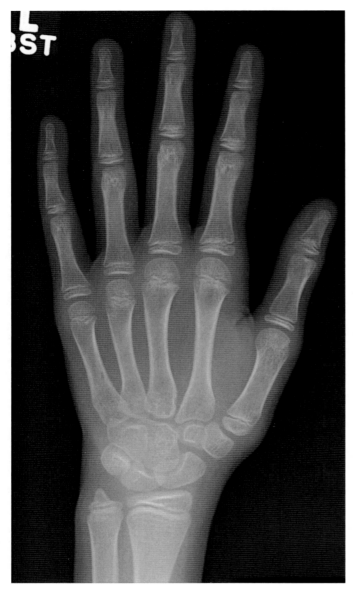

Figure 9.33 Anteroposterior radiograph showing Mild coarsening of trabecular pattern in the tubular bones of the hand.

Hemosiderosis, on the other hand, is associated with increased iron deposition in the reticuloendothelial cells (Kupffer cells) of the liver as well as other organs such as the spleen and bone marrow. It usually spares the rest of the organs and does not lead to complications, unlike hemochromatosis.

Imaging findings

Osteoporosis is mostly seen in hemochromatosis. Bones of the axial as well as appendicular skeleton may be involved. Altered metabolic state may lead to generalized osteopenia with reinforcement of the secondary trabecular pattern (Figure 9.33).

Various articular manifestations, e.g. calcification of the intervertebral disc (called chondrocalcinosis; typically seen in outer fibers of annulus fibrosus), symphysis pubis and wrist, are seen in 20–60% of cases. Synovial membrane abnormalities may include increased iron deposition (also seen in rheumatoid arthritis, degenerative disease [Figure 9.33], pigmented villonodular synovitis, hemophilia and hemarthrosis). Gross structural joint damage or arthropathy may be present in 25–50% of cases.

Some peculiar features useful for diagnosis of hemochromatosis include:

1. Unusual sites – metacarpophalangeal joints (mostly second and third), midcarpal and radiocarpal compartments, elbows and glenohumeral joints.
2. Formation of large subchondral cysts.
3. Symmetric loss of articular cartilage.
4. Joint space narrowing, bony eburnation, osteophytosis.
5. Involvement of the pancreatic parenchyma which differentiates it from hemosiderosis.
6. May lead to complications like organ fibrosis or hepatocellular carcinoma.

Hemosiderosis usually manifests as hepatosplenomegaly. The characteristic MRI appearance of a patient with iron overload in the reticuloendothelial system is low signal intensity in the liver and spleen on spin echo T2-weighted images with a normal pancreas (Figure 9.34). The affected bone marrow is low in signal and contains less fat. Extraskeletal findings pertaining to the underlying cause, such as hemolytic anemias, may also be seen, e.g. cholelithiasis (Figure 9.35). Initiation of chelation therapy may also lead to mild loss of vertebral height (Figure 9.36).

Scurvy

Scurvy refers to the clinical syndrome of deficiency of vitamin C. Clinically manifest disease is typically preceded by an asymptomatic prodrome of four to six months.

Pathophysiology

The basic defect responsible for scurvy lies in the normal cellular activity of growing bones. At the cartilage–shaft junction, proliferating cartilage cells are markedly diminished in number and rate of mitoses. On the epiphyseal side of the zone of provisional calcification, deposition of mineral continues, while, on the diaphyseal side, destruction of the same stops, disturbing this dynamic equilibrium.

Imaging findings

Radiographs show a thickened zone of provisional calcification which is not structurally strong. Being brittle, it gives way to fissures and fractures. Thus the trabeculae are disorganized; transverse fractures occur through this brittle zone, and the heavy zones of provisional calcification project beyond the diaphyseal limits, giving rise to the most typical finding, that of metaphyseal spurs. The "scurvy line" refers to atrophic

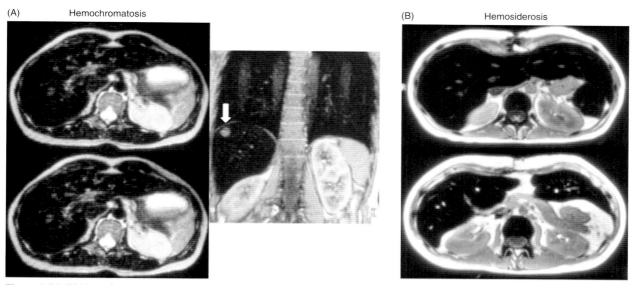

Figure 9.34 (A) Hemochromatosis: T2-weighted MR scans show iron deposition-related signal loss in liver, pancreas and heart muscle (the last not shown). A small HCC is noted on the coronal scan (arrow). (B) Hemosiderosis: T2-weighted MR scans show iron deposition-related signal loss in the reticuloendothelial system, in liver, spleen, and bone marrow.

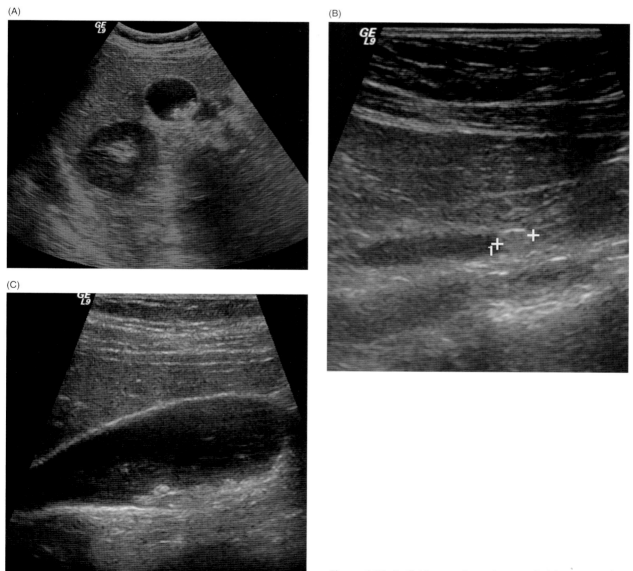

Figure 9.35 (A–C) Ultrasound examination of abdomen reveals cholelithiasis and choledocholithiasis, due to underlying hemolytic anemia.

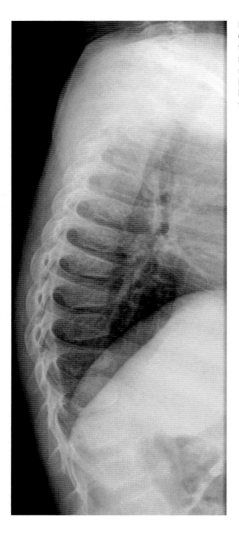

Figure 9.36 Hemosiderosis. Lateral view of thoracic spine shows anterior wedging at T10 and mild loss of vertebral height of the T11 vertebral body, following chelation therapy.

Table 9.5 Abdominal imaging features in hemochromatosis and hemosiderosis

	Liver	Spleen	Pancreas	Bone marrow
Hemosiderosis	Low signal	Low signal	Usually normal, can be reduced	Low signal
Hemochromatosis	Low signal	Normal	Low signal	Normal

Signal refers to T2 star weighted MRI sequences.
Adapted from Siegelman *et al.* (1991).

Table 9.6 Radiographic and pathological correlation of common features of scurvy

Radiographic features	Pathological finding
Transverse metaphyseal line of increased density	Prominent thickened zone of provisional calcification
Transverse metaphyseal line of decreased density – "scurvy line"	Decrease in trabeculae and detritus in junctional area of metaphysic (Trummerfeldzone)
Metaphyseal beaks or excrescences	Lateral extensions of the heavy zone of provisional calcification with periosteal elevation and stimulation
Subepiphyseal infractions (corner or angle sign)	Decreased, brittle trabeculae in junctional area, with fracture and hemorrhage
Periostitis	Subperiosteal hemorrhage with elevation and stimulation of periosteum
Epiphyseal shell of increased density with central lucency (Wimberger sign)	Prominent thickened provisional zone of calcification with atrophy of central spongiosa

bone between the heavy zone of provisional calcification and heavier spongiosa in the shaft. Subepiphyseal marginal clefts, due to incomplete separation of the physeal plate from the shaft, are also seen, referred to as the "corner" or "angle" sign. All metaphyseal changes appear earlier and are more marked in sites of rapid growth: distal end of femur, proximal end of humerus, distal ends of radius and ulna, and both ends of tibia and fibula.

Ossification centers show a thickened, peripheral rim of calcified cartilage, due to persistence of a thick zone of transition accompanied by central rarefaction – giving rise to the "Wimberger sign." Diaphyseal spongiosa becomes atrophic, causing "ground-glass" texture. Subperiosteal hemorrhage is common in long tubular bones, but may also form on flat bones of the shoulder girdle, orbit and calvarium. However, hemarthrosis is exceedingly rare.

Optimum sites for detection and evaluation of scorbutic changes are the knees and wrists, the earliest signs being generalized bony atrophy with thickened zones of provisional calcification.

Signs of healing

These are: thickening of cortex, spongiosa is clearly defined, scurvy lines disappear, and the thickened zone of calcification is buried within the shaft as a "transverse line."

Almost complete catch-up growth is seen in all adequately treated cases, with time.

Further reading

Bennett DL, El-Khoury GY Imaging hyperparathyroidism and renal osteodystrophy. In *Imaging of Arthritic and Metabolic Bone Disease*, ed. BN Weissman (Philadelphia: Saunders, 2009) pp. 642–56.

Bosch AM (2006) Classical galactosaemia revisited. *J Inherit Metab Dis* **29**(4), 516–25.

Chanson P, Salenave S (2008) Acromegaly. *Orphanet J Rare Dis* **3**, 17.

Chew FS (1991) Radiologic manifestations in the musculoskeletal system of miscellaneous endocrine disorders. *Radiol Clin North Am* **29**(1), 135–47.

El Hage S, Ghanem I, Baradhi A *et al.* (2008) Skeletal features of primary hyperoxaluria type 1, revisited. *J Child Orthop* **2**(3), 205–10.

Fregonese L, Stolk J (2008) Hereditary alpha-1-antitrypsin deficiency and its clinical consequences. *Orphanet J Rare Dis* **3**, 16.

Kottamasu SR Bone formation and metabolic bone disease. In *Caffey's Pediatric Diagnostic Imaging*, ed. JP Kuhn, TL Slovis, JO Haller (Philadelphia: Mosby, 2004) pp. 2232–68.

Pastores GM (2008) Musculoskeletal complications encountered in the lysosomal storage disorders. *Best Pract Res Clin Rheumatol* **22**(5), 937–47. Review.

Pezeshk P, Carrino JA Hypoparathyroidism and PTH resistance. In *Imaging of Arthritic and Metabolic Bone Disease*, ed. BN Weissman (Philadelphia: Saunders, 2009) pp. 657–9.

Pezeshk P, Carrino JA Rickets and osteomalacia. In *Imaging of Arthritic and Metabolic Bone Disease*, ed. BN Weissman (Philadelphia: Saunders, 2009) pp. 660–7.

Pezeshk P, Carrino JA Hypophosphatasia. In *Imaging of Arthritic and Metabolic Bone Disease*, ed. BN Weissman (Philadelphia: Saunders, 2009) pp. 668–77.

Pitt MJ Rickets and osteomalacia. In *Bone and Joint Imaging*, ed. D Resnick (Philadelphia: WB Saunders Company, 1996) pp. 511–24.

Resnick D Parathyroid disorders and renal osteodystrophy. In *Bone and Joint Imaging*, ed. D Resnick (Philadelphia: WB Saunders Company, 1996) pp. 552–71.

Siegelman ES, Mitchell DG, Rubin R *et al.* (1991) Parenchymal versus reticuloendothelial iron overload in the liver: distinction with MR imaging. *Radiology* **179**, 361–6.

Slovis TL *Caffey's Pediatric Diagnostic Imaging*, 11th edn. (St. Louis: Mosby, 2007).

Chapter

10

Skeletal dysplasias and syndromes

Keith A. Kronemer and Thomas E. Herman

The approach to the skeletal dysplasias and syndromes taken here is based primarily on radiographic findings, with the addition of pertinent clinical data, including inheritance patterns. Owing to a rapidly expanding knowledge of the human genome, a chromosomal map classification of skeletal dysplasias and syndromes is increasingly valuable. However, because some osteochondrodysplasias do not yet have a confirmed genetic locus, a workable chromosomal classification of these conditions does not exist.

Achondroplasia group

The achondroplasia group can also be called the FGFR 3 disorders. These are conditions including achondroplasia with mutations in the *FGFR 3* (fibroblast growth factor receptor 3) gene located at genetic locus 4p16.

Thanatophoric dysplasia

Affected children are usually stillborn or die shortly after birth owing to hypoplastic lungs. The fetus or infant has marked short-limbed dwarfism, a large head with frontal bossing, and a depressed nasal bridge. Numerous skinfolds are present. The child has a relatively long trunk.

Radiographic findings include marked rhizomelic shortening of the long bones with metaphyseal flaring and osseous bowing and widening. Pronounced flattening of the vertebral bodies, with more constriction of their mid-portions and wide intervertebral disc spaces, is evident, giving the appearance of an inverted U or H to each vertebra on frontal radiographs. The thorax is slender, owing to short ribs with flared anterior ends. Small, rectangular iliac bones, small sacroiliac notches and short, wide pubic and ischial bones are seen (Figure 10.1).

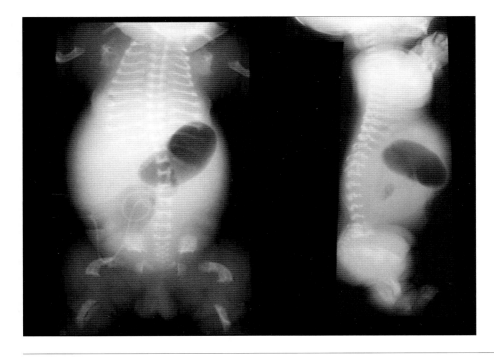

Figure 10.1 Thanatophoric dysplasia: frontal and lateral radiographs of the chest and abdomen in a stillborn infant after attempted resuscitation. Diffuse platyspondyly is present. The square iliac bones are seen with small sacrosciatic notches. The femurs have a characteristic telephone-receiver appearance. Striking micromelia is present.

Essentials of Pediatric Radiology, ed. Heike E. Daldrup-Link and Charles A. Gooding. Published by Cambridge University Press.
© Cambridge University Press 2010.

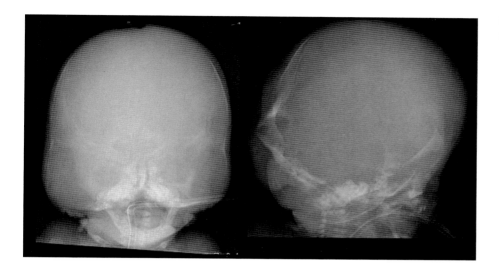

Figure 10.2 Thanatophoric dysplasia: thanatophoric dwarf with cloverleaf skull.

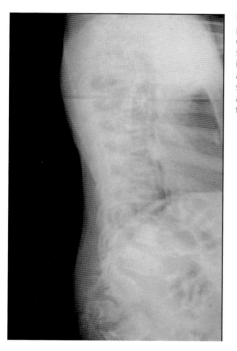

Figure 10.3 Achondroplasia: lateral radiograph of the thoracolumbar spine. L1 vertebral body is abnormal with marked anterior hypoplasia, with significant retrolisthesis and resulting in a low thoracolumbar kyphosis.

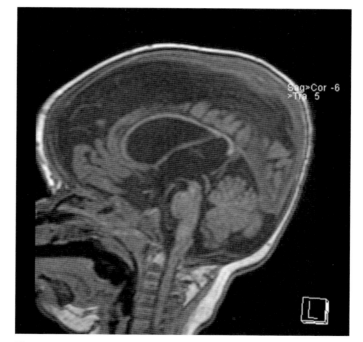

Figure 10.4 Achondroplasia: sagittal T1-weighted image of the brain of a three-month-old infant. There is macrocrania with prominent ventricles and subarachnoid spaces, but a very narrow cranial base and foramen magnum.

The phalanges are short, relatively broad, and cupped. The base of the skull is short, and the foramen magnum is small. A cloverleaf skull may be seen (Figure 10.2).

Classic (heterozygous) achondroplasia

Classic achondroplasia, a relatively common type of dwarfism of autosomal dominant inheritance, is evident at birth. Clinical manifestations include short limbs, especially of the proximal portions (rhizomelic micromelia); a large head, with a prominent forehead and a depressed nasal bridge; thoracolumbar kyphosis in infancy (Figure 10.3); and exaggerated lumbar lordosis, with prominent buttocks in children and adults. The hands are stubby and trident. Because of the constricted basicranium, foramen magnum and spinal canal, persons with

achondroplasia may develop compression of the spinal cord, lower brain stem, cauda equina and nerve roots at any age.

Radiographic findings include a large cranium and a small foramen magnum (Figure 10.4). The interpediculate distances of the lower lumbar vertebrae, which normally increase proceeding distally, remain the same at all levels or decrease in the lower lumbar region. The pedicles are short, the backs of the vertebral bodies are often concave, and the spinal canal is small. The vertebral bodies are flattened and appear bullet shaped in infancy and early childhood. The iliac bones are squared, with small sacrosciatic notches and flat acetabular angles (Figure 10.5). Shortening of

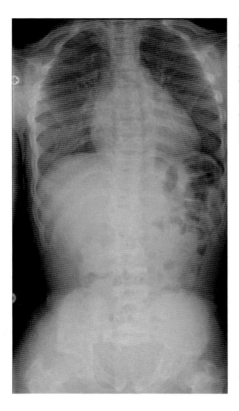

Figure 10.5 Achondroplasia: frontal radiograph of the chest, abdomen and pelvis. Lumbar stenosis with narrowed interpedicular distance with small iliac wings is present. There is also a champagne-glass configuration to the true pelvis with small sacrosciatic notches.

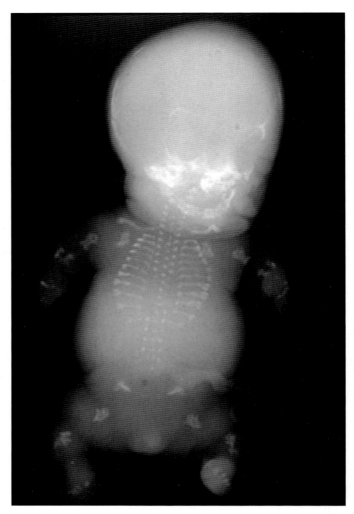

Figure 10.6 Achondrogenesis type I: frontal radiograph of stillborn infant with type I achondrogenesis shows a poorly ossified pelvis, spine and marked limb shortening.

the tubular bones, especially the proximal ones, and metaphyseal flaring are seen. The fibulae may be long. Shortening of the tubular bones in the hands and feet is evident. The ribs are shortened.

Hypochondroplasia

Hypochondroplasia, an autosomal dominant disorder has clinical and radiographic findings similar but less severe than those of achondroplasia. Radiographic findings include narrowing of the interpediculate distances distally and exaggerated posterior concavity of vertebral bodies in the lumbar region, mild platyspondyly, small spinal canals, shortening of the tubular bones, and a short, broad femoral neck. Mild metaphyseal flaring occurs. The iliac bones are shortened, with flattened acetabular roofs and small sciatic notches. The fibulae may be slightly long, and the distal ends of the ulnae are short, with prominent ulnar styloid processes.

Achondrogenesis group

This group can also be called the COL2A1 and SLC26A2 disorders. These are disorders of cartilage formation. The *COL2A1* (collagen type 2, alpha 1) gene at gene locus 12q13.11 is responsible for producing the collagen that is present in cartilage. The *SLC26A2* (solute carrier 26, A2) gene located at gene locus 5q31–q34 is responsible for cartilage formation.

Achondrogenesis/hypochondrogenesis

Achondrogenesis is characterized by a disproportionately large head, short trunk, protuberant abdomen, severe micromelia,

and hydrops. It has been divided into types I and II. Type I (Figure 10.6) is subdivided into IA (Houston-Harris) with rib fractures and IB (Fraccaro) without rib fractures. Type II (Langer-Saldino), or hypochondrogenesis (Figure 10.7), represents the severe end of the spondyloepiphyseal dysplasia congenita spectrum. The gene mutation in achondrogenesis type IA is not known; type IB has a mutation in the *SLC26A2* gene, and type II in the *COL2A1* gene.

Radiographic findings common to both types include severe lack of ossification of the vertebral bodies (especially caudally); small, deformed iliac bones; absent or poor ossification of the pubic and ischial bones, calcaneus and talus; tubular bones that are strikingly short and malformed, with wide, cupped ends; and short ribs with cupped and flared ends.

Spondyloepiphyseal dysplasia congenita

This short-trunk dwarfism is characterized by mild shortening of the limbs, flat face, cleft palate, short neck, increased

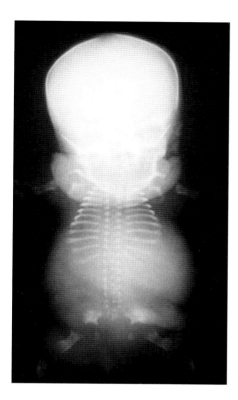

Figure 10.7 Achondrogenesis type II: frontal radiograph of entire stillborn infant. Normal calvarial ossification, and better spinal and pelvic ossification than in type I. Marked micromelia.

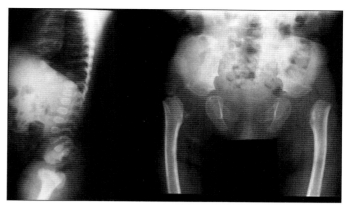

Figure 10.8 Spondyloepiphyseal dysplasia congenita: lateral radiograph of the lumbar spine and frontal radiograph of the pelvis. The vertebral bodies have a somewhat oval appearance, and platyspondyly in the lower lumbar region. There is characteristic absent ossification of the femoral heads and almost absent ossification of the femoral necks.

anteroposterior chest diameter, and joint restriction. Patients develop progressive kyphoscoliosis, dorsal kyphosis, or lumbar lordosis. The hands and feet are often normal except for the presence of equinovarus deformity. Important additional features include myopia and retinal detachment, which can lead to blindness, and atlantoaxial instability. The pattern of inheritance is usually autosomal dominant. Spondyloepiphyseal dysplasia (SED) congenita is caused by various mutations in the COL2A1 gene.

Radiographic findings include a decreased height of the vertebral bodies and, in infancy, pear-shaped vertebrae. In childhood, anterior wedging, irregularity and generalized flattening of the vertebral bodies occur. The interpediculate distances in the lower lumbar vertebrae may be narrowed. Hypoplasia of the odontoid process may be associated with atlantoaxial dislocation. Typical radiographic findings include a marked delay in the ossification of the pubic bones and proximal portion of the femora. The femoral heads often ossify from multiple centers, and a progressive coxa vara develops, with premature osteoarthritis. The long tubular bones have delayed epiphyseal ossification, with irregular epiphyses, and metaphyseal irregularity and flaring (Figure 10.8).

Diastrophic dysplasia

Diastrophic dysplasia is characterized by the short stature, progressive scoliosis and kyphosis, clubfeet, multiple contractures and dislocations, and distinctive abnormalities of the hands, feet and ears. In addition to short and broad hands and feet, the thumbs and great toes may be held in a hitchhiker's position. The ear lobes are deformed from cystic masses appearing in the first few months of life. A cleft palate is common. Diastrophic dysplasia is caused by various mutations in the SLC26A2 gene.

Radiographic findings include marked shortening of the tubular bones with metaphyseal widening and rounding. The epiphyses are delayed in appearance, especially the proximal femoral epiphysis, and are flattened and deformed. Flattening is particularly marked in the outer portion of the distal femoral epiphysis. The tibial ossification center in infancy is located medially. Disproportionate shortening of the ulna and the fibula occurs. The radial heads may be dislocated. The bones of the hands and feet are small, especially the first metacarpal, which may be round or oval. The epiphyses in the hands may be irregular, distorted and wide. The carpal bones may ossify prematurely, appear deformed, or reveal accessory ossification centers. The feet show similar findings in addition to equinovarus deformity. The most common finding in the foot is hindfoot valgus deformity and metatarsus adductus. Femora may have broad intertrochanteric regions with short femoral necks. Scoliosis sometimes is evident at or soon after birth and tends to be progressive and rigid. The cervical vertebrae may reveal defective development, which can lead to kyphosis, spinal instability and cord compression. Calcification of the pinna of the ear and airway cartilages is sometimes seen.

Metatropic dysplasia

Metatropic dysplasia is characterized by short extremities and a normal or elongated trunk at birth and by a short trunk with kyphoscoliosis later in life. At birth, the ends of the long tubular bones are prominent, and the joint movement is limited. In infancy, the thorax appears to be long and narrow; a small, soft tissue fold resembling a tail may be present over the sacrum.

The tubular bones of the extremities are short and have marked metaphyseal widening, resembling a trumpet or dumbbell

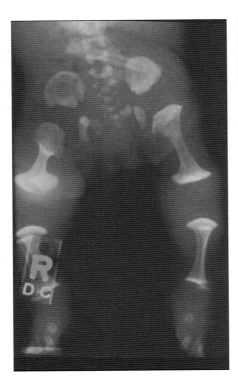

Figure 10.9 Metatropic dysplasia: very broad metaphyses are present with dumbbell configuration particularly of the femurs.

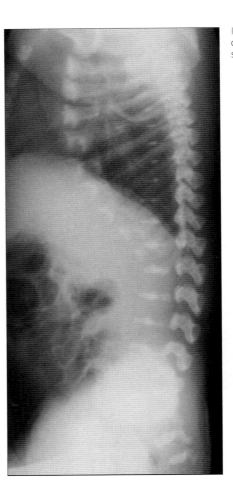

Figure 10.10 Metatropic dysplasia: marked platyspondyly is present.

(Figure 10.9). The trochanters are particularly large, typically the lesser trochanter, and the appearance simulates that of a battle-ax, especially in infancy. The appearance of the epiphyses is delayed, and they are small, flat and deformed. The vertebral bodies are rectangular or diamond-shaped in infancy and markedly reduced in height, and the intervertebral disc spaces appear large (Figure 10.10). The pelvis is characterized by shortened ilia with curved lateral margins, flat acetabular roofs, and small sacrosciatic and lateral iliac notches. In infancy, the thorax is elongated and has a decreased anteroposterior diameter as a consequence of the short ribs. The tubular bones of the hands and feet have metaphyseal expansion and delayed and irregular epiphyseal ossification. The carpal and tarsal bones are also irregular, with delayed ossification.

Asphyxiating thoracic dystrophy (Jeune syndrome)

Initial reports of this autosomal recessive condition described infants with constricted chests and mild shortening of the extremities who died from pulmonary hypoplasia. Later reports included patients with less severe respiratory symptoms, although those who survive to childhood have a progressive nephritis. Asphyxiating thoracic dystrophy is due to various mutations in the *IFT80* gene (intraflagellar transport 80 homolog gene) at gene locus 3q26.1. This gene is concerned with proteins for normal cilia. It is unclear how this gene mutation results in the skeletal and hepatorenal manifestations.

The radiographic features are a narrow thorax and short, horizontally oriented ribs with wide, irregular costochondral junctions (Figure 10.11). The clavicles may have a high, handlebar appearance. The neonatal pelvic findings are short iliac, pubic and ischial bones, with the lateral borders of the ilia being rounded. The acetabular roofs are flat, with downward spike-link projections at the medial, lateral and sometimes central aspects of the acetabulum. The pelvis normalizes with age, but the proximal femoral metaphyses may become progressively irregular. Infants have mild digital shortening, especially in the distal phalanges, and inconstant polydactyly. There may be cone-shaped epiphyses that fuse prematurely.

Asphyxiating thoracic dystrophy has similar features to chondroectodermal dysplasia, but has a higher prevalence of progressive renal disease, hepatic fibrosis, less prominent nail changes, and less frequent polydactyly.

Chondroectodermal dysplasia (Ellis-van Creveld dysplasia)

Ellis-van Creveld dysplasia, a short-limbed dwarfism, is characterized by ectodermal dysplasia, polydactyly and congenital heart disease. The condition is inherited as an autosomal recessive trait and is evident at birth. The disease is due to

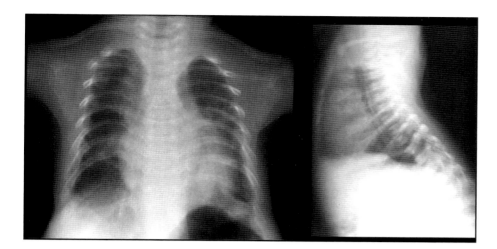

Figure 10.11 Jeune syndrome: frontal and lateral radiographs of chest. Hypoplastic ribs extending only laterally with relative cardiomegaly and thoracic hypoplasia are shown. A bicycle handlebar configuration of the clavicles is present.

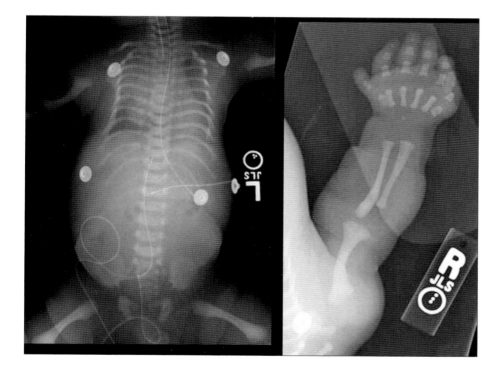

Figure 10.12 Ellis-van Creveld syndrome: frontal radiograph of the chest and abdomen and frontal radiograph of the right upper extremity. Short ribs are present, producing a conical, small thorax. The iliac wings are small with a trident configuration. Post-axial polydactyly is present in the hand.

mutations in the two Ellis-van Creveld genes *EVC* and *EVC2*, located at 4p16 and 4p16.2 respectively. Short stature, distal shortening of limbs, polydactyly (especially in the hands), absent or hypoplastic fingernails or toenails, dysplastic teeth, and upper lip abnormalities are common findings. Cardiac defects, renal abnormalities and hydrocephalus may be seen. In addition, some patients have shortening of the tubular bones (especially the phalanges), carpal fusion, an extra carpal bone, cone-shaped epiphyses, enlargement of the proximal end of the ulna and distal end of the radius (drumstick appearance), and anterior dislocation of the radial heads. A wider but hypoplastic lateral aspect of the proximal end of the tibia, medial tibial diaphyseal exostoses, genu valgum and fibular shortening are typical (Figure 10.12).

Pseudoachondroplasia

Pseudoachondroplasia is a type of short-stature dwarfism that clinically resembles achondroplasia, except for a normal-appearing head. The hands and feet are shorter than those seen in true achondroplasia. The disorder is due to mutations in the *COMP* gene (cartilage oligomeric protein gene) located at gene locus 19q31.

Radiographic findings become apparent in late infancy and are modified throughout childhood. Initially, the epiphyses are small and flattened, and the metaphyses are wide. In adults, the tubular bones are short and expanded at their ends. The epiphyses remain abnormal, and premature degenerative arthritis develops as the metaphyseal irregularity resolves

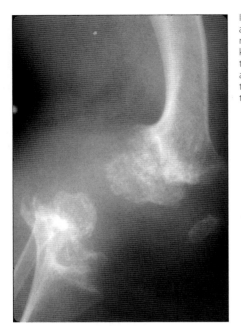

Figure 10.13 Pseudo-achondroplasia: lateral radiograph of the right knee. Severe fragmentation of the metaphyses and epiphyses of the distal femur and proximal tibia are present.

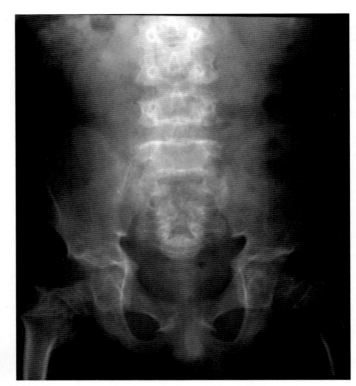

Figure 10.14 Pseudoachondroplasia: frontal radiograph of the pelvis and hips. The metaphyses and epiphyses of the proximal femurs are fragmented. The hips are varus.

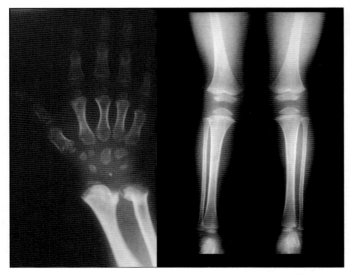

Figure 10.15 Multiple epiphyseal dysplasia: frontal radiographs of the hand and lower extremities. All of the epiphyses are small and flattened. The apparent deformity of the distal radius and ulna is due to flexion of the wrist. The metaphyses are normal.

(Figure 10.13). The vertebral bodies are initially oval or biconvex, with central tongue-like anterior projections; later they become wedged or flattened, but the vertebral bodies can have a more normal appearance in adulthood. The inferior border of the ilium has a sloping acetabular angle and a spiked appearance. The iliac wings may be slightly underdeveloped. There is coxa vara and deformity of the femoral heads (Figure 10.14).

Multiple epiphyseal dysplasia

The autosomal dominant disorders have been divided into Ribbing (hip) and Fairbanks (long bones). The appearance of the former resembles bilateral Legg–Perthes. In the latter, all the long bones show epiphyses that are small, fragmented, flattened and delayed. The carpals and tarsals are small (Figure 10.15). There may be a "double" patella with another form of the disease. Degenerative joint disease is the result, and the spine may show multiple Schmorl's nodes. This disorder, like pseudoachondroplasia, is due to mutations in the *COMP* gene.

Chondrodysplasia punctata (stippled epiphyses)

There is variability of the clinical findings and associated disorders in patients with stippled epiphyses, leading to multiple subtypes. We will discuss two.

Rhizomelic type

The rhizomelic type, the most clearly recognized type, is an autosomal recessive disorder that is characterized by marked rhizomelic shortening of the extremities, a flat face, a depressed nasal bridge, microcephaly, lymphedema of the cheeks, psychomotor retardation, cataracts and joint contractures. Most infants die from failure to thrive or from recurrent infections. Rhizomelic chondrodysplasia punctata is a peroxisomal disorder caused by mutations in the *PEX7* gene (peroxisome biogenesis factor 7) located at gene locus 6q22.

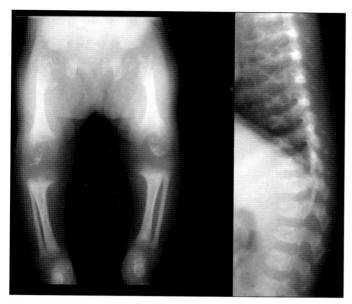

Figure 10.16 Chondrodysplasia punctata: frontal radiograph of both lower extremities and lateral radiograph of the lumbar spine. Punctate calcifications are seen in the patella, proximal femurs and vertebral spinous processes, as well as coronal cleft vertebral bodies. Slight rhizomelic shortening is present in the lower extremities with a relatively shortened femur.

Radiographic findings include severe, symmetric rhizomelic shortening of the tubular bones, with metaphyseal splaying and abundant stippled calcification in the ends of the long bones (Figure 10.16). Epiphyseal ossification is delayed. Calcifications are seen adjacent to the spine, especially in the cervical and sacral regions, and adjacent to the pubic, ischial, tarsal and carpal bones, patellae and ribs. The airway can be narrowed by abnormal calcification in the laryngeal and tracheal cartilages. Lateral radiographs of the spine show anterior and posterior ossification centers separated by a lucent band, so-called coronal cleft. The vertebral bodies are irregular, and kyphoscoliosis may develop. The iliac wings lack normal flaring. The stippling tends to resolve, especially in the patients who survive beyond infancy, and the bones become more osteopenic.

Conradi-Hünermann or Conradi's type

The Conradi-Hünermann form, also called Conradi's type, is autosomal dominant in its inheritance pattern. It may be apparent at birth, owing to facial characteristics. Some degree of limb shortening occurs in the majority of patients but may be asymmetric. Limitation of articular motion and joint contractures are common. Other findings include clubfeet, dislocated hips, genu valgum, kyphoscoliosis and short stature. Cutaneous manifestations of the disease are present in approximately 20% of patients; these include cutaneous thickening and scaling, an orange-peel appearance of the skin, sparse eyebrows and eyelashes, and alopecia. Congenital cardiac malformations are found in approximately 10% of the patients.

Radiographic findings consist of calcific deposits in and around epiphyses and other cartilaginous areas, such as the

trachea. These calcifications often resolve by early childhood. Areas that are commonly involved include the acetabulum, proximal portion of the femur, patella, spine, and carpal and tarsal bones. Shortening of the long tubular bones in a unilateral or bilateral distribution is seen. The metaphyseal regions appear normal. In addition to stippling, the spine may show scoliosis, which may be partly attributable to limb shortening. Coronal cleft vertebrae are infrequent. In more severe cases, epiphyseal dysplasia and early degenerative changes are often evident.

Epiphyseal stippling can also be found in infants born to mothers taking warfarin sodium or phenytoin and in patients with the fetal alcohol syndrome, chromosomal abnormalities, prenatal rubella infection, the CHILD syndrome (congenital hemidysplasia with ichthyosiform nevus and limb defects), and Zellweger syndrome. The last-mentioned disorder is characterized by manifestations that include craniofacial dysmorphism, profound hypotonia, dysgenesis of the brain, renal cortical cysts, and soft tissue calcifications, especially about the patella and hip.

Metaphyseal dysplasias

The term metaphyseal dysplasia applies to a number of conditions in which the greatest involvement occurs in the metaphyses, which are flared and irregular; the epiphyses and diaphyses may also be abnormal, however. The spine is normal or involved minimally. There are several types, the most common of which are discussed here.

Jansen's type

The Jansen type of metaphyseal dysplasia is a rare but severe disorder characterized by marked dwarfism, swelling of the joints, and bowed forearms and legs. In infancy, radiographs reveal marked irregularity of the metaphyses, widening of the growth plates, diffuse osteopenia, and mild bowing of the long tubular bones. The metaphyseal changes are also apparent in the short tubular bones. In childhood, the metaphyses become cupped, with wide zones of irregular calcification that eventually disappear as the growth plate closes in adulthood. The resultant bones are shortened and bowed and have metaphyseal flaring. The spine shows minimal platyspondyly, and the anterior ends of the ribs are flared.

Schmid's type

These patients have short stature of variable severity and bowed legs; the disorder usually manifests after infancy. Radiographically, metaphyseal irregularity, flaring, and growth plate widening are present, most obviously about the knees and hips. Proximal femoral metaphyseal involvement with resultant coxa vara is common (Figure 10.17).

McKusick's type

This metaphyseal dysplasia is called cartilage-hair hypoplasia. Patients are of normal intelligence and are very short; they

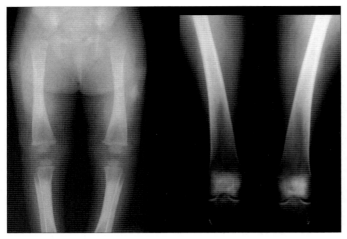

Figure 10.17 Metaphyseal dysplasia: frontal radiographs of bilateral femurs at 1 year and at 15 years. Metaphyseal broadening is present, producing an Erlenmeyer flask-like deformity to the long bones, more pronounced on the later radiograph. The thin cortices of the metaphyses produce lucent metaphyses, somewhat more marked at the younger age.

have fine, light-colored hair, small hands, bowed legs and joint laxity. Complex immune deficiencies are seen. Radiographic findings include minimal epiphyseal flattening with metaphyseal cupping and flaring. Metaphyseal abnormalities are most prominent in the lower extremities and, when severe, are associated with a short stature. The bones in the hands and feet are small, and the carpal bones appear irregular. The vertebral bodies are small. Additional vertebral abnormalities include atlantoaxial subluxation with odontoid hypoplasia. This disorder is due to a mutation in the *RMRP* gene (RNA component of mitochondrial RNA processing endoribonuclease) located at gene locus 9q21.

Dyschondrosteosis

Dyschondrosteosis, also called Léri-Weill syndrome, is characterized by a mild mesomelic type of limb shortening with Madelung's deformity of the forearm. The term mesomelic indicates that limb shortening results primarily from changes in the forearms and lower legs. The inheritance pattern is autosomal dominant, and the disease expresses itself more frequently and more severely in female patients. Radiographic findings include a shortened radius that is bowed dorsally and laterally, and a distal segment of the ulna that is often subluxed or dislocated dorsally. Lack of development of the distal radial epiphysis, with premature fusion of the medial side of the physis, is the most characteristic finding in dyschondrosteosis. The carpal bones fit into the resulting V-shaped deformity of the radius and ulna. Dyschondrosteosis is due to mutations in the *SHOX* gene (short stature homeobox gene) located at gene locus Xpter-p22.32.

Cleidocranial dysplasia

Cleidocranial dysplasia, an autosomal dominant disorder with high penetrance, has a wide range of clinical manifestations.

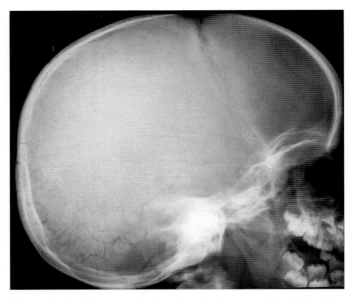

Figure 10.18 Cleidocranial dysplasia: lateral radiograph of the skull in eight-year-old male with multiple Wormian bones along lambdoid sutures, and a persistent large anterior fontanelle.

The head is large and brachycephalic, with a small face and bossing of the frontal and parietal bones. The sutures are wide, and their closure delayed (Figure 10.18). Genu valgum and short fingers may be seen. Cleidocranial dysplasia is due to mutations in the *RUNX2* gene (runt related transcription factor 2) located at gene locus 6p21.

Radiographic findings include poor ossification of the skull, with wide sutures and multiple Wormian bones (Figure 10.19). Parietal bone ossification may be absent at birth. The mandible may be broad, with persistence of its synchondrosis. Although total clavicular absence is uncommon, any portion of the clavicle may be absent; the middle or outer portion is affected most commonly. The scapula is hypoplastic, with a small glenoid cavity, and the thorax may be bell shaped, especially in patients with more severe clavicular abnormalities. Pelvic alterations consist of a delay in ossification of the pubic bones, a wide symphysis pubis, and narrow iliac wings (Figure 10.20). Coxa valga deformity is frequent, unilateral or bilateral coxa vara deformity may develop. The spinal changes consist primarily of spina bifida occulta. The findings in the hand include small, tapered distal phalanges; slightly small middle phalanges; pseudo epiphyses in the metacarpal bones; cone-shaped epiphyses; and retarded ossification of the carpal bones.

Osteodysplasty (Melnick-Needles syndrome)

The clinical appearance of affected patients is characteristic. Typically, the face is small, with large ears, protruding eyes, micrognathia and malaligned teeth; the upper portions of the arms are short, and the thorax is narrow. The inheritance pattern of the disorder is X-linked autosomal dominant, and it is lethal in most male subjects.

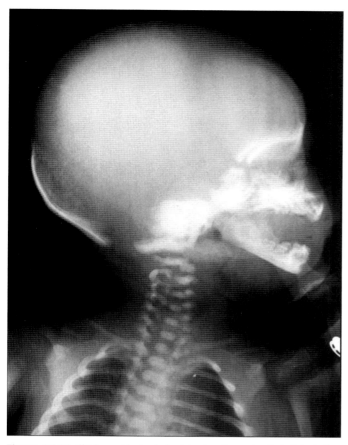

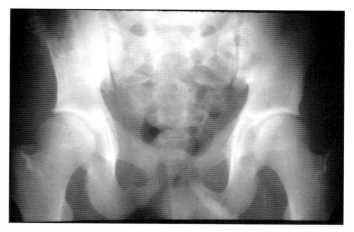

Figure 10.20 Cleidocranial dysplasia: frontal radiograph of the pelvis in a 15-year-old male. Poor ossification of the symphysis pubis is present.

Figure 10.19 Cleidocranial dysplasia: lateral radiograph of skull including frontal view of the clavicles. The sutures are widely patent with multiple Wormian bones in the lambdoid sutures. The lateral third of the clavicles is hypoplastic and not united to the medial clavicles.

Radiographically, the cortex of the tubular bones is irregular, with an undulating contour and multiple constrictions of the medullary cavities. Lateral bowing of the tibia is typical. The ribs have a ribbon-like appearance and cortical irregularity. The normal curvature of the clavicle is accentuated, and it may have cortical irregularity and wide medial ends. Sclerosis appears at the base of the skull and mastoid bones, and the anterior portion of the cranial fossa is small. The mandible is thin and small, with an obtuse angle and hypoplastic coronoid processes. In the spine, the vertebral bodies show an increased height and anterior concavity; in the lumbar region, the spinal canal may be enlarged, and the laminae appear thinned. Scoliosis or kyphoscoliosis can occur. The disorder is due to a mutation in the *FLNA* gene (filamin A alpha) located at gene locus Xq28.

Osteogenesis imperfecta

This dysplasia has a type 1 collagen abnormality and is generally broken down into five types. Type II is the severe form seen in utero, and is lethal (Figure 10.21). The skull has poor ossification and Wormian bones. The chest is small and shows ribs that may have multiple fractures (Figure 10.22). The spine

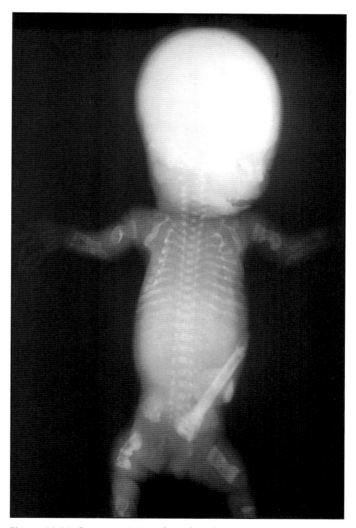

Figure 10.21 Osteogenesis imperfecta: frontal radiograph of entire stillborn infant with type II OI. Beaded ribs and shortened, fractured, concertina-like femurs are seen. Poor calvarial ossification is also noted.

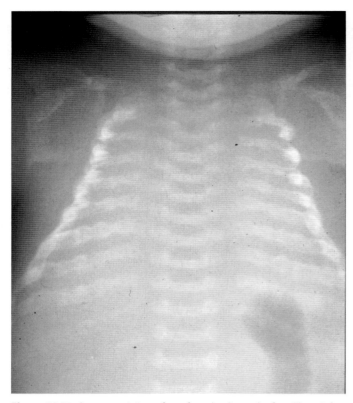

Figure 10.22 Osteogenesis imperfecta: frontal radiograph of a stillborn infant with type II OI. There are fractures of the ribs producing a beaded appearance.

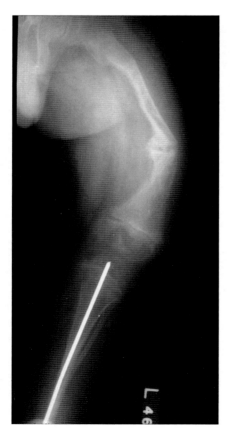

Figure 10.24 Osteogenesis imperfecta: frontal radiograph of the left leg. There is a healing fracture of the left mid-femur. The tibia is internally fixed from prior fracture. The bones are diffusely osteopenic.

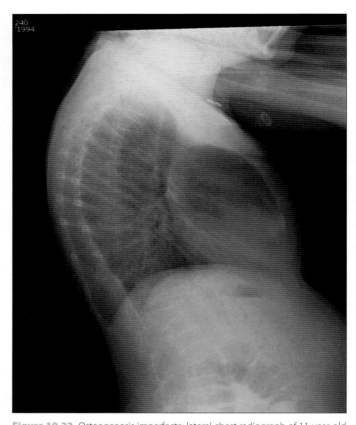

Figure 10.23 Osteogenesis imperfecta: lateral chest radiograph of 11-year-old with type I OI. The vertebral bodies are osteopenic with compression fractures.

has multiple compression fractures. The extremities have multiple fractures and can be thin or accordion-like with wide bones, especially the femurs. Other milder forms of osteogenesis imperfecta (OI) such as type I may show generalized osteoporosis, Wormian bones, vertebral collapse (Figure 10.23), thin tubular bones, bowing (Figure 10.24), rib fractures (Figure 10.25) and hyperplastic callus (type V). Almost all types of OI are due to mutations in the *COL1A1* gene (collagen type 1 alpha 1) located at gene locus 17q21.3 or the *COL1A2* gene (collagen type 1, alpha 2) located at gene locus 7q22.1. Type 1 collagen is involved in formation of normal bone osteoid and normal sclera.

Osteopetrosis

Osteopetrosis is a complex disease with at least four different types that have distinct features.

Autosomal recessive malignant type

The precocious type of osteopetrosis is an autosomal recessive form, also called the lethal form; however, some patients survive for a number of years. Clinical abnormalities include failure to thrive, hepatosplenomegaly, and cranial nerve dysfunction, especially blindness and deafness. The head may be large owing to hydrocephalus. Obliteration of the marrow cavity by abnormal bone leads to anemia and thrombocytopenia and predisposes to recurrent infections, with early death occurring

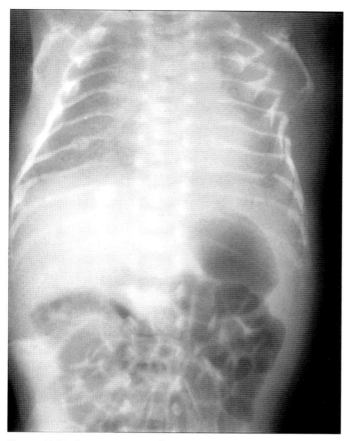

Figure 10.25 Osteogenesis imperfecta: frontal radiograph of the chest in a newborn infant with type III OI. The ribs are thin, osteopenic with multiple fractures, some acute while others are healing. There is post-traumatic deformity of both scapulae.

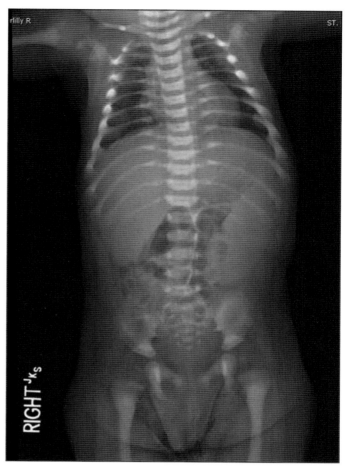

Figure 10.26 Osteopetrosis recessive type: frontal radiograph of the chest and abdomen in an infant with autosomal recessive osteopetrosis. The bones are sclerotic with metaphyseal lucency and rickets-like appearance. Splenomegaly is also present.

in most patients. There are multiple gene mutations in various sites accounting for some heterogeneity.

The radiographic findings are characterized by generalized osteosclerosis (Figure 10.26). Tubular bones show a failure of differentiation between the cortex and the medullary cavity. Modeling in these bones is defective and may lead to a club-like appearance. There may be longitudinal striations and "bone-within-bone" (or "endobone") appearance, which is characteristic. Periostitis may be seen, particularly in infants, and fractures, which generally heal, are common. The entire skull is involved, but the cartilaginous portion at its base is affected most frequently and severely. The teeth may be malformed, and the mastoid regions and paranasal sinuses are poorly developed. In the spine, the vertebral bodies tend to be uniformly radiodense, with a prominent anterior vascular notch. There may be a form called petro rickets in which there are rickets-like changes (Figure 10.27).

Autosomal dominant type

The delayed type, an autosomal dominant variety of osteopetrosis, is also called Albers-Schönberg disease. Affected persons

may be relatively asymptomatic. The disease may be detected because of a pathological fracture, problems after tooth extraction, mild anemia, or cranial nerve palsies. The radiographic findings are similar to, but less severe than, those in the precocious form of the disease. The bones are diffusely osteosclerotic, with defective tubulation and a thickened cortex (Figure 10.28). The vertebral endplates become accentuated, especially with advancing age (Figure 10.29). A "bone-within-bone" appearance or radiolucent bands in the ends of the diaphyses are sometimes seen. Type 1 autosomal dominant (with calvarial sclerosis but without a rugger-jersey spine) osteopetrosis is due to mutations in the *LRP5* gene (low density lipoprotein receptor related protein 5) located at locus 11q13. Type 2, with a rugger-jersey spine, is due to mutation in the *CLCN7* gene (chloride channel 7) located at 16p13.

Autosomal recessive intermediate

A milder, recessive form of osteopetrosis is distinct from both the more severe recessive form seen in infants and the less severe autosomal dominant form. Affected patients are often

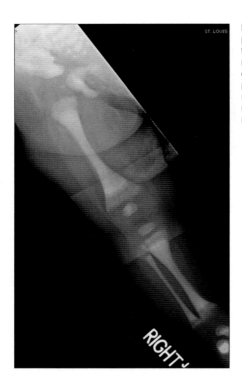

Figure 10.27 Osteopetrosis recessive type: frontal radiograph of the right lower extremity. Sclerosis of the pelvis and diaphyses is present with metaphyseal lucency and rickets-like changes in the metaphyses.

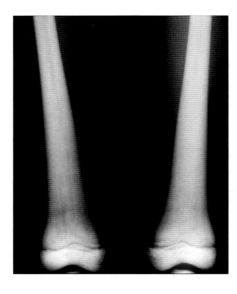

Figure 10.28 Osteopetrosis dominant type: frontal radiographs of the distal femurs. There is diffuse sclerosis of the bones without cortical–medullary distinction and an Erlenmeyer flask deformity.

of short stature, with pathological fractures, anemia and hepatomegaly. The radiographic findings are characterized by diffuse bone sclerosis, interference with normal bone modeling, a "bone-within-bone" appearance, and retained primary and impacted permanent teeth.

Tubular acidosis type

This variety, also called "marble brain" disease or Sly's disease, consists of osteopetrosis, renal tubular acidosis and cerebral calcifications. Radiographic findings are detected throughout the skeleton and include osteosclerosis, obliteration of the medullary cavity, and pathological fractures. An unusual aspect of this disease is the occurrence of progressive improvement in the radiographic abnormalities. Intracranial calcification can be located anywhere in the brain, but generally it is found in the basal ganglia and periventricular areas.

Pyknodysostosis

The syndrome of pyknodysostosis consists of osteosclerosis; short stature; frontal and occipital bossing; a small face with a receding chin; short, broad hands; and hypoplasia of the nails. Radiographic findings include generalized and uniform osteosclerosis. Metaphyseal modeling is only mildly abnormal, and the medullary cavities may be narrowed. The bones of the hands and feet are short, with hypoplasia or osteolysis of the distal phalanges. In the skull, a marked delay in closure of the sutures is evident, and the anterior fontanelle may remain open, even in adults. Wormian bones are common, especially in the lambdoid sutures. The mandible is hypoplastic, without normal angulation. The vertebral bodies are sclerotic, and errors in vertebral segmentation may be present in the upper portion of the cervical spine. The acromial ends of the clavicles may be resorbed. Multiple fractures may occur. Pyknodysostosis is due to mutations in the *CTSK* gene (cathepsin K gene) located at gene locus 1q21.

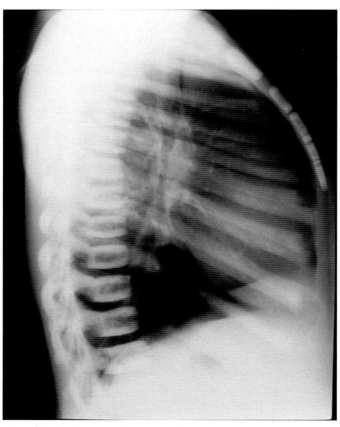

Figure 10.29 Osteopetrosis autosomal dominant type: lateral radiograph of chest. Osteosclerosis of the ribs and sternum is present, as well as endplate sclerosis of the vertebrae, producing rugger-jersey appearance.

Diaphyseal dysplasia (Camurati-Engelmann disease)

Camurati-Engelmann disease is a generalized, bilaterally symmetrical dysplasia of bone that is characterized by cortical thickening, narrowing of the medullary cavity, and a sclerotic and expanded diaphyseal segment that results from periosteal and endosteal bone formation (Figure 10.30). The epiphyses are spared. Diaphyseal dysplasia is an autosomal dominant disorder with considerable variability of expression. In some patients, the presenting symptoms appear in the first decade of life, whereas in others, the disease is not discovered until the second, third, or fourth decade of life. In order of decreasing frequency, the tibia, femur, humerus, ulna, radius, and bones of the hands and feet are affected. A symmetrical distribution is typical. Sclerosis of the base of the skull is common.

The course of this disease is variable. Progressive findings are common, but spontaneous improvement in adolescence has also been recognized. Increased intracranial pressure and encroachment on cranial nerves can lead to significant complications in some patients. Camurati-Engelmann disease is due to mutations in the *TGFB1* gene (transforming growth factor beta 1) located at gene locus 19q13.2.

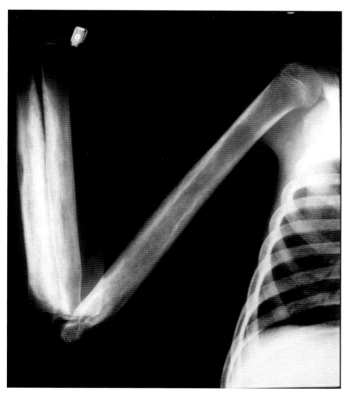

Figure 10.30 Camurati-Engelmann disease: lateral radiograph of right upper extremity. Marked cortical thickening is present along the shafts of the radius and ulna.

Craniometaphyseal dysplasia

The basic features of both the autosomal dominant and recessive forms of craniometaphyseal dysplasia are facial deformity, cranial hyperostosis, and failure of normal modeling of tubular bones. The recessive forms of the disease are accompanied by more severe facial involvement, which in some cases leads to striking abnormalities consisting of a broad mass at the base of the nose and hypertelorism. Dental malocclusion and facial paralysis often occur. Deafness results, in part, from foraminal constriction, with encroachment on the auditory nerve, and from direct involvement of the ossicles in the inner ear.

Radiographically, progressive sclerosis of the base of the skull and about the cranial sutures, obliteration of the paranasal sinuses, and loss of the lamina dura about the teeth are seen. In infancy, osteosclerosis in the diaphysis of the tubular bones, similar to that observed in diaphyseal dysplasia, is evident; it subsequently disappears and is replaced by a severe modeling defect manifesting as metaphyseal expansion, cortical thinning, and club-shaped epiphyses. Craniometaphyseal dysplasia is due to mutations in the *ANHK* gene (ankylosis, progressive mouse homolog) located at locus 5p15.1.

Pyle's dysplasia

Pyle's (or metaphyseal) dysplasia is a rare disorder that demonstrates either recessive or dominant transmission; it manifests at a variable age with mild clinical symptoms and signs. The radiographic abnormalities include marked expansion of the metaphyseal segments of tubular bones with an Erlenmeyer flask appearance, especially in the distal portion of the femur and proximal portions of the tibia and fibula. The spine may show platyspondyly or biconcave vertebrae. The bones on the pelvis, medial portions of the clavicles, and sternal ends of the ribs are expanded.

Multiple hereditary exostoses

This disease is characterized by cartilage-capped exostoses that usually arise near the diaphyseal side of the physeal line. The patients, usually boys, develop painless lumps near the ends of the long tubular bones and have mild shortness of stature. This disorder is due to mutations in the exostosis genes *EXT1* located at 8q24.11 and *EXT2* located at 11p12.

The radiographic appearance and size of the exostoses are extremely variable and, in part, depend on their sites of origin. They arise in the metaphyseal side of the growth plate, and the apex of the exostosis points away from the epiphysis. Associated metaphyseal expansion and deformity are evident adjacent to the base of the exostosis, except when the lesions are small.

The bones of the forearm are frequently deformed, with ulnar angulation of the distal articular surface of the radius, bowing of the radius, ulnar shift of the carpus, shortening of the ulna, and dislocation of the radial head (Figure 10.31). The fibula may also be shortened, with lateral obliquity of the ankle joint. Although the ends of the long tubular bones are involved

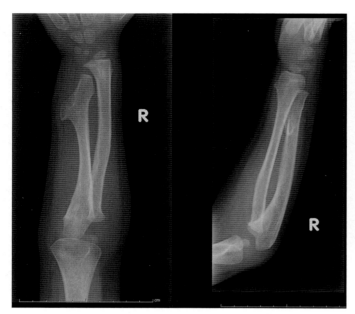

Figure 10.31 Multiple hereditary exostoses: frontal and lateral radiographs of the right forearm with large distal ulnar exostosis and smaller distal radial metaphyseal exostosis. The shortened ulna produces a "bayonet" configuration in the forearm.

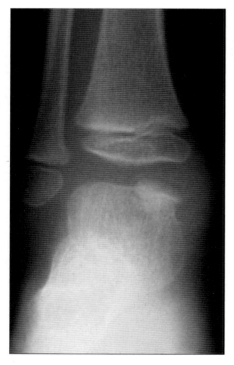

Figure 10.33 Trevor's disease: frontal radiographs of the ankle demonstrating a medial exostosis from the talar dome.

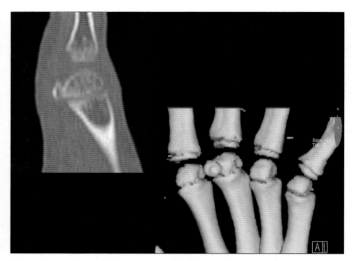

Figure 10.32 Trevor's disease: sagittal reformatted image and 3D reformatted CT scan of third finger, right hand. A small exostosis is present volarly from the third metacarpal epiphysis.

including vessels, nerves, and tendons. The incidence of malignant transformation is low. The findings that suggest malignant transformation are: continued growth of the osteochondroma after cessation of normal growth, a changing appearance of calcifications in the cartilage cap, and an irregular outline of the osteochondroma.

Trevor's disease

In dysplasia epiphysealis hemimelica, or Trevor's disease, the patients present with hard lumps around a joint, usually the ankle, but it can be any major joint, especially in the lower extremity (Figure 10.32). A function of that joint may be disturbed. Radiographs show a calcified mass coming off an epiphysis (Figure 10.33). The mass may have a cartilaginous cap.

Enchondromatosis (Ollier's disease)

Ollier's disease, a nonhereditary condition, is characterized by multiple enchondromas distributed throughout the tubular and flat bones of the body (Figure 10.34). The presenting clinical manifestations are masses that increase in size as the child grows, asymmetric limb shortening, and either genu varum or genu valgum deformity. The femur and tibia are affected most commonly. Radiographically, the lesions are seen clearly in infancy and consist of radiolucent masses that can be round, triangular or linear. The tubular bones may exhibit considerable expansion, especially in the hands. Pathological fractures may occur. Focal areas of calcification may appear within the mass. Cartilaginous areas that extend from the physis can lead to considerable interference with growth, resulting in osseous shortening and deformity. Angular deformities are most common in the distal position of the femur and are associated with nonuniform metaphyseal involvement. In the pelvis, V-shaped radiolucent areas appear in the iliac crest.

most frequently, the ribs, scapula and iliac bone often are affected. Vertebral involvement, although uncommon, can lead to spinal cord and nerve root compression. Small lesions in the metaphyseal region of the phalanges or the metacarpal bones may lead to V-shaped physeal lines.

Complications related to the osteochondromas are interference with growth: compression of surrounding structures,

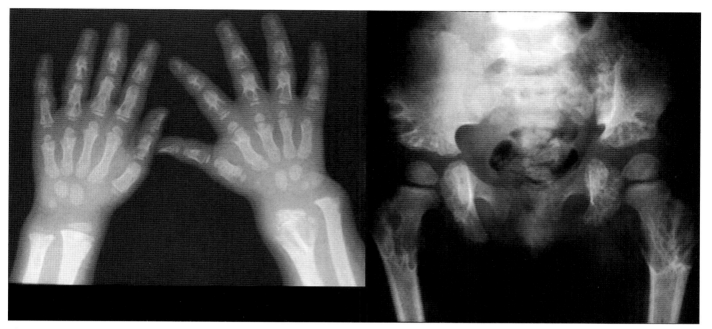

Figure 10.34 Ollier's syndrome: frontal radiographs of hands and frontal pelvic radiograph. Multiple lucent enchondromas are present in the short bones of the hands, pelvic bones and long bones.

The enchondromas typically stabilize or even regress in adulthood. Malignant transformation to chondrosarcoma may occur in up to 25% of the patients by the age of 40 years.

Enchondromatosis with hemangiomas (Maffucci's syndrome)

Maffucci's syndrome represents the combination of enchondromatosis and soft tissue hemangiomas. The hemangiomas are detected at birth or shortly thereafter and are of variable size and number. They can produce large masses and distortion of bone growth, including scoliosis. The distribution of the hemangiomas does not correlate with that of the enchondromas. Hemangiomas may occur in other organs, including those of the gastrointestinal tract. Hemangiomas in the head and neck may distort the trachea and produce dysphagia or epistaxis. CT scanning and MR imaging are useful in the evaluation of the nature, extent, and vascularity of the soft tissue and bony lesions.

The radiographic features in Maffucci's syndrome are similar to those of Ollier's disease, with the addition of phleboliths and soft tissue masses. Involvement of the hands and feet is frequent and severe. A higher frequency of malignant transformation of the enchondroma is seen in Maffucci's syndrome than in Ollier's disease.

Metachondromatosis

Metachondromatosis, an autosomal dominant condition, is characterized by multiple cartilaginous exostoses and enchondromas with prominent marginal calcifications. The principal sites of the exostoses are the hands and feet, although the entire skeleton, including the spine, may be affected. In contrast to typical cartilaginous exostoses, the exostoses in this syndrome point towards the growth plate, are small, and may decrease in size or resolve completely. The enchondromas are seen in the iliac crests and the metaphyses of the tubular bones and appear as irregular, calcified lesions. Extra-articular calcification and ossification are common.

Hypophosphatasia

There are six forms of the disease. The lethal perinatal and severe infantile disease, and the autosomal dominant adult type will be discussed. The former has profound defective ossification of the skull, ribs that show fractures, are thin and poorly ossified. The spine has multiple fractures. The long bones have poor irregular and mottled ossification at the bone ends and bowing. There may be Bowdler spurs. The disorder is due to mutations in the *ALPL* gene (alkaline phosphatase liver/bone/kidney gene) located at locus 1q36.

The adult form has ricketic-like changes with physeal widening, radiolucent tongues in the metaphyses, and osteopenia.

Dysostosis multiplex group

This group includes all the mucopolysaccharidoses (MPSs) and mucolipidoses. These are lysosomal disorders due to deficiency of specific proteins needed to break down glycosaminoglycans and various other lysosomal carbohydrates and fats.

The radiographic abnormalities of these disorders are designated dysostosis multiplex. The skull is usually large and dolichocephalic, with premature closure of the sagittal suture. The mastoids and paranasal sinuses are poorly developed. An elongated J-shaped sella turcica, prominent adenoids,

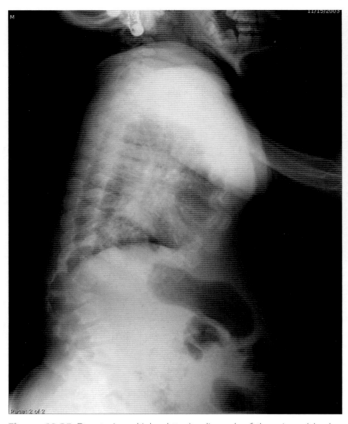

Figure 10.35 Dysostosis multiplex: lateral radiograph of thoracic and lumbar spine. A hypoplastic anteriorly beaked L1 vertebral body is present. The ribs are broad.

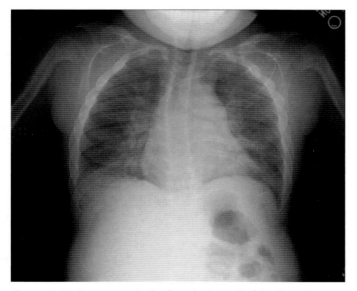

Figure 10.37 Dysostosis multiplex: frontal radiograph of the chest. Characteristic findings of dysostosis multiplex are present, with broad ribs particularly laterally, broad medial clavicles, varus shoulders. The patient has bilateral interstitial infiltrates and a central venous line in place.

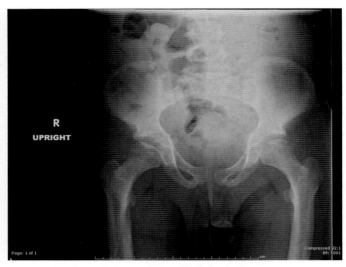

Figure 10.36 Dysostosis multiplex: frontal radiograph of the pelvis. Superiorly flared ilia, narrowed distally at supracetabular region. Flattened capital femoral epiphyseal centers.

malformed teeth, flattened mandibular condyles, large tongue, and thick diploic space are common. In the spine, there is defective development of the anterosuperior portion of the vertebral bodies at the thoracolumbar junction, with gibbus formation owing to the presence of hook-shaped vertebrae. The vertebral bodies are oval, slightly diminished in height, or flattened (Figure 10.35). In the pelvis, the superior acetabular region is underdeveloped, resulting in a widened acetabular roof and wide acetabular angle. Coxa valga is frequent, and development of the femoral heads is delayed, causing them to become dysplastic (Figure 10.36). In the chest, the ribs are widened but taper near their vertebral margins. The clavicles are thick, short and widened (Figure 10.37). The changes in the long tubular bones are greater in the upper extremities than in the lower extremities. Constriction of the humeral and femoral necks, with resultant varus deformities, may occur. In the hand, diffuse osteopenia, cortical thinning, and proximal tapering of the second to fifth metacarpal bones are observed. The proximal and middle phalanges are short and wide, and the terminal phalanges are hypoplastic. The carpal bones are small and deformed. Similar but less dramatic changes occur in the foot.

A precise diagnosis also requires clinical information, including the pattern of genetic transmission, and biochemical data, including the pattern of increased urinary excretion of acid mucopolysaccharides.

The mucopolysaccharidoses include: (I) Hurler/Scheie, (II) Hunter, (III) Sanfilippo, (IV) Morquio, (VI) Maroteaux-Lamy and (VII) Sly. Type V has been found to be a form of the type I syndrome and is thus not used any more. Patients with Hurler syndrome and Morquio syndrome (which includes subtypes A and B) show osseous abnormalities. Patients with Hurler syndrome show less-severe findings and, in early infancy, an inferior "beak" of the vertebral bodies on lateral radiographs. Patients with Morquio disease show more severe skeletal manifestations with vertebral bodies that are slightly rounded, with a small anterior beak, universal vertebra plana (platyspondyly), constricted iliac bones with elongated pelvic inlet ("wine glass" pelvis) and proximally pointed short metacarpals.

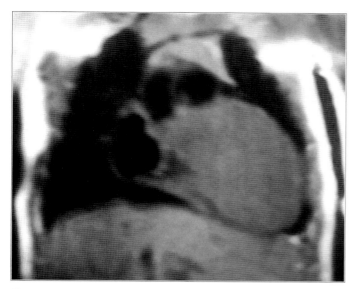

Figure 10.38 Basal cell nevus syndrome: T1-weighted MR image of the heart. A large cardiac fibroma is present.

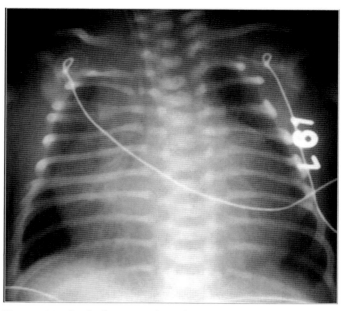

Figure 10.39 Basal cell nevus syndrome: frontal chest radiograph of the same patient as Figure 10.38. Cardiomegaly is present as well as multiple bifid ribs.

With subsequent growth, a central tongue or projection appears, protruding from the anterior surface of the vertebral bodies. In adulthood, the vertebrae are flat and rectangular, with irregular margins. Hypoplasia of the odontoid process, leading to atlantoaxial instability, may result in upper spinal cord damage during anesthesia. In the pelvis, increased obliquity in the lateral aspect of the acetabular roofs and considerable flaring of the iliac wings are observed. Progressive dysplasia of the capital femoral epiphysis is also seen in Morquio.

Syndromes

Basal cell nevus syndrome

Basal cell nevus syndrome, or Gorlin syndrome, is an autosomal dominant condition characterized by basal cell skin carcinomas, odontogenic keratocysts of the jaw, and lamellar calcifications in the falx cerebri, the diaphragma sellae and the tentorium cerebelli. In addition to basal cell carcinoma, there is increased incidence of multiple neoplastic conditions including medulloblastoma, Hodgkin's disease, fibrosarcoma, bilateral calcified ovarian fibromas, intra-abdominal lymphangioma and cardiac fibroma (Figure 10.38). Associated skeletal malformations include bifid anterior ribs, cervical spine segmentation anomalies, Sprengel deformity, spotty sclerotic skeletal lesions and phalangeal cysts (Figure 10.39). Odontogenic keratocysts are much more common in the mandible than the maxilla, are infrequently symptomatic and begin to appear between the ages of 7 and 40 years. Basal cell nevus syndrome is due to mutations in the *PTCH1* (patched homolog 1) gene at locus 9q22.3. *PTCH1* is a tumor suppressor gene.

Beckwith-Wiedemann syndrome

Beckwith-Wiedemann syndrome (BWS) is a condition characterized by exomphalos (anterior abdominal wall defects),

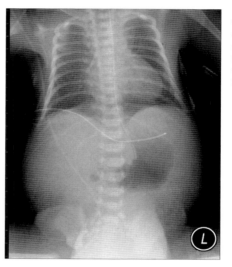

Figure 10.40 Beckwith-Wiedemann syndrome: frontal supine radiograph of chest and abdomen in large newborn infant with omphalocele overlying pelvis.

macroglossia, hemihypertrophy, nephromegaly, islet cell hyperplasia, nephroblastomatosis, adrenal cytomegaly, neonatal adrenal macrocysts, intestinal malrotation and an increased incidence of benign and malignant tumors (Figure 10.40).

Originally, BWS was described as a triad of exomphalos, macroglossia and gigantism. The most characteristic of these abnormalities is macroglossia, which occurs in 99% of patients and often requires surgical reduction due to feeding and respiratory difficulties. Gigantism, defined as postnatal size over the 90th percentile, is present in almost 90% of patients. Anterior abdominal wall defects occur in 50–70% of patients. Hemihypertrophy is found in 25% and is the only clinical feature highly associated with the development of malignancy.

The risk of malignant tumor in patients with BWS is approximately 7%. The most common malignant tumors are Wilms tumor, adrenal carcinoma, hepatoblastoma and neuroblastoma. Other reported tumors which may occur include rhabdomyosarcoma, pancreatoblastoma, breast fibroadenoma, gastric teratoma, hepatic hemangioendothelioma and splenic hemangioma (Figure 10.41). Tumor surveillance screening in BWS is widely practiced, with current recommendations for abdominal sonography to evaluate for renal, adrenal, pancreatic and hepatic masses every three to six months until six to eight years. Beckwith-Wiedemann syndrome is due to abnormal regulation of genes at the 11p15.5 locus, including several nonprotein encoding sites and the *IGF2* gene (insulin-like growth factor 2).

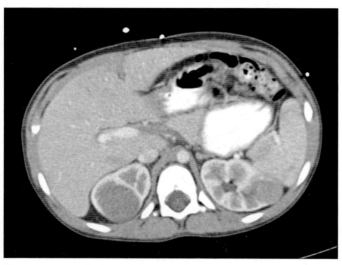

Figure 10.41 Beckwith-Wiedemann syndrome: axial CT image through both kidneys demonstrating bilateral renal cortical masses which are small Wilms tumors.

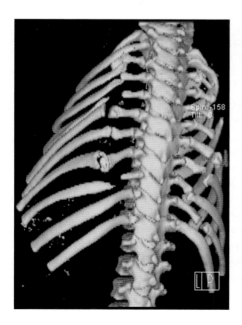

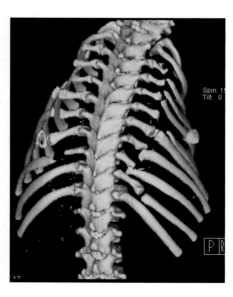

Cerebrocostomandibular (rib-gap) syndrome

Cerebrocostomandibular syndrome, also called rib-gap syndrome, is characterized by a small mandible, cleft palate, glossoptosis, and posterior rib gaps. Neonatal respiratory distress is the usual presenting sign. Mental retardation is seen in one half of the patients and microcephaly in 20%. Rib gaps are filled with fibrovascular tissue, can be symmetric, and are usually seen in the third through the seventh ribs (Figure 10.42). Eventually the rib gaps may partially heal. Miscellaneous findings may include stippled epiphyses, clubfoot, elbow dysplasia, scoliosis, progressive kyphosis, multiple ossification centers of the calcaneus, vesicoureteral reflux, and renal cysts. The diagnosis has been made prenatally.

Congenital insensitivity to pain

Congenital insensitivity to pain is an autosomal recessive syndrome characterized by decreased sensitivity to pain without affecting touch or proprioception. The typical clinical presentation is an insidious progressive joint swelling. The foot and ankle tend to be the most common areas of involvement. Subperiosteal hemorrhages may occur in neonates, with later development of fractures, epiphyseal separations, periosteal new bone formation and dislocations of weight-bearing joints. Avascular necrosis, Charcot arthropathy, and heterotopic ossification can occur. Skin ulcerations or surgical interventions may lead to osteomyelitis. Child abuse has been misdiagnosed in patients with congenital insensitivity to pain.

Currarino triad

Currarino triad consists of congenital anal stenosis or low imperforate anus, scimitar hemisacrum, and a presacral mass (Figure 10.43). The presacral mass may be a teratoma (two-thirds of cases), a lipoma, a dermoid cyst, an enteric cyst, or an

Figure 10.42 Cerebrocostomandibular syndrome: 3D reformatted CT images of the ribs, viewed from the posterior. Bilateral unossified gaps are present in the ribs.

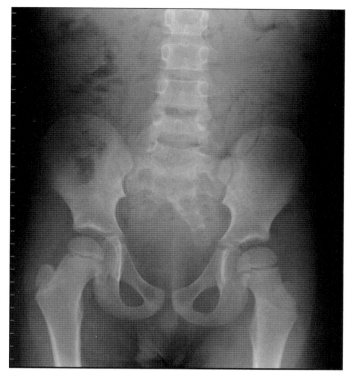

Figure 10.43 Currarino triad: frontal radiograph of the pelvis and lower lumbar spine. A scimitar sacrum is present with absence of almost all ossification below S3 on the right.

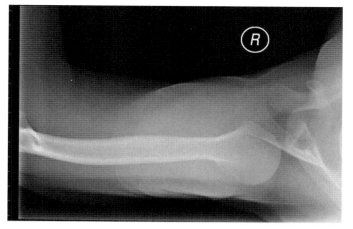

Figure 10.44 Ehlers-Danlos syndrome: axillary view of the right shoulder demonstrating a posterior dislocation of the right shoulder.

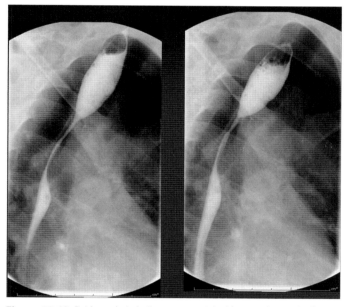

Figure 10.45 Epidermolysis bullosa: sequential oblique radiographs from a barium swallow demonstrating a long segment proximal esophageal stricture just below the level of the carina.

anterior meningocele. An intact first sacral segment and a sickle-shaped sacrum is a distinctive anomaly to this syndrome. Myelodysplasia with tethered cord and intradural lipoma also occurs frequently.

Approximately one-third of patients with anal stenosis have Currarino triad. Although constipation is the most frequent symptom, life-threatening meningitis and sepsis may occur, particularly with presacral anterior meningoceles. Approximately 50% of presacral tumors communicate with the spinal canal in Currarino triad.

Ehlers-Danlos syndrome

Ehlers-Danlos syndrome (EDS) is a heterogeneous group of inherited anomalies of connective tissue characterized by varying degrees of skin hyperextensibility, joint hypermobility and connective tissue fragility (Figure 10.44).

Joint dislocation or subluxation may involve any joint and be acute or chronic. The hip may be dislocated at birth. Premature polyarticular arthritis is the result of dislocations. Flatfoot, clubfoot and hallux valgus are common. Round subcutaneous soft tissue calcifications are characteristic of EDS. Patients may have scoliosis, kyphosis, spondylolisthesis, and a widened spinal canal. Aneurysms and spontaneous arterial rupture may be seen. Supporting structures of the colon, bladder and uterus may be weakened by defective collagen, and may spontaneously rupture. Recurrent inguinal hernias should raise the suspicion for EDS, as should unexplained bladder or bowel diverticula in children.

Other clinical manifestations of EDS include mitral valve prolapse, aortic and mitral valvular insufficiency, recurrent pneumothorax, and cystic lung disease.

Epidermolysis bullosa dystrophica

Epidermolysis bullosa (EB) is manifest by extreme fragility of the skin because of breakdown of tissues at the junction between the epidermis and dermis. EB is associated with severe cutaneous and gastrointestinal involvement including pseudo-syndactyly of hands and feet (mitten hands), microstomia, esophageal strictures, and constipation and bladder outlet obstruction due to perianal and periurethral scarring. Esophageal strictures often in the upper esophagus may cause high-grade obstruction and malnutrition (Figure 10.45). Congenital pyloric atresia is associated with EB.

Fanconi anemia

Fanconi anemia is a rare, usually autosomal recessive, disease characterized by multiple congenital abnormalities, pancytopenia and cancer susceptibility, especially leukemia (Figure 10.46). The mean age of onset is eight years. Skeletal abnormalities are seen in 70% of patients, with 50% having radial ray abnormalities ranging from bilateral absent thumbs and radii to a unilateral hypoplastic thumb or bifid thumb (Figure 10.47). Renal abnormalities occur in about one-third of the patients and include unilateral renal agenesis, horseshoe kidney, hypoplasia, double ureters and hydronephrosis. Microcephaly, microphthalmia, mental retardation, ear malformations, syndactyly, brachydactyly, Sprengel deformity, Klippel-Feil deformity, clubfoot, hip dislocation, scoliosis, kyphosis, brown pigmentation of the skin and short stature are features of this condition. Fanconi anemia is due to mutations in one of 13 genes involved in synthesis of a single complex protein involved in repair of DNA. These genes are called *FANC- A, B, C, D1, D2, E, F, G, I, J, L, M* and *N*. All mutations are associated with autosomal recessive inheritance, except that due to *FANCB* which is X-linked.

Fibrodysplasia ossificans progressiva

Fibrodysplasia ossificans progressiva is characterized by progressive swelling and ossification of the soft tissues of the extremities. Patients typically have microdactyly of the great toes and thumbs from a monophalangeal great toe and shortening of the first metatarsal and metacarpal, hallux valgus, tibial osteochondromas, and shortening of the femoral neck. Beginning in early childhood, patients develop painful episodes of soft tissue swelling, often following minor trauma, with subsequent heterotopic ossification in the musculature and connective tissues. Heterotopic ossification typically progresses from the axial to the appendicular skeleton, and causes progressive limitation of motion, including respiratory excursions. Fibrodysplasia ossificans progressiva is due to mutations in the *ACVR1* gene which codes for a bone morphogenic protein type 1 receptor, located at gene locus 2q23.

Goldenhar syndrome

Goldenhar syndrome, also known as oculoauriculovertebral dysplasia, is a complex of unilateral craniofacial and systemic abnormalities associated with first and second branchial arch derivatives (Figure 10.48). In addition to temporal, maxillary and mandibular hypoplasia, there may be cleft lip and palette, ipsilateral microglossia, and characteristic epibulbar dermoid tumors of the orbit. Ear abnormalities range from periauricular skin tags to anotia. Vertebral segmentation anomalies are variable, usually in the cervical and thoracic regions (Figure 10.49). Intracranial abnormalities can include encephalocele, aqueductal stenosis, and agenesis of the corpus callosum or vermis. Systemic abnormalities may include ventriculoseptal defects, tetralogy of Fallot, dextrocardia, tracheoesophageal fistula, renal duplication, and vesicoureteral reflux.

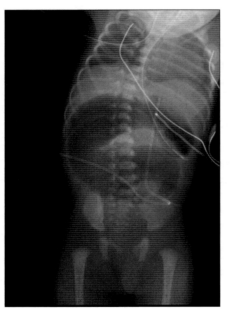

Figure 10.46 Fanconi anemia: frontal radiograph of the chest and abdomen. Jejunal atresia is present. There is also a left-sided hemivertebral body between L5 and S1.

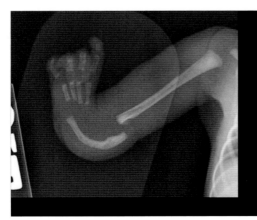
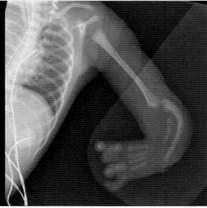

Figure 10.47 Fanconi anemia: frontal radiographs of bilateral upper extremities demonstrate absent radius and thumb on the right, and hypoplastic radius with absent thumb on the left.

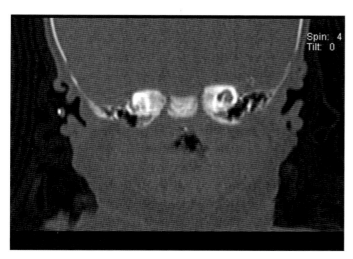

Figure 10.48 Goldenhar syndrome: coronal reformatted cranial CT scan. Absent external auditory canals.

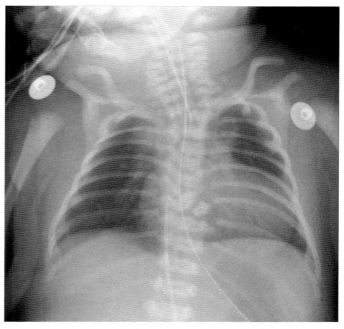

Figure 10.49 Goldenhar syndrome: frontal radiograph of the chest. Multiple mid-thoracic vertebral body segmentation errors are present. The heart is at the upper limits of normal with a right aortic arch. An umbilical artery catheter, endotracheal tube and nasogastric tube are in place. D-transposition of the great arteries and pulmonary stenosis are present.

Hajdu-Cheney syndrome

Hajdu-Cheney syndrome is an autosomal dominant disorder with characteristic facial features, osteolysis of the distal phalanges of the hands and feet and multiple Wormian bones. In addition to multiple Wormian bones, the craniofacial findings include bathrocephaly, cranial suture persistence, hypoplastic sinuses, an elongated sella, progressive basilar impression, and syringomyelia and Arnold-Chiari malformation. In over 90% of the patients, the hands and feet show band-like osteolysis in the mid-portion of the distal phalanges, especially the hands. This finding may be seen as early as age three, but typically occurs in later childhood. Osteolysis may also be seen in the radial heads. Cardiovascular abnormalities include valvular disease and heart block. The disease may respond to bisphosphonates.

Cystic kidney disease resembling adult polycystic disease can be seen in up to 10% of the patients, as can glomerulo-nephritis, which can lead to chronic renal failure.

Holt-Oram syndrome

Holt-Oram syndrome is an autosomal dominant condition in which anomalies of the upper extremities and shoulders are associated with congenital heart disease (Figure 10.50). The disease is familial in 60–70% of cases, with new mutations accounting for the remainder. The most common limb anomalies are radial ray anomalies including triphalangeal thumb, hypoplastic thumb, abnormal scaphoid, extra carpal bones, absent or hypoplastic radii, phocomelia and laterally hooked clavicles. The limb anomalies tend to be bilateral and asymmetrical, more severe on the left. Cardiac anomalies occur in up to 95% of patients (Figure 10.51). The most common anomalies are atrial septal defects (60%), ventricular septal defects (30%) and conduction defects. More severe anomalies such as tetralogy of Fallot, atrioventricular defect, hypoplastic

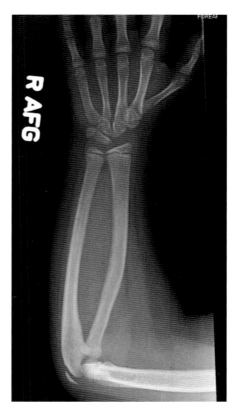

Figure 10.50 Holt-Oram syndrome: frontal radiograph of the forearm and hand. There is a hypoplastic scaphoid with fusion of the lunate and triquetrum.

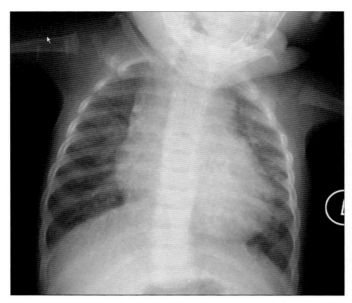

Figure 10.51 Holt-Oram syndrome: frontal radiograph of the chest. Cardiomegaly with increased vascularity secondary to a large ASD is present. Lateral clavicular hooking is also present.

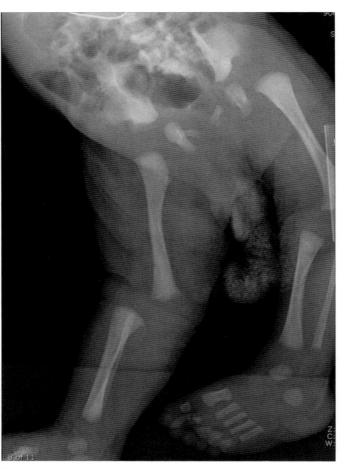

Figure 10.52 Larsen syndrome: oblique radiographs of both lower extremities demonstrating anterior knee dislocations and superolateral left hip dislocation with pseudoacetabular formation.

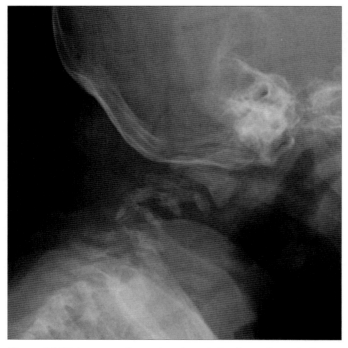

Figure 10.53 Larsen syndrome: lateral cervical spine radiograph demonstrates cervical kyphosis.

left heart, truncus arteriosus and total anomalous pulmonary venous return may occur. Holt-Oram syndrome is caused by a mutation in the *TBX5* gene (T-box 5 gene) at location 12q24.1. T-box genes are involved in tissue formation during fetal development.

Larsen syndrome

Larsen syndrome is characterized by multiple joint dislocations, especially knees, hips and elbows, and a typical facies with a prominent forehead, flat nasal bridge and hypertelorism. In knee dislocations, which are the most frequent, the tibia is displaced anteriorly (Figure 10.52). Considerable epiphyseal deformity can occur secondary to the dislocations. Other osseous abnormalities include clubfoot, accessory carpal bones, bifid calcaneus, delayed epiphyseal ossifications, coronal vertebral clefts and retarded bone age.

Cervical kyphosis can be seen as a result of dysplastic midcervical vertebrae, and anteroposterior subluxation in the cervical spine (Figure 10.53). Kyphosis may be life threatening due to cord compression.

Marfan syndrome

Marfan syndrome is a connective tissue disorder caused by mutations in a component of elastin. The typical patient is tall with disproportionate long, slender limbs and digits. Common

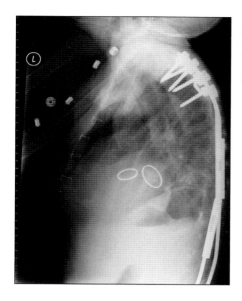

Figure 10.54 Marfan syndrome: lateral radiograph of the chest. Residual thoracic hyperkyphosis is present following posterior fixation.

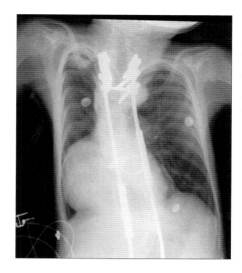

Figure 10.55 Marfan syndrome: frontal radiograph of the chest. Striking cardiomegaly is present status post-aortic and mitral valve prosthesis. A thoracolumbar scoliosis is present following posterior fixation with growing rods.

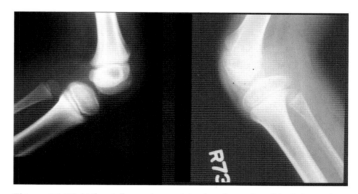

Figure 10.56 Nail patella syndrome: lateral radiographs of both knees in a six-year-old female without patella or patellar ossification identified.

defects include pectus deformities (excavatum or carinatum), joint laxity, ocular problems (usually ectopia lentis from lax suspensory ligaments and myopia) and spinal deformity (scoliosis, which may be severe and progressive, kyphosis and spondylolisthesis) (Figure 10.54).

Cardiovascular manifestations, which are the most devastating aspect of Marfan syndrome, result from loss of tensile strength of the supporting tissue of the aortic and cardiac valves. These include aortic dilatation, regurgitation and aortic dissection and mitral valve prolapse. A measurement of aortic root growth may have prognostic value for aortic complications. Serious cardiovascular abnormalities may be present at birth (Figure 10.55).

Other findings include dural ectasia occurring in the majority of patients, diaphragmatic and intestinal hernias, diverticulosis coli and Zenker's diverticulum, arachnodactyly, spinal arachnoid cysts or diverticula, protrusio acetabuli, joint laxity, reduced arm span to height ratio, and osteopenia. Joint laxity can result in joint dislocations. Marfan syndrome is due to mutations in the *FBN1* gene (fibrillin 1 gene) located at locus 15q21.1, involved in the formation of the proteins of the intercellular matrix.

Meckel-Gruber syndrome

Meckel-Gruber syndrome is an autosomal recessive malformation syndrome characterized by developmental defects in the central nervous system and kidneys, and post-axial polydactyly. Intracranial anomalies are most commonly occipital encephalocele or Dandy-Walker anomaly. Renal abnormalities include cysts, nephromegaly and corticomedullary dysplasia. Other findings include hepatic ductal dysplasia and cysts, fibrosis and hamartomas of visceral organs, cleft lip and palate, and visceral heterotaxy. Other skeletal changes include dysplastic hips, micrognathia, limb bowing, short limbs and vertebral

anomalies. Prenatal sonographic evaluation demonstrates oligohydramnios and typical morphological findings in the second trimester.

Nail patella syndrome

Nail patella syndrome or Fong syndrome is an autosomal dominant condition mapped to the long arm of chromosome 9, characterized by dysplastic finger and toe nails and hypoplastic or absent patellae (Figure 10.56). Additionally the radial head and capitellum may be hypoplastic. The pelvis typically shows flaring of the iliac wings with a characteristic conical horn (Fong's horn) arising from the dorsal iliac surface (Figure 10.57).

Noonan syndrome

Noonan syndrome is an autosomal dominant condition associated with proportionate short stature, dysmorphic facial features and either pulmonic stenosis or hypertrophic cardiomyopathy. The facial features of Noonan syndrome are hypertelorism, down-slanted palpebral fissures, ptosis and neck

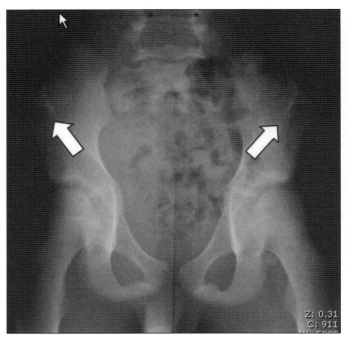

Figure 10.57 Nail patella syndrome: pelvis of 12-year-old male with bilateral Fong's horns from central iliac wings (arrows).

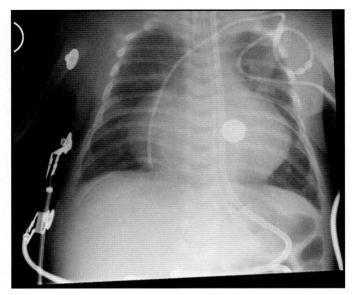

Figure 10.58 Noonan syndrome: frontal radiograph of the chest of a child with Noonan syndrome and severe cardiomyopathy, awaiting cardiac transplantation.

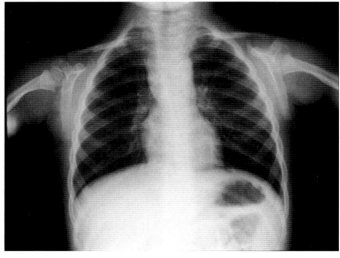

Figure 10.59 Osteolysis syndrome: frontal radiograph of the chest. Clavicular osteolysis is present bilaterally.

pterygia. Approximately 20% of Noonan syndrome patients have lymphatic abnormalities such as pulmonary lymphangiectasia, intestinal lymphangiectasia and/or lymphedema. Bleeding diathesis occurs in 50% of Noonan syndrome patients. Patients may have thoracic deformity (especially pectus carinatum), cubitus valgus, and low set ears. Other, less typical cardiac lesions may occur in Noonan syndrome, including atrial septal defect, atrioventricular canal and tetralogy of Fallot (Figure 10.58).

Osteolysis syndromes

The osteolysis syndromes are difficult to classify but can be roughly divided based on the areas of bone absorption and associated malformations (Figure 10.59).

Hereditary multicentric osteolysis involving the carpal and tarsal bones starts by age three or four years, with arthritis-like symptoms of wrists and feet (Figure 10.60). There develops a progressive absorption of the carpal and tarsal bones that become crenated and eventually disappear, with marked narrowing of the carpal and tarsal areas. The adjacent metacarpals and metatarsals are often involved, showing erosions and pencilling. Unlike rheumatoid arthritis, the mineral content of the bones remains good.

The forms principally involving the distal phalanges are also progressive and can be called acro-osteolysis. The lesions may stabilize in adult life. The more proximal phalanges can also exhibit absorption.

Gorham syndrome, or "vanishing bone disease", is a condition usually starting gradually or abruptly before the age of 40 years which has striking radiographic findings of massive osteolysis and with proliferation of vascular and lymphatic vessels which involve soft tissues and bones. The destructive process may involve a whole region (i.e. shoulder or hip), with the adjacent bones being severely affected. The shoulder region is the most commonly affected.

Poland syndrome

Poland syndrome is characterized by partial or complete absence of the pectoral muscles, associated with anomalies of the ipsilateral upper extremity (Figure 10.61). It is occasionally associated with the development of neoplasm, and may have familial inheritance. Extremity changes range from syndactyly,

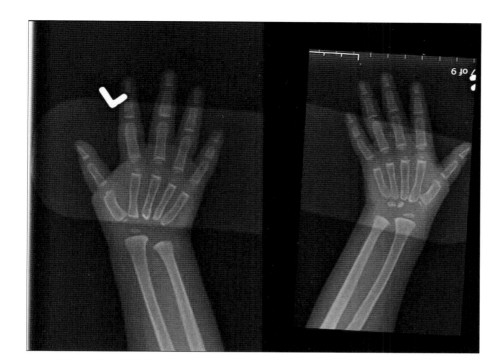

Figure 10.60 Osteolysis, carpal-tarsal: five-year-old male with proteinuria. Frontal radiographs of both hands. The carpal area is markedly diminished on the left with absent carpal bone ossification; on the right, ossification centers of the capitate and hamate have an unusual crenated contour and the carpal area is small.

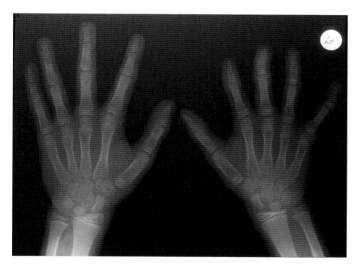

Figure 10.61 Poland syndrome: frontal radiographs of both hands. There is striking shortening of the middle phalanges of the left hand. The left pectoral muscles were also absent.

polydactyly or phalangeal hypoplasia to radial ray anomalies and shoulder girdle anomalies. Other reported anomalies include scoliosis, rib anomalies and renal hypoplasia/agenesis. Plain radiographs demonstrate relative thoracic hyperlucency as well as skeletal extremity changes. CT and MR better demonstrate the musculoskeletal anomalies and also possible breast hypoplasia. Poland syndrome is thought to arise from subclavian arterial compromise in fetal life.

Rubinstein-Taybi syndrome

Rubinstein-Taybi Syndrome is a sporadic condition characterized by facial dysmorphism, mental retardation and broadening of the thumbs and great toes. Characteristic broadening of the distal phalanges of the thumb and great toe is a diagnostic marker for the syndrome. Additional radiographic findings include delayed skeletal maturation and dislocations, flared iliac wings, large foramen magna, and cervical instability with odontoid malformation. Visceral malformations include malrotation and vesicoureteral reflux. Intracranial lesions include agenesis of the corpus callosum and Dandy-Walker malformation.

Shwachman-Diamond syndrome

Shwachman-Diamond syndrome is a metaphyseal chondrodysplasia with associated pancreatic insufficiency and fatty replacement of the pancreas, and cyclic neutropenia (Figure 10.62). Skeletal changes are seen in more than 75% of patients, and include metaphyseal widening with patchy lucent and sclerotic changes adjacent to the zone of provisional calcification, osteopenia, delayed skeletal maturity, and irregular rib ends with broad and short ribs. Less common skeletal changes include clinodactyly, syndactyly, overtubulation of long bones, genu valgum, coxa vara and supernumery metatarsals (Figure 10.63). Shwachman-Diamond syndrome is due to mutations in the *SBDS* gene (Shwachman-Bodian-Diamond gene), which has an unknown function, located at gene locus 7q11.

Thrombocytopenia—absent radius (TAR) syndrome

Thrombocytopenia with absent radius is a congenital malformation syndrome characterized by bilateral absence of radii and thrombocytopenia. The thrombocytopenia is early onset,

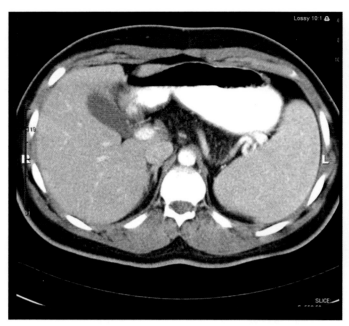

Figure 10.62 Shwachman-Diamond syndrome: axial CT scan through the pancreas demonstrating diffuse fatty replacement of the pancreas.

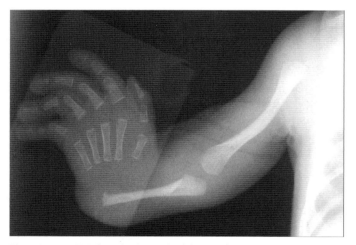

Figure 10.64 TAR: frontal radiograph of the right forearm. There is absence of the radius but a normal biphalangeal thumb.

but usually transient, and may be associated with a marked leukemoid reaction. A distinguishing feature from other absent radius conditions is the presence of the thumb (Figure 10.64). Other upper extremity abnormalities may be present in TAR syndrome, including phocomelia, hypoplasia or absence of any of the other bones, and shoulder anomalies.

Up to 50% of patients with TAR syndrome may have very significant lower extremity abnormalities including absent fibula, phocomelia, dislocated knees, ankles and hips, fusion of the femur and tibia, short long bones and clubfeet. Approximately 30% have congenital heart disease, primarily tetralogy of Fallot and septal defects.

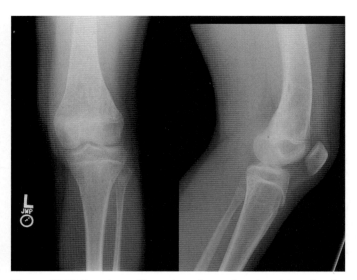

Figure 10.63 Shwachman-Diamond syndrome: frontal and lateral radiographs of the left knee. A metaphyseal dysplasia is present, most noticeable in the distal femur with a conical lucency within the medial aspect of the distal femoral metaphysis.

Trisomy 13 syndrome (Patau syndrome)

Trisomy 13 is characterized by low birthweight, craniofacial dysmorphism and mental retardation. Prenatally detected sonographic abnormalities are common, including structural abnormalities of the face and of the central nervous system, most often ventriculomegaly and holoprosencephaly. Other intracranial abnormalities include agenesis of the corpus callosum and Dandy-Walker malformation. Cardiovascular anomalies are common. There may be thin ribs, hypoplasia of the pelvis with high acetabular and iliac angles, and a variety of hand and foot anomalies including post-axial polydactyly and rocker-bottom feet. Prenatal sonography can detect many of the morphological findings of trisomy 13, as well as echogenic intracardiac foci, increased nuchal translucency and echogenic bowel, suggesting further evaluation or karyotyping.

Trisomy 18 syndrome (Edwards syndrome)

Trisomy 18 is characterized by low birthweight, hypotonia followed by hypertonia, craniofacial dysmorphism and mental retardation. The three most common clinical findings are clenched hands, rocker-bottom feet and low-set or malformed ears. Common radiographic findings include gracile ribs, congenital heart disease (ventricular septal defect, patent ductus arteriosus, atrial septal defect) and a small pelvis with narrow iliac crests with high iliac and acetabular angles (Figure 10.65). Other radiographic findings include thinning of the calvarium, hypoplasia of the mandible and maxilla, dolichocephaly, aplasia of the medial thirds of the clavicles, and other changes of the hand including short thumb and index finger with ulnar deviation of the digits. Intracranial findings include gyral and lobar dysplasia often involving the hippocampus, cerebellum and midbrain, cerebellar hypoplasia, choroid plexus cysts and an enlarged cisterna magna.

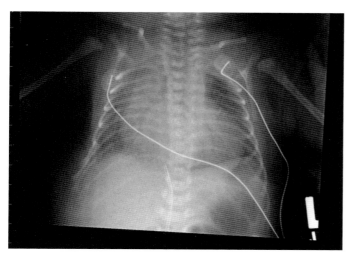

Figure 10.65 Trisomy 18: frontal radiograph of the chest in a neonate. The ribs are thin in this infant with a broad chest. Marked cardiomegaly is present. The patient had multivalvular heart disease.

Trisomy 21 syndrome (Down syndrome)

Trisomy 21 is the most common chromosomal syndrome. The syndrome is characterized by mental retardation, low birth-weight, craniofacial dysmorphism and a host of anomalies involving virtually all organ systems.

Pelvic radiographs demonstrate characteristics of trisomy 21 early in life. Flaring of the iliac wings and flattening of the acetabular roofs are seen and can be quantified by measuring the iliac index. The iliac index is the sum of the acetabular angle (the angle between the roof of the acetabulum and a line drawn through the triradiate cartilages) and the iliac angle (the angle between the iliac wing and a line drawn through the triradiate cartilages). In trisomy 21 patients, the iliac index is less than 60°.

Skeletal abnormalities include brachycephaly with micrognathia, hypoplastic atlas, cervical spondylosis in older patients, a systemic arthropathy similar to JRA, hypersegmentation of the sternum, gracile ribs, 11 ribs, bell-shaped thorax, congenital hip dislocation, absence of widening of the interpediculate distance of the lumbar spine and slightly diminished bone mass. The occipito-atlantal instability found in Down syndrome is controversial both for diagnosis and therapy. Antero-posterior occipito-atlantal instability is defined as more than 2 mm of motion on extension of the occipito-atlantal joints. An MRI of the neck is recommended to evaluate for signal changes in the cord if the motion is greater than 2 mm. An atlantoaxial distance of 4.5 mm or less is considered normal. However, from 4.5 to 10 mm and with a normal neurological exam, avoidance of high risk sports (driving, football) is recommended. If more than 4.5 mm with a neurological deficit, activities are restricted and MRI recommended to evaluate for cord changes. Greater than 10 mm, surgical fusion is recommended.

Other radiographic findings in trisomy 21 include congenital heart disease, most often endocardial cushion defect or

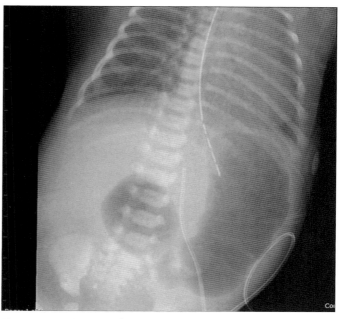

Figure 10.66 Trisomy 21: frontal radiograph of the abdomen demonstrates a "double-bubble" sign diagnostic of duodenal atresia. Note is also made of an enlarged heart due to cardiac disease, and flared iliac wing with flattened acetabular roof typical of trisomy 21.

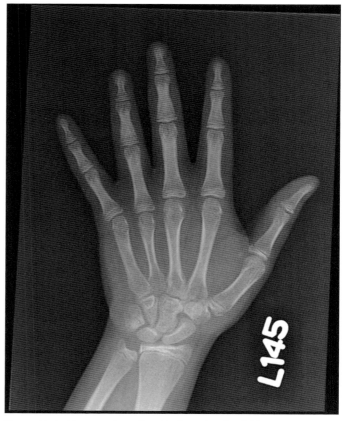

Figure 10.67 Turner syndrome: frontal radiographs of the left hand demonstrate a short fourth metacarpal, and a relatively small carpus with a lacy trabecular pattern of osteopenia in the carpal bones.

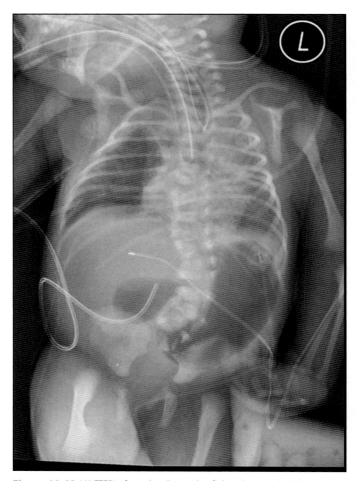

Figure 10.68 VACTERL: frontal radiograph of the chest and abdomen in a newborn with esophageal atresia with a distal fistula, with nasogastric tube coiled in the proximal esophagus, duodenal atresia and numerous thoracolumbar vertebral segmentation anomalies, costal anomalies, absence of the sacrum and bilateral dislocated hips.

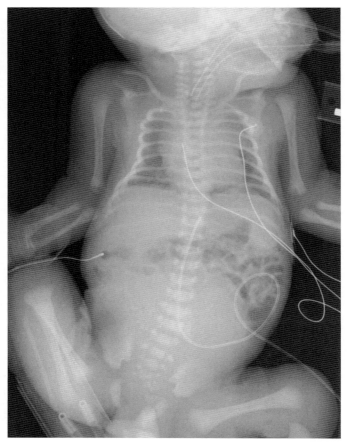

Figure 10.69 VACTERL: frontal radiograph of the chest and abdomen in a neonate. Esophageal atresia and imperforate anus with a rectourethral fistula are present. The nasogastric tube ends in the proximal esophagus. Enterolithiasis is present in the right colon and splenic flexure associated with the rectourethral fistula. There is a large abdominopelvic mass: a large urinary bladder due to massive bilateral vesicoureteral reflux.

ventricular septal defect, duodenal atresia or stenosis, malrotation, tracheoesophageal fistula, imperforate anus, Hirschsprung disease, and peripheral lung cysts (Figure 10.66). Patients with trisomy 21 have an increased incidence of leukemia, most commonly acute lymphocytic leukemia (ALL).

Turner syndrome

Turner syndrome, or isochromosome X, was initially described as a triad of infertility, web neck and cubitus valgus deformity of the elbow. There is valgus deformity of the elbow, brachycephaly, thin lateral clavicles, hypoplasia of the sacrum, pectus carinatum, platyspondyly, overtubulation of long bones, and flattening of the medial tibial condyle with associated patellar dislocation and proximal tibial exostosis. Hand radiographs demonstrate typical changes, with osteopenia, shortening of the fourth and fifth metacarpals, delayed maturation, phalangeal predominance, a V-shaped deformity of the distal radiocarpal joint and drumstick-shaped distal phalanges (Figure 10.67). Cardiovascular findings include

septal defects, aortic coarctation and mitral valve prolapse. Renal anomalies include rotational anomalies, bifid renal pelvis, horseshoe kidney and multicystic dysplastic kidney. Autoimmune conditions, including hypothyroidism, diabetes, and juvenile rheumatoid arthritis have been associated with Turner syndrome. Genital abnormalities include ovarian and uterine absence or hypoplasia. Other abnormalities include intestinal telangiectasia, lymphedema, and lymphangioma.

VACTERL association

The acronym VATER (later expanded to VACTERL) describes the anomalies in multiple organ systems believed to arise from mesodermal defects occurring by the fifth week of fetal life, probably from a defect in blastogenesis. VACTERL is believed to be a primary, polytopic, developmental field defect which is causally heterogeneous and rarely familial. The mnemonic acronym denotes the following: V – vertebral anomalies, A – anorectal anomalies, C – cardiac lesions, TE – tracheoesophageal anomalies, especially esophageal atresia, R – renal anomalies,

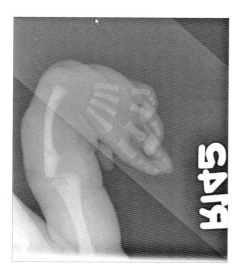

Figure 10.70 VACTERL: frontal radiographs of the forearm and hand in a neonate with esophageal atresia. There is absence of the radius and a hypoplastic thumb without phalangeal ossification.

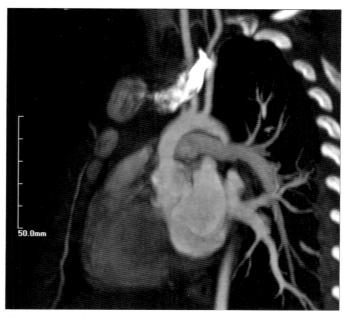

Figure 10.71 Williams syndrome: 3D reformatted CT angiogram demonstrating supravalvular narrowing of the aorta above the sinuses of Valsalva and the origins of the carotid arteries.

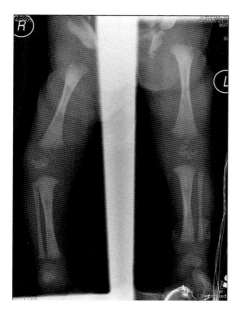

Figure 10.72 Zellweger syndrome: frontal radiograph of both legs. Punctate calcifications are present within the patella bilaterally, as well as in both greater trochanters, the left triradiate cartilage and ischial tuberosity cartilage.

Cardiovascular anomalies include isolated ventriculoseptal defect (most frequent), atrial septal defect, tetralogy of Fallot and transposition of the great arteries. Central nervous system anomalies are not included in the VACTERL acronym but are not uncommon in affected patients. As much as one-third of patients with imperforate anus have spinal dysraphism, including tethered cord, intradural lipoma and lipomeningocele. Hydrocephalus associated with the VACTERL association is known to have a high rate of recurrence in subsequent pregnancies. This is referred to as VACTERL-H association, with hydrocephalus added to the acronym. VACTERL-H is frequently an X-linked disorder, particularly when aqueductal stenosis is present and the prognosis is poor.

Williams syndrome

Williams syndrome is a rare autosomal syndrome related to partial deletion of chromosome 7. Patients present with a characteristic elfin facies, mental retardation, supravalvular aortic stenosis and infantile hypercalcemia (Figure 10.71). Skeletal changes include osteosclerosis in infancy, often associated with hypercalcemia, pectus excavatum, radioulnar synostosis and delayed bone age. Williams syndrome is due to deletion of genes in the locus 7q11, including the *ELN* gene (Elastin gene).

Zellweger syndrome

Zellweger (cerebrohepatorenal) syndrome is the result of mutation of genes involved in peroxisome biogenesis. Findings include characteristic flat facies with a high forehead, severe hypotonia, seizures, mental retardation, liver enlargement and

L – limb anomalies, especially radial ray anomalies (Figure 10.68). Defects in at least three organ systems of the VACTERL acronym should be present in order to apply the diagnosis. If any of these features are present, a genetic condition associated with either esophageal atresia or with imperforate anus needs to be excluded.

The vertebral anomalies may occur in any part of the spine, although sacral anomalies are most common in patients with imperforate anus (Figure 10.69). Thirteen rib-bearing vertebral bodies is the most common skeletal anomaly in some series of esophageal atresia patients. Hemivertebra and hypoplastic vertebra are the next most common. Limb anomalies are variable, including radial segment hypoplasia, proximal focal femoral deficiency, fibular hemimelia and amelia (Figure 10.70). Renal anomalies include agenesis, dysplasia, hypoplastic kidneys, horseshoe kidney and pelvic kidney.

dysfunction, stippled epiphyses and renal cysts. The most helpful radiographic findings seen at birth are stippled calcifications, typically affecting the patellae and the Y-cartilages of the pelvis (Figure 10.72). The calcifications may involve many other areas and may be periarticular. The renal cysts tend to be small and in the periphery of the kidneys.

Within the central nervous system, findings include microgyria, pachygyria, heterotopic dysplasia, ventricular dilatation, periventricular cysts, and leukoencephalopathy. Skull findings include widened cranial sutures and dolichocephaly.

Gastrointestinal abnormalities include anorectal malformations, intestinal lymphangiectasia, and hepatomegaly with abnormal liver function studies. Extremity abnormalities include contractures, clubfoot, and retarded skeletal maturation. Fetal hypokinesia and increased nuchal translucency have been noted in utero. Zellweger syndrome is a peroxisomal disorder due to mutation in one of 12 genes coding for peroxins (PEX genes) which are needed for normal peroxisomal assembly, although more than half of cases are due to mutations in the *PEX1* gene.

Further reading

Ansell BM (2000) Rheumatic disease mimics in childhood. *Curr Opin Rheumatol* **12**(5), 445–7.

Azouz EM, Teebi AS, Eydoux P, Chen MF, Fassier F (1998) Bone dysplasias: an introduction. *Can Assoc Radiol J* **49**(2), 105–9.

Baujat G, Legeai-Mallet L, Finidori G, Cormier-Daire V, Le Merrer M (2008) Achondroplasia. *Best Pract Res Clin Rheumatol* **22**(1), 3–18.

Brusin JH (2008) Osteogenesis imperfecta. *Radiol Technol* **79**(6), 535–48; quiz 549–51.

Dighe M, Fligner C, Cheng E, Warren B, Dubinsky T (2008) Fetal skeletal dysplasia: an approach to diagnosis with illustrative cases. *Radiographics* **28**(4), 1061–77.

Faden MA, Krakow D, Ezgu F, Rimoin DL, Lachman RS (2009) The Erlenmeyer flask bone deformity in the skeletal dysplasias. *Am J Med Genet A* **149A**(6), 1334–45.

Finn CT, Vedolin L, Schwartz IV *et al.* (2008) Magnetic resonance imaging findings in

Hunter syndrome. *Acta Paediatr Suppl* **97**(457), 61–8.

Glass RB, Fernbach SK, Norton KI, Choi PS, Naidich TP (2004) The infant skull: a vault of information. *Radiographics* **24**(2), 507–22.

Job-Deslandre C (2004) Inherited ossifying diseases. *Joint Bone Spine* **71**(2), 98–101.

Kant SG, Grote F, de Ru MH *et al.* (2007) Radiographic evaluation of children with growth disorders. *Horm Res* **68**(6), 310–15.

Lachman RS (1997) The cervical spine in the skeletal dysplasias and associated disorders. *Pediatr Radiol* **27**(5), 402–8.

Laor T, Jaramillo D (2009) MR imaging insights into skeletal maturation: what is normal? *Radiology* **250**(1), 28–38. Review.

Lemyre E, Azouz EM, Teebi AS, Glanc P, Chen MF (1999) Bone dysplasia series. Achondroplasia, hypochondroplasia and thanatophoric dysplasia: review and update. *Can Assoc Radiol J* **50**(3), 185–97.

Levin TL, Berdon WE, Lachman RS *et al.* (1997) Lumbar gibbus in storage diseases

and bone dysplasias. *Pediatr Radiol* **27**(4), 289–94.

Markowitz RI, Zackai E (2001) A pragmatic approach to the radiological diagnosis of pediatric syndromes and skeletal dysplasias. *Radiol Clin North Am* **39**(4), 791–802.

Morcuende JA (1993) Orthopedic aspects of skeletal dysplasia in children. *Curr Opin Pediatr* **5**(3), 363–7.

Mortier GR (2001) The diagnosis of skeletal dysplasias: a multidisciplinary approach. *Eur J Radiol* **40**(3), 161–7.

Papageorghiou AT, Fratelli N, Leslie K, Bhide A, Thilaganathan B (2008) Outcome of fetuses with antenatally diagnosed short femur. *Ultrasound Obstet Gynecol* **31**(5), 507–11.

Sheridan BD, Gargan MF, Monsell FP (2009) The hip in osteochondrodysplasias: general rules for diagnosis and treatment. *Hip Int* **19**(Suppl. 6), S26–34.

Wiggins GC, Shaffrey CI, Abel MF, Menezes AH (2003) Pediatric spinal deformities. *Neurosurg Focus* **14**(1), e3.

Chapter 11

Transplant imaging in children

Govind Chavhan and Paul Babyn

Introduction

Transplantation has become an established treatment for many conditions and indeed is often the last resort for patient survival. The number of transplantations is increasing as improved surgical techniques, immunosuppression, and post-operative care have increased success rates. The common types of transplant are reviewed in Table 11.1. The most common transplantation performed in children at our institution is bone marrow transplantation (approximately 100 cases per year). Commonly transplanted organs in children in decreasing order of frequency include kidney, liver, heart, lungs, bowel and pancreas (Table 11.2). With the increasing number of transplants of various organs come new challenges for the radiologist in terms of pre- and post-transplant imaging. Preoperative imaging is done to evaluate the potential donor to exclude any significant pathology and to obtain anatomical information for operative planning. Following transplantation, imaging is mainly performed to evaluate complications, which may be acute or chronic.

This chapter outlines principles of pre- and post-transplant imaging of organs such as liver, kidney, lung, heart, small bowel and bone marrow in children, with illustrative examples. Also discussed is post-transplantation lymphoproliferative disorder (PTLD), which can complicate any transplantation. Rejection of the transplanted organ or tissue occurs when the recipient's immune system attacks the transplant, causing damage to the organ, and can have systemic effects. Transplant rejection is one of the commonest complications but does not have specific radiological features.

Table 11.1 Types of transplant

Autograft	Transplant of tissues/organ in the same person. Patient's own tissues are transplanted to another place
Allograft	Transplant of organ or tissue from a genetically nonidentical member of the same species e.g. human to human
Isograft	Subset of allograft. Transplant between genetically identical twins. Same as autograft in terms of recipient's immune response
Xenograft	Transplantation from one species to another e.g. porcine heart valve transplant
Split transplant	A single organ, e.g. liver, from a deceased donor can be split and transplanted into two recipients
Domino transplant	Sequential transplants – an organ from a deceased donor is transplanted into the first recipient. The first recipient's organ then is transplanted into a second recipient. For example, a donor's heart and lungs are transplanted into a second person whose heart, in turn, is transplanted into a third person. Domino transplant has been performed for liver as well
Orthotopic transplant	Diseased organ is removed and donor's organ is placed in that place, e.g. liver and heart transplants
Heterotopic transplant	Transplantation of an organ to a site that is different from the location that the organ would ordinarily occupy within the body. Diseased organ is usually not removed from the body, e.g. heart transplant and renal transplant

Table 11.2 Commonly performed pediatric transplants

Organs	Sources of organ
Bone marrow	Living donor or autograft
Kidney	Deceased or living donor
Liver	Deceased or living donor
Heart	Deceased donor only
Enbloc heart and lung transplant	Deceased donor or domino transplant
Lung	Deceased or living donor
Intestine	Deceased or living donor
Pancreas	Deceased donor only

Essentials of Pediatric Radiology, ed. Heike E. Daldrup-Link and Charles A. Gooding. Published by Cambridge University Press.

(A)

(B)

(C)

(D)

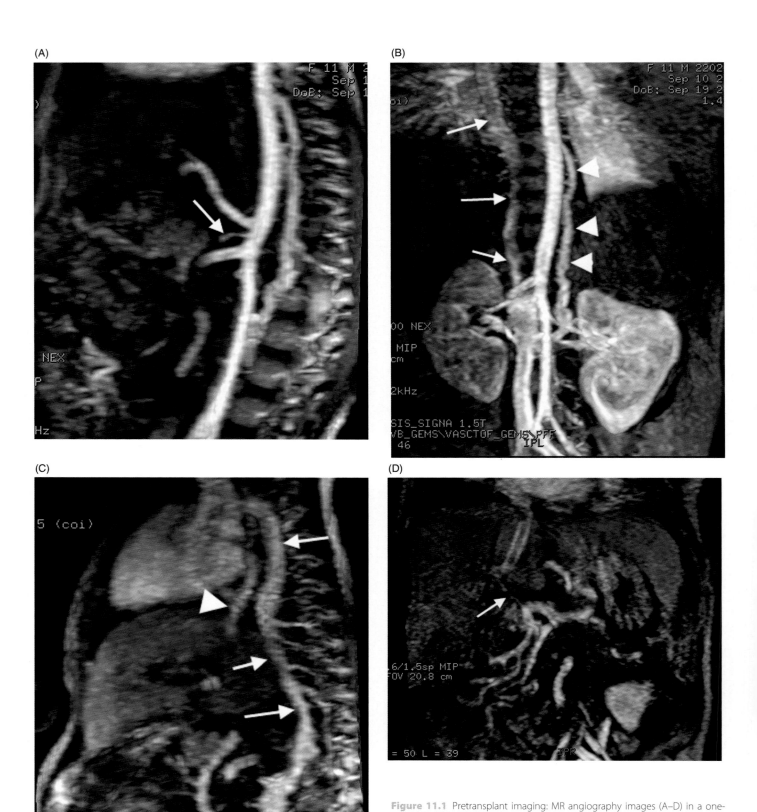

Figure 11.1 Pretransplant imaging: MR angiography images (A–D) in a one-year-old child with failed Kasai procedure for biliary atresia. The splenic artery arises directly from the aorta (arrow on A). There is interruption of intrahepatic IVC with azygous continuation of IVC (arrows on B and C) and prominence of hemiazygous vein (arrowheads on B). Note the short segment of suprahepatic IVC (arrowhead on C) available for anastomosis. The portal vein is atretic (arrow on D). Pretransplant MRA (E) in another child shows anomalous origin of the right hepatic artery from the superior mesenteric artery (arrow).

(E)

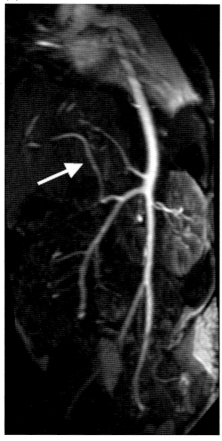

Figure 11.1 (Cont.)

Pretransplant imaging

Pretransplant imaging is often performed to evaluate the donor as well as recipient. Live donor organ imaging may be performed to evaluate organ anatomy and its vasculature for suitability for transplant. Length, caliber and anatomical variations of vessels are important for surgical planning (Figure 11.1). Similar information about the biliary, bronchial and urinary tract is required for transplantation. The usual modalities used include US, CT, MR and angiography.

Liver transplant

Liver transplant is an established therapy for end-stage pediatric liver disease. Common indications in children include biliary diseases, such as biliary atresia, sclerosing cholangitis, cystic fibrosis, primary biliary cirrhosis; metabolic diseases, such as alpha-1 antitrypsin deficiency, glycogen storage disease, Wilson's disease, hemochromatosis; and cirrhosis from any cause. Presently used grafts include pediatric cadaveric whole organ graft, segmental or split adult cadaveric grafts, and living related adult segmental graft (segments II and III or II–IV). Use of split cadaveric graft and living donor segmental graft has increased the donor pool. Usually

the donor hepatic artery, portal vein, suprahepatic IVC and infrahepatic IVC are anastomosed end-to-end to the respective recipient vessels. If the vascular pedicle is short, especially in split and segmental grafts, autologous iliac artery conduit or donor conduit from the infrarenal aorta can be used. However, this increases the risk of vascular complications. When recipient vena cava is kept as it is and donor hepatic vein is attached end-to-side to it, the technique is called "piggyback" technique. Biliary anastomosis is end-to-end fashion except in biliary atresia where hepato-jejunostomy is performed. US is the primary modality for evaluation of the liver transplant. Comprehensive assessment of parenchymal, biliary and vascular complications can be done by MRI combined with MR cholangiography and contrast-enhanced MR angiography.

Vascular complications usually occur in the early postoperative period and are discussed in Table 11.3 (Figures 11.2–11.8). The hepatic artery is the sole supply to the biliary epithelium of transplanted liver, hence its patency is vital for survival of the graft. Caliber difference between donor and recipient vessels may normally be seen (Figure 11.4B). Hemodynamically significant stenosis is diagnosed when a three- to fourfold increase in velocity is seen at the site of narrowing. Intrahepatic parvus tardus pattern may be normally seen in the first 72 hours after transplant because of edema at the anastomotic site; hence, early on, this finding should be interpreted with caution.

Biliary complications are the most common complications seen after pediatric liver transplant (in up to 27% of cases) and the majority of them occur in the first three months following surgery. They include anastomotic leakage (Figure 11.9A–C), stenosis with proximal dilatation (Figure 11.9D, E), bile duct stones, sludge, bilioma and rare mucocele of cystic duct remnant. Bile duct leak or stricture can lead to cholangitis, sepsis and abscess. Nonanastomotic strictures are probably related to hepatic arterial insufficiency. Post-transplantation biliary leak should prompt a search for hepatic artery thrombosis.

Liver parenchymal abnormalities such as infarction, biliomas or abscess can complicate transplantation. Infarction can be seen as round or geographical hypoechoic solid lesion on ultrasound. It is seen as irregular, peripherally located wedge-shaped hypoattenuating lesions on CT images. A periportal area of low echogenicity on US and hypodensity on CT, called the "periportal collar sign," can be seen normally and is thought to result from dilatation of lymphatic channels. It usually resolves within a few weeks. Organ rejection is a common complication; however, it does not have specific imaging features.

Other complications include localized collections (Figure 11.10), extrahepatic biliomas and PTLD.

Renal transplant

The kidney is one of the most commonly transplanted organs in children as well as adults. The renal graft is usually

Table 11.3 Vascular complications of liver transplant

	Incidence	Risk factors	Clinical features	Imaging features	Treatment
Hepatic artery stenosis	14%	Clamp injury, intimal trauma. Commonly at anastomotic site	Can lead to biliary ischemia, hepatic failure	US 80–90% sensitive in detection. Velocity >2 m sec^{-1}, parvus tardus with low resistive index (RI) in distal circulation	Balloon dilatation, surgical
Hepatic artery thrombosis	5%	Split and segmental grafts. Prolonged cold ischemia, caliber difference, conduits	Elevated liver enzyme, bile leak, fulminant hepatic necrosis, failure	US detection in up to 90% of cases. Complete absence of flow, collaterals. MR/CT angiography useful for evaluation	Thrombectomy, intra-arterial thrombolysis, angioplasty.
Portal vein (PV) stenosis	4%	Usually at anastomosis. Reduced size grafts, short length PV	Asymptomatic or portal hypertension	>50% reduction in lumen suggestive of stenosis. Three- to fourfold increase in velocity at narrowed segment suggests hemodynamically significant stenosis	Percutaneous stent placement, balloon angioplasty
Portal vein thrombosis	3.2%	Reduced size graft. Surgical difficulties, presence of portosystemic shunt, prior splenectomy, conduits	New onset massive ascites, varices, elevated liver function tests (LFTs), splenomegaly	Acute thrombus is usually anechoic. Echogenic thrombus with absent color flow. Thrombus can be non-lumen occlusive. MRA provides excellent details	Thrombectomy, segmental resection, stent, balloon angioplasty. Extension of thrombus into peripheral branches usually requires retransplantation
IVC stenosis	Common in children	Partial liver transplant. More frequent in superior anastomosis. Size difference, kinking	Pleural effusion, edema, ascites, hepatomegaly. Budd-Chiari syndrome	Reduced caliber at anastomosis, three- to fourfold increase in velocity with aliasing	Balloon angioplasty, stent. Pressure gradient measurement done for functional significance
IVC thrombosis	<1%	At anastomoses. Use of catheters, compressing fluid collection	Lower limb edema	Anechoic or echogenic thrombus without color flow. MRA is excellent in depiction and extent	—

Data from Berrocal et al. (2006).

placed heterotopically in the extraperitoneal space in one of the iliac fossae. The right donor kidney is placed in the left iliac fossa and vice versa. The donor renal artery is anastomosed end-to-end to the internal iliac artery or end-to-side to the external iliac artery. In cadaveric transplant, the portion of donor aorta around the origin of the renal artery is used and is known as a Carrel patch. The donor renal vein is almost always anastomosed end-to-side to the recipient external iliac vein. The donor ureter is anastomosed to the bladder by ureteroneocystostomy or to the recipient ureter or pelvis. In small children with small iliac fossae the renal allograft is placed more cephalad with anastomosis to the aorta and vena cava.

Postoperative complications can be seen in up to 12–20% of adult and pediatric renal transplants. Complications can be broadly divided into four categories: rejection, vascular,

urological and fluid collections. Rejection can be hyperacute (within hours to 2 days), acute (24 hours to 3–4 days) or chronic (months to years). Acute rejection is the most common rejection and is indicated by an increased resistive index (RI) of more than 0.80. However, it is a nonspecific finding and can be seen in cyclosporine toxicity and acute tubular necrosis. Chronic rejection is the leading cause of late graft loss and may show thin cortex and mild hydronephrosis. Graft biopsy is required for the diagnosis of rejection and prognosis.

Vascular complications can be seen in 3 to 15% of cases in adults and children and include renal arterial thrombosis (Figure 11.11), renal artery stenosis (Figure 11.12), renal vein thrombosis (Figure 11.13), pseudoaneurysm and arteriovenous fistula (Figure 11.14). Renal artery stenosis can be seen in 3–10% of cases in pediatric renal transplant. It can cause hypertension

(A)

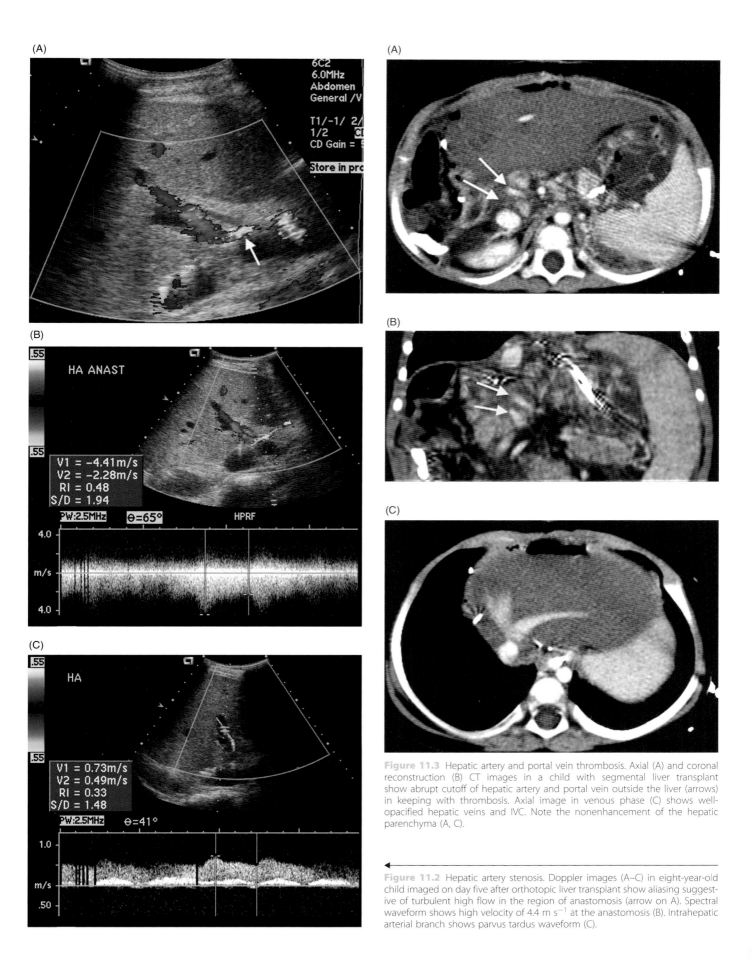

(A)

(B)

HA ANAST

V1 = -4.41m/s
V2 = -2.28m/s
RI = 0.48
S/D = 1.94

(B)

(C)

HA

V1 = 0.73m/s
V2 = 0.49m/s
RI = 0.33
S/D = 1.48

(C)

Figure 11.3 Hepatic artery and portal vein thrombosis. Axial (A) and coronal reconstruction (B) CT images in a child with segmental liver transplant show abrupt cutoff of hepatic artery and portal vein outside the liver (arrows) in keeping with thrombosis. Axial image in venous phase (C) shows well-opacified hepatic veins and IVC. Note the nonenhancement of the hepatic parenchyma (A, C).

Figure 11.2 Hepatic artery stenosis. Doppler images (A–C) in eight-year-old child imaged on day five after orthotopic liver transplant show aliasing suggestive of turbulent high flow in the region of anastomosis (arrow on A). Spectral waveform shows high velocity of 4.4 m s^{-1} at the anastomosis (B). Intrahepatic arterial branch shows parvus tardus waveform (C).

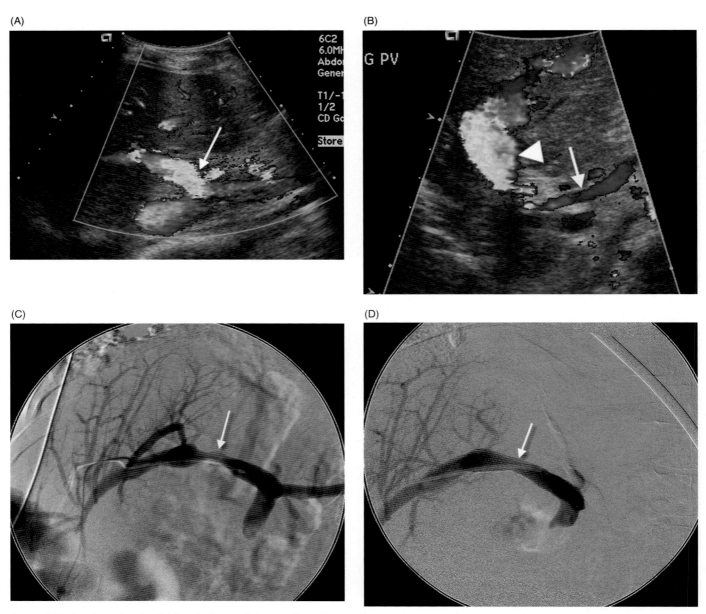

Figure 11.4 Portal vein imaging. (A) Doppler image of the transplanted liver on day one shows normal portal vein with some aliasing in the anastomosis region (arrow). (B) Portal vein in another child with segmental liver transplant shows caliber difference in recipient (arrow) and donor (arrowhead) portal veins. (C, D) Percutaneous portal venogram in an eight-year-old child performed six years after liver transplant for biliary atresia shows stricture of the vein at the porta (arrow on C). A stent is placed across the stricture that improves the caliber of the vein (arrow on D).

and progressive renal insufficiency. Stenosis is commonly seen at the anastomosis, though it can also be seen in donor or recipient arterial segments. Predisposing factors include suture techniques, trauma, kinking, rejection and infection. Ultrasound is the initial modality for evaluation. Aliasing and increased peak systolic velocity of more than 200 cm sec^{-1} in the narrowed segment, velocity gradient of 2 : 1 between pre- and poststenotic segment, and dampening of distal flow with parvus tardus waveforms are the suggestive features of stenosis. MR angiography can be useful for evaluation when US is inconclusive or difficult to perform because of body

habitus. Percutaneous transluminal angioplasty, stenting and surgical revision are the treatment options. Arterial or venous thrombosis is seen in 1% of cases and usually occurs in the early (<1 week) post-transplant period. Faulty surgical technique, kinking, compression of the vessel by fluid collection, hypercoagulable state and rejection are the predisposing factors for thrombosis. It can cause segmental infarction of the graft. US shows absent flow in the thrombosed segment of artery and vein. Increased RI or diastolic reversal in intrarenal arteries with enlarged echogenic kidney can be seen in venous thrombosis. If thrombosis extends to the intrarenal vessels, the

(A)

(B)

(C)

(D)

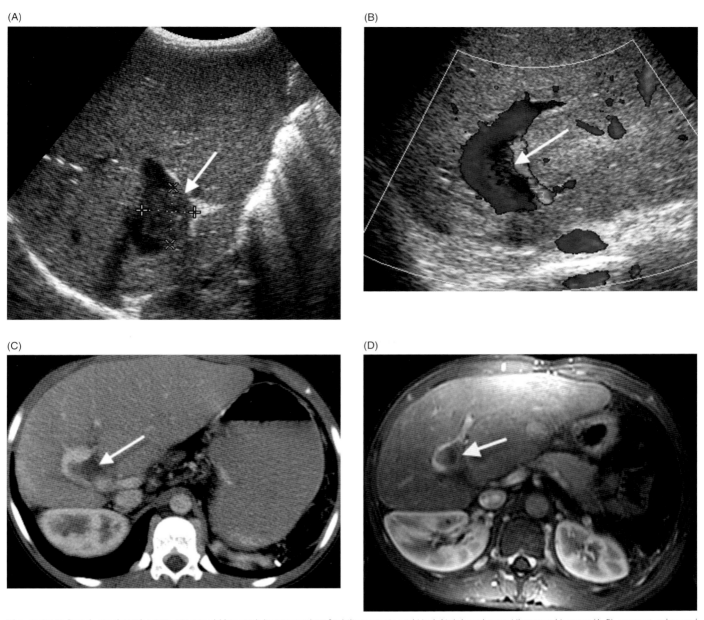

Figure 11.5 Portal vein thrombosis in 15-year-old boy with liver transplant for biliary atresia and Hodgkin's lymphoma. Ultrasound images (A, B), contrast-enhanced axial CT (C) and MR (D) images show non-lumen-occlusive thrombus in the portal vein (arrows).

graft is usually nonsalvageable. Arteriovenous fistulas (AVFs) are usually the result of vascular trauma from renal biopsy. They can present as hypertension, hematuria or high-output cardiac failure. Most of the small asymptomatic AVFs (70%) resolve spontaneously within one to two years. Large AVFs require transcatheter embolization or surgical repair. US can easily detect AVF, and findings include increased arterial flow with characteristic high-velocity/low-impedance waveform, arterialization of venous flow and fistulous communication between artery and vein. Pseudoaneurysm can occur from anastomosis, biopsy or mycotic infection, and can easily be detected by US. Pseudoaneurysm is rare but can cause devastating bleeding and shock from rupture.

Urological complications are seen in 1–10% of pediatric transplant cases and include ureteral obstruction (Figure 11.15) and urine leak. Transplant ureter, especially the terminal segment at the ureterovesical junction, is prone to ischemia. Causes of ureteral obstruction include clot, calculi, stricture and extrinsic compression from fluid collection. Mild dilatation of the pelvicalyceal system and ureter is common in the early postoperative period due to denervation and edema at the ureteric anastomosis. If the dilatation seen on US is associated with elevated serum creatinine or oliguria it is suggestive of obstruction. Urine leak is a potentially life-threatening complication because of the risk of infection in immunosuppressed patients. The most frequent site of

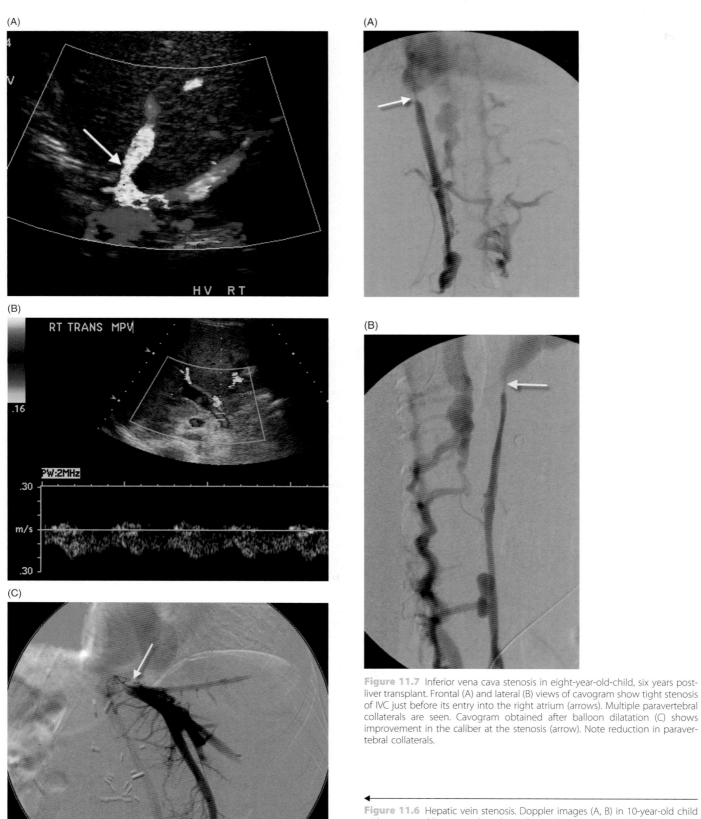

(A)

(B)

(C)

(A)

(B)

Figure 11.7 Inferior vena cava stenosis in eight-year-old-child, six years post-liver transplant. Frontal (A) and lateral (B) views of cavogram show tight stenosis of IVC just before its entry into the right atrium (arrows). Multiple paravertebral collaterals are seen. Cavogram obtained after balloon dilatation (C) shows improvement in the caliber at the stenosis (arrow). Note reduction in paravertebral collaterals.

Figure 11.6 Hepatic vein stenosis. Doppler images (A, B) in 10-year-old child with segmental liver transplant show aliasing (arrow on A) and high velocity up to 2.7 m s^{-1} (B) at the anastomosis of hepatic vein and IVC, suggestive of anastomotic narrowing. This was confirmed on percutaneous transhepatic venography (arrow in C).

(C)

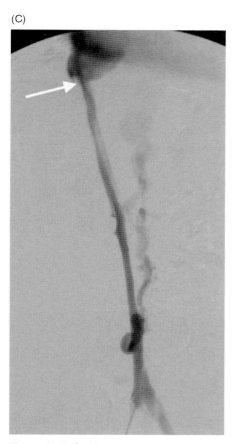

Figure 11.7 (Cont.)

(A)

(B)

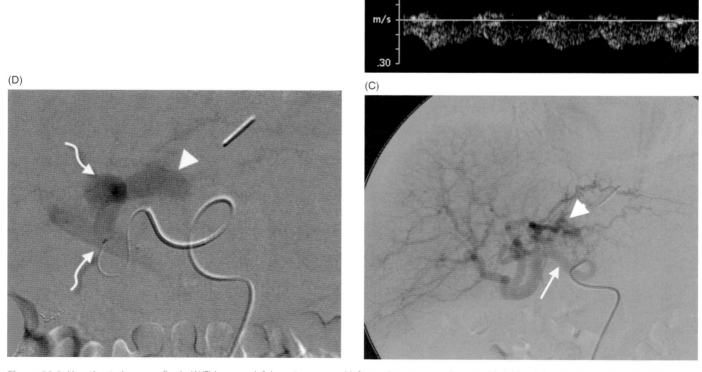

(D)

(C)

Figure 11.8 Hepatic arteriovenous fistula (AVF) between left hepatic artery and left portal vein in an eight-year-old child with liver transplant. (A) Color Doppler US image shows prominence of left hepatic artery with turbulence (arrow) and left portal vein (curved arrow). Communication between the two is shown with the arrowhead. (B) Spectral waveforms in the portal vein show reversed hepatofugal flow that is "arterialized." (C, D) Hepatic artery (arrow on C) injection shows tortuous vessels on the left side (arrowhead) and opacification of the left and main portal vein (curved arrows) suggestive of AVF.

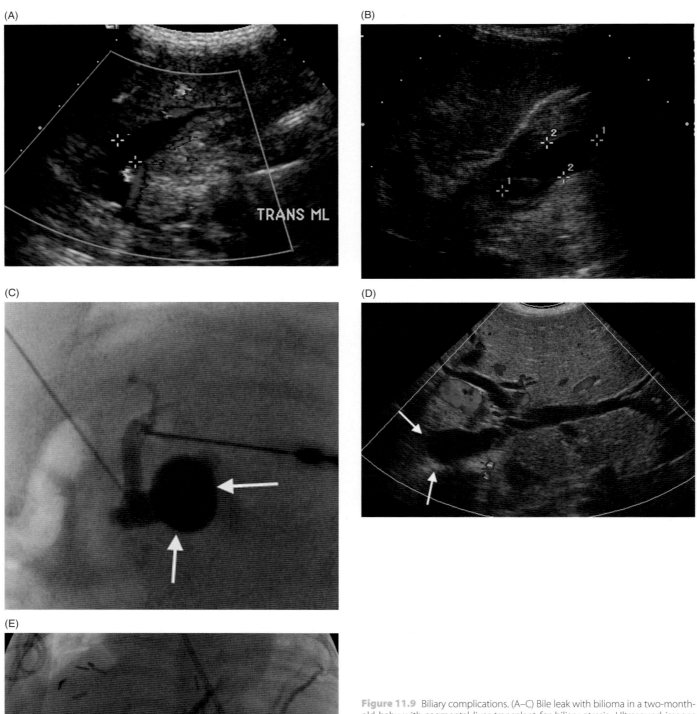

Figure 11.9 Biliary complications. (A–C) Bile leak with bilioma in a two-month-old baby with segmental liver transplant for biliary atresia. Ultrasound images (A, B) show marked dilatation of intrahepatic bile duct (cursor on A) and a complex collection on inferior aspect of the liver (cursors on B). Percutaneous transhepatic cholangiogram (C) confirmed the bile leak communicating with the collection, suggestive of bilioma (arrows). (D, E) Biliary anastomotic stricture in three-year-old child with segmental liver transplant for biliary atresia. US image shows marked dilatation of bile ducts up to the neoporta (arrows on D). PTC shows no contrast passage into the bowel, suggestive of anastomotic stricture (arrows on E). External biliary drainage was placed subsequently (not shown).

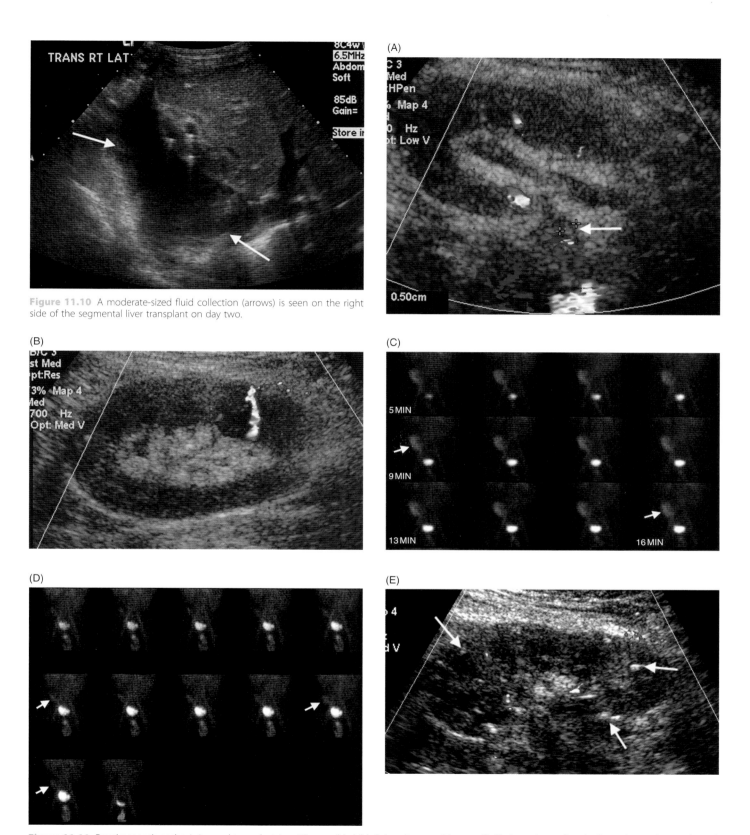

Figure 11.10 A moderate-sized fluid collection (arrows) is seen on the right side of the segmental liver transplant on day two.

Figure 11.11 Renal artery thrombosis in renal transplant in a 12-year-old child. Color ultrasound images (A, B) show absent flow in the main renal artery (arrow). Marked hypoperfusion of the renal graft is seen with loss of corticomedullary differentiation. (C) Renal DTPA (diethylene triamine pentaacetic acid) image shows reduced perfusion of the renal graft (arrow). (D) Follow-up DTPA scan done after one year shows little perfusion of the graft (arrow). Follow-up ultrasound image (E) shows smaller kidney with little flow and lost corticomedullary differentiation and multiple foci of calcification (arrows).

(A)

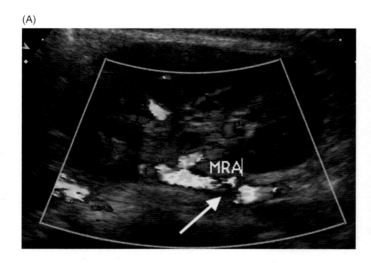

(B)

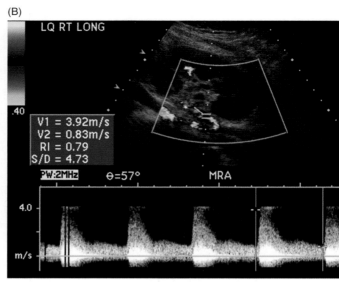

(C)

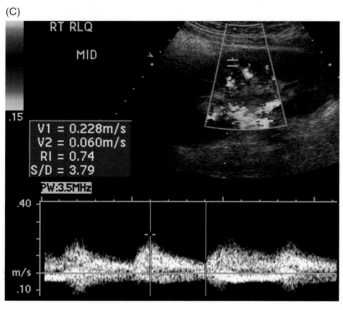

Figure 11.12 Renal artery anastomotic stenosis in a 16-year-old boy with renal transplant for Caroli's disease. Aliasing is seen in the region of anastomosis (arrow on A). Spectral waveforms (B) show high velocity of 3.9 m s^{-1} in the region of anastomosis. Intrarenal spectrum (C) displays parvus tardus waveforms suggesting significant stenosis at anastomosis.

leak is the distal ureter, particularly one affected by ischemia. Antegrade contrast study or radionuclide study can detect the leak.

Perigraft fluid collections can be seen in approximately 50% of renal transplant patients, and 15–20% of these are clinically significant. Fluid collections include lymphocele, urinomas, hematoma (Figure 11.16) and abscess. Lymphoceles are the most common collections and usually occur weeks to months after transplantation. They commonly show internal septations, as opposed to urinomas that rarely show septations. US detects fluid collections, but their appearance is nonspecific. They can be reliably differentiated by aspiration and chemical analysis.

Bone marrow transplantation

Bone marrow transplantation (BMT) is an established form of treatment for many conditions including leukemia, lymphoma, solid tumors such as neuroblastoma, bone marrow failure, immunodeficiencies and many genetic disorders. Stages of BMT include pretransplantation period, transplantation, and post-transplantation period. Pretransplantation period includes four to six days before transplantation in which chemotherapy or whole body radiation is given to eradicate tumor cells. During transplantation, intravenous infusion of donor stem cells is done. These cells then gradually migrate to marrow spaces. The post-transplantation period can be divided into engraftment (first 15–30 days, during which stem cells grow in the marrow spaces), early postengraftment period (from 15–30 days to 100 days after transplantation) and late postengraftment period (more than 100 days). During engraftment there is severe marrow aplasia with pancytopenia. Common complications in the early postengraftment period include infections (Figure 11.17), acute graft-versus-host disease (GVHD) and graft failure. Late complications include

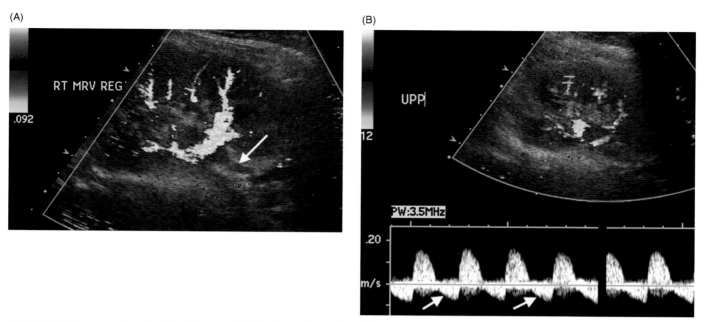

Figure 11.13 Renal vein thrombosis in a 14-year-old child with renal transplant. Color Doppler US images of the transplant kidney show absent flow in the renal vein (arrow on A) and reversed diastolic flow in intrarenal arteries (arrows on B). The kidney is enlarged and echogenic.

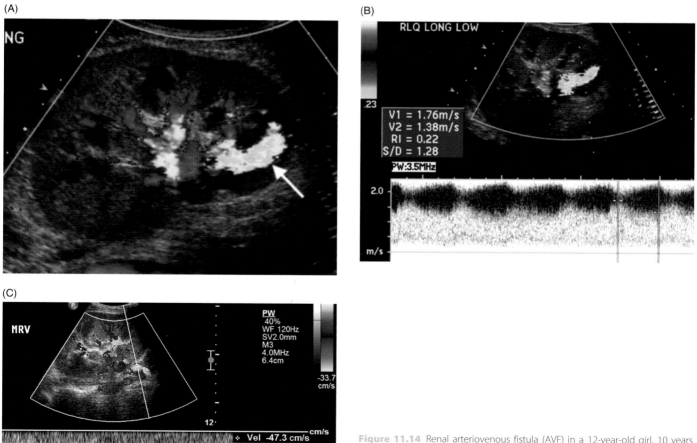

Figure 11.14 Renal arteriovenous fistula (AVF) in a 12-year-old girl, 10 years post-liver transplant and 1 month post-renal transplant. Doppler images of the transplant kidney (A–C) show findings suggestive of AVF in the lower pole. Aliasing is seen in the lower pole artery (arrow on A). High-velocity, low-resistance flow, classic for AVF, is seen on spectral waveform (B). The renal vein shows high-velocity "arterialized" flow (C).

(A)

(B)

(C)

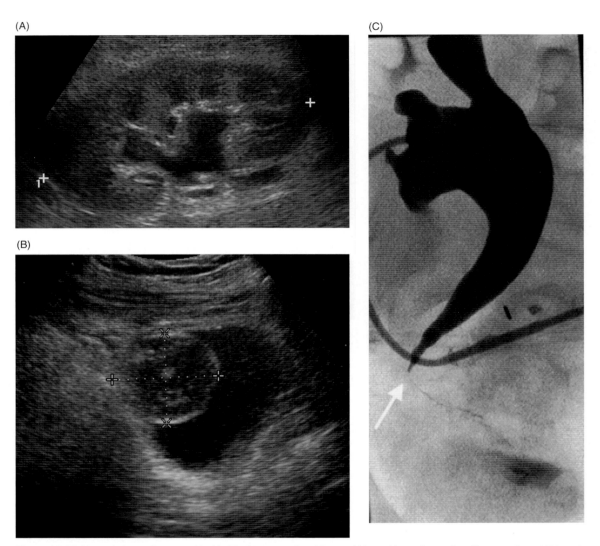

Figure 11.15 Ureteral obstruction caused by bladder hematoma in a 16-year-old boy with renal transplant. The transplanted kidney shows mild hydronephrosis (A). A round soft tissue lesion is seen on the right side in the bladder (measured on B). Percutaneous nephrostomy was performed after one week. Contrast injection through nephrostomy (C) shows severe narrowing of the ureter at the ureterovesical junction (arrow) with proximal dilatation.

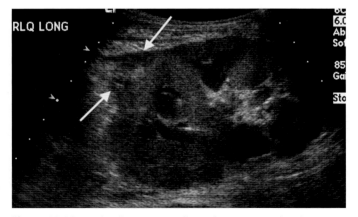

Figure 11.16 Renal collection. A small post-biopsy perinephric hematoma (arrows) is seen at the upper pole of the transplant kidney in the right lower quadrant.

recurrence of primary disease, chronic GVHD, avascular necrosis and secondary malignancies.

Pulmonary complications are common and affect more than 50% of patients. Interstitial pneumonitis can be idiopathic or infectious from cytomegalovirus, respiratory syncytial virus, adenovirus and *Pneumocystis jiroveci* infection. Radiological appearance is nonspecific and includes increased lung markings, areas of ground-glass and nodular densities on CT. Pulmonary infection by fungi such as *Aspergillus*, *Candida* and *Mucor*, and bacteria such as *Klebsiella* and *Streptococcus* are commonly seen early on. Other pulmonary complications including pulmonary edema, hemorrhage, bronchiolitis obliterans with organizing pneumonia (BOOP) and pulmonary calcifications can occur.

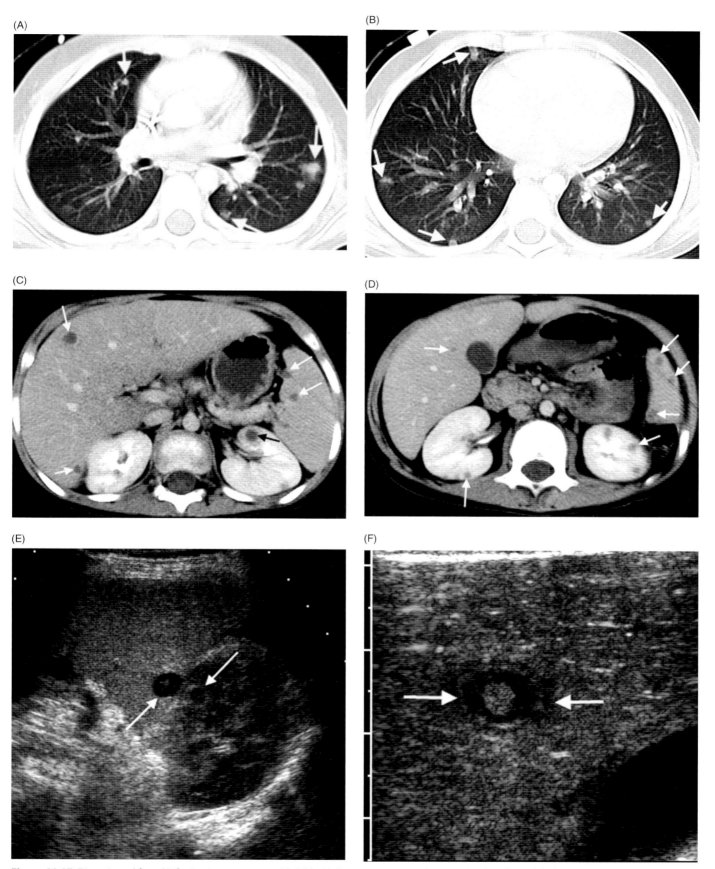

Figure 11.17 Disseminated fungal infection in a seven-year-old child with bone marrow transplantation (BMT) performed for leukemia. Axial CT images of lungs (A, B) and abdomen (C, D), and ultrasound images of spleen and left kidney (E) and liver (F) show round, varying sized nodules (arrows) suggestive of fungal granulomas. Some of the pulmonary nodules show a typical "halo" due to perilesional hemorrhage (A, large nodule in left lung). Ultrasound images (E, F) show target appearance of the granulomas with central echogenic focus.

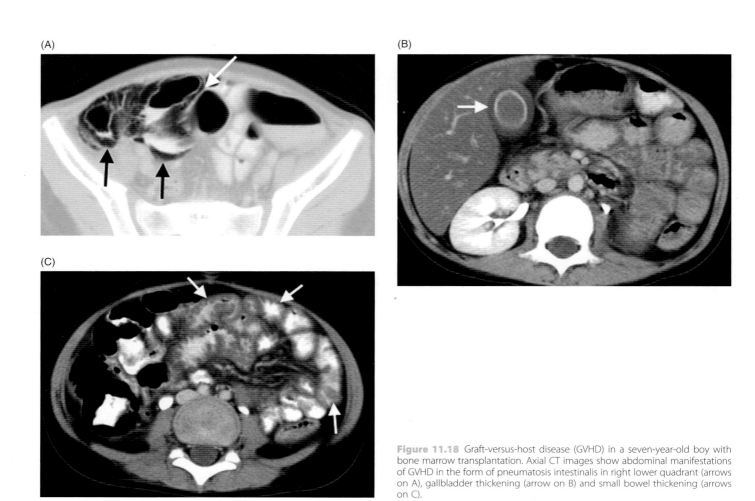

Figure 11.18 Graft-versus-host disease (GVHD) in a seven-year-old boy with bone marrow transplantation. Axial CT images show abdominal manifestations of GVHD in the form of pneumatosis intestinalis in right lower quadrant (arrows on A), gallbladder thickening (arrow on B) and small bowel thickening (arrows on C).

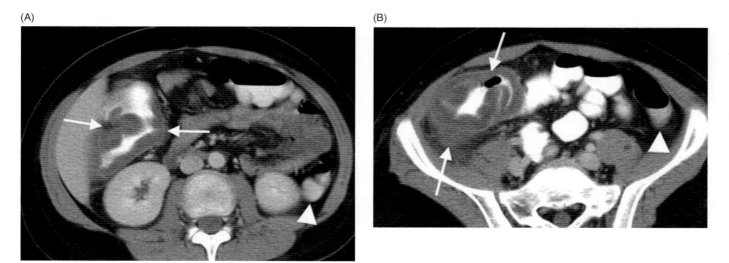

Figure 11.19 Neutropenic colitis/typhlitis in a nine-year-old child with bone marrow transplantation performed for leukemia. Axial CT images (A, B) show circumferential thickening of cecum and ascending colon up to the hepatic flexure (arrows). The descending colon (arrowhead) is not thickened.

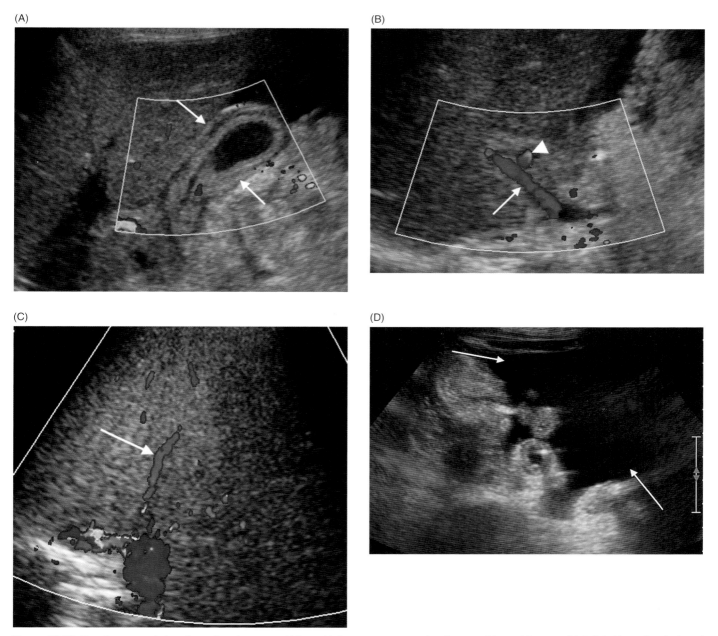

Figure 11.20 Hepatic veno-occlusive disease in a three-year-old boy with bone marrow transplant for stage IV neuroblastoma. (A) Gallbladder wall is thickened (arrows on A). (B) Portal vein flow is reversed (arrow) and opposite of the hepatic arterial flow (arrowhead). (C) Hepatic veins are patent but show narrow caliber (arrow on C). (D) Generalized ascites is seen (arrows on D).

Common abdominopelvic complications include graft-versus-host disease (GVHD) (Figure 11.18), neutropenic colitis (Figure 11.19), pneumatosis intestinalis, hepatic veno-occlusive disease (VOD) (Figure 11.20), fungal and bacterial infections and PTLD. GVHD is a multisystem complication resulting from donor T-lymphocytes damaging epithelium of skin, liver, gastrointestinal tract and other organs. GVHD presents with rash, increased bilirubin, hepatic dysfunction and diarrhea. It can be seen in 30–50% of allogenic BMT but GVHD does not occur in autologous BMT. On CT it may demonstrate increased enhancement of bowel wall, gallbladder wall and urinary bladder wall.

Pneumatosis intestinalis is probably related to high doses of steroid. It usually has a benign course unless it is associated with neutropenic colitis in which case it can be worrisome for necrosis of the bowel. VOD results from concentric narrowing of terminal hepatic venules with necrosis of hepatocytes, and is usually seen in the first two weeks. Ultrasound shows periportal hypoattenuation, hepatosplenomegaly, increased intrahepatic RI, small caliber hepatic veins, GB wall thickening, ascites and, in severe cases, reversal of portal venous flow. Liver can also be affected by fungal disease, PTLD, focal nodular hyperplasia and iron deposition in the BMT patient. Cyclophosphamide can cause hemorrhagic cystitis.

(A)

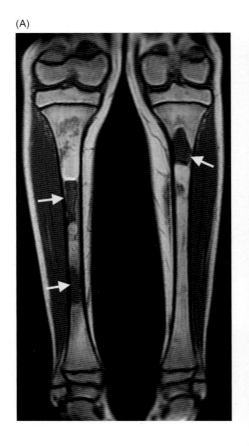

(B)

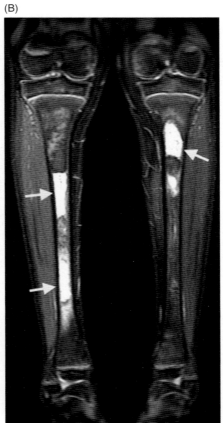

(C)

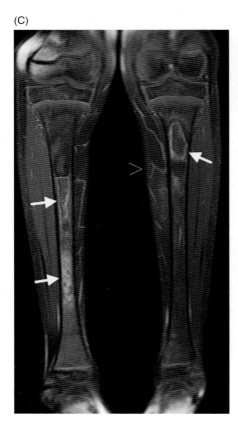

(D)

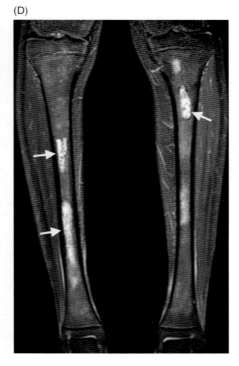

Figure 11.21 Bone infarcts in a 14-year-old boy with bone marrow transplant. Coronal T1W (A), T2W (B), and post-gadolinium T1W (C) images show T1-hypointense (A) and T2-hyperintense (B) well-defined areas of bone marrow signal abnormality (arrows) in both tibiae. These areas show peripheral enhancement (C). On follow-up MR imaging (T2W coronal image) after three years, these infarcts demonstrate a persistent abnormal T2 signal with serpiginous borders (arrows).

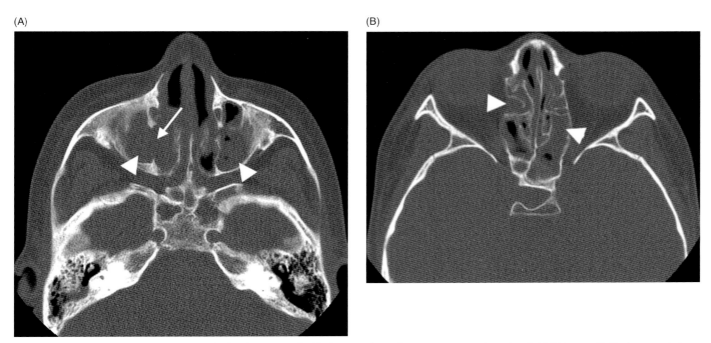

Figure 11.22 Fungal sinusitis in a 10-year-old girl with acute myeloid leukemia and post-bone marrow transplantation. Axial CT images (A, B) of paranasal sinuses show diffuse mucosal thickening with fluid accumulation in bilateral maxillary, ethmoid and sphenoid sinuses (arrowheads). There is destruction of the medial wall of the right maxillary antrum (arrow).

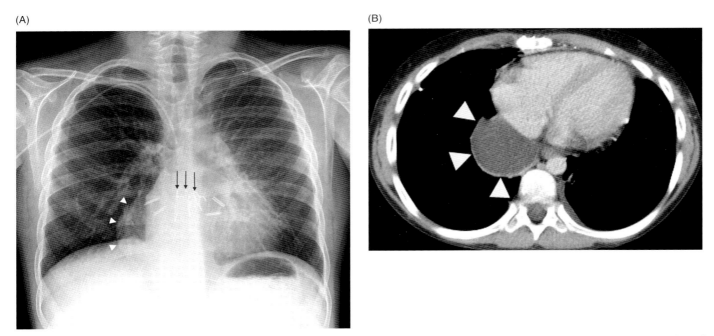

Figure 11.23 Mediastinal collection in a 12-year-old boy with lung transplant for cystic fibrosis. (A) Frontal radiograph of the chest shows right paracardiac soft tissue density (arrowheads). Vertical sutures (black arrows) are seen closing the typical transverse sternotomy (clamshell) performed for lung transplantation. (B) Axial contrast-enhanced CT image of the chest shows the fluid collection (arrowheads) posterior to the heart.

Musculoskeletal complications of BMT include bone infarction (Figure 11.21) and avascular necrosis. Infections, infarction, hemorrhage and drug toxicity are some of the complications seen in the CNS in BMT patients. GVHD does not directly affect the CNS, probably because of its lack of lymphatics. Nearly one-third of patients are affected by paranasal sinusitis within two years of BMT (Figure 11.22), and this is one of the common causes of fever. Sinusitis may be due to fungal infection from *Aspergillus* or bacterial infection such as *Streptococcus* and *Haemophilus influenzae*. CT may show air–fluid level and mucosal thickening. Invasive sinusitis (usually *Aspergillus*) shows periantral soft tissue invasion, bone erosion and orbital invasion.

(A)

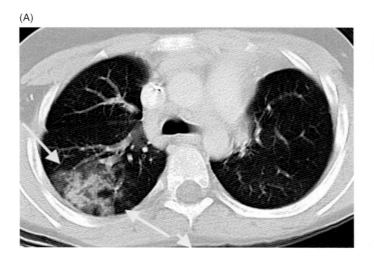

(B)

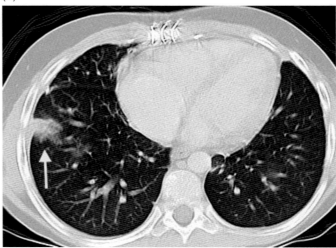

(C)

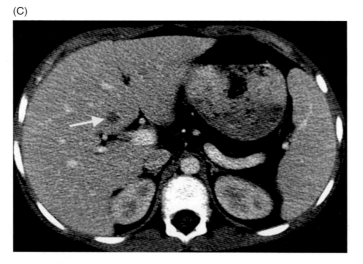

Figure 11.24 Atypical mycobacterial infection in a 10-year-old boy with lung transplantation for cystic fibrosis. Axial CT images (A, B) show nonspecific airspace opacities in the periphery of the right lung (arrows). Axial CT image of the abdomen (C) shows a small hypodense lesion in the liver (arrow).

Lung transplant

Lung transplantation is performed in children with irreversible and disabling end-stage pulmonary disease including cystic fibrosis, Eisenmenger complex, pulmonary fibrosis and bronchopulmonary dysplasia. Unilateral lung transplant is usually performed through a posterolateral thoracotomy, while sequential bilateral transplant (as for cystic fibrosis) is performed through a transverse sternotomy (Figure 11.23). Donor pulmonary arteries and mainstem bronchi are joined end-to-end to recipient pulmonary arteries and mainstem bronchi. The donor's left atrial cuff is attached to the recipient's left atrium.

Complications seen in lung transplant patients include acute rejection (within three weeks of transplantation), chronic rejection (after three months of transplantation), infections (Figure 11.24), PTLD and bronchial complications. Plain chest radiographs and especially CT scans of the chest play important roles in the evaluation of these complications. Radiological findings, however, are nonspecific and include ground-glass densities, interlobular septal thickening and small nodules in acute rejection. Similar findings are seen in chronic rejection

that is characterized by bronchiolitis obliterans (Figures 11.25, 11.26). Infection can be bacterial (*Enterobacter, Pseudomonas, Staphylococcus aureus, H. influenzae*), viral (CMV, herpes, Epstein-Barr) or fungal (*Candida, Aspergillus*). Radiological findings in infection are nonspecific and may include ground-glass areas, nodules, airspace disease, abscesses and mediastinal lymphadenopathy. Bronchial stenosis (usually at anastomosis), stent migration and bronchial dehiscence are some of the bronchial complications seen (Figure 11.27). They can be evaluated by bronchoscopy and CT scan.

Cardiac transplant

Cardiac transplant has become an established form of treatment in many end-stage cardiac diseases, with one-year post-transplant survival exceeding 80%. Common indications for heart transplantations include cardiomyopathy, congenital cardiac disease including hypoplastic left heart syndrome, and unresectable malignant cardiac tumors. Orthotopic cardiac transplant in children involves end-to-end anastomosis of donor and recipient aorta and pulmonary arteries. The donor left atrium is

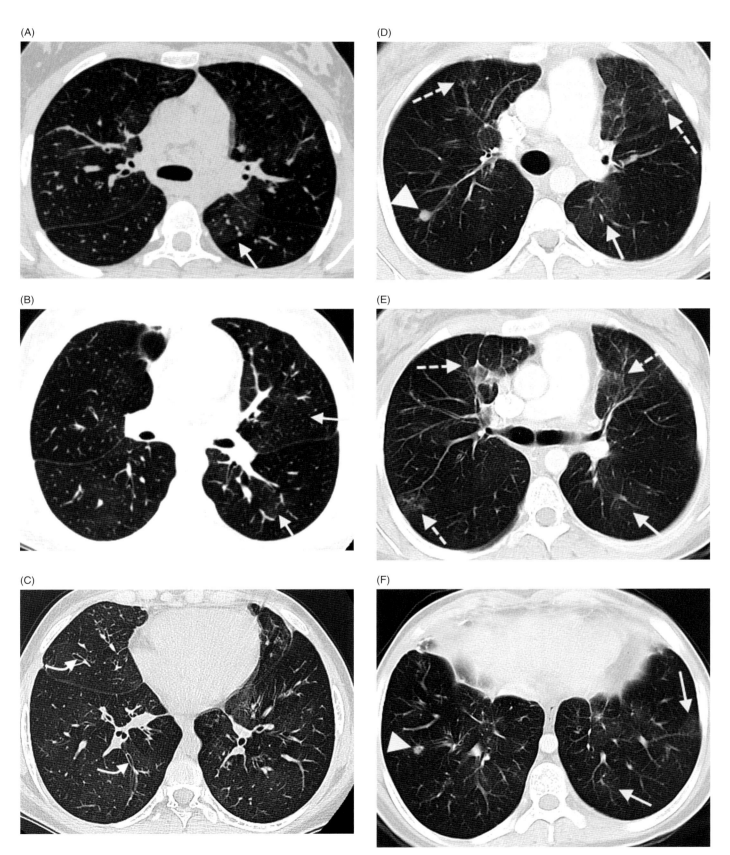

(A)

(B)

(C)

(D)

(E)

(F)

Figure 11.25 Bronchiolitis obliterans organizing pneumonia (BOOP) in a 14-year-old boy with lung transplant. Initial axial images of the lungs (A, B, C) show ill-defined areas of ground-glass opacities (arrows) alternating with lucent areas of air-trapping and few bronchiectatic changes (curved arrows). Follow-up CT images after six months (D, E, F) show persistent ground-glass opacities (arrows), a few more dense airspace opacities (hatched arrows) and nodules (arrowheads).

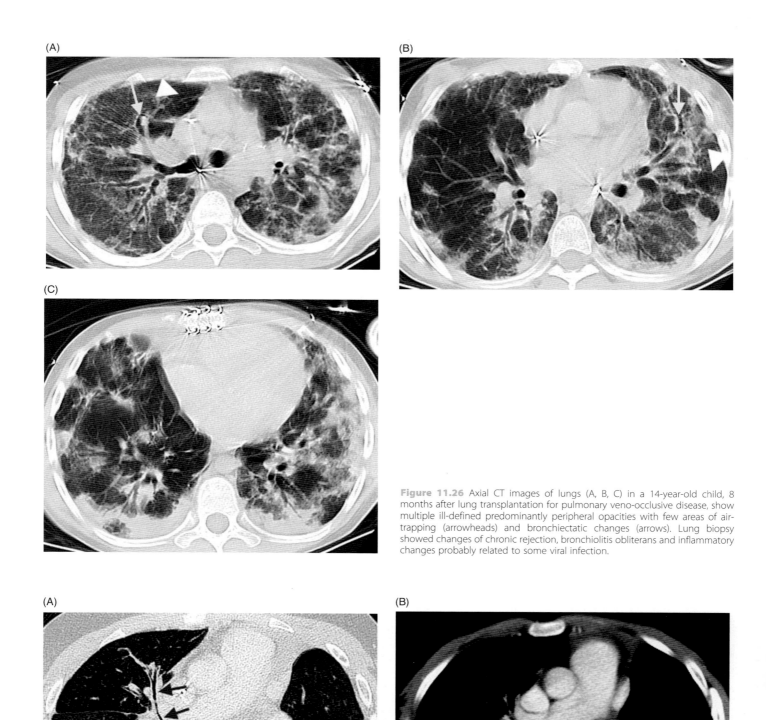

(A)

(B)

(C)

Figure 11.26 Axial CT images of lungs (A, B, C) in a 14-year-old child, 8 months after lung transplantation for pulmonary veno-occlusive disease, show multiple ill-defined predominantly peripheral opacities with few areas of air-trapping (arrowheads) and bronchiectatic changes (arrows). Lung biopsy showed changes of chronic rejection, bronchiolitis obliterans and inflammatory changes probably related to some viral infection.

(A)

(B)

Figure 11.27 (A) Axial high-resolution CT image of transplanted lungs shows diffuse narrowing of the right middle lobe bronchus (arrows) with hyperexpansion of the lobe. (B) Axial contrast-enhanced CT image in the same patient shows mild narrowing at the right pulmonary artery anastomosis (arrow).

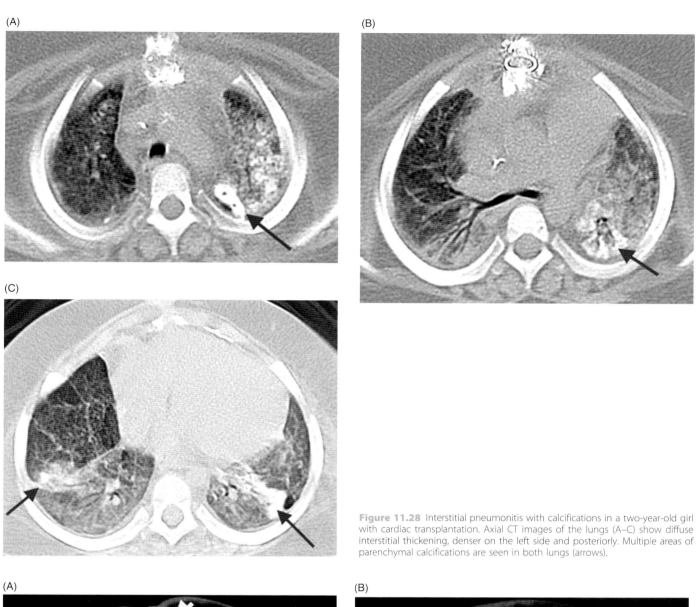

(A)

(B)

(C)

Figure 11.28 Interstitial pneumonitis with calcifications in a two-year-old girl with cardiac transplantation. Axial CT images of the lungs (A–C) show diffuse interstitial thickening, denser on the left side and posteriorly. Multiple areas of parenchymal calcifications are seen in both lungs (arrows).

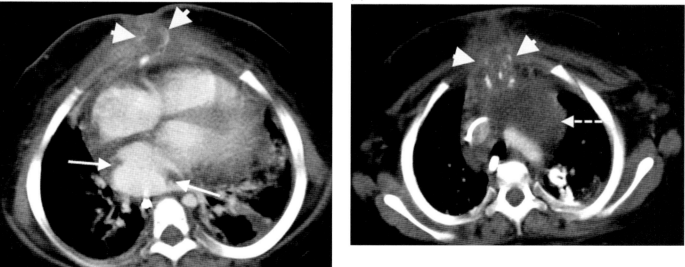

(A)

(B)

Figure 11.29 Sternal osteomyelitis in a two-year-old girl with cardiac transplantation. Axial CT images (A, B) of the chest show peripherally enhancing collection associated with sternal destruction (arrowheads). There is also an anterior mediastinal collection (hatched arrow on B). Notch representing right atrial anastomosis is indicated by arrows on A.

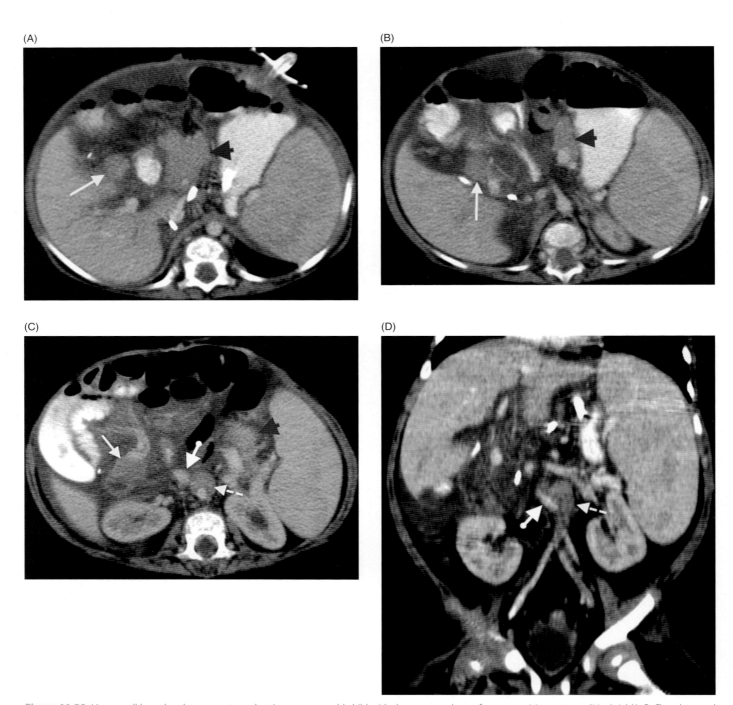

(A) (B) (C) (D)

Figure 11.30 Liver, small bowel and pancreas transplant in a one-year-old child with short gut syndrome from necrotizing enterocolitis. Axial (A, B, C) and coronal reconstruction (D) CT images of the abdomen show free fluid in the abdomen. Transplanted pancreas is seen on the right side of the abdomen (arrows). The native pancreas is indicated by arrowheads. A conduit from the infrarenal aorta (arrow with rounded end) supplies the transplanted liver. A small hematoma is seen at the anastomosis of the conduit and the aorta (hatched arrow).

attached to the recipient's left atrial cuff. The donor right atrium is attached to the recipient's right atrium. The technique may vary with the anatomy of the congenital heart disease.

Infection, rejection and lymphoproliferative disease such as PTLD are the common complications seen in the post-transplant period. Pneumonia is the leading infectious complication and usually occurs within the first three to four months

(Figure 11.28). Complications related to surgical procedure are seen in the immediate postoperative period and include mediastinal fluid collections, hematoma, and sternal osteomyelitis (Figure 11.29). However, these should be differentiated from the common postoperative appearances such as enlarged cardiac silhouette, double atrial contour from atrial anastomosis, and postoperative pneumopericardium, pneumothorax and

(A)

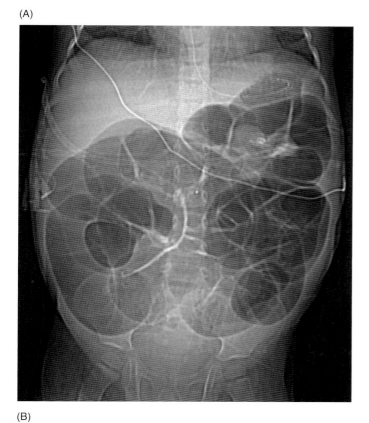

(B)

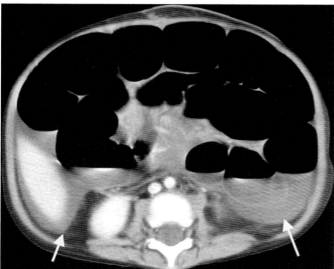

(C)

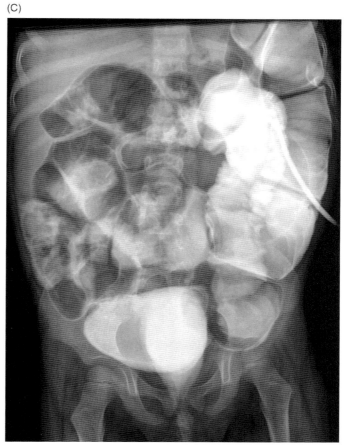

Figure 11.31 Ileus in a five-year-old child with small bowel transplantation for microvillous inclusion disease. CT scout (A), axial CT image (B) and GI contrast study (C) show diffuse dilated bowel loops. CT shows ascites (arrows) but no cause of bowel obstruction was seen. GI contrast study shows unobstructed passage of contrast up to the rectum.

pneumomediastinum, which may persist for a few days following surgery. Delayed mediastinal widening may be related to steroid-induced fat deposition.

Small bowel transplant

Small bowel transplantation is performed in children for short gut syndrome and intestinal failure. Short gut syndrome is a malabsorption disorder caused by surgical removal of small intestine (more than two-thirds of its length) or from complete dysfunction of a large segment of bowel. Common causes of short gut syndrome in children include gastroschisis, necrotizing enterocolitis, midgut volvulus and intestinal atresia. Children with short gut syndrome, who cannot tolerate total parenteral nutrition or have complications related to it, are candidates for bowel transplantation. Small bowel can be transplanted isolated, or it can be combined with liver or as a part of multivisceral transplantation that includes small bowel, liver, pancreas, stomach and duodenum (Figure 11.30).

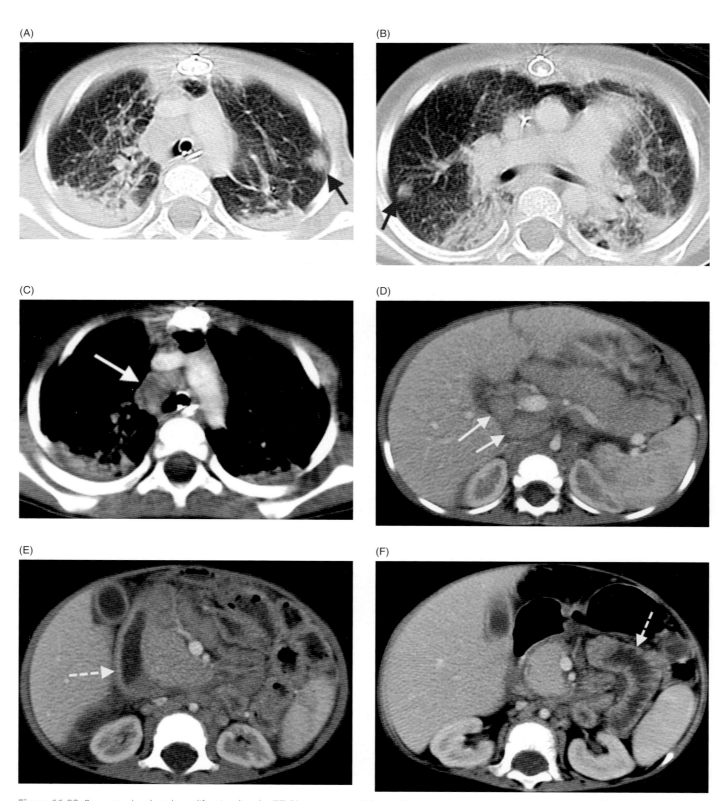

Figure 11.32 Post-transplant lymphoproliferative disorder (PTLD) in a two-year-old girl with cardiac transplant. Axial images of the lungs (A, B) show nodules (black arrows) and posterior airspace opacities. Axial images of the chest (C) and abdomen (D, E) show enlarged lymph nodes (white arrows), bowel wall thickening (hatched arrow) and ascites. Follow-up CT images after reduction of chemotherapy (F, G) show some reduction in lymph node enlargement (arrows); however, bowel wall thickening (hatched arrows) is persistent.

(G)

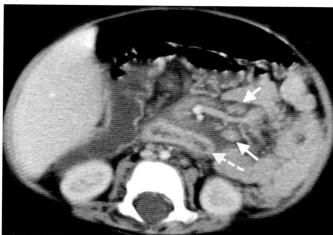

Figure 11.32 (Cont.)

Transplantation of small bowel can be complicated by acute or chronic rejection, infection, obstruction, anastomotic stenosis or leakage, perforation, enterocutaneous fistula, motility disorder (Figure 11.31), collection or abscess, PTLD, GVHD, internal or external hernias and thrombosis of mesenteric vessels. Gastrointestinal contrast studies are performed for evaluation of anastomotic integrity, postsurgical anatomy of the bowel, small bowel transit time, gastric emptying and enterocutaneous fistulas. Mucosal fold thickening suggestive of submucosal edema is a nonspecific finding and can be a normal finding in the initial postoperative period. It is important to discuss the surgical anatomy with the surgeon before performing the contrast study. US and CT are performed for evaluation of bowel thickening, abscesses, collections and PTLD.

Post-transplantation lymphoproliferative disorder

PTLD is a complication seen in post-transplantation patients in whom a spectrum of unregulated lymphoid expansion occurs that ranges from polyclonal hyperplasia to monoclonal malignant lymphoma. It is related to chronic immunosuppression and, in most cases, results from Epstein-Barr virus (EBV)-induced B-cell lymphoproliferation. The overall frequency of PTLD is around 2% but is seen with higher frequency (approximately 8%) in children. Three major risk factors include allograft type, EBV infection or reactivation and intense immunosuppressive regimens. PTLD is seen more frequently in liver, lung and heart transplant, and less frequently in renal transplant patients. About 85% of PTLD cases are of B-cell origin and contain EBV. Most cases of PTLD are seen in the first year after transplantation and present with a variety of clinical manifestations. PTLD can involve any organ system including the allograft. In descending order of frequency it involves the abdomen, chest, head and neck, and brain (Figure 11.32). Histologically, three forms are seen: hyperplastic (early lesion), polymorphic, and monomorphic (lymphomas). The polymorphic form has a better prognosis and is more likely to respond to a reduction in immunosuppressive therapy.

CT is the main modality for evaluation of PTLD in terms of presence, extent and biopsy guidance. Hypodense nodular masses or diffuse infiltration and enlargement can be seen in liver, spleen and kidneys. Circumferential wall thickening, dilatation, ulceration and intussusception can be seen in the bowel with the small bowel being most frequently involved. Abdominal lymphadenopathy including omental and mesenteric involvement are other manifestations. PTLD in the chest can manifest as discrete nodular parenchymal lung masses, airspace consolidation that does not respond to antibiotic therapy, and mediastinal lymphadenopathy. Diffuse enlargement of the pharyngeal and palatine tonsils and cervical lymphadenopathy is seen in head and neck PTLD. Sinonasal involvement in PTLD cannot be distinguished from an infective process radiologically. Solitary brain lesion is the most frequent manifestation of brain PTLD.

Further reading

Berrocal T, Parron M, Alvarez-Luque A, Prieto C, Santamaria ML (2006) Pediatric liver transplantation: a pictorial essay of early and late complications. *Radiographics* **26**, 1187–209.

Crossin JD, Muradali D, Wilson SR (2003) US of liver transplants: normal and abnormal. *Radiographics* **23**, 1093–114.

Duro D, Kamin D, Duggan C (2008) Overview of pediatric short bowel syndrome. *J Pediatr Gastroenterol Nutr* **47**, S33–6.

Hollingsworth CL, Frush DP, Kurtzburg J, Prasad VK (2008) Pediatric hematopoietic stem cell transplantation and the role of imaging. *Radiology* **248**, 348–65.

Knisely BL, Mastey LA, Collins J, Kuhlman JE (1999) Imaging of cardiac transplantation complications. *Radiographics* **19**, 321–39.

Kobayashi K, Censullo ML, Rossman LL et al. (2007) Interventional radiologic management of renal transplant dysfunction: indications, limitations, and technical considerations. *Radiographics* **27**, 1109–30.

Levine DS, Navarro OM, Chaudry G, Doyle JJ, Blaser SI (2007) Imaging the complications of bone marrow transplantation in children. *Radiographics* **27**, 307–24.

Medina LS, Siegel MJ (1994) CT of complications of pediatric lung transplantation. *Radiographics* **14**, 1341–9.

Pecchi A, De Santis M, Torricelli P et al. (2005) Radiologic imaging of the transplanted small bowel. *Abdominal Imaging* **30**, 548–63.

Pickhardt PJ, Siegel MJ, Hayashi RJ, Kelly M (2000) Posttransplantation lymphoproliferative disorder in children: clinical, histopathological, and imaging features. *Radiology* **217**, 16–25.

Surratt JT, Siegel MJ, Middleton WD (1990) Sonography of complications in pediatric renal allografts. *Radiographics* **10**, 687–99.

Tjang YS, Stenlund H, Tenderich G, Hornik L, Körfer R (2008) Pediatric heart transplantation: current clinical review. *J Card Surg* **23**(1), 87–91.

Chapter 12

Iatrogenic devices

Soni C. Chawla

The word "iatrogenic" comes from the Greek roots "iatros" meaning "the healer or physician" and "gennan" meaning "as a product of." Hence "iatrogenic" means due to the action of a physician or a therapy and "iatrogenic devices" are any objects, tubes, catheters and lines introduced or placed in a patient for therapy or diagnosis or to serve a particular purpose.

In this chapter we will review CSF shunts, endotracheal tubes (ETTs) and feeding tubes (FTs), intravenous and intra-arterial catheters, cardiac devices and orthopedic devices.

CSF shunts

CSF flow dynamics
Cerebrospinal fluid (CSF) is an ultra-filtrate of plasma and is produced by the choroid plexus (CP) of the lateral and fourth ventricles and the ependymal lining of the ventricles. CSF flows from the lateral ventricle through the foramen of Monro into the third ventricle and then into the fourth ventricle

through the sylvian aqueduct. The CSF exits the ventricular system via the foramina of Luschka (lateral) and Magendie (medial) situated in the fourth ventricle. CSF then ascends into the basal cisterns and around the cerebral convexities where it is reabsorbed by the arachnoid villi which project into the dural venous sinuses (Flowchart 12.1; Figure 12.1).

Hydrocephalus is defined as excess volume of CSF and is caused by an obstruction to the normal CSF flow dynamics described above. It is primarily caused by obstruction to the flow of CSF within the ventricular system.

CSF produced in choroid plexus and ependymal lining in the ventricles
↓ a
Foramen of Monro
↓ b
Third ventricle
↓ c
Cerebral aqueduct
↓ d
Fourth ventricle
↙ ↘ e
Foramen of Luschka (Lateral)   Foramen of Majendie (Medial)
↙ ↘ f
Basal cisterns and cerebral convexities
↓ g
Absorbed by arachnoid villi
↓ h
Dural venous sinuses

Flowchart 12.1 CSF flow dynamics.

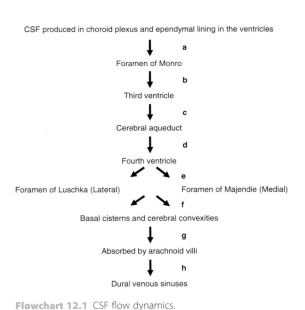

Figure 12.1 CSF flow dynamics. Schematic diagram shows flow of CSF, as described in the text. CP = choroid plexus; LV = lateral ventricle.

Essentials of Pediatric Radiology, ed. Heike E. Daldrup-Link and Charles A. Gooding. Published by Cambridge University Press.
© Cambridge University Press 2010.

(A)

(B)

(C)

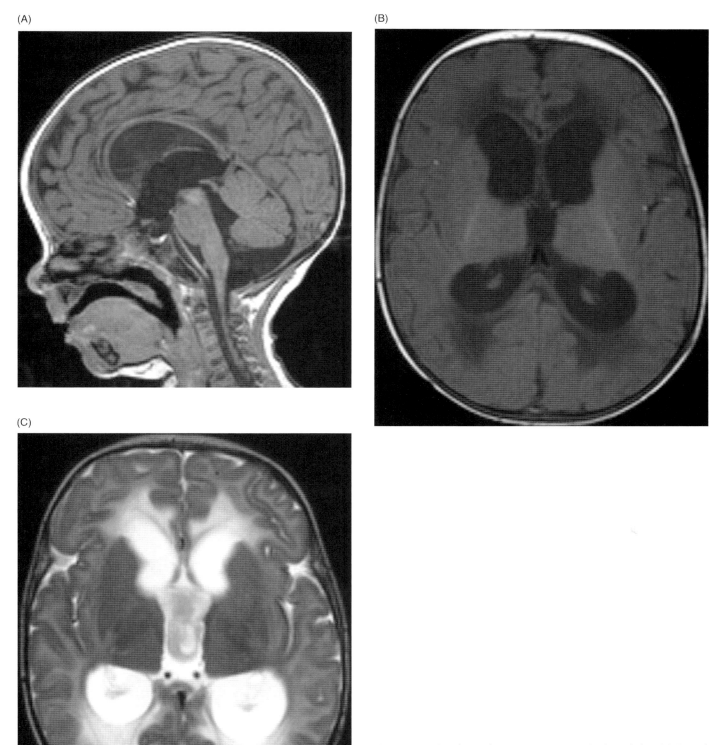

Figure 12.2 Post-hemorrhagic communicating hydrocephalus. (A) Sagittal T1WI MR shows dilated lateral, third and fourth ventricles in a three-month-old baby. (B) Axial T1WI MR shows dilated lateral and third ventricles with periventricular hypointensity consistent with interstitial edema caused by transependymal migration of CSF in a three-month-old baby. (C) Axial T2WI MR shows post-hemorrhagic communicating hydrocephalus with periventricular hyperintensity consistent with interstitial edema caused by transependymal migration of CSF in a three-month-old baby.

- Due to blockage of arachnoid villi and decreased reabsorption into the dural venous sinuses and
- Due to overproduction by the choroid plexus (rare and controversial).

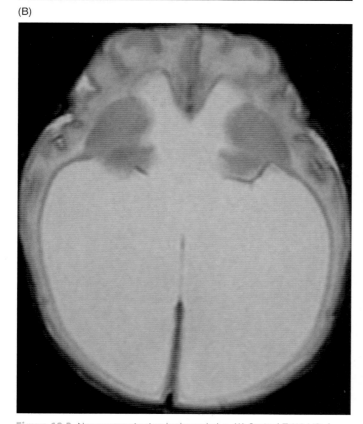

Figure 12.3 Noncommunicating hydrocephalus. (A) Sagittal T1WI MR shows dilated lateral and third ventricles and normal-sized fourth ventricle in a case of aqueductal stenosis. (B) Axial T2WI MR shows significantly dilated lateral ventricles in a case of aqueductal stenosis.

Hydrocephalus is primarily classified into two types: communicating or extraventricular, and noncommunicating or intraventricular.

Communicating or extraventricular hydrocephalus is caused by extraventricular obstruction at the level of the arachnoid villi and decreased absorption of the CSF mainly caused by prior hemorrhage, meningitis or obstruction of the dural venous sinuses (Step g and h in Flowchart 1; Figure 12.2).

Noncommunicating or intraventricular hydrocephalus is induced by obstructive lesions at various levels (Steps a to f in Flowchart 1; Figure 12.3) due to various causes such as third ventricular tumors, e.g. colloid cyst, subependymal giant cell astrocytoma, glioma, or aqueductal stenosis, or fourth ventricular tumors, e.g. medulloblastoma, cerebellar pilocytic astrocytoma.

Types of diversionary shunts

Hydrocephalus is an endemic condition in the pediatric population. CSF diversionary procedures like shunt placement are some of the most common pediatric neurosurgical procedures. Types of shunt include ventriculoperitoneal (VP), ventriculopleural (VPL), ventriculoatrial (VA), ventriculolumbar (VL), and ventriculovenous and ventriculo-gallbladder (Table 12.1). The VP shunt is by far the commonest type of shunt used in the pediatric population. The ventriculolumbar shunts are mainly reserved

Table 12.1 Types of diversionary shunt

Ventriculoperitoneal[a]
Ventriculolumbar
Ventriculopleural
Ventriculoatrial
Ventriculovenous
Ventriculo-gallbladder

[a] Commonest

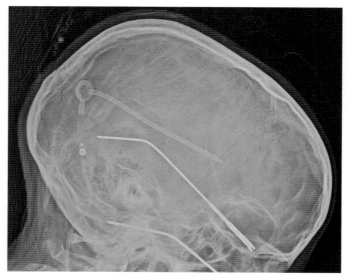

Figure 12.4 Ventriculoperitoneal (VP) shunt. Lateral radiograph of the skull shows the proximal end of the VP shunt terminating in the expected region of the lateral ventricle. A Codman Hakim valve is seen connected to the shunt.

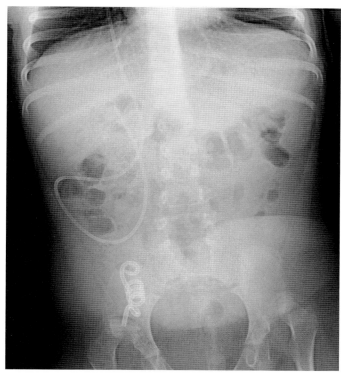

Figure 12.5 Ventriculoperitoneal (VP) shunt. Frontal radiograph of the abdomen shows the distal end of the VP shunt terminating in the right upper quadrant. There is no obvious kinking or discontinuity of the VP shunt. A cecostomy tube is seen in the right lower quadrant.

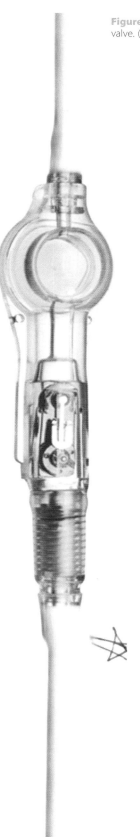

Figure 12.6 Codman Hakim programmable valve. (Courtesy of Johnson and Johnson.)

for adults with normal pressure hydrocephalus and patients with small slit ventricles or recurrent VP shunt malfunction.

Ventriculoperitoneal (VP) shunts

Each shunt has a proximal intracranial segment inserted through the frontal, parietal or temporal bone, so that the tip and the side holes of the catheter lie within the frontal horn of the lateral ventricle (Figure 12.4). Care is taken by the neurosurgeons to avoid proximity of the shunt catheter tip to the choroid plexus, to prevent the occlusion of the catheter by the growth of choroid plexus into the tip and side holes of the shunt catheter. The distal tip of the catheter is tunneled through the skin of the neck, thorax and abdomen into the peritoneal cavity for the drainage of CSF (Figure 12.5).

Today neurosurgeons have a wide variety of shunts with programmable valves to choose from for a particular patient. One of the commonly used valves is the Codman Hakim programmable valve (Figures 12.6 and 12.7), which has 18 pressure settings ranging between 30 and 200 mm H_2O. The neurosurgeon selects one of the settings at the time of shunt placement and is also able to make precise pressure adjustments to help control intracranial pressure and the ventricle size at any time in the future (as per the need of the patient). Various valve configurations are available (Figure 12.8), with a prechamber reservoir or a siphonguard. A plain radiograph is used to verify valve pressure at placement and whenever the valve is reprogrammed or if the patient undergoes an MRI. Proper technique as shown in

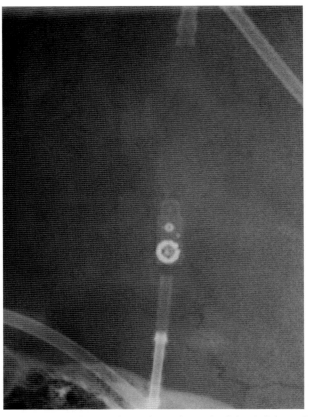

Figure 12.7 Codman Hakim valve. Radiograph of the skull shows Codman Hakim valve below a lucent reservoir along the VP shunt. The valve pressure is set at 40 and 60 mm of H$_2$O.

Figure 12.9 is mandatory for the correct assessment of the valve pressure. The setting of the valve is easily determined by comparing the position of the radiopaque marker on the valve cam to the fixed position of the radiopaque right-hand-side indicator on the base plate of the valve. Comparing the radiographs of the valve to the diagram on the programming unit panel (Figure 12.10) indicates the valve pressure. Pressure settings of 70, 120 and 170 mm of H$_2$O align with the cross in the center of the valve.

Clinical studies have not conclusively shown that any particular kind of shunt valve system performs better over others in terms of infection, malfunction (Table 12.2) and other complications. However, Tuli and coworkers have conclusively shown in a large prospective study that the timing of the previous shunt procedure is significant: a revision performed in less than six months results in an increased risk of failure. Also, age at first shunt insertion and the time interval since last revision are important predictors of repeated shunt variables. Patients less than 40 weeks of age, and those from 40 weeks to 1 year of age had a hazard ratio (HR) of 2.49 and 1.77, respectively, in comparison with shunt insertions performed in patients greater than 1 year of age. Also, concurrent other surgical procedures were associated with an increased risk of failure.

Investigation of shunt malfunction (Table 12.3)

If a child with a shunt presents acutely with the classical clinical triad of raised ICP with headaches, vomiting and papilledema,

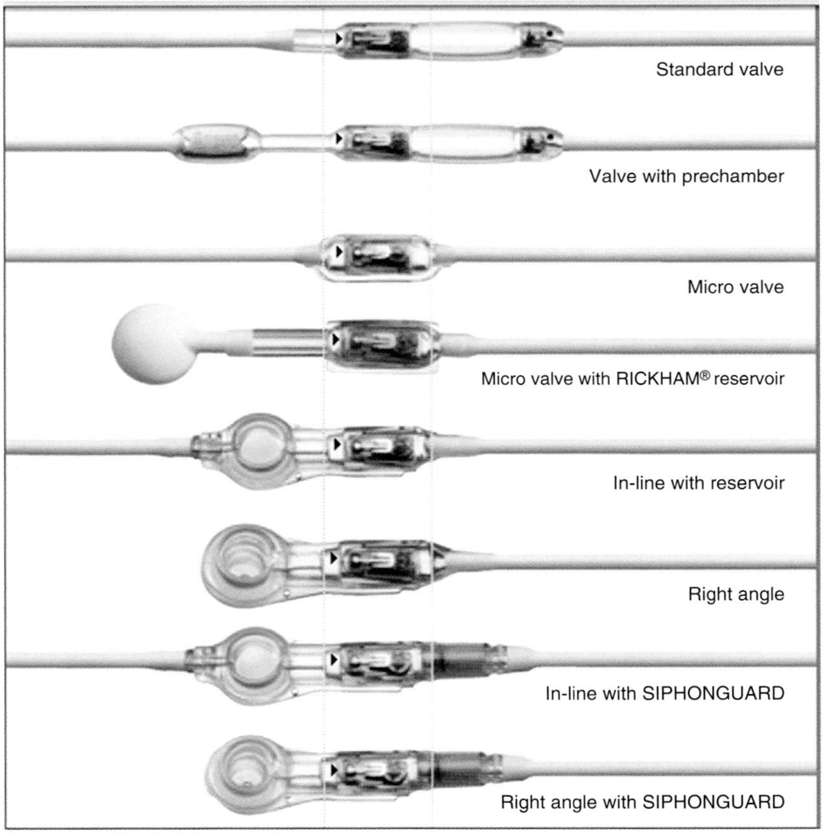

Figure 12.8 Various valve configurations. (Courtesy of Johnson and Johnson.)

Standard valve

Valve with prechamber

Micro valve

Micro valve with RICKHAM® reservoir

In-line with reservoir

Right angle

In-line with SIPHONGUARD

Right angle with SIPHONGUARD

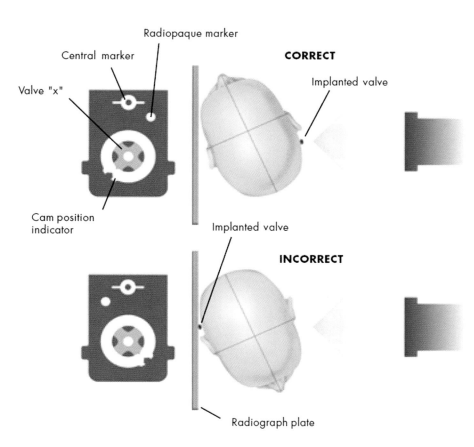

Central marker

Radiopaque marker

Valve "x"

CORRECT

Implanted valve

Cam position indicator

Implanted valve

INCORRECT

Radiograph plate

Figure 12.9 Diagrammatic representation of the radiographic technique to evaluate valve pressure. A proper radiograph is generated when the film is shot with the X-ray beam perpendicular to the plane of the valve. (Courtesy of Johnson and Johnson.)

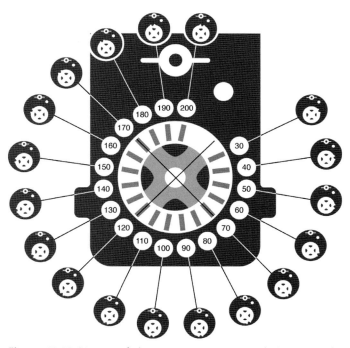

Figure 12.10 Diagram of the programming unit panel. Comparing the patient's radiographs taken with proper technique as shown in Figure 12.9 to this diagram on the programming unit panel indicates the valve setting. The pressure settings of 70, 120 and 170 mm H₂O align with the cross in the center of the valve. (Courtesy of Johnson and Johnson.)

Table 12.2 Causes of shunt malfunction

- Mechanical causes
  - Kinking
  - Discontinuity/disconnection
  - Break/fracture
  - Functional failure of the valve/shunt apparatus
  - Migration
- Overdrainage
  - Epidural, subdural and intracranial hematoma
  - Slit ventricle syndrome
- Infection

Table 12.3 Investigation of shunt malfunction

- Shunt series
- CT scan of brain
- MRI brain
- Nuclear imaging

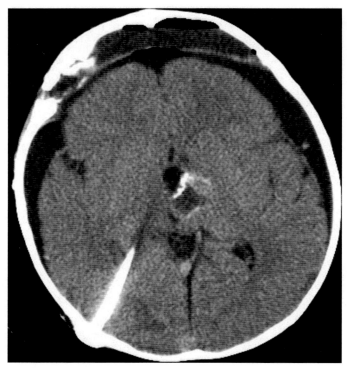

Figure 12.11 Acute complications of shunt revision. Axial noncontrast CT scan shows bilateral subdural collection and epidural hematoma with pneumocephalus in a 14-month-old boy with craniopharyngioma. Calcified mass is seen in the suprasellar region.

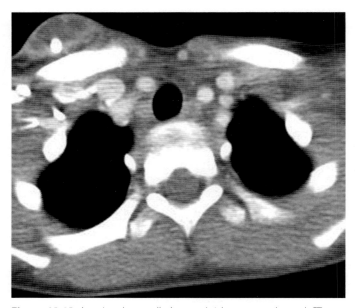

Figure 12.12 Anterior chest wall abscess. Axial contrast-enhanced CT scan shows small rim-enhancing fluid collection around the VP shunt in the anterior chest wall on the right side consistent with an abscess in an eight-year-old boy.

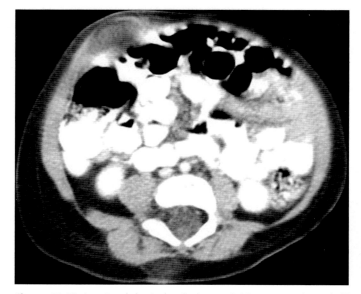

Figure 12.13 Anterior abdominal wall abscess. Axial contrast-enhanced CT scan shows small rim-enhancing fluid collection in the anterior abdominal wall consistent with an abscess in a 19-month-old baby with meningomyelocele and shunt removal.

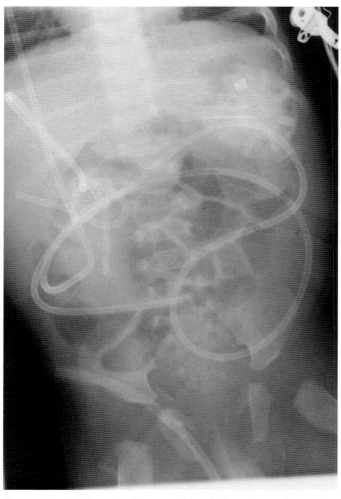

Figure 12.14 Mechanical malfunction of the VP shunt due to a knot. Radiograph of the abdomen shows a VP shunt with a knot in the right mid-abdomen. The other patent VP shunt is seen terminating in the lower abdomen.

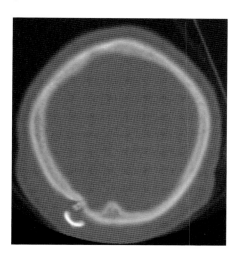

Figure 12.15 Mechanical malfunction of the VP shunt due to disconnection. Axial CT scan of the brain in bone window shows the VP shunt detached from its reservoir, causing subgaleal CSF collection in a six-year-old child with bilateral open-lipped schizencephaly.

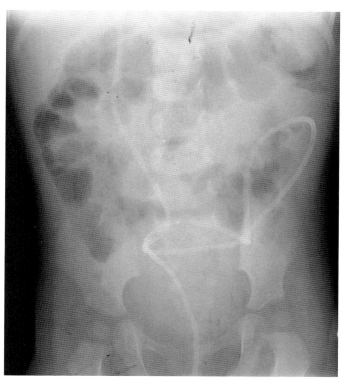

Figure 12.16 VP shunt migration. Radiograph of the abdomen shows VP shunt which perforated the descending colon and is seen exiting out through the rectum in a six-month-old baby.

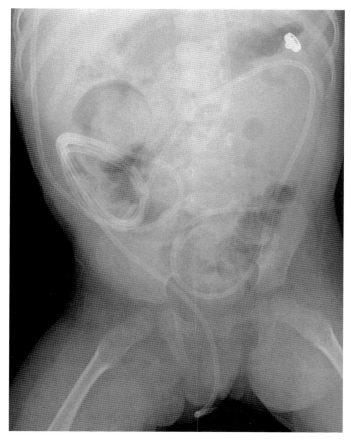

Figure 12.17 VP shunt migration. Radiograph of the abdomen shows two VP shunts, one exiting out through the vagina and the other terminating in the left lower abdomen.

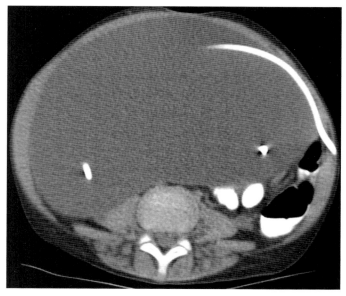

Figure 12.18 CSF pseudocyst. Axial contrast-enhanced CT scan shows large low-attenuation fluid collection in the abdomen in a four-year-old boy with VP shunt which is seen coursing into the fluid collection.

shunt malfunction is investigated. Acute complications related to shunt insertion occur soon after insertion, such as focal sensory/motor deficit, intracranial bleed, subdural/epidural hematoma (Figure 12.11), pneumocephalus (Figure 12.11), etc. The other causes of shunt malfunction are mainly mechanical and infection (Figures 12.12 and 12.13). Mechanical malfunction could be due to knots (which is very rare; Figure 12.14),

kinking, discontinuity, break/fracture of the tubing, functional failure or disconnection of the shunt valve/apparatus (Figure 12.15) and migration (Figures 12.16 and 12.17).

Shunt series comprising of frontal and lateral radiographs of the skull and neck and frontal radiographs of the chest and

(A)

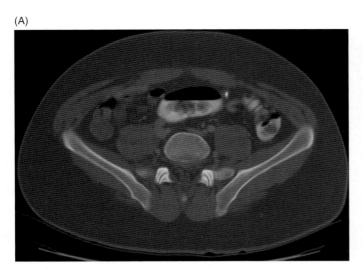

(B)

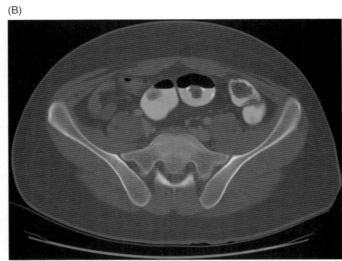

Figure 12.19 (A) Axial CT of the lower abdomen in bone window shows shunt catheter traversing alongside the sigmoid colon. (B) Axial CT of the lower abdomen in bone window shows shunt catheter within the lumen of the sigmoid colon consistent with bowel perforation.

abdomen are obtained to evaluate for obvious kinks, discontinuity or disconnection. The commonest site of disconnection is between the valve apparatus and the distal shunt tubing (Figure 12.15). Most shunts have translucent areas that one should be aware of to avoid being mistaken for abnormal disconnection. Comparison with prior shunt series is recommended. Also, fixity of the distal catheter in a particular position is worrisome and is concerning for the possibility of an infectious process or a peritoneal CSF pseudocyst formation (Figure 12.18). Rarely, bowel perforation may be caused by the shunt (Figure 12.19).

CT scan of the brain is mainly done to assess the size of the ventricles. Worsening hydrocephalus (Figure 12.20) and overdrainage with epidural, subdural and intraventricular hematomas and slit ventricles are easily identified on a CT brain study.

Further evaluation with magnetic resonance imaging (MRI) of the brain is done to evaluate the status of preexisting processes like tumors or congenital abnormalities. As mentioned earlier, the programmable valves are susceptible to magnetic disturbances due to their ferromagnetic properties, and hence evaluation of valve pressure is necessary after a diagnostic MRI.

Nuclear scintigraphy

Radionuclide VP shunt studies are mainly used for assessment of patency of the peritoneal catheter. After successful withdrawal of CSF from the shunt reservoir, a small amount of ^{99m}Tc DTPA (1 mCi) is injected into the reservoir. Dynamic and static images of the head, neck, chest, abdomen and pelvis are acquired.

A region of interest is drawn around the reservoir and a time–activity curve (TAC) is generated and halftime ($t_{1/2}$) is calculated.

Three scintigraphic patterns are observed:

- Patent: $t_{1/2} < 7$ min, entire length of peritoneal catheter is visualized, and free dispersion in the peritoneal cavity (Figure 12.21).

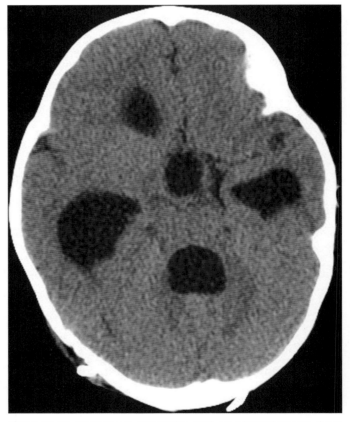

Figure 12.20 Worsening hydrocephalus. Axial nonenhanced CT scan shows dilated lateral, third and fourth ventricle in an 11-month-old girl with shunt malfunction.

- Partial obstruction: $t_{1/2} > 7$ min, entire/partial length of peritoneal catheter visualized, and with/without tracer in peritoneal cavity:

(A)

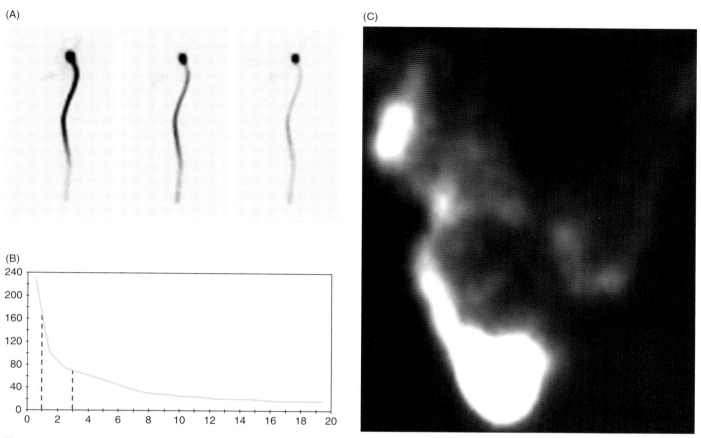

(B)

(C)

Figure 12.21 Patent pattern in nuclear scintigraphy. (A) Dynamic images show prompt peritoneal catheter and reservoir clearance. (B) TAC [x axis: time (min), y axis: counts min^{-1}] shows $t_{1/2}$ of 1.4 min. (C) Static anterior image of the abdomen: peritoneal dispersion. (Courtesy of H. Eslamy, MD.)

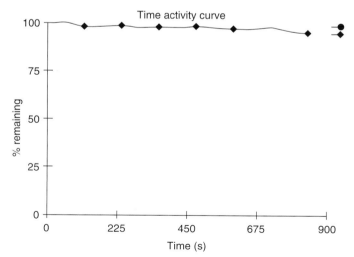

Figure 12.22 Complete obstruction pattern in nuclear scintigraphy. $t_{1/2}$ is markedly prolonged at 227 minutes, and there was lack of visualization of the peritoneal catheter and dispersion in the peritoneal cavity in a 15-year-old boy with spina bifida presenting with worsening headache.

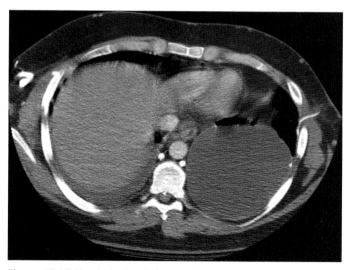

Figure 12.23 Ventriculopleural shunt malfunction. Axial contrast-enhanced CT scan shows a large low-attenuation fluid collection in the left pleural space. The shunt catheter is seen coursing into the pleural cavity through the left lateral chest wall.

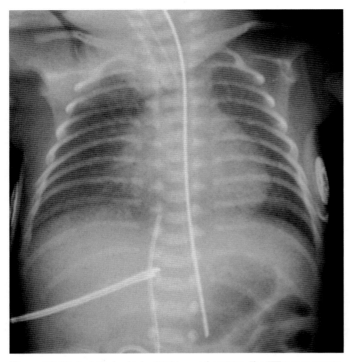

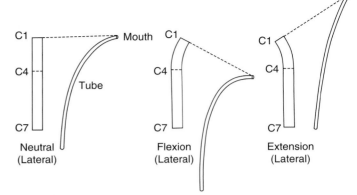

Figure 12.25 ETT changes position with the position of the neck. With chin-down position, which causes neck flexion, the ETT moves down toward the carina, and with chin-up position, which causes extension of the neck, the ETT moves up toward the thoracic inlet. In other words, chin down – ETT down, and chin up – ETT up. (Courtesy of R. Brasch, MD.)

Figure 12.24 Endotracheal tube (ETT) in good position. The ETT is seen terminating at T2 level in a 2-day-old baby boy born at 28 weeks of gestation with respiratory distress syndrome (RDS). The umbilical venous catheter (UVC) terminates at the junction of the inferior vena cava (IVC) and the right atrium in good position. The orogastric tube terminates in the stomach in good position.

- Free dispersion: generalized distribution of tracer in peritoneal cavity.
- Loculation: lack of free dispersion.
- Complete obstruction: $t_{1/2}$ typically >20 min, lack of visualization of the peritoneal catheter and dispersion in the peritoneal cavity (Figure 12.22).

Other shunts

Ventriculoatrial shunts have the distal tip in the right atrium. Complications like sepsis, thromboembolic events, shunt nephritis and pulmonary hypertension have led to the decline of their use except as a last resort. Ventriculopleural shunts are also not favored due to inadvertent life-threatening complications like pneumothorax, pleural effusion (Figure 12.23) and infection.

Other proposed shunts have also failed due to various complications and are rarely used in clinical practice.

Endotracheal tubes (ETTs) and feeding tubes (FTs)

The most common use of plain radiography in the neonatal intensive care unit (NICU) is to evaluate the position of the tubes, lines and assist devices. This includes ETTs, orogastric tubes (OGTs), peripherally inserted central catheters (PICCs),

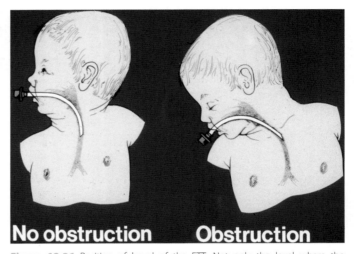

Figure 12.26 Position of bevel of the ETT. Not only the level where the ETT ends but also the position of the bevel is very important. If the bevel is against the tracheal wall, it can cause damage to the mucosa of the trachea and cause obstruction to the flow of air and aeration of the lungs. (Courtesy of R. Brasch, MD.)

umbilical catheters (UACs) and umbilical venous catheters (UVCs), and extracorporeal membrane oxygenation (ECMO) catheters.

Endotracheal tubes (ETTs)

It is very important to accurately assess the position of the ETT to ensure proper ventilation for the infant. The tip of the ETT should be between the thoracic inlet (level of the T1 vertebral body) and the carina (usually at the level of the T4 vertebral body) (Figure 12.24). In older infants, it is advisable that the ETT tip be at approximately 1.5 cm above the carina; however, it is very difficult in neonates, especially in premature babies, as the trachea is short and measures only a couple of centimeters. Also, the ETT changes position with the position of the neck (Figure 12.25); with chin-down position, which causes neck flexion, the ETT moves down toward

Table 12.4 Recommendations of the National Resuscitation Program (NRP) for ETT sizes by age and weight

Age	NB[a]	NB	NB	NB	1 mo	6 mo	1 y	2–3 y	4–5 y	6–8 y	10–12 y	>14 y
Weight	<1	1–2	2–3	>3	4	7	10	12–14	16–18	20–26	32–42	>50
ETT	2.5	3.0	3–3.5	3.5	4	4	4–4.5	4.5	5–6	6–6.5	7	7.5–8.5

[a] NB = Newborn.

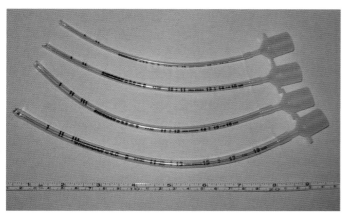

Figure 12.27 ETTs of varying sizes used in infants.

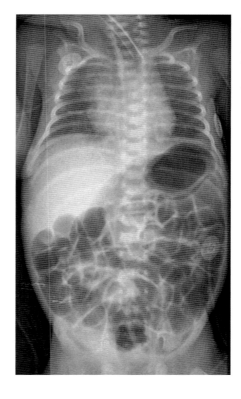

Figure 12.28 Esophageal intubation. The ETT is seen coursing posterior to the tracheal air column with copious amounts of bowel gas in the abdomen consistent with esophageal intubation in a 13-day-old baby.

the carina, and with chin-up position, which causes extension of the neck, the ETT moves up towards the thoracic inlet. In other words, chin down – ETT down, and chin up – ETT up. This happens as the ETT is fixed at the nose or the mouth, only the tip can move with flexion and extension of the head and neck. With maximum extension (inferior border of mandible above C4), the ETT can ascend by 2 cm. With flexion (inferior border of mandible over upper thoracic spine), the tip can descend by 2 cm.

Not only the level but also the position of the bevel is very important. If the bevel is against the tracheal wall, it can cause damage to the mucosa of the trachea and cause obstruction to the flow of air and aeration of the lungs (Figure 12.26). Once such a complication is recognized, turning the infant's head to one side or extending the neck and then keeping the neck in neutral position relieves the obstruction.

Different sizes of ETTs are used as per the recommendations of the National Resuscitation Program (NRP) (Table 12.4). Commonly used sizes in the NICU are 2.5–4F depending upon the gestational age (Figure 12.27). The correct length of insertion (lip to ETT tip distance) can be estimated by using the formula

Insertion depth (cm) = 6 + weight (kg)

The correct ETT size and length of insertion is estimated by the neonatalogist before insertion.

It is vital to confirm the position of the ETT after placement and recognize esophageal intubation (Figures 12.28 and 12.29). The ETT is seen terminating in an air-filled distended esophagus separate from the tracheal air column in the case of

an esophageal intubation. Also, the stomach and proximal small bowel segments are distended with air.

Once it is confirmed that the ETT is terminating in the trachea, its position is ascertained by counting the vertebral bodies and the ribs. ETTs above the thoracic inlet (Figure 12.30) or extending into the main stem bronchi (Figure 12.31) warrant repositioning. Recommendations for minor excursions are worthless, especially in neonates and young infants wherein the small size of the trachea makes it a difficult task for the neonatalogist.

Significant hyperinflation with flattening of the diaphragm is noted with high frequency oscillator ventilation (HFOV) when a small volume of oxygen is administered at a higher frequency. An ETT may rarely make its way into the tracheal bronchus.

Prolonged intubation with a cuffed ETT causes mucosal damage and leads to tracheal stricture/stenosis (Figure 12.32). Strictures are also seen at the site of the tracheostomy stoma (Figure 12.33), especially with prolonged placement of a tracheostomy tube (Figure 12.34). Malpositioned tracheostomy tubes

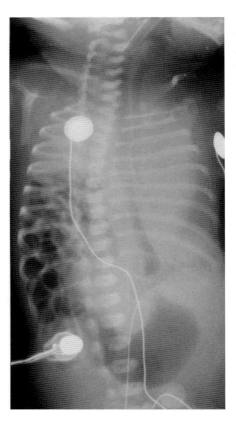

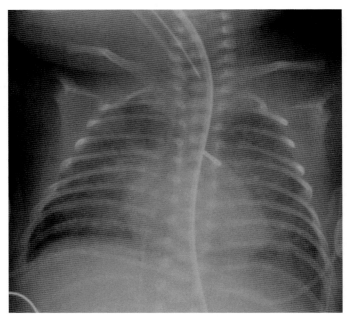

Figure 12.29 Esophageal intubation. The ETT is seen coursing posterior to the tracheal air column with copious amounts of bowel gas in the stomach and proximal small bowel, which is seen herniated in the right lower chest, in a newborn with congenital diaphragmatic hernia. The esophagus is also seen filled with air.

Figure 12.30 High position of ETT. The ETT is seen terminating at C6–7 level in an infant with bronchopulmonary dysplasia. A PDA clip is seen in the mediastinum. The feeding tube courses into the stomach.

(A)

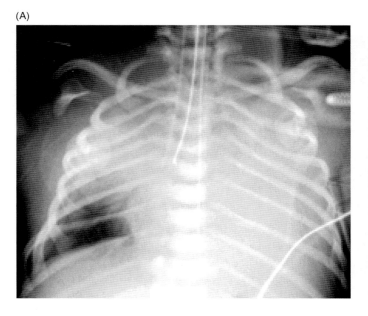

(B)

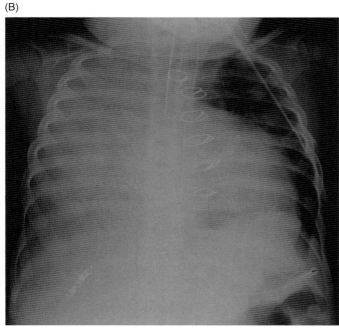

Figure 12.31 Low position of ETT. (A) Frontal radiograph of the chest shows ETT terminating in the right lower lobe bronchus in a newborn with respiratory distress. There is opacification in the left lung and right upper lobe consistent with atelectasis caused by ETT malposition. (B) Frontal radiograph of the chest shows ETT terminating at the carina in a six-month-old baby with complex congenital heart disease. There is right lung atelectasis caused by ETT malposition. Multiple sternal sutures are seen in place. Coils noted in the right upper quadrant were placed to obliterate the transhepatic access tract by the interventional pediatric cardiologist.

(A)

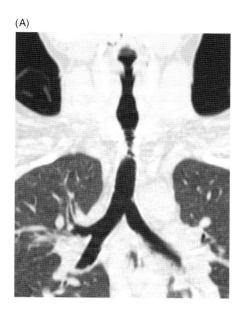

(B)

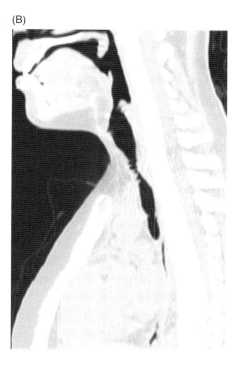

Figure 12.32 Tracheal stricture. Coronal (A) and sagittal (B) CT scan in lung window shows mid-tracheal stenosis about 6.5 cm below the vocal cords and measuring 3.3 × 0.5 × 0.5 cm with irregularity of the mucosal lining consistent with granulation tissue after intubation for drug over-dose in an 18-year-old boy.

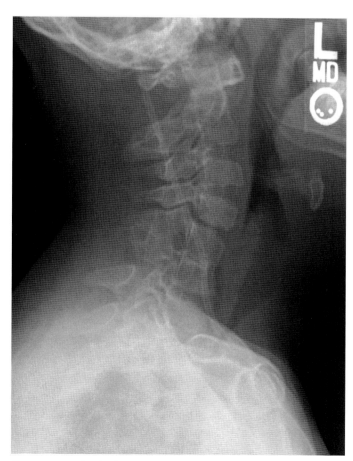

Figure 12.33 Tracheal stenosis. Lateral radiograph of the neck shows narrowing of the trachea at the level of C7 after tracheostomy.

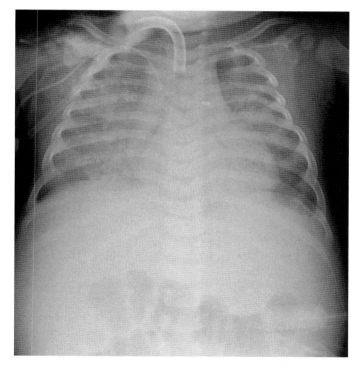

Figure 12.34 Tracheostomy. Frontal radiograph of the chest shows tracheostomy cannula terminating at T2 level in a three-month-old premature infant with oxygen dependence due to bronchopulmonary dysplasia. A central venous catheter is seen terminating in the superior vena cava. A gastrostomy tube (GT) is seen in the left upper quadrant.

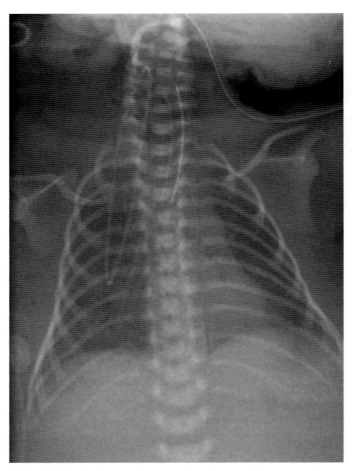

Figure 12.35 Direct cannulation. Frontal radiograph of the neck and chest shows direct cannulation in a seven-day-old girl with status post-surgery of a cervical teratoma and atretic proximal airway.

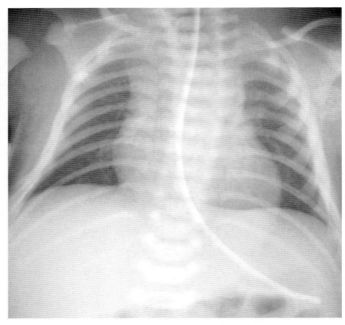

Figure 12.36 Feeding tube. Frontal radiograph of the chest and upper abdomen shows the feeding tube terminating in the stomach in a two-day-old premature baby. Note the dense radiopaque tip of the enteral feeding tube.

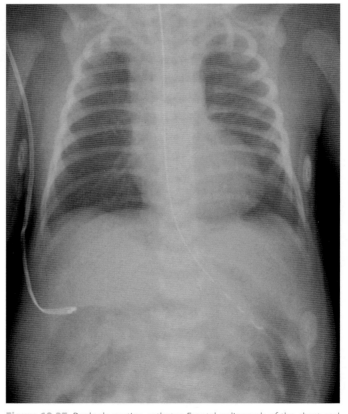

Figure 12.37 Replogle suction catheter. Frontal radiograph of the chest and upper abdomen shows the Replogle terminating in the stomach in a nine-day-old baby with gastroschisis status postsurgery. Note all the ports of the Replogle are within the stomach. A temperature probe is seen placed in the right upper quadrant.

(see Figure 12.38) should be repositioned promptly to ensure adequate lung aeration. Direct cannulation of the trachea is done in cases of upper airway obstruction or atresia (Figure 12.35).

Feeding tubes (FTs)

A wide variety of feeding tubes are used in the pediatric population. In newborn babies and young infants, a feeding tube (Figure 12.36) or Replogle (Figure 12.37) is inserted through the oral cavity and hence they are called orogastric tubes (OGTs). In older children and teenagers, feeding tubes are placed through the nose and hence are referred to as nasogastric tubes (NGTs).

OGTs and NGTs are widely used for short-term rehabilitation. If long-term nutritional management is necessary, enteral feeding tubes are used. Nasojejunal tubes (NJTs; Figure 12.38) are commonly used for enteral feeding when needed for a finite period. The gastrostomy tubes (GTs), gastrojejunostomy tubes (GJTs) and jejunostomy tubes (JTs) are placed when the child needs enteral feeding for prolonged periods or indefinitely.

The Replogle suction catheters/tubes (RTs) are widely used for gastric decompression in infants with abdominal distension. An 8F RT is used for infants less than 1500 g, and 10F RT is used for infants weighing more than 1500 g

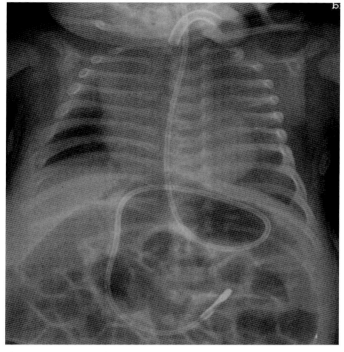

Figure 12.38 Enteral feeding tube. Frontal radiograph of the chest and upper abdomen shows the nasojejunal tube (NJT) terminating in the fourth portion of the duodenum in a six-week-old baby. The tip of the tracheostomy cannula is at C7 level.

(Figure 12.39). The RT is connected to suction apparatus if necessary in cases of gastrointestinal (GI) obstruction. The RT has two ports (Figure 12.40): the colored (vented) port is flushed with air to maintain patency and also it prevents the RT from attaching to the gastric mucosa, and the clear port is irrigated with saline to maintain patency. The volume of the aspirated contents is monitored and assessed for the presence of blood in cases of GI hemorrhage and bile in cases of GI obstruction.

Once the RT is inserted, the position is determined by plain radiography of the chest and the upper abdomen. The RT is well positioned when all the ports are within the stomach (Figure 12.37). If there are ports noted in the esophagus, at the gastroesophageal junction (Figure 12.41), in the pylorus or duodenum, repositioning is suggested.

The appropriate-sized NJT is placed by the radiologist under direct fluoroscopic guidance. The position is confirmed by injecting a small amount of contrast and is considered to be optimal if it terminates in the proximal jejunum. Feeds through the NJT are given as slow continuous infusions or timely boluses as per the metabolic requirements of the child. The GTs (Figures 12.34 and 12.42), GJTs and JTs are also commonly placed by the interventional radiologist rather than gastroenterologist or surgeon.

Once the feeding tube is inserted, the position is verified by plain radiography. Commonly, 5F and 8F feeding tubes are used in the NICU (Figure 12.39). The FT may enter the no-entry pathway and make its way into the airway and reach the right or left main stem or the lower lobe bronchus (Figure 12.43). Occasionally, the feeding tube or the Replogle, after entering the correct pathway into the esophagus may perforate the esophagus, and cause pneumomediastinum, or

(A)

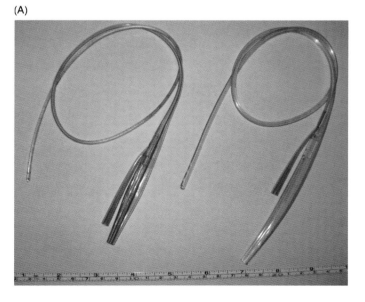

(B)

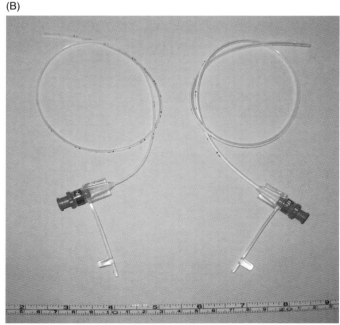

Figure 12.39 (A) Replogle suction catheters 8F and 10F. (B) Feeding tubes 5F and 8F.

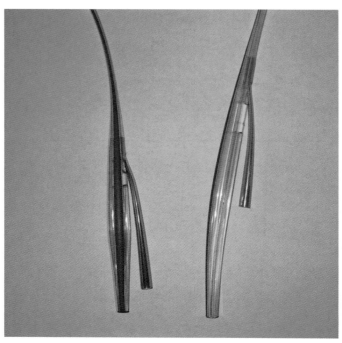

Figure 12.40 Ports of Replogle suction catheter (RT). The RT has two ports: the colored (vented) port is flushed with air to maintain patency and also it prevents the RT from attaching to the gastric mucosa, and the clear port is irrigated with saline to maintain patency.

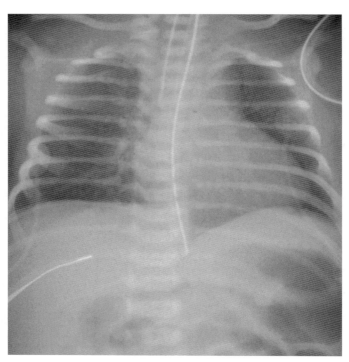

Figure 12.41 Malpositioned Replogle suction catheter. Frontal radiograph of the chest shows the Replogle terminating at the gastroesophageal junction with its ports in the esophagus in a seven-day-old baby after gastroschisis repair. Note the mildly prominent bowel segments in the upper abdomen.

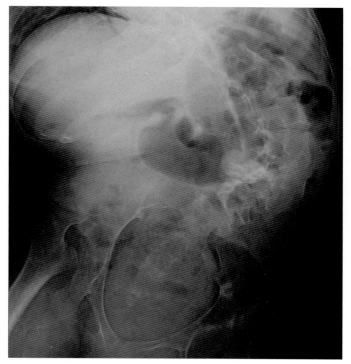

Figure 12.42 Gastrostomy tube (GT). Plain radiograph of the abdomen shows a GT along the greater curvature of the stomach, which is filled with air, in a 13-year-old boy with cerebral palsy, severe scoliosis, bilateral coxa valga and hip dislocation.

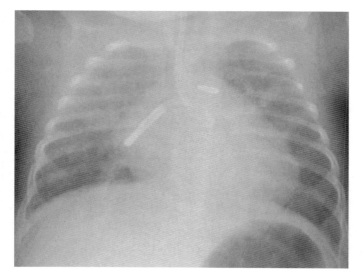

Figure 12.43 Malpositioned feeding tube. Frontal radiograph of the chest shows the feeding tube terminating in the right lower lobe bronchus. Coarse granular opacities in the lung are due to bronchopulmonary dysplasia. A PDA clip is seen in the mediastinum.

(A)

(B)

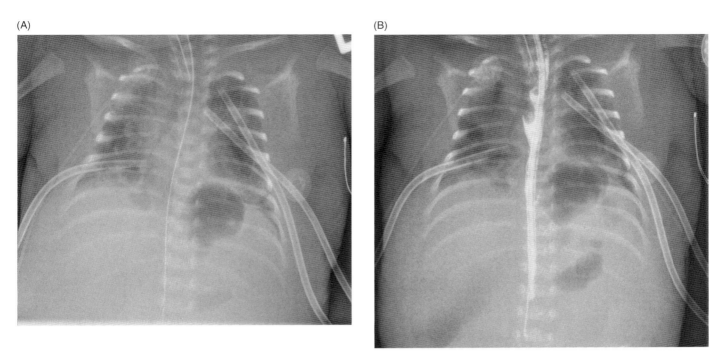

Figure 12.44 Esophageal perforation. (A) Frontal plain radiograph of the chest shows the Replogle catheter coursing straight into the abdomen without turning leftward to reach the stomach in a two-week-old baby with cavitary pneumonia and septicemia. (B) Frontal radiograph of the chest post-administration of 10 ml of nonionic iodinated contrast media shows opacification of the proximal esophagus with free contrast in the mediastinum consistent with esophageal perforation. The stomach is filled with air. Multiple chest tubes were placed due to recurrent pneumothoraces. There is marked soft tissue swelling (anasarca).

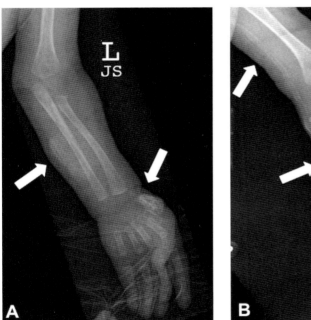
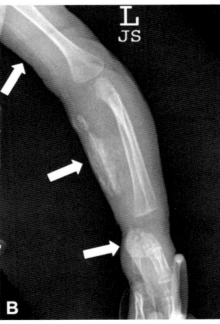

Figure 12.45 Calcium gluconate extravasation. (A) Anteroposterior (ap) and (B) lateral radiograph of the left hand shows increased densities/concretions (arrows) along the medial border of the distal ulna and lateral border of the first metacarpal consistent with calcium gluconate extravasation in a newborn. Note the carpal bones are not ossified at birth.

make its way through the mediastinum into the abdomen (Figure 12.44).

Intravenous and intra-arterial catheters

A wide variety of intravenous and intra-arterial catheters are used in the pediatric population, the commonest being an intravenous (IV) catheter placement which usually doesn't require imaging for confirmation of placement. Rarely, a hard swelling around an IV catheter may be evaluated by plain

radiography; these are due to extravasation of calcium gluconate solution, seen as a concretion of increased density around the injection site (Figure 12.45).

The next most common vascular access is a peripherally inserted central venous catheter (PICC), which is placed to retain vascular access for at least a few weeks. This is accomplished with a catheter placed through a peripheral vein of the upper extremity or the lower extremity (especially in newborns and infants) and advanced into one of the great veins: superior

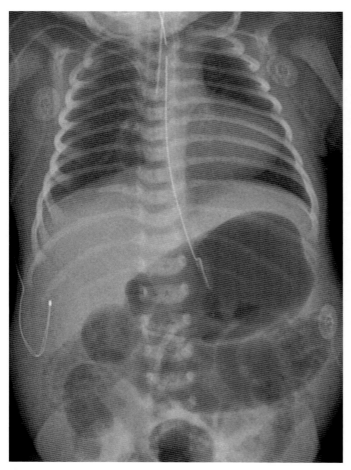

Figure 12.46 Properly positioned upper extremity peripherally inserted central venous catheter (PICC). Frontal radiograph of the chest and abdomen shows right upper extremity PICC terminating in the superior vena cava (SVC) in good position in a premature infant with necrotizing enterocolitis. Note the diffuse intramural air in the abdomen. ETT terminates at T4.

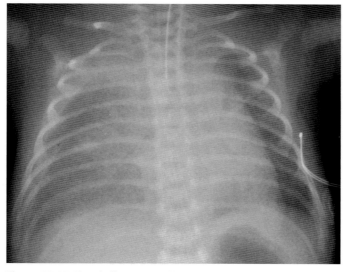

Figure 12.48 Pleural effusion caused by PICC placement. Frontal radiograph of the chest shows small apical right pleural effusion which appeared after PICC placement. The PICC was removed.

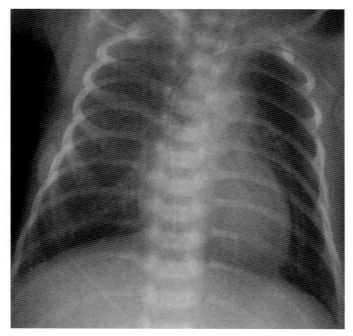

Figure 12.47 Malposition of upper extremity peripherally inserted central venous catheter (PICC). Frontal radiograph of the chest shows left upper extremity PICC terminating in the low right atrium. This needs prompt repositioning to avoid complications.

vena cava (SVC) for upper extremity PICCs and the inferior vena cava (IVC) for lower extremity PICCs.

Figure 12.46 demonstrates proper positioning of a PICC inserted through an upper extremity vein. However, for practical purposes, an upper extremity PICC is considered to be deep if it overlies the lateral two-thirds of the clavicle and is considered as central if it terminates over the medial one-third of the clavicle. Similarly, for all practical purposes, the clinician considers a lower extremity PICC deep if it terminates within the pelvic cavity and considers it as central if it is at or is superior to L3. The PICC within the cardiac silhouette needs repositioning, whether it is an upper or lower extremity PICC (Figure 12.47).

Malposition (Figure 12.47) and infection are two of the most common complications of PICC placement, among others such as thrombosis, occlusion, arrhythmias (due to stimulation of the sinus node in the right atrium; Figure 12.47), pleural effusion (Figure 12.48) and breakage (Figure 12.49). Cardiac tamponade is very rare and can be fatal. The PICC pierces the right atrial wall or the left atrial appendage and causes sudden cardiac tamponade. A sudden deterioration of the cardiovascular status in a patient with a PICC should raise the suspicion of a cardiac tamponade. PICC may rarely become looped or knotted (Figure 12.50) at the time of insertion. Sometimes the PICC takes an unusual course, thus revealing vascular anomalies like left-sided superior vena cava (SVC) (Figure 12.51). PICCs may course through shunts and reach unusual locations, as seen in Figure 12.50, which shows a left jugular PICC coursing

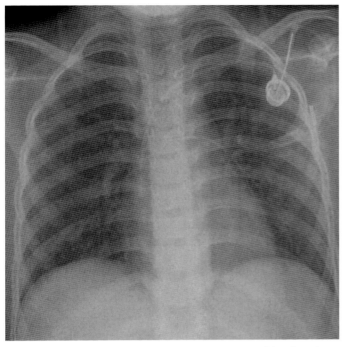

Figure 12.49 Broken/transected PICC. Frontal radiograph of the chest shows the broken fragment of the PICC which is seen looped in the left pulmonary artery in a nine-year-old boy. Left-sided portacath is seen terminating in the upper right atrium.

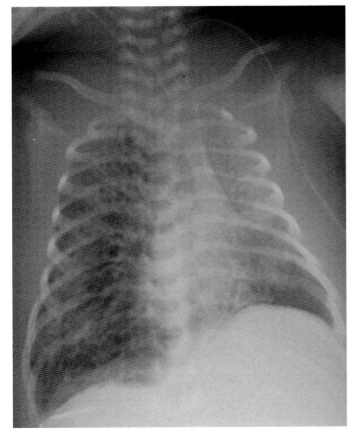

Figure 12.51 Left-sided superior vena cava. Frontal radiograph of the chest shows left-sided jugular PICC terminating in the left-sided SVC in a four-day-old premature baby with respiratory distress syndrome and pulmonary interstitial emphysema in the right lung. The ETT terminates at C7.

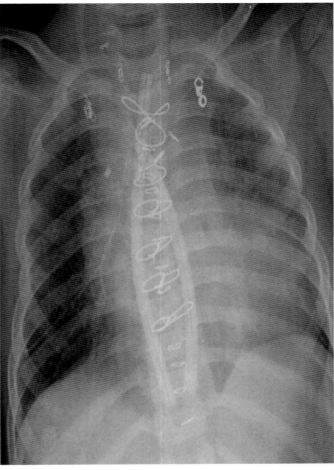

Figure 12.50 Loop/knot of left upper extremity PICC. Frontal radiograph of the chest shows a left jugular PICC coursing from the left brachiocephalic vein into the superior vena cava, and through the stent placed at the Glenn shunt (from the superior vena cava to the right pulmonary artery) and appears to make a loop or knot in a branch of the right pulmonary artery in the right lower lobe, in a four-year-old boy with complex congenital heart disease.

through the SVC into the Glenn shunt and terminating in a branch of the right pulmonary artery in the lower lobe of the right lung. If the vascular access is needed for a prolonged time, the PICC is replaced by tunneled central venous catheters (Broviac or Hickman) (Figure 12.52). The central venous catheters are mainly used to prevent the numerous needle sticks that would be needed during treatment of patients with malignancies.

Peripheral arterial lines (PAL) are placed to monitor arterial blood gases, acid–base status and blood pressure. These are placed in the radial or the posterior tibial artery. Allen's test is performed before insertion to ensure adequate collateral circulation between the radial and ulnar artery. Complications like thromboembolism due to PAL placement may lead to ischemia of the distal extremities: finger tips or toes. Infection and hemorrhage are other occasional complications with a remote role of radiography for evaluation.

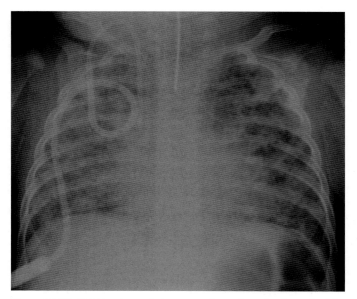

Figure 12.52 Right jugular central venous catheter. Frontal radiograph of the chest shows right-sided jugular venous Broviac catheter terminating in the SVC in a three-month-old premature baby with bronchopulmonary dysplasia (BPD). Note bilateral diffuse coarse interstitial granular opacities with cystic lucencies consistent with BPD. The ETT terminates at T2.

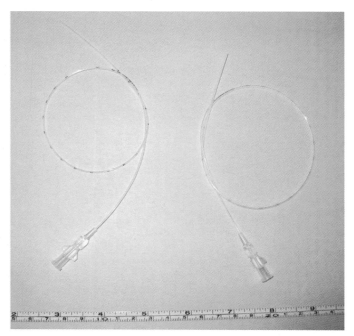

Figure 12.53 Umbilical vessel catheters. A 3.5F catheter is used for infants weighing less than 1250 g, and a 5F catheter is used for infants weighing over 1250 g, for umbilical artery catheterization. A 5F catheter is used for all infants for umbilical vein catheterization.

Umbilical vessel catheters are placed through the umbilical artery and vein and are referred to as umbilical arterial catheters (UACs) and umbilical venous catheters (UVCs), respectively, in a newborn that is either of low birthweight, premature, large for gestational age or in acute respiratory distress due to various causes.

Umbilical arterial catheters (UACs) are used primarily to monitor arterial blood gases, acid–base status and blood pressure. A 3.5F catheter is used for infants weighing less than 1250 g and a 5F catheter is used for infants weighing over 1250 g (Figure 12.53). The UAC follows the course of the umbilical arteries, which are the direct continuation of the internal iliac arteries, and enter the aorta through the iliac arteries. Hence the UAC from the umbilicus is initially directed inferiorly and posteriorly (overlying the sacroiliac joint) and then courses superiorly into the common iliac artery and finally into the abdominal aorta (Figure 12.54). In the aorta, there are two potential positions for the UAC, described as "high line" or "low line." The high line is placed between the T5 and T8 thoracic vertebral bodies (Figure 54A), well below the arch of the aorta and its branches and the ductus arteriosus, and well above the main branches of the abdominal aorta, namely the celiac artery at T10 level. The low line is placed at the level of the L3–L4 lumbar vertebral bodies (Figure 12.55), below the origin of the inferior mesenteric artery at L3 and above the aortic bifurcation (L4–L5). At our institution, high line is the standard of practice. The Cochrane systematic review suggests that high positioning of UAC in babies in NICU leads to fewer complications and reduced need for replacement and reinsertion of catheters compared to low positioning.

High positioning is achieved by inserting the catheter 1 cm more than the infant's umbilical to shoulder length or by estimating the length with the following equation:

$$(\text{Weight in kg} \times 3) + 9 \text{ cm}$$

The position of the UAC is always confirmed by plain radiography. One of the most dreaded complications of the UAC placement is thrombosis leading to an ischemic limb, evidenced by blanching, cyanosis (Figure 12.56) or mottling. Other complications include embolism, vasospasm, hypertension, traumatic aneurysm (Figure 12.57), necrotizing enterocolitis, hemorrhage, infection and hematuria, among others. The contraindications for UAC placement include omphalitis, omphalocele, necrotizing enterocolitis and peritonitis.

Umbilical venous catheters (UVCs) are used primarily for infusion of resuscitation fluid in a critically ill infant or for administration of fluids, parenteral nutrition, intravenous medications, central venous pressure measurement, exchange transfusion in cases of severe unconjugated hyperbilirubinemia and for diagnosis of infradiaphragmatic total anomalous pulmonary venous return (TAPVR type III).

A 5F umbilical vessel catheter is used for all infants, regardless of infant size and gestational age (Figure 12.53). The UVC follows the course of the single umbilical vein which extends from the umbilicus to the left portal vein in the liver. The umbilical recess is a focal dilatation of the umbilical vein just proximal to its junction with the left portal vein. The blood from the umbilical vein is directed to the

(A)

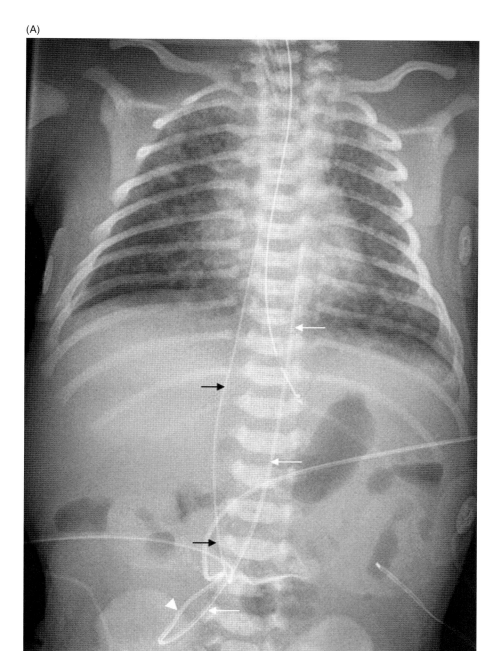

(B)

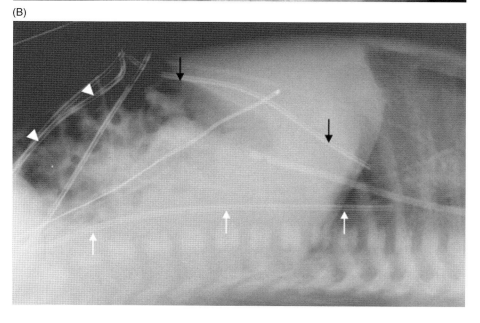

Figure 12.54 Normal radiographic appearance of umbilical arterial catheter (UAC) and umbilical venous catheter (UVC). (A) Frontal radiograph of abdomen shows UAC entering the abdomen at the umbilicus and coursing in the caudad direction (white arrowhead) and posteriorly into the right iliac artery before coursing superiorly in the aorta (white arrows). The UVC is also seen entering the abdomen at the umbilicus but coursing in the cephalad direction (black arrows) into the umbilical vein, through the left portal vein and ductus venosus, into the inferior vena cava, and terminating in the upper right atrium. The UAC terminates at T8 in proper position for a "high line." The ETT terminates at T1. Bilateral coarse opacities in the lung are due to meconium aspiration syndrome. (B) Cross-table lateral radiograph of abdomen shows UAC entering the abdomen at the umbilicus and coursing inferiorly (white arrowheads) and posteriorly as it courses through the umbilical artery and then ascending into the posteriorly located aorta (white arrows). The UVC (black arrows) also enters the abdomen at the umbilicus and runs superiorly and anteriorly until it reaches the inferior vena cava and right atrium.

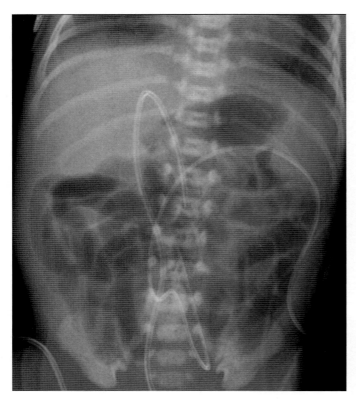

Figure 12.55 Normal radiographic appearance of a "low UAC" Frontal radiograph of the abdomen shows the UAC entering the abdomen at the umbilicus, coursing in the caudad direction and terminating in the aorta at the L3/4 level. The UVC is coursing inferiorly not in a correct position; it is likely into the mesenteric vein.

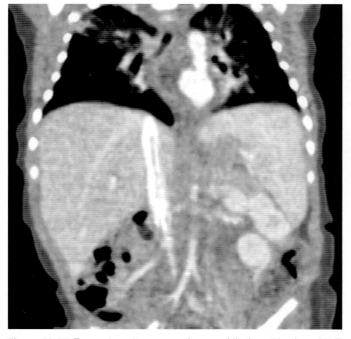

Figure 12.57 Traumatic aortic aneurysm due to umbilical arterial catheter (UAC) placement. Coronal CT scan shows fusiform aneurysm in the thoracic aorta in a two-year-old premature baby with history of UAC placement and septic joints. (Courtesy of R. Brasch, MD.)

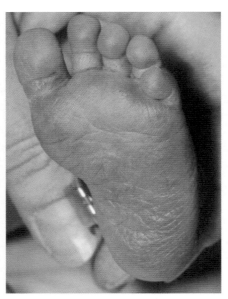

Figure 12.56 Photograph of a newborn baby with blue toes, with arterial compromise post-UAC placement due to arterial thrombosis, one of the most dreaded complications of the UAC placement. (Courtesy of R. Brasch, MD.)

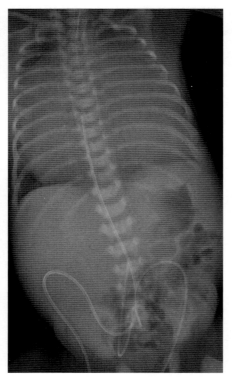

Figure 12.58 UVC malposition. Frontal radiograph of the chest and the abdomen shows UVC terminating in the right atrium in a newborn with significant cardiomegaly due to Ebstein's anomaly. The UAC terminates at L4, in the proper position for a "low line."

inferior vena cava (IVC) through the ductus venosus. The tip of the UVC is placed at the IVC/RA junction for administration of fluids (Figure 12.54B). This can be achieved by inserting the catheter two-thirds of the shoulder-to-umbilicus distance. Thus, the UVC follows the course of the single umbilical vein along the anterior abdominal wall and into the left portal vein and finally through the ductus venosus into the IVC (Figure 12.54). For emergency situations, the UVC is advanced only until there is a free flow of blood and never more than 8 cm in a term infant.

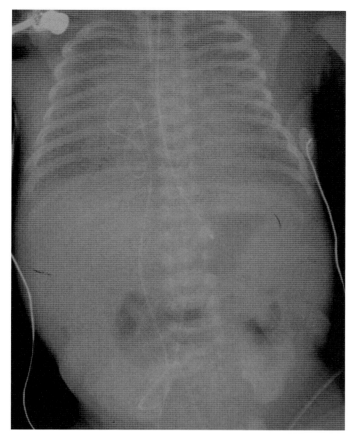

Figure 12.59 UVC malposition. Frontal radiograph of the chest and the abdomen shows the UVC coiled in the right atrium and terminating in the region of the foramen ovale in a newborn with significant pulmonary interstitial edema due to transient tachypnea. The UAC terminates at T4, high for a "high line." (Courtesy of M. Sims, MD.)

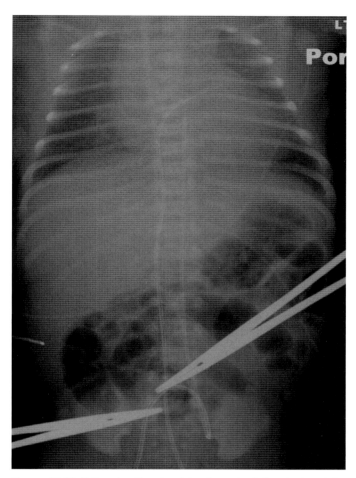

Figure 12.60 UVC malposition. Frontal radiograph of the chest and the abdomen shows UVC coursing through the right atrium and foramen ovale and terminating in the left superior pulmonary vein. The UAC terminates at T7, in good position for a "high line."

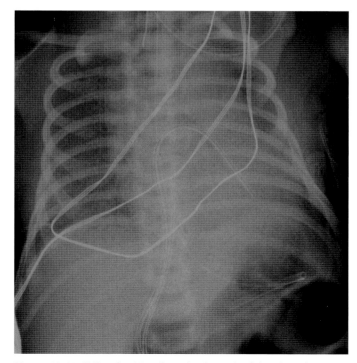

Figure 12.61 UVC malposition. Frontal radiograph of the chest shows one UVC coursing through the right atrium and foramen ovale, left atrium and finally terminating in the left ventricle in a newborn with respiratory distress syndrome. The other UVC terminates in the right atrium.

The position of the UVC is always confirmed by plain radiography. Malpositioning of the UVC occurs frequently as it is inserted by a neonatologist or nurse practitioner without fluoroscopic guidance. Repositioning of the UVC is suggested if it terminates in the right atrium (Figure 12.58) or within the cardiac silhouette (Figure 12.59). If the UVC is advanced even further in a normal infant, it may pass through the foramen ovale and reach the left atrium or a pulmonary vein (usually left upper lobe) (Figure 12.60). Occasionally the UVC from the left atrium crosses through the mitral valve and reaches the left ventricle (Figure 12.61).

The catheter may not reach the IVC or the RA, however, but may reach the left (Figure 12.62) or right portal vein (Figure 12.63). The catheter may get coiled in the umbilical recess (Figure 12.64) just proximal to its junction with the left portal vein.

Occasionally the UVC may have an anomalous position due to congenital heart disease or due to various shunts performed for treating congenital heart diseases. The UVC may exit through the right atrium into the coronary sinus and end in the persistent left superior vena cava (SVC) or into the left subclavian or internal jugular vein.

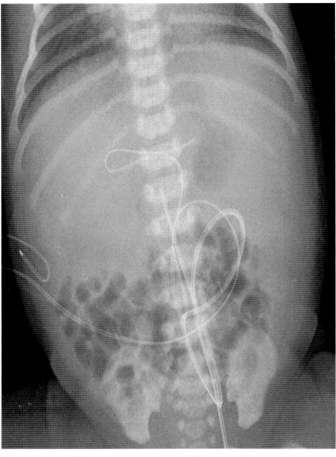

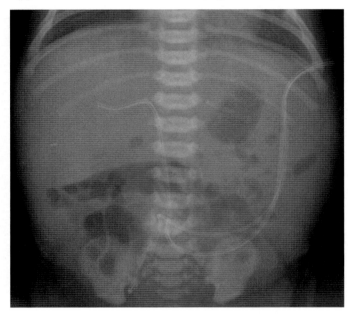

One of the most dreaded complications of UVCs is perforation of the right atrial or left atrial wall. This may cause pericardial effusion leading to cardiac tamponade and a sudden deterioration of the infant's hemodynamic status, and may be fatal (Figure 12.65).

Rarely the UVC may perforate the portal vein and cause a hematoma within the liver. The hematoma has a variable appearance depending on the age. The hematoma may appear anechoic (Figure 12.66), heterogeneous or echogenic on US. Hypodense low-attenuation lesions (Figure 12.67) are chronic,

Figure 12.62 UVC malposition. Frontal radiograph of the abdomen shows UVC terminating in the left portal vein. The UAC terminates at L1, too high for an attempted "low line."

Figure 12.63 UVC malposition. Frontal radiograph of the abdomen shows UVC terminating in the right portal vein.

(A)

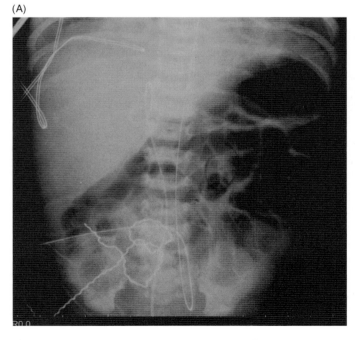

(B)

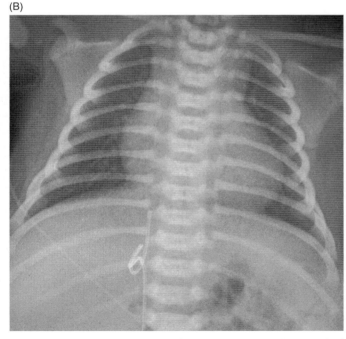

Figure 12.64 UVC malposition. (A) Frontal radiograph of the abdomen shows UVC coiled in the umbilical recess. (Courtesy of M. Sims, MD.) (B) Frontal radiograph of the chest shows UVC coiled in the umbilical recess.

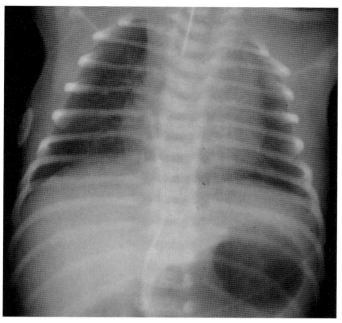

Figure 12.65 UVC malposition. Frontal radiograph of the chest shows UVC terminating in the upper right atrium. The baby deteriorated post-placement and pericardial effusion was found on autopsy. (Courtesy of M. Sims, MD.)

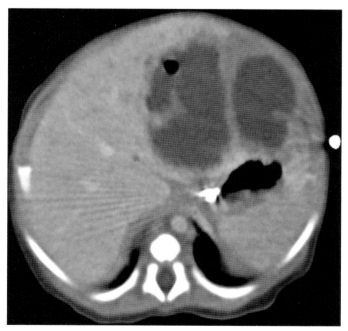

Figure 12.67 Complication due to UVC. Axial contrast-enhanced CT shows low-attenuation lesions with bubbles of air. Bloody fluid was aspirated and culture of the fluid was negative, consistent with a hematoma. (Courtesy of S. Ghahremani, MD.)

and hyperdense are acute, on CT. The hematoma eventually calcifies and is well evaluated on CT, rather than US, as these cause significant acoustic shadowing on US. UVC placement may cause thrombosis in the IVC, ductus venosus or the portal vein, which may also become calcified.

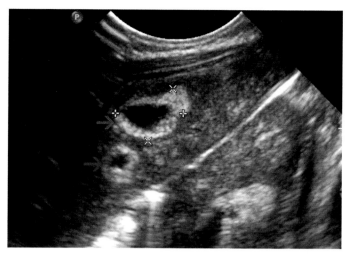

Figure 12.66 Complication due to UVC. Ultrasound image of the liver shows thick-walled anechoic lesions consistent with hematomas. There were no signs of infection. (Courtesy of S. Ghahremani, MD.)

Thus, due to the high prevalence of malposition, the position of the UVC is always confirmed by plain radiography immediately after placement and before anchoring it, to allow repositioning if needed.

Cardiac devices

On November 29, 1944, Drs. Blalock and Taussig decided to proceed with the anastomosis of the subclavian artery to the pulmonary artery in a cyanotic child with tetralogy of Fallot: the shunt now known as the Blalock-Taussig (B-T) shunt. This surgery led to the treatment of blue babies, and revolutionized the field of pediatric-cardiac surgery. Early palliation and elective repair at five to six years of age was the trend for treatment of pediatric congenital heart diseases up to 1970. Then came the trend of primary repairs in infancy and finally in neonates in the mid 1980s.

With the advent of transcatheter cardiac devices (TCCDs), the treatment of congenital heart disease has been further revolutionized and the use of surgery for certain types of shunts has declined considerably. Today TCCDs are used for closure of certain types of septal defects, both atrial (ASD) and ventricular (VSD); and for occlusion of patent ductus arteriosus (PDA) and collateral vessels in complex congenital heart disease; and for stenting various stenotic lesions. The increasing use of the TCCD by the pediatric cardiologist has led to the need for understanding the appearance of such devices on plain radiography. We no longer only have to verify the position of the tubes and lines, but also the position of the cardiac devices. Malposition or embolization and change in position of cardiac devices are very critical information for the pediatric cardiologist. If one is well acquainted with the normal appearance and location of various cardiac devices in different clinical scenarios, it becomes easy to recognize the aberrant location. In this section, we will review the normal appearance of the commonly used cardiac devices.

(A)

(B)

(C)

(D)

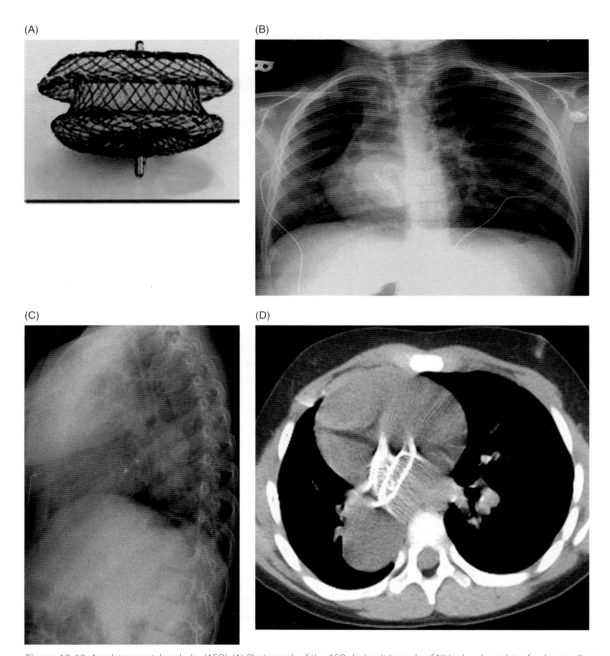

Figure 12.68 Amplatzer septal occluder (ASO). (A) Photograph of the ASO device. It is made of Nitinol and consists of polyester discs connected by a waist in the center. (B) Frontal radiograph of the chest shows an ASO within the cardiac silhouette in the region of the atrial septum. The oval soft tissue density lesion seen around the ASO is a bronchogenic cyst. (C) Lateral radiograph of the chest shows an ASO within the cardiac silhouette in the region of the atrial septum. The oval soft tissue density lesion seen posterior to the heart is a bronchogenic cyst. (D) Axial CT scan shows ASO placed in the atrial septum. There is a dense streak artifact caused by the device. The oval low-attenuation lesion seen posteriorly is a bronchogenic cyst.

Atrial septal defect (ASD)

The four types of ASD are based on the location of the septal defect: ostium primum, ostium secundum, foramen ovale and sinus venosus defect. For appropriate placement of a cardiac device the defect should be surrounded by the septum, and hence only ostium secundum and foramen ovale defects, which are surrounded by the interatrial septum, are treated by the pediatric cardiologist. The Amplatzer septal occluder (ASO) is used for closure of ASDs. The device is made of Nitinol and consists of polyester discs connected by a waist in the center. Figure 12.68 shows the normal appearance of an ASO on plain radiography and CT in a child after ASD closure.

Although rare, embolization of ASD devices does occur immediately or, rarely, late. Thus any change or malposition should be recognized on plain radiography.

(A)

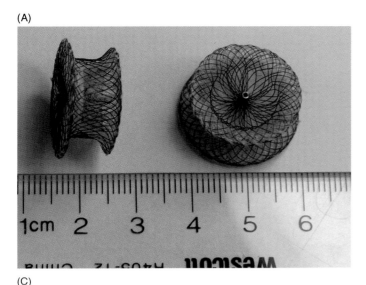

(B)

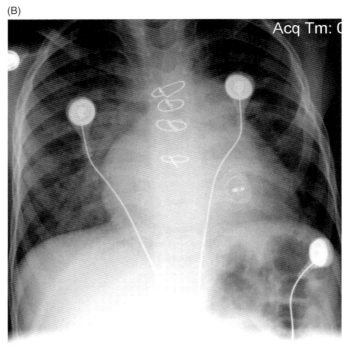

(C)

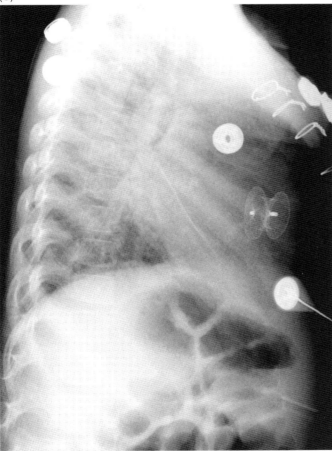

Figure 12.69 Amplatzer ventricular septal occluder (AVSO). (A) Photograph of the AVSO device. It is made of Nitinol and polyester discs connected with a thick waist to anchor well at the thick interventricular septum. (B) Frontal radiograph of the chest shows AVSO to the left of midline along the course of the interventricular septum. (C) Lateral radiograph of the chest shows AVSO in profile along the course of the interventricular septum. (Courtesy of M. I. Boechat, MD.)

Ventricular septal defect (VSD)

There are four types of VSDs recognized based on the location of the septal defect: membranous or perimembranous, inlet, outlet or supracristal, and muscular or trabecular. Membranous and muscular VSDs are treated by interventional pediatric cardiologists due to the presence of circumferential septal

tissue around the septal defect, which anchors the closure device. The currently available Amplatzer ventricular septal occluder (AVSO) is not FDA (Food and Drug Administration) approved. ASO or PDA occluder devices have also been used for VSD closure. The AVSO is also made of Nitinol and polyester discs connected with a thick waist to anchor well at

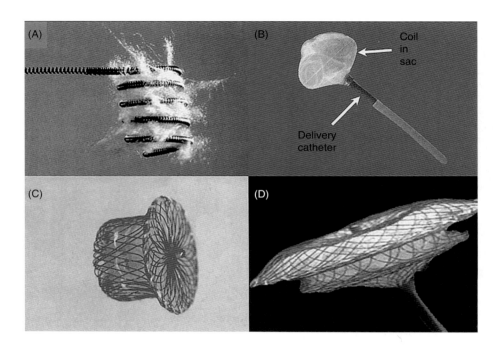

Figure 12.70 PDA occlusion devices. (A) Gianturco coils; (B) Grifka sac; (C) Amplatzer duct occluder; (D) Nit-Occlud coils. (Courtesy of M. I. Boechat, MD.)

the thick interventricular septum (Figure 12.69). Figure 12.69 shows the normal appearance of muscular AVSO in a child after VSD closure.

Patent ductus arteriosus (PDA)

PDA causes left-to-right shunt from the aorta to the pulmonary artery and causes increased pulmonary vascularity and congestive heart failure in the newborn period. Surgery is necessary for neonatal cases and for rare large PDAs, due to technical difficulties. A PDA ligation clip is placed surgically in small infants. Various PDA occlusion devices are available: Gianturco coil (GC), Ivalon plug (IP), Gianturco-Grifka vascular occlusion device (GGVOD), Rashkind duct occluder (RDO), Amplatzer duct occluder (ADO) and Nit-Occlud coil (NOC) (Figure 12.70).

The GC is made of stainless steel and Dacron fibers, and is used for closure of small and medium-sized PDAs. GGVODs made of stainless steel and nylon sac were introduced for closure of tubular PDAs.

Rashkind introduced the Rashkind duct occluder, a double umbrella device or the button device in the 1970s. It was used for occlusion of PDAs up to 8 mm in diameter and is not used commonly today as the deployment technique is rather complex and some studies have shown a considerable incidence of residual leak. It is made of a stainless steel wire frame and is covered by polyurethane fabric.

Porstman reported the first nonsurgical closure of PDA with an Ivalon plug in 1967. The main disadvantage of this technique is the use of a large delivery system and it cannot be used in infants and young children.

Amplatzer duct occluder (ADO)

In 1998, Masura reported his experience with ADO and it has since then been used for closure of long tubular, and moderate to large PDAs.

The ADO has a Nitinol wire framework and is filled with polyester fabric. Figure 12.71 shows the appearance of ADO on plain radiography.

Nit-Occlud coils (NOCs) or Nit-Occlud PDA occlusion system

These are currently under FDA study and are used for occlusion of PDAs up to 4 mm in diameter. They are designed for transcatheter occlusion of PDA of all types and shapes, and sizes up to 5 mm. Figure 12.72 shows the appearance of a NOC placed in a child with PDA.

Vascular embolization

Arterial and venous collaterals develop in many congenital heart diseases, sometimes as part of the physiology of the heart disease (such as major aortopulmonary collateral arteries [MAPCAs], and internal mammary to pulmonary arteries in cases of pulmonary atresia) or as a result of a surgical procedure like Glenn shunt where venous collaterals develop between the superior vena cava (SVC) and the pulmonary arteries. Such collaterals are embolized using Gianturco coils, the Amplatzer plug, and Amplatzer duct occluder among others. Figure 12.73 shows embolization of the internal mammary arteries in a child with Ebstein's anomaly and pulmonary atresia. Coils are also used to plug the transhepatic access.

(A)

(B)

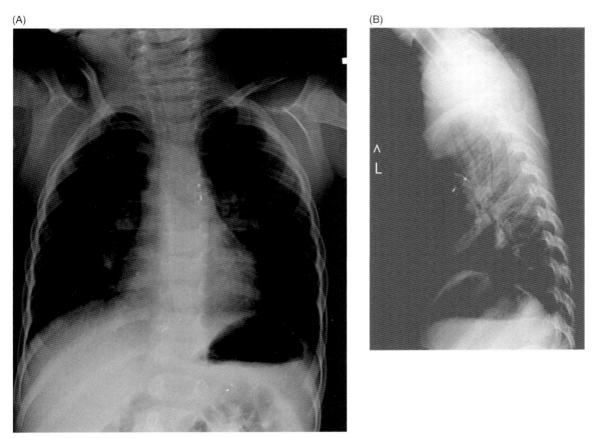

Figure 12.71 Normal appearance of Amplatzer duct occluder. (A) Frontal radiograph of the chest shows ADO in the region of the PDA between the aortic arch and the pulmonary artery. (B) Lateral radiograph of the chest shows ADO in profile in the region of the PDA.

(A)

(B)

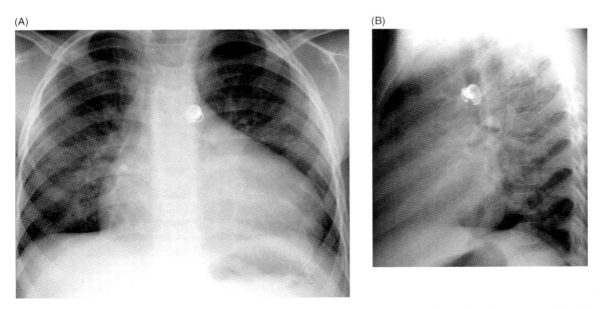

Figure 12.72 Normal appearance of Nit-Occlud coils (NOCs). (A) Frontal radiograph of the chest shows NOC in the region of the PDA between the aortic arch and the pulmonary artery. (B) Lateral radiograph of the chest shows NOC almost in profile in the region of the PDA. (Courtesy of M. I. Boechat, MD.)

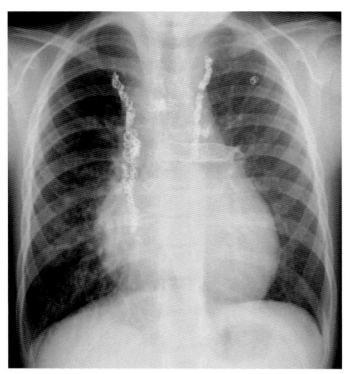

Figure 12.73 Frontal radiograph of the chest shows multiple coils used for embolization of collaterals between pulmonary arteries and the internal mammary arteries in a child with Ebstein's anomaly and pulmonary atresia. A stent is seen in the left pulmonary artery. (Courtesy of M. I. Boechat, MD.)

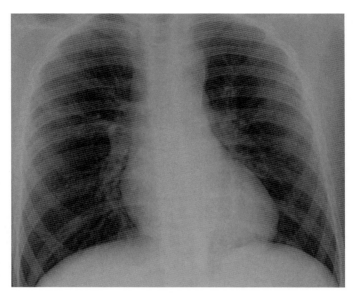

Figure 12.74 Frontal radiograph of the chest shows an aortic stent in a teenager with coarctation of the aorta. (Courtesy of M. I. Boechat, MD.)

Vascular and intracardiac stenting

Stents are used in cases of stenotic lesions of the pulmonary artery and vein, aorta, SVC, etc. Coronary stents are used for stenting. Figure 12.73 shows a stent in the left pulmonary artery in a child with Ebstein's anomaly and pulmonary atresia.

Stents are also used to create or maintain the ASD as a communication between the right and left atrium in cases of single ventricle physiology.

Patency of PDA is maintained by PDA stenting in some cases of congenital heart disease like pulmonary atresia where PDA is vital to maintain blood flow to the lungs for oxygenation.

Aortic stenting is used in early childhood or adolescent age instead of surgery in patients with congenital postductal aortic stenosis. Figure 12.74 shows an aortic stent in a teenager with coarctation of the aorta. Aortic dissection is also treated with stent grafts.

In conclusion, knowledge of the normal appearance and expected location of the various cardiac devices placed by the interventional pediatric cardiologist helps one to recognize possible complications and warrant prompt management.

Orthopedic devices

Orthopedic devices are commonly used for treating trauma, fractures, joint reconstruction, limb preservation, spinal conditions, congenital abnormalities and deformities. "Children

are not miniature adults; however, adults are grown up children," and also because children are still growing, their bodies' response to injuries, infections and deformities can be quite different than an adult's.

The challenges currently faced by many orthopedic companies dealing with developing implants for children seem obvious, as children grow continuously and there is also a true difference with gender, as a girl's skeleton typically matures ahead of a boy's. All secondary ossification centers appear earlier in girls as well as fuse earlier than in boys. In addition, the immature skeletons of children have vulnerable growth plates which, when disturbed, cause severe growth disturbances and limb length discrepancies. Today some hardware companies are really striving hard to provide anatomically appropriate orthopedic implants for children, with the aid of collaborative input from orthopedic surgeons. In this section we will review some of the commonly used orthopedic devices in the pediatric population.

Trauma and fractures

Fractures are treated nonsurgically with closed reduction (CR) under anesthesia; or surgically with open reduction and internal fixation (ORIF), wherein screws, pins, nails and plates are used to transfix a fracture; or surgically with open reduction and external fixation, wherein surgical pins placed through the skin are attached to an external metal frame. Bone grafts are occasionally used. Pins and screws can also be placed without an incision under direct vision.

Cannulated screws available in various lengths and thread patterns are widely used in treating fractures in the pediatric population for physeal injuries including Salter II, III and IV and nonphyseal injuries mainly of the distal tibia in the maturing skeleton (Figure 12.75). A cortical screw is fully threaded

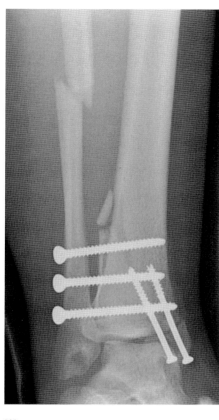

Figure 12.75 Anteroposterior radiograph shows three cortical screws affixed at the fractures through the distal fibula and tibia, and two cortical screws transfixed at the medial malleolar fracture in a 15-year-old girl who was injured in a car accident.

and a cancellous screw is threaded at the distal end. Generally cortical screws should not be used in cancellous bone. However, cancellous screws may be used only in cancellous bone.

Pins or K-wires (Kirschner wires) are usually used to transfix supracondylar, radial and phalangeal fractures (Figures 12.76 and 12.77) in pediatrics. Several studies have shown a decreased incidence of cubitus varus (so-called gunstock deformity) in the patients with supracondylar fractures treated by percutaneous pinning versus only closed reduction. The range of elbow motion is also found to be better in the group treated with pin fixation. Also, the costs and hospital stays were significantly less in those treated by pinning.

Intramedullary nails (IM) are used for comminuted and displaced long bone shaft fractures. Typically a single IM nail is introduced into the medullary canal through the fracture site and fixed with screws at both ends (Figure 12.78). Today, several studies have shown that the elastic/flexible intramedullary nail fixation is a minimally invasive and effective surgical approach for treatment of extremity fractures in children and is associated with fewer complications. It also allows early postoperative mobility and secures a satisfactory bone union and effective functional recovery. Typically two nails are introduced into the medullary canal with the unique advantage of a closed reduction in order to create an elastic fixation that resists deformity. The nails are introduced above and below

(A)

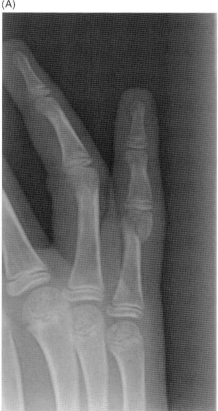

(B)

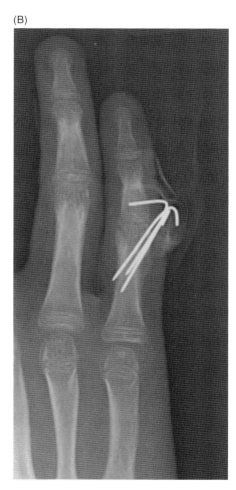

Figure 12.76 (A) Radiograph shows minimally displaced fracture through the distal aspect of the proximal phalanx of the fifth digit of the right hand in a 12-year-old boy. (B) Anteroposterior radiograph shows three K-wires transfixed at the fracture site.

(A)

(B)

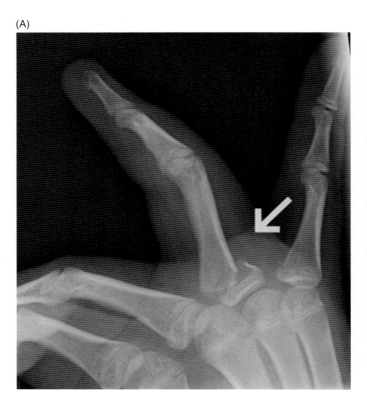

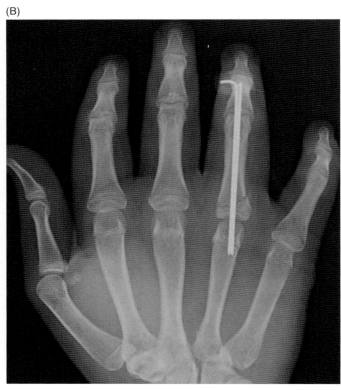

Figure 12.77 (A) Radiograph shows displaced Salter II fracture through the proximal aspect of the proximal phalanx of the fourth digit of the right hand in a 14-year-old boy. (B) Anteroposterior radiograph shows two K-wires transfixed at the fracture site.

(A)

(B)

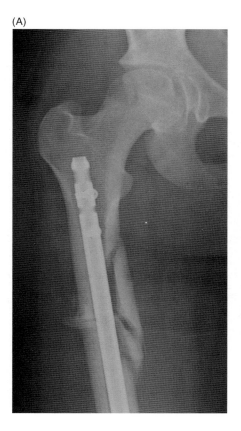

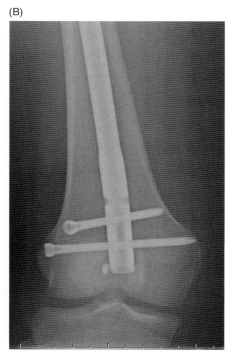

Figure 12.78 (A) Anteroposterior radiograph shows the proximal end of an intramedullary nail used for internal fixation of the comminuted fracture through the proximal right femur. (B) Anteroposterior radiograph shows the distal end of an intramedullary nail fixed with two screws through the distal femur in a 15-year-old girl who was injured in a motor-vehicle accident.

the growth plates to avoid interference with the growth plates and hence significantly reduce growth disturbances.

Displaced fractures at the ends of the long bones in the immature and mature skeleton are fixed with plates and screws (Figure 12.79), or screws only.

Slipped capital femoral epiphysis (SCFE) is a Salter-Harris type I fracture due to the repetitive stress of weight-bearing leading to posteromedial displacement of the femoral epiphysis. This is treated by insertion of screws to immobilize the

femoral epiphysis on the growth plate without attempting reduction (Figure 12.80). A higher incidence of avascular necrosis (AVN) is reported with open reduction and fixation. Complications of SCFE, like avascular necrosis (Figure 12.80), chondrolysis leading to joint-space narrowing and hardware failure, are diagnosed by plain film radiography.

For Salter-Harris type I and II injuries in children younger than 10 years of age, angulations of up to 30° can be accepted, as a greater degree of remodeling occurs in young children. In children older than 10 years, up to 15° of angulation is generally acceptable. Children younger than 10 years of age with angulation of more than 30°, and older children (10 years and above) may be better treated as adults, with plates and screws.

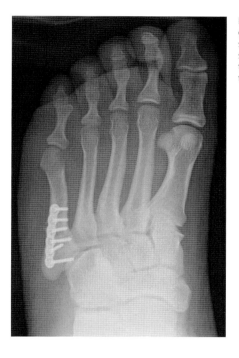

Figure 12.79 Radiograph of the left foot shows a small plate and six screws transfixed at the displaced fifth metatarsal fracture.

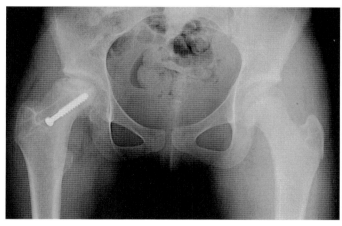

Figure 12.80 Slipped capital femoral epiphysis (SCFE). Radiograph shows a screw inserted through the femoral neck to immobilize the femoral epiphysis on the growth plate. Note the lucent crescent in the femoral epiphysis consistent with avascular necrosis.

(A)

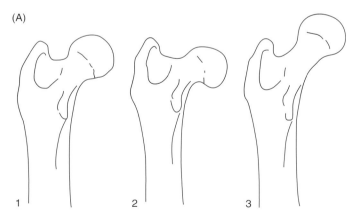

(B)

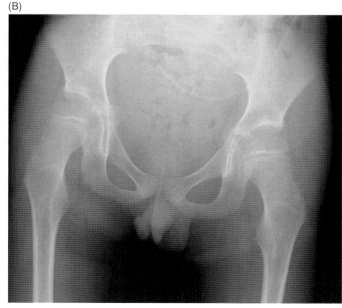

Figure 12.81 (A) Line diagrams demonstrate: (1) normal neck–shaft angle (120–150°); (2) coxa vara (<120°); and (3) coxa valga (>150°). (B) Anteroposterior radiograph shows bilateral coxa valga, right greater than left with partial subluxation of the right hip.

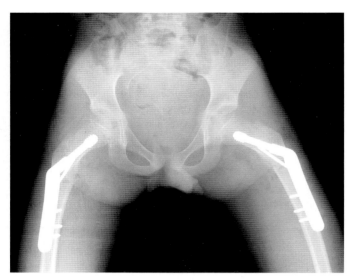

Figure 12.83 Anteroposterior radiograph of the pelvis with both hips shows bilateral coxa valga corrected by varus osteotomy and angled blade plate fixation to prevent hip dislocation.

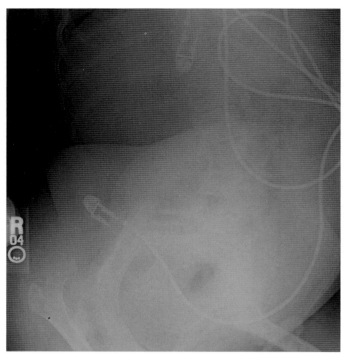

Figure 12.82 Coxa valga with right hip dislocation. Radiograph of the pelvis shows coxa valga and right hip dislocation caused by abnormal muscular forces and spasticity in a teenager with cerebral palsy.

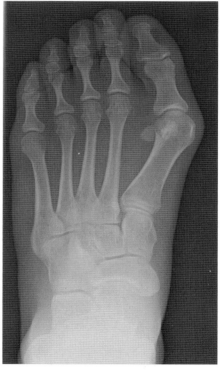

Figure 12.84 Hallux valgus or bunion deformity. Anteroposterior radiograph of the left foot shows medial deviation of the first metatarsal and lateral deviation of the hallux, with mild medial soft tissue enlargement of the first metatarsal head in a 17-year-old girl.

Deformity correction

The normal femoral neck–shaft angle at any age is between 120 to 150°. When the neck–shaft angle is decreased to less than 120° it is coxa vara, and when it is increased over 150° it is coxa valga (Figure 12.81). Both entities can be congenital or acquired and may be progressive when acquired. In clinical practice, most cases of coxa valga are more symptomatic as compared to coxa vara. The commonest cause of significantly progressive coxa valga is cerebral palsy and other neuromuscular disorders, caused mainly by the nonambulatory and non-weight-bearing condition. The increased pull on the femoral head due to abnormal muscular forces and spasticity causes coxa valga and, eventually, subluxation or dislocation of the femoral head (Figure 12.82). This is corrected by varus osteotomy and angled blade plate fixation to prevent hip dislocation (Figure 12.83).

The hallux is the first or innermost digit of the foot of humans, the great toe or the big toe. Valgus is a lateral displacement away from the midline of the body. Hallux valgus or bunion deformity (Figure 12.84) is defined as medial deviation of the first metatarsal and lateral deviation and/or rotation of the hallux, with or without medial soft tissue enlargement of the first metatarsal head. Hallux valgus is caused by various etiologies, including biomechanical, traumatic, genetic and metabolic factors. No definite association of the entity with the use of high-heeled shoes is yet to be confirmed. This condition can lead to painful motion of the joint or difficulty with footwear and presents in females during adulthood 10 times more frequently than males. An angle of over 20° with painful movements at the first metatarsophalangeal joint (MTPJ) and difficulty with footwear with or without associated foot disorders needs surgical correction. Medical, physical and orthotic treatment options are tried first before opting for surgical

Displaced metacarpal, metatarsal and phalangeal fractures are treated with closed reduction and immobilization. However, displaced intra-articular metacarpal, metatarsal and phalangeal fractures (Figures 12.76 and 12.77), and open fractures are treated with ORIF using K-wires, plates and screws.

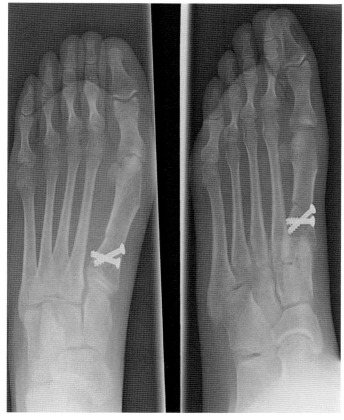

Figure 12.85 Correction of hallux valgus deformity. Anteroposterior and oblique views of the left foot show osteotomy at the base of the first metatarsal with partial excision of the head of the first metatarsal in a 17-year-old girl with hallux valgus deformity.

correction. Surgical treatment depends on various factors like the intermetatarsal angle, hallux valgus angle, mobility of the first ray, and status of the first MTPJ, and there are over 100 different options. Osteotomy of the shaft and/or base of the first metatarsal is performed with an intermetatarsal angle of over 15° and a hallux valgus angle of less than 40° (Figure 12.85). MTPJ arthrodesis with osteotomy of the base of the first metatarsal is performed with intermetatarsal angle of over 15° and hallux valgus angle of greater than 40° (Figure 12.85). Osteotomy/partial excision of the head of the first metatarsal is performed in cases with an incongruent joint with degenerative joint disease involving the first MTPJ (Figures 12.85 and 12.86).

Pes planus or flat foot has various causes, such as tarsal coalition, congenital vertical talus, etc. This is treated by various surgical options; one of them is the conical subtalar implant (CSI), which is a cylindrical metallic implant placed in the subtalar joint for correction of flat foot (Figure 12.87). If no history is provided, one may mistake this for a bullet on plain radiography.

Codivilla first described the method of distraction osteogenesis in 1905 to elongate a femur. In 1951, a Russian orthopedic surgeon, Gavriil Abramovich Ilizarov, developed a technique for

treating complex fractures and nonunion of the long bones. During the treatment of a patient with a short amputation stump, Ilizarov performed an osteotomy and fixed an external fixator to lengthen the bone with the intention of placing a bone graft at a later date; however, to his surprise he discovered new bone formation at the osteotomy site. He demonstrated that controlled tension and stress effects caused an increase in metabolic activity and caused cellular proliferation, neovascularization and osteogenesis. Ilizarov is the father of modern distraction osteogenesis. Today this technique is widely used in the pediatric population for correcting limb length discrepancies (Figure 12.88) and angular deformities, and for treating fractures with nonunion. Radiographs are done at regular intervals to assure adequate osteogenesis at the osteotomy site and also to rule out any evidence of hardware failure or loosening. Distraction osteogenesis is also used in the treatment of mandibular hypoplasia in cases of micrognathia and in treatment of upper airway obstruction, as in obstructive sleep apnea.

Scoliosis is spinal curvature in the coronal plane with a rotational component, with the apex of the curve towards the right known as dextroconvex scoliosis or towards the left known as levoconvex scoliosis. Plain radiography (Figure 12.89) is widely used for diagnosis and follow-up of scoliosis. The Cobb angle (Figure 12.90) is measured between the upper endplate of the upper end vertebral body and the lower endplate of the lower end vertebral body. The end vertebrae are the most tilted vertebrae at the ends of the curve. Perpendiculars are drawn to the tangents through the vertebral endplates and the angle is measured on plain radiographs. However, on PACS it is easily measured by using the angle tool and drawing tangents through the endplates of the end vertebrae. Care should be taken to perform posteroanterior (pa) views of the spine instead of anteroposterior (ap) views with adequate breast and gonadal shielding. The pa views have considerably less radiation to the breasts than ap views. CT scans of the spine with sagittal, coronal and 3D reformations are excellent for surgical planning. However, these are not done routinely as they involve a significant amount of radiation. MR is indicated in cases of congenital, levoconvex or painful scoliosis to rule out an intraspinal abnormality like tethered cord, diastematomyelia, etc.

Scoliosis can be one of two types: postural/flexible, or structural. Postural scoliosis is due to faulty posture as the name suggests, and can be corrected by lateral bending towards the convex side of the curve. However, structural scoliosis cannot be corrected by lateral bending or change in position. There are various causes of structural scoliosis, the most common being idiopathic which is a diagnosis of exclusion. The other causes include congenital, neuromuscular, infection, trauma, tumors, dysplasias, etc. In cerebral palsy up to 25% of patients have severe scoliosis and the spinal curve is C-shaped (Figure 12.91).

Idiopathic scoliosis is classified into three types based on age of onset: infantile idiopathic, juvenile, and adolescent.

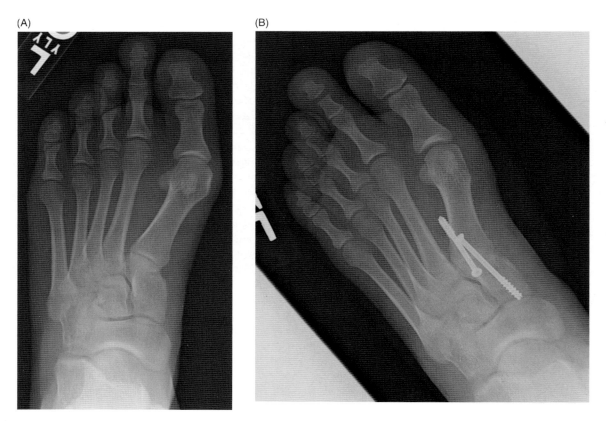

Figure 12.86 (A) Anteroposterior radiograph of the left foot shows hallux valgus deformity in an 18-year-old girl. (B) Anteroposterior radiograph of the left foot shows arthrodesis of the first metatarsophalangeal joint (MTPJ) and osteotomy of the base of the first metatarsal. There is partial excision of the head of the first metatarsal.

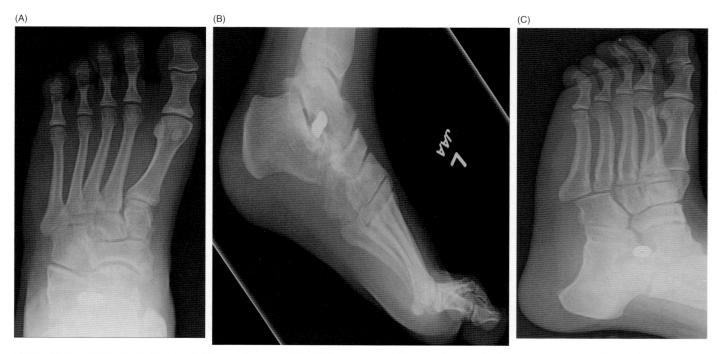

Figure 12.87 Anteroposterior, lateral and oblique radiographs of the left foot show a metallic conical subtalar implant inserted in the subtalar joint for correction of pes planus.

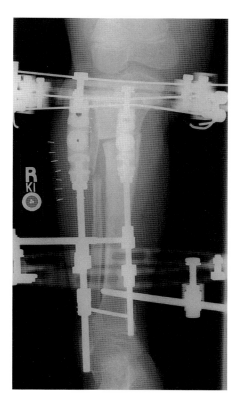

Figure 12.88 Ilizarov technique or distraction osteogenesis. Anteroposterior radiograph of the tibia and fibula shows osteotomies through their proximal shafts with an Ilizarov external fixator for correction of limb length discrepancy.

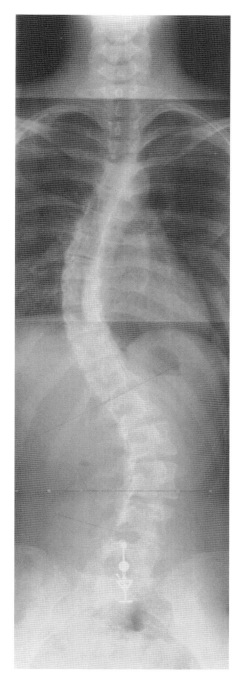

Figure 12.89 Scoliosis. Posteroanterior radiograph of the spine shows S-shaped curve of the spine in a teenage girl. The thoracic curve is the primary curve and the lumbar curve is a secondary compensatory curve.

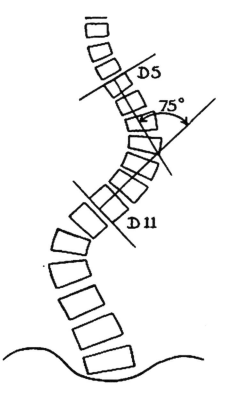

Figure 12.90 Line diagram for measurement of Cobb angle. The Cobb angle is measured between the upper endplate of the upper end vertebral body and the lower endplate of the lower end vertebral body. The end vertebrae (D5 and D11) are the most tilted vertebrae at the ends of the curve. Perpendiculars are drawn to the tangents through the endplates of the end vertebrae, and the angle is measured on plain radiographs.

The infantile type presents at an early age, less than three years, and is common in boys, with a tendency to progress. The juvenile type presents between 3 and 10 years of age and is common in girls. The adolescent type presents in children 10 years and older and occurs in both boys and girls. The spinal curve is usually S-shaped. This type has a tendency to progress rapidly in girls and close follow-up and timely interventions are recommended. Overall, three to five children out of 1 000 require treatment.

The management of scoliosis depends mainly on two important factors: maturity of the skeleton and the degree of spinal curvature. In an immature skeleton with curves less than 20°, or less than 25° in a mature skeleton, management is conservative and includes regular follow-up and radiography.

However, rapidly progressive curves, even if less than 25°, require active management. Curves between 25 and 40° are treated with orthotic devices like spinal braces to prevent progression. The orthotist is a specialist who fits, adjusts and supervises the use of braces. One of the commonly used braces is the thoracolumbosacral brace (TLSO; Figure 12.92). A TLSO is custom made for each patient and is made of plastic that fits the torso mainly to prevent progression of the spinal curve. The braces are not used if the patient has respiratory or neurological compromise. With curves of greater than 50°, especially in a growing child (girls less than 15 years and boys less than

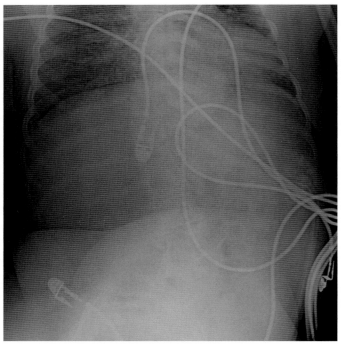

Figure 12.91 Scoliosis due to cerebral palsy. Frontal radiograph shows C-shaped scoliosis caused by abnormal muscular forces and spasticity in a teenager with cerebral palsy.

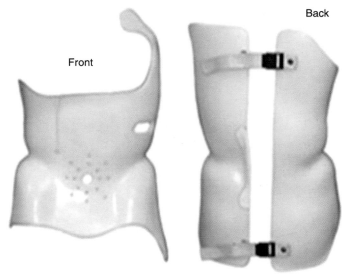

Figure 12.92 Thoracolumbosacral brace (TLSO).

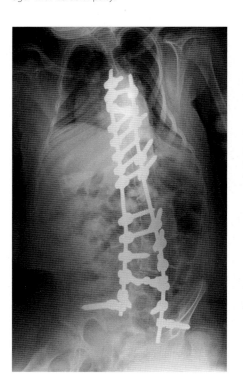
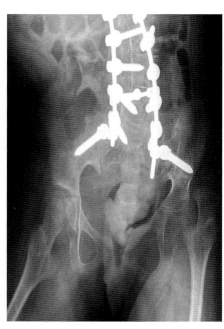

Figure 12.93 Posterior spinal fusion. Frontal radiographs of the spine and pelvis show two rods and multiple screws used for fixation of the spine and correction of severe scoliosis in a boy with cerebral palsy. Note there is diffuse osteopenia and significant constipation.

17 years), and in patients with respiratory or neurological compromise, spinal fusion is performed.

Posterior spinal fusion was first performed by Russell Hibbs for tuberculous spinal deformity in 1911 and for correction of scoliosis in 1914. He primarily corrected the scoliosis by bony fusion of the vertebral column in better anatomical alignment. With his technique he could partially correct the scoliosis and, more importantly, prevent the progression of the scoliosis. Most surgeons then performed Hibbs-type fusion procedures with additional bone grafts. In the 1960s Paul Harrington refined the scoliosis surgery by introducing the Harrington rods for correction of scoliosis. Soon, posterior spinal fusion with Harrington rods became the most acceptable treatment for scoliosis.

Today, posterior spinal fusion (Figure 12.93) with bone grafting is usually performed, and the spine is stabilized by using internal fixation devices, such as Harrington rods, a Luque system, Cotrel-Dubousset system, or Zielke instrumentation with screws or wires or hooks. Aims of surgery are to treat curves of greater than 40–50° in a growing child, to prevent curve progression, to preserve respiratory and neurological function and to improve cosmetic appearances.

Further reading

Donoghue VB, Bjørnstad PG *Radiological Imaging of the Neonatal Chest,* 2nd edn. (New York: Springer, 2007).

Eichhorn JG, Jourdan C, Hill SL, *et al.* (2008) CT of pediatric vascular stents used to treat congenital heart disease. *AJR Am J Roentgenol* **190**(5), 1241–6.

Eichhorn JG, Long FR, Jourdan C, *et al.* (2008) Usefulness of multidetector CT imaging to assess vascular stents in children with cogential heart disease: an in vivo and in vitro study. *Catheter Cardiovasc Interv* **72**(4), 544–51.

Hunter TB, Yoshino MT, Dzioba RB, *et al.* (2004) Medical devices of the head, neck and spine. *Radiographics* **24**, 257–85.

Musgrave DS (2002) Pediatric orthopedic trauma: principles in management. *Crit Care Med* **30**(11), S431–43.

Quasney MW, Goodman DM, Billow M *et al.* (2001) Routine chest radiographs in pediatric intensive care units. *Pediatrics* **107**(2), 241–8.

Strauss KJ, Kaste SC (2006) The ALARA concept in pediatric interventional and fluoroscopic imaging: striving to keep radiation doses as low as possible during fluoroscopy of pediatric patients—a white paper executive summary. *AJR Am J Roentgenol* **187**, 818–19.

Strive JL (2006) Pediatric cardiac imaging: the beat goes on! *Pediatr Radiol.* **36**(7), 578–80.

White E, Lu D, Eyer B *et al.* (2010) Gallery of uncommon orthopedic implants: a guide for emergency radiologist. *Emerg Radiol* **17**(3), 227–47.

Information on MR safety of medical devices: www.mrisafety.com

Chapter 13

Radiation protection in children undergoing medical imaging

Donald P. Frush

Introduction

The discovery of the X-ray was one of the most significant advances in medicine. Use of X-ray modalities in medical care, including radiography, fluoroscopy and angiography, and computed tomography, account for the vast majority of diagnostic imaging procedures performed in adults and children. Despite the benefits, the principle concerns for medical imaging that uses X-rays are the real and potential biological consequences. The fundamental issues with the ALARA (as low as reasonably achievable) principle as it relates to the cost (or risk) benefit ratio have been discussed in depth previously. Suffice it to say that even while the benefits of medical imaging are often not well defined or understood, the decision to perform medical imaging must weigh heavily in favor of the benefit side of this equation. While the radiation risk cannot be eliminated, it can be reduced by familiarity with, and ultimately adaption of, strategies to reduce radiation exposure in children.

There are some fundamental considerations when addressing the topic of radiation protection. First there is the underlying assumption that there is no safe level of radiation. This is the ALARA (as low as reasonably achievable) principle. The ALARA principle is a consequence of the linear no-threshold model, where what we know occurs (e.g., a significantly increased *risk* of developing cancer) at higher levels of radiation exposure is extrapolated to lower levels of radiation. The next point is that the following material will address the stochastic (versus deterministic) risks of radiation. Stochastic effects, predominantly cancer, are those where the risk is higher with higher radiation doses; the effect (i.e., cancer) is not worse. This is in distinction to deterministic effects, where there is a threshold well above ranges of radiation doses in diagnostic imaging, and the severity of the effect itself increases as the radiation dose increases. Deterministic effects include epilation and dermal burns. Virtually all radiation doses for diagnostic imaging fall below the threshold for deterministic effects. Higher dose procedures are seen in the setting of complex interventional procedures, particularly

when image-guided therapy is warranted. In addition, discussion will focus on those strategies which are, in general, under the direct control of the radiologist. While technical developments and technology assessment will continue to provide new opportunities for dose reduction and radiation protection, these are a result of often protracted cooperation between the scientific/medical community and industry, and do not have an immediate and direct benefit to the child. Furthermore, material provided here is meant to serve as a guideline only. The application of various strategies for radiation protection will depend on factors such as expertise, available resources and standards of practice. Finally, and perhaps most importantly, this discussion of radiation protection will be based on the concept of adequate image quality rather than optimal image quality. That is, the objective should be a radiation dose resulting in image quality that is sufficient to establish a diagnosis.

The practice of radiation safety, whether in children or adults, assumes a responsibility of all stakeholders. This includes, but is not limited to, radiologists, medical and health physicists, radiological technologists, radiation safety officers, and administration. It is a shared responsibility. On a more global basis, industry, regulatory agencies and health care organizations also have a duty to foster technical development and innovation, as well as education, for radiation protection. Moreover, radiation protection is the responsibility of *anyone* who performs medical imaging. It must be recognized that specialists who are not radiologists may perform this imaging, and they have the same responsibility for the safety and welfare of children as do those in the radiology specialty.

The two major goals of radiation protection are to ensure that the appropriate imaging modality or imaging strategy is indicated and, when indicated, that the imaging technique is appropriate: the *right test* done in the *right way*. It is not the intent of the material in this chapter to discuss the appropriateness of imaging. Suffice it to say that while the subject of inappropriate use of imaging has been raised in the United States, this has also been highlighted as a global issue that needs to be addressed. In addition, there is some contention with the process of guideline

Essentials of Pediatric Radiology, ed. Heike E. Daldrup-Link and Charles A. Gooding. Published by Cambridge University Press.
© Cambridge University Press 2010.

establishment. To this end, guidelines for appropriate imaging are available through the American College of Radiology (ACR) Appropriateness Criteria^{TM}, as well as Practice Guidelines and Standards (www.acr.org). Examples of additional guidelines are available through the National Guideline Clearing House (www.guideline.gov). In addition, the increased penetration of electronic order entry systems provides an opportunity for imaging strategies at the order level. Guidance at order entry is an important step in imaging management since, often, once an examination has been ordered, it is simply performed without further consideration as to whether it is appropriate or not.

With this background in mind, the following material will first briefly introduce the potential bioeffects of radiation, and subsequently provide a pragmatic approach to techniques that can be employed to control radiation dose in radiography, fluoroscopy and angiography, and computed tomography in children.

Biological effects of radiation

X-rays are composed of photons which are high-energy particles. As photons pass through tissue, energy is transferred which causes ionizations at the nuclear level that can disrupt DNA. While high levels of radiation will result in cellular death, lower levels can affect DNA itself as well as regulatory mechanisms, leading to uncontrolled growth such as cancer. When there is a break in DNA, this can be single or double stranded. With single-stranded disruption, the break is often repaired; however some double-stranded breaks cannot be properly repaired, which may lead to either cell death, or they may be improperly repaired, which can lead to altered replication. The development of cancer, however, is likely a multistep process, of which direct effect on DNA is just one step.

Unique issues in children include that their tissues are more vulnerable to radiation; this is not due to inherently increased *sensitivity* of the cells as far as is known, but is likely due in part to cellular division and tissue growth. While this increased vulnerability (despite the prior distinction, this is often referred to as sensitivity) has been stated to be as high as 10-times, this is probably more in the order of 2- to 4-times that of adult tissue. Since the induction of solid cancer may take decades – and recent data suggest that this risk may be lifelong – radiation exposure is therefore more of a concern in children given their longer potential lifetime. Finally, it is important to consider that similar exposure levels between adults and children can result in a higher dose given the smaller cross-sectional area in children. For example, the same CT protocol in a 90 kg adult will provide a higher organ, and thus effective dose (as a population estimate), to a 9 kg child, even though the amount of radiation from the tube is identical.

The risk of induction of a fatal cancer by low-level radiation exposure is not certain, is based on estimations of what is understood at higher levels of exposure, and is small if there is a risk at all. Low-level radiation exposure is generally under about 100 mSv (mSv is the SI derived unit of dose equivalent,

i.e., the absorbed dose, in grays, multiplied by a *dimensionless* "quality factor" Q, dependent upon radiation type, and by another dimensionless factor N, dependent on all other pertinent factors, such as body part irradiated, the time and volume over which the dose was spread, and the species of the subject). Above this level of radiation, there are scientific data demonstrating a significantly increased risk of cancer. Risks below this level are more debatable, although recent reports support the premise that doses to the level of about 50 mSv have a significant risk of cancer induction. Not only does the estimation of risk for diagnostic imaging using ionizing radiation depend on the model used, such as the linear no-threshold model, but also on the age of the individual, size (including amount of excess fat), gender, tumor type, duration of exposure (e.g., acute vs. protracted), the region of exposure, individual susceptibility (e.g., genetic or syndromic considerations) and the dose. One example is that a pelvic CT with an effective dose of 10 mSv has very little, if any, risk of inducing breast cancer as compared with a 10 mSv exposure from a chest CT. Therefore, extreme caution should be taken when considering global discussions of risks for an individual examination such as CT, or radiography, given the uncertainties of estimations. Rather, it is better to address the risks in general terms as small, at most, and (presumably) much smaller than the potential benefit of the diagnostic imaging study. The epidemiology of cancer risks with diagnostic imaging in children was recently comprehensively discussed.

A rule of thumb is that there is a 5% increase in the risk of developing a fatal cancer for every Sv of exposure. This means that for an acute exposure resulting in an effective dose of 100 mSv, the risk would be 0.5% (5 in 1000 – or 1 in 200); for a 10 mSv exposure, this would be 0.05% (5 in 10 000 – or 1 in 2000).

This estimation is actually going to be higher in children, estimated to be 15%, especially in females, although the 5% estimate is often employed across all ages and genders.

Doses from diagnostic imaging modalities that deliver ionizing radiation will vary, depending on the technique used (i.e., multiple projections versus single projection), region of the body (i.e., wrist versus lumbar spine), and modality (i.e., radiography versus computed tomography). A comparison of some radiation doses is provided in Table 13.1. Since the unit of sieverts is not well understood by clinical colleagues, and is very unlikely to be recognized by patients, the discussion of dose equivalence based on the number of chest X-rays is often helpful in providing relative radiation amounts during discussions.

One final comment regarding radiation exposure is warranted. The individual dose for pediatric CT exam, obviously, can be quite high, ranging from <2 mSv to more than 25 mSv. Because CT is used frequently and the use has been increasing both in adults and children, this provides a relatively high collective dose to the US population. Recently, in Report 160 by the National Council of Radiation Protection and Measurement (NCRP), it is stated that the radiation exposure to the United States population has increased 5.7 times from the early

1980s to 2006. Medical imaging now accounts for nearly half of the exposure to the population, with the remainder coming from background radiation, where previously about 80–85% of radiation exposure to the population was from background sources. Background radiation is about 3–3.5 mSv per year, and medical imaging now accounts for about 3.0 mSv (Figure 13.1), as well.

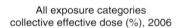

Table 13.1 Typical medical radiation doses: five-year-old (mSv)

	Radiation dose (mSv)	CXR equivalents
Three-view ankle	0.0015	1/14th
Two-view chest	0.02	1
99mTc radionuclide gastric emptying	0.06	3
99mTc radionuclide cystogram	0.18	9
99mTc radionuclide bone scan	6.2	310
FDG PET-CT	10–15	750
Fluoroscopic cystogram	<0.33	16
Chest CT	up to 3	150
Abdomen CT	up to 5	250

Notes: Borrowed with permission from the American Academy of Pediatrics. Modified from Brody *et al.* (2007).

There is a growing recognition of the importance of dose estimation and recording in diagnostic imaging. Currently, in the United States, there is no national regulation of patient dose for diagnostic imaging. Regional strategies for tracking the number of CT scans a patient has had and notification (which includes education) of referring care providers once a threshold for CT scans is met or exceeded has met with some success.

Strategies for radioprotection in children

Technical considerations

The same general technical considerations of adequate patient preparation are critical for all modalities. First, the patient should be appropriately immobilized (including judicious use of sedation), if necessary. This will improve diagnostic quality and decrease additional exposures with concomitant unnecessary additional radiation dose (Figure 13.2). In addition, for all modalities, but especially with fluoroscopy and computed tomography, understanding the clinical indications will help to configure the examination, conceivably reducing the radiation dose. Communication of any technical modifications in CT that deviate from protocol is the responsibility of the supervising radiologist. This responsibility of communication is also important in fluoroscopy. For example, during fluoroscopy, dialogue will minimize administration of contrast when fluoroscopy is not activated (potentially missing important information) or will minimize the activation of fluoroscopy before the technologist knows that the contrast should be administered. Simply stated, there must be ongoing dialogue between the radiologist

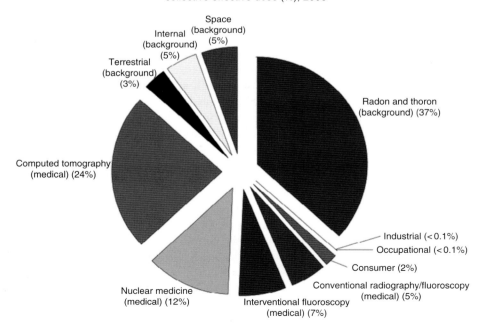

Figure 13.1 Contributions to radiation exposure to the United States population in 2006, including exposure from diagnostic imaging modalities (Mettler *et al.*, 2008). With permission from the NCRP.

All exposure categories collective effective dose (%), 2006

Space (background) (5%)
Internal (background) (5%)
Terrestrial (background) (3%)
Radon and thoron (background) (37%)
Computed tomography (medical) (24%)
Industrial (<0.1%)
Occupational (<0.1%)
Consumer (2%)
Conventional radiography/fluoroscopy (medical) (5%)
Interventional fluoroscopy (medical) (7%)
Nuclear medicine (medical) (12%)

(A)

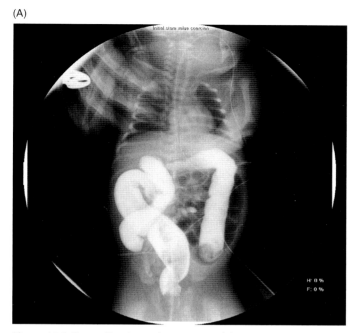

(B)

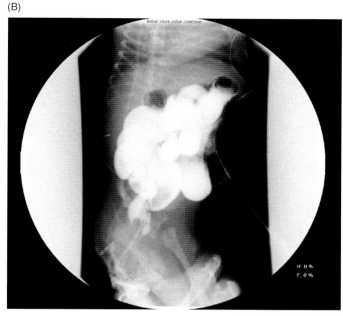

Figure 13.2 Poor collimation and patient immobilization during fluoroscopic evaluation for a neonate with failure to pass meconium. In both ap (A) and oblique (B) projections, there is poor collimation including regions outside those of interest, including a participant's hands. Hands that hold the infant should not be in the radiation field.

performing the fluoroscopic procedure and the technologist or other assistant, so that the examination is coordinated.

With all the equipment, whether it is radiography, fluoroscopy and angiography, or CT, it is important to have individuals who are familiar with that particular piece of equipment. Incorrect pediatric parameters for radiography, unfamiliarity with controls (and other methods for radioprotection) during fluoroscopy, and uncertainty over appropriate settings for CT can all result in unnecessary radiation exposure. Ignorance, despite the ever increasing technical complexity of much of diagnostic imaging, is not an acceptable excuse. Finally, with all modalities, quality assessment by qualified personnel, including technologists and medical and health physicists, is critical to assure proper equipment functioning.

Radiation protection in radiography

Radiography is still the most commonly performed imaging procedure in children. While there is still some older screen film radiography performed, the technology is evolving toward computed radiography (CR) and digital radiography (DR) exclusively, and discussion of digital technologies will be emphasized.

There are multiple strategies for radiation protection which can be used for radiography in infants and children, including establishment of optimal technique, minimization of unnecessary additional exposures, and appropriate collimation. Technical exposure factors can vary substantially in adults and children. The range of exposure factors for diagnostic examinations and interventional procedures has been reported to vary up to 88 fold. This type of variation potentially could be modulated using *diagnostic reference levels*, although these have not been established nationally in the United States. Pediatric protocols for CR and DR have greater demands on the range of techniques than with adult imaging, given the wide ranges of sizes in children (e.g. weights of 1.0 kg to more than 100 kg). Pediatric protocols are best established with the initial assistance of the application specialist with the particular vendor. It is important to review image quality shortly after the installation of new equipment to assure that image quality and dose estimates are within acceptable standards (Figure 13.3). This type of quality review is important with any imaging modality. With radiography, for example, it is possible to manually collimate the image to look as if the exposure was limited to the appropriate region. This was not possible with screen film radiography, where the exposure served as quality control. This type of exposure outside the field is important to monitor, but is not readily evident on daily clinical viewing of digital radiographic images.

There is a small amount of scatter radiation that occurs from radiography. The importance of the scatter is nominal and will not be reduced by shielding. With appropriate collimation, shielding is not a requisite for radiography. However, as with fluoroscopy and angiography and computed tomography, placement of shields beyond the level of exposure assures the child and the family that all measures are taken for radioprotection. However, the routine use of shields will have to be based on individual practice standards. Placing shields on areas of increased radiation vulnerability/sensitivity, such as the gonads for pelvic radiography, will depend on the clinical indication. For females, the benefit of gonadal

(A) 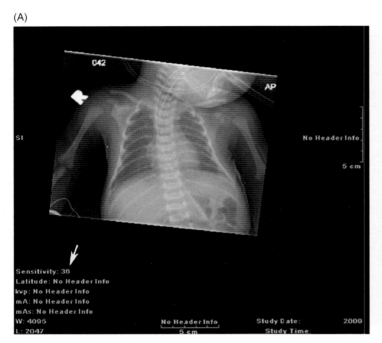 (B)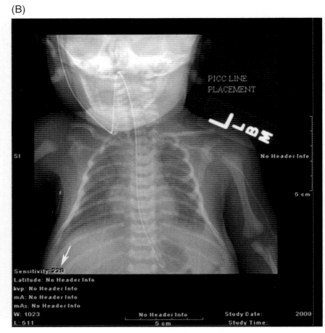

Figure 13.3 Installation of a new digital radiography system. (A) Initial neonatal chest radiograph had an exposure index ("S" value 39) (arrow) which was very low, indicating a relatively high exposure. (B) Following review of manufacturer-supplied protocols, adjustments were made to the existing exposure factors, which were able to be reduced, resulting in a more appropriate index ("S" value 220) (arrow). The left arm was included since assessment was for PICC placement. Note very similar image quality as in (A), despite lower dose.

(A)　　　　(B)　　　　(C)

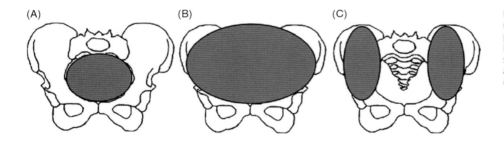

Figure 13.4 Conventional (A), theoretical/optimal (B), and investigator-recommended (C) options for placement of gonad shielding of ovaries. The left image provides the highest likelihood of ovarian shielding while minimizing obscuration of pelvic anatomy. Borrowed with permission from Springer (Bardo *et al.*, 2009).

shielding during radiography is not predictable given the variable location of the ovaries (Figure 13.4).

Digital radiography was heralded as technology that would reduce the overall radiation dose to children. This is in large part due to the wider range of latitudes of the detector with more tolerance of under- and over-exposure. In addition, digital technology nearly eliminates the previous substantial problem of film loss and possible repeat examinations. However, it has not been universally recognized that digital technology has reduced the dose. This is partly due to the fact that relatively high exposures (i.e., blackening due to over-exposures) do not result in poor image quality as they did with film screen technology (Figure 13.3). In addition, annotation such as mAs and kVp for CR and DR is not consistently presented on digital image display (Figure 13.5) (nor is it known by the vast majority of radiologists what exposure factors are reasonable for neonates vs. older children) and cannot be assessed during routine clinical examination interpretation. For CR, exposure factors used by the technologist have to be entered if they are to be archived. With DR, this can occur automatically. In addition, descriptors of exposure indices, such as the "S" value, on CR and DR displays are not understood by radiologists, nor do they always represent the same magnitude between vendors. These "S" values are, under increasing regulation, now more closely tied to the direction of change (e.g., lower values mean higher exposure factors) although this is not the case with all vendors. Documentation of dose on the images is becoming increasingly important as efforts are underway for tracking patients' cumulative dose record. For example, for radiography or fluoroscopy, the dose area product (DAP) could be placed on the image in consistent units. For fluoroscopy this could be $\mu Gy \cdot m^2$. However, this is not a convention. As radiology experts, it is important to continue to advocate for this standardization of annotation for the benefit of patient

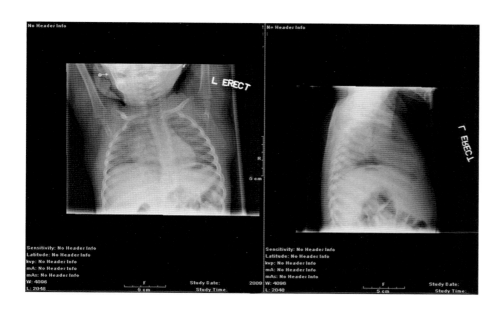

Figure 13.5 Annotation on frontal and lateral computed radiographic images in an infant does not include tube current or kilovoltage. In addition, the requisition history for this study was "well child check," without other clear indication, and the examination had low lung volumes, limiting the diagnostic potential.

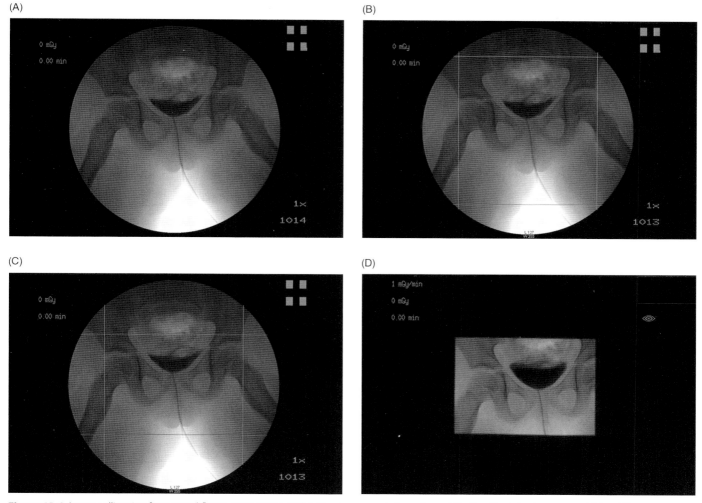

Figure 13.6 Image collimation from stored fluoroscopic image. Collimation is progressively performed (A–D) without having to use additional fluoroscopy.

dose index (or estimate) recording and dose tracking, as well as the ability to more easily perform quality assessment.

Radiation management for fluoroscopy and angiography

While the equipment and use varies between these two modalities, they will, for the purposes of this discussion, be considered together. Just as with other modalities using ionizing radiation, considerations should first be given to other modalities which may provide the same or similar diagnostic information. For example, diaphragm fluoroscopy may be performed by sonography, especially in infants and young children. Sonographic surveillance during intussusception reduction techniques has also been promoted. For interventional procedures, ultrasound-guided imaging offers the advantage of real-time localizations without the need to worry about cumulative radiation dose. In addition, sonography equipment is portable and this image guidance is less costly in terms of resources than either CT fluoroscopy or conventional angiography. MR enterography can be performed instead of the traditional fluoroscopy and radiography in the

Pediatrics

Examination report

Figure 13.7 An example during a hypothetical examination showing archiving of dose–area product and fluoroscopic time, yielding an overall dose record.

Patient name:	Pattern^Patty
Date of birth:	Dec 10, 2001
Gender:	Female

Patient ID:	FRNA46YF.1
Accession number: Request Identification:	A12345

Examination1 :	Date/time:	Feb 26, 2009 1:40:08 PM

Exam description:	Voiding cystogram Voiding cystogram
Exam ID:	E-FRNA6VV5.1
Performing physician: Requesting physician:	Dr. Frush
Total fluoroscopy time:	0:27 mm:ss
DAP (fluoroscopy):	15.08 μGy m^2
DAP (exposure):	37.50 μGy m^2
Total dose–area product:	52.58 μGy m^2
Skin dose:	3 mGy
Glandular dose:	mGy
Number of exposure runs:	6
Total number of exposures:	9

Run	APR	Time hh:mm	kV	mAs	ms	II-format	No. of images
1	Bladder ap, digital	1:40:54 PM	79	3.9	49.8	12"	1
2	Bladder ap, digital 2fps	1:40:59 PM	78	3.8	48.1	12"	4
3	Bladder ap, digital	1:41:02 PM	79	4.0	49.9	12"	1
4	Bladder ap, digital	1:41:33 PM	79	6.3	49.9	8"	1
5	Bladder ap, digital	1:41:36 PM	79	4.9	49.7	10"	1
6	Abdomen ap, TB	1:42:08 PM	63	3.2	8.8		1

Patient name: Pattern^Patty
Patient ID: FRNA46YF.1   Accession number: A12345

Figure 13.7 (Cont.)

Examination2:	Date/time:	Feb 26, 2009 1:43:03 PM

Exam description:	Ureter
	Ureter
Exam ID:	E-FRNHJOBZ.1
Performing physician:	
Requesting physician:	
Total fluoroscopy time:	0:00 mm:ss
DAP (fluoroscopy):	0.00 µGy m^2
DAP (exposure):	6.15 µGy m^2
Total dose–area product:	6.15 µGy m^2
Skin dose:	0 mGy
Glandular dose:	mGy
Number of exposure runs:	2
Total number of exposures:	2

Run	APR	Time hh:mm	kV	mAs	ms	II-format	No. of images
1	Ureter,, TB	1:43:21 PM	69	5.0	12.8		1
2	Ureter,, TB	1:43:23 PM	69	5.0	12.8		1

evaluation of inflammatory bowel disease. The doses of a combined fluoroscopic and radiographic procedure in the setting of inflammatory bowel disease can approach that of CT examinations.

Fluoroscopic and angiographic radiation protection centers most on reducing fluoroscopic time and maximizing distance. Reducing fluoroscopic time is the easiest and the single most effective way to reduce radiation exposure. For trainees, this strategy is easily taught but does require supervision to be effective. Alarms may be set to remind the performer of cumulative fluoroscopy time. These may be set based on individual preferences, but an alarm occurring somewhere between each one to three minutes of fluoroscopy time should be considered. Additionally, if possible, especially for prolonged fluoroscopy or angiography, changing the patient position (or imaging equipment position) will spread the dose between superficial areas while still being able to look at the structure in question. Fluoroscopy should be activated only when obtaining either anatomical or functional information, or a combination of both. Collimation limited to the area of interest will reduce unnecessary radiation exposure (Figure 13.2). The use of active fluoroscopy during collimation and localization of the region of interest for the examination should be minimized. There is some equipment available where collimation can be performed based on the image hold mode on the screen, rendering collimation during active fluoroscopy unnecessary (Figure 13.6). Other dose reduction measures include using the smallest magnification factor. Magnifying the area in question can increase radiation dose several fold. Image quality will be improved by having the image intensifier as close to the patient as possible. This also reduces dose. For example, a 10 cm air gap can increase radiation dose by 38% versus no air gap. In addition, the X-ray *source* should be as far from the patient as tenable. The lowest photon flux should be employed. As a rule, in pediatric fluoroscopy, the lowest flux (noisiest image) should be the default setting, with adjustments based on individual patient needs, such as small anatomy or a large (thick) patient.

Technical advancements in fluoroscopy include pulsed fluoroscopy, with improvements in both dose and image quality, as well as assessment of radiation risks with these advancements. Additional technologies include image hold (to review images instead of performing real-time fluoroscopy), image (or fluoro) store or capture for archiving, and video recording. This latter technology will allow review of complicated cases without having to perform additional fluoroscopic evaluation. The recent advances in fluoroscopic radiation management were recently very well addressed by Hernanz-Schulman. As with both radiography and CT, capturing and archiving exposure data is important, although there is not a single set of standards for such. This could include fluoroscopic time, and dose–area product, both for the fluoroscopy and the CR or DR images obtained (Figure 13.7). These CR and DR images are an additional radiation cost compared with the fluoro capture

(A)

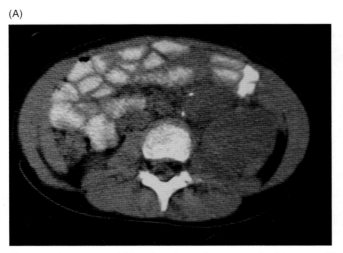

(B)

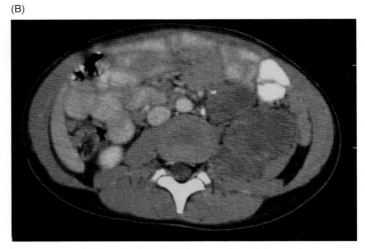

Figure 13.8 Four-year-old female with ganglioneuroma. Pre-IV-contrast (A) and post-contrast administration (B) axial CT images of the abdomen demonstrate a paraspinal mass with calcifications that are evident during both phases. No additional information was gained with the pre-contrast study. Borrowed with permission from Elsevier (Frush, 2005).

images, although the latter are typically noisier. For pulsed fluoroscopy, the lowest frame rate possible should also be employed for fluoroscopic evaluation. For example, 2 frames per second would substantially lower the dose over fluoroscopy using 15–30 frames per second. However, if more continuous functional information (such as video fluoroscopic swallows) is necessary, the slower frame rates may not provide brief but critical dynamic information, such as aspiration. With current grid-controlled pulse fluoroscopy, the image quality benefit obtained by having a grid in place during the entire pediatric examination may outweigh the small dose penalty, which was quite high with continuous fluoroscopic units in the past. These decisions about the routine or selective use of grids will have to be made following discussions with the application specialists from individual vendors, with review of dose data and image quality including that obtained from phantom evaluations.

Radiation management in computed tomography

Of all those modalities using ionizing radiation, CT provides the highest dose (Table 13.1). Adjustments for CT scanning in children include limiting coverage to the area in question, minimizing overlapping scans (which in adults can account for a decrease in the dose index of 17%), minimizing the use of multiphase examinations, and adjusting technical parameters (especially the tube current and kVp) based on scan indication, region scanned, and the size of a child. Considerations for protocols for CT examinations in body CT MDCT examinations for children can be found in several sources.

Technical factors including tube current (mA) and peak kilovoltage (kVp) can be reduced during scanning of several regions in children. For example, due to the high intrinsic contrast of the aerated lungs in chest CT, bones in skeletal

CT, and opacified vessels in CT angiography, both of these parameters can be lowered to reduce patient dose (Figure 13.8). In our practice, less than 5% of all body CT examinations should be multiphase examinations. Multiphase examinations tend to be more common and protocol-driven in adults. When a multiphase examination may be necessary in children, for example evaluation of both venous and arterial anatomy, or for assessment of enhancement characteristics of lesions such as those seen in a kidney, or extravasation of contrast such as from the renal collecting system in the setting of trauma, then individual parameters can be adjusted for the different phases (Figure 13.9). For example, for extravasation of contrast from the renal collecting system, delayed (10–15 minutes) images may be obtained at both lower kVp and lower mA given the intrinsic high attenuation of the contrast media. Adjustments can be made based on the clinical indication. Examples include follow-up bowel obstruction or abscess, particularly if a baseline CT has been performed. Examinations in these situations may and can have higher noise with the use of reduced tube current. In addition, assessment for renal calculi, given the densely attenuating stones, can be considered especially in follow-up cases.

The technical advancement of tube current modulation, a form of automatic exposure control, can reduce patient dose based on modifications of tube current for patient geometry (in the x, y axis) as well as organ attenuation and resultant image noise (in the longitudinal plane of the body – z axis). This technology has been reported to reduce dose estimates in children by 45%. The basis subserving this technology will differ between vendors and one must exercise judgment in applying these without a full understanding of the technical components. For example, without understanding how one vendor's tube current modulation works, it is conceivable that a higher dose could be delivered to a child than if a standard size-based fixed tube current is used. With any CT examination, including those using tube current modulation,

(A)

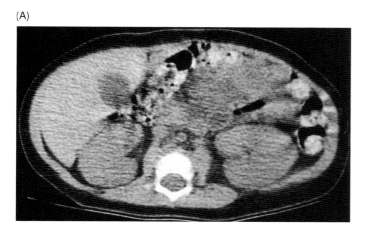

(B)

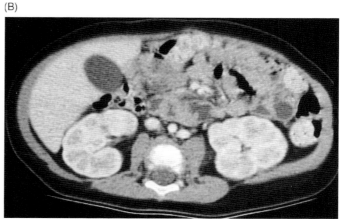

(C)

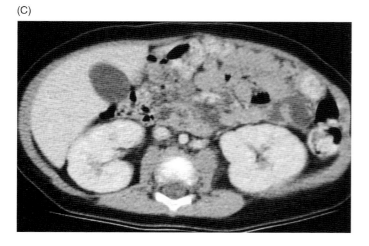

Figure 13.9 Infant with possible nephroblastomatosis that was not resolved by sonography. (A) Low dose (10 mAs) pre-contrast study to localize extent of kidneys, followed by (B) arterial (32 mAs) and (C) nephrographic phase (24 mAs with a larger pitch) was normal. The total dose of this three-phase exam was approximately 1.5-times that of a single phase examination appropriate for this age. The examination was normal. Borrowed with permission from Elsevier (Frush, 2005).

the child should be adequately centered in the scanner, as tube current modulation does not work as effectively with patients who are off-centered. One recent innovation is a more sophisticated modulation where the tube current is reduced when the X-ray source is over sensitive anterior organs (e.g., lens, breast) of the body. However, this technology has yet to be systematically assessed for dose reduction and image quality in children.

Shielding considerations for CT are the same as with fluoroscopy and angiography and digital radiography. That is, shielding will do nothing to minimize the internal scatter. As with these other modalities, the primary beam is very well collimated, as a rule. However, there is an additional consideration in computed tomography. Because of the need to have a consistent and sufficient photon flux for image reconstruction through the beginning and end of the scan region, the tube will need to rotate more than the expected scan coverage. This is called over ranging and can increase patient dose by upwards of 16%; this over-ranging dose can be greater in children. In addition, there is a "tail" of radiation that extends beyond the effective beam width. While there is technology that is currently reducing this over-ranging exposure by collimating the scan at the beginning and the end, this is not universally available. Over ranging is more of

a problem with higher effective beam widths (i.e. ≥ 64-slice scanners), where over ranging will be greater than with 4-slice or 16-slice scanners. In these settings, shielding sufficiently below the area of coverage so as not to encroach on the region of the diagnostic scan will reduce some of this over-ranging dose. One must be aware, however, of shielding close to the area of interest in CT, as shields may move, and repeat scanning defeats the purpose of the reduction in over-ranging dose.

In-plane shielding, where the shield, usually of a bismuth material, is in the field of scanning, has been shown to reduce surface dose. This is in the order of about 60% (four-ply shield) in adults and 30% (two-ply shield) in children. There is some debate about whether the benefits of shielding are greater than the benefits of simply reducing the tube current alone. However, data from pediatric breast shield studies does support the fact that breast dose is reduced substantially, and the benefits of attenuating the primary beam (approximately 30%) are far in excess of the small cost (6%) of local capture of scatter by the tissues under the shield.

There are additional needs for CT, as well as all ionizing radiation modalities, with respect to dose assessment. It is important to realize that dose assessment on imaging modalities does not represent individual patient dose but is an *index* or an *estimate* of that dose. Whether what is represented is an air dose, surface dose, skin dose, or, with CT, CT dose index or dose–length product, this does not necessarily equate to the dose for that child. However, this information can be helpful in terms of adjusting techniques for that individual patient, such as on the CT scanner with changes of CT dose index, or in review of protocols to assure that dose estimates and indices are within reasonable standards. With CT examinations, the CT dose index and dose–length product are not necessarily representative of the pediatric patient, being more appropriate for adult body and head imaging. Current efforts are underway for improving dose assessment, display, and archiving in CT examinations in children.

Conclusions

Diagnostic imaging is an extremely valuable component of healthcare. However, with those modalities that use ionizing radiation, there is potential radiation risk. Examinations which are obtained inappropriately, or performed using exposure factors which are excessive, increase the potential radiation risk, and may increase the cost of medical care as well. The specialty of radiology is dedicated to image quality and safety. Therefore, it is incumbent upon radiology personnel, especially radiologists and technologists, to be aware of those strategies which can be undertaken to use only as much radiation as is needed to perform diagnostic-quality imaging.

Further reading

Amis E, Butler P, Applegate K et al. (2007) American College of Radiology paper on radiation dose in medicine. *J Am Coll Radiol* **4**, 272–84.

Bader D, Datz H, Bartal G et al. (2007) Unintentional exposure of neonates to conventional radiography in the neonatal intensive care units. *J Perinatol* **27**, 579–85.

Bai YZ, Qu RB, Wang GD et al. (2006) Ultrasound-guided hydrostatic reduction of intussusceptions by saline enema: a review of 5218 cases in 17 years. *Am J Surg* **192**, 273–5.

Bardo D, Black M, Schenk K et al. (2009) Location of the ovaries in girls from newborn to 18 years of age: reconsidering ovarian shielding. *Pediatr Radiol* **39**, 253–9.

Birnbaum S (2008) Radiation safety in the era of helical CT: a patient-based protection program currently in place in two community hospitals in New Hampshire. *J Am Coll Radiol* **5**, 714–18.

Brenner DJ, Doll R, Goodhead DT et al. (2003) Cancer risk attributable to low doses of ionizing radiation: assessing what we really know. *Proc Natl Acad Sci USA* **100**, 13761–6.

Brody AS, Frush DP, Huda W et al. (2007) American Academy of Pediatrics Section on Radiology. Radiation risk to children from computed tomography. *Pediatrics* **120**(3), 677–82.

Cook JV, Kyriou JC, Pettet A et al. (2001) Key factors in the optimization of paediatric X-ray practice. *Br J Radiol* **74**, 1032–40.

Coursey C, Frush D, Yoshizumi T et al. (2008) Pediatric chest MDCT and tube current modulation: effect on radiation dose with breast shielding. *Am J Roentgenol* **190**, 54–61.

Dixon RL (2003) A new look at CT dose measurement: beyond CTDI. *Med Phys* **30**, 1272–80.

Dixon RG Special procedures (angiography): clinical practice. In *2006 Syllabus—Categorical Course in Diagnostic Radiology Physics: From Invisible to Visible—The Science and Practice of X-Ray Imaging and Radiation Dose Optimization*, ed. DP Frush, W Huda (Oak Brook, IL: Radiological Society of North America, 2006) pp. 203–9.

Fricke BL, Donnelly LF, Frush DP et al. (2003) In-plane bismuth breast shields for pediatric CT: effects on dose and imaging quality using experimental and clinical data. *AJR Am J Roentgenol* **180**, 407–11.

Frush DP Practical approach to manage radiation exposure. In *Pediatric Imaging*, 2nd edn., ed. H Carty, F Brunelle, D Stringer, S Kao (Berlin: Elsevier, 2005) pp. 33–44.

Frush DP Radiation dose and image quality for pediatric CT: clinical considerations. In *2006 Syllabus—Categorical Course in Diagnostic Radiology Physics: From Invisible to Visible—The Science and Practice of X-Ray Imaging and Radiation Dose Optimization*, ed. DP Frush, W Huda (Oak Brook, IL: Radiological Society of North America, 2006) pp. 167–82.

Frush DP MDCT in children: scan techniques and contrast issues. In *MDCT from Protocols to Practice*, ed. MK Kalra, S Saini, GD Rubin (Milan: Springer Verlag Italia, 2008) pp. 333–54.

Frush DP, Frush KS, Oldham KT et al. (2009) Imaging of acute appendicitis in children: EU versus US ... or US versus CT? A North American perspective. *Pediatr Radiol* **39**, 500–5.

Gaca AM, Jaffe TA, Frush DP et al. (2008) Radiation doses from small-bowel follow-through and abdomen/pelvis MDCT in pediatric Crohn disease. *Pediatr Radiol* **38**(3), 285–91.

Geleijns J, Salvadó Artells M, Veldkamp WJ et al. (2006) Quantitative assessment of selective in-plane shielding of tissues in computed tomography through evaluation of absorbed dose and image quality. *Eur Radio*, **16**, 2334–40.

Goske MJ, Applegate KE, Frush DP et al. (2008) The image gently campaign: working together to change practice. *Am J Roentgenol* **190**, 273–4.

Greess H, Lutze J, Nomayr A et al. (2004) Dose reduction in subsecond multislice spiral CT examination of children by online tube current modulation. *Eur Radiol* **14**, 995–9.

Hall EJ (2002) Lessons we have learned from our children: cancer risks from diagnostic radiology. *Pediatr Radiol* **32**, 700–6.

Hall EJ (2009) Radiation biology for pediatric radiologists. *Pediatr Radiol* **39**(Suppl. 1), S57–64.

Hernanz-Schulman M Fluoroscopy clinical practice: controlling dose and study quality—new challenges and opportunities. In *2006 Syllabus—Categorical Course in Diagnostic Radiology Physics: From Invisible to Visible—The Science and Practice of X-Ray Imaging and Radiation Dose Optimization*, ed. DP Frush, W Huda (Oak Brook, IL: Radiological Society of North America, 2006) pp. 133–9.

Hintenlang KM, Williams JL, Hintenlang DE (2002) A survey of radiation dose associated with pediatric plain-film chest X-ray examinations. *Pediatr Radiol* **32**, 771–7.

Hollingsworth CL, Yoshizumi TT, Frush DP *et al.* (2007) Pediatric cardiac-gated CT angiography: assessment of radiation dose. *AJR Am J Roentgenol* **189**(1), 12–18.

Hopper KD, King SH, Lobell ME, TenHave TR, Weaver JS (1997) The breast: in-plane X-ray protection during diagnostic thoracic CT—shielding with bismuth radioprotective garments. *Radiology* **205**, 853–8.

Kalra MK, Dang P, Singh S *et al.* (2007) Automatic patient centering for MDCT: effect on radiation dose. *AJR Am J Roentgenol* **188**(2), 547–52.

Kalra MK, Maher MM, Toth TL *et al.* (2004) Techniques and applications of automatic tube current modulation for CT. *Radiology* **233**, 649–57.

Karmazyn B, Frush D, Applegate K *et al.* (2009) CT with a computer-simulated dose reduction technique for detection of pediatric nephroureterolithiasis: comparison of standard and reduced radiation doses. *AJR Am J Roentgenol* **192**, 143–9.

Kim S, Yoshizumi TT, Frush DP, Anderson-Evans C, Toncheva G (2009) Dosimetric characterisation of bismuth shields in CT: measurements and Monte Carlo simulations. *Radiat Prot Dosimetry* **133**(2), 105–10.

Lee CI, Forman HP (2008) The hidden costs of CT bioeffects. *J Am Coll Radiol* **5**(2), 78–9.

Levin DC, Rao VM, Parker L *et al.* (2008) Ownership or leasing of CT scanners by nonradiologist physicians: a rapidly growing trend that raises concern about self-referral. *JACR* **5**, 1206–9.

Linet MS, Kim KP, Rajaraman P (2009) Children's exposure to diagnostic medical radiation and cancer risk: epidemiologic and dosimetric considerations. *Pediatr Radiol* **39**(Suppl. 1), S4–S26.

McCollough CH, Bruesewitz MR, Kofler JM (2006) CT dose reduction and dose management tools: overview of available options. *Radiographics* **26**, 503–12.

Medical News Today (Nov 26, 2008) Article: New CT scanner from Siemens Healthcare sets the bar higher. MediLexicon International Ltd. www.medicalnewstoday.com/articles/130930.php (last accessed Jan 22, 2010).

Mettler FA Jr, Thomadsen BR, Bhargavan M *et al.* (2008) Medical radiation exposure in the U.S. in 2006: preliminary results. *Health Phys* **95**, 502–7.

Miller DL, Blater S, Cole PE *et al.* (2003) Radiation doses in interventional radiology procedures: the RAD-IR study: part I: overall measures of dose. *Vasc Interv Radiol* **14**(6), 711–27.

Molen AJ, Geleijns J (2007) Overranging in multisection CT: quantification and relative contribution to dose – comparison of four 16-section CT scanners. *Radiology* **242**(1), 208–16.

Muhogora WE, AhmedNA, Almosabihi JS *et al.* (2008) Patient doses in radiographic examinations in 12 countries in Asia, Africa, and Eastern Europe: initial results from IAEA projects. *AJR Am J Roentgenol* **190**, 1453–61.

National Council on Radiation Protection and Measurements *Implementation of the Principle of As Low As Reasonably Achievable (ALARA) for Medical and Dental Personnel*, 2nd reprinting, report no. 107 (Bethesda, MD: NCRP, 1997).

National Council on Radiation Protection and Measurements (Jul 10, 2008) Press release: NCRP Executive Director, David A. Schauer, Participated in a WHO Global Initiative on "Radiation Safety in Health Care Settings." NCRP, 7910 Woodmont Avenue, Bethesda, MD. www.ncrponline.org/Press_Rel/WHO_June2008.pdf (last accessed Dec 14, 2009).

Paolantonio P, Ferrari R, Vecchietti F, Cucchiara S, Laghi A (2009) Current status of MR imaging in the evaluation of IBD in a pediatric population of patients. *Eur J Radiol* **69**(3), 418–24.

Paterson A, Frush DP (2007) Dose reduction in paediatric MDCT: general principles. *Clin Radiol* **62**(6), 507–17.

Paterson A, Frush DP, Donnelly LF (2001) Helical CT of the body: are settings adjusted for pediatric scanning? *AJR Am J Roentgenol* **176**(2), 297–301.

Preston DL, Cullings H, Suyama A *et al.* (2008) Solid cancer incidence in atomic bomb survivors exposed in utero or as young children. *J Natl Cancer Inst* **100**, 428–36.

Ptak T, Rhea JT, Novelline RA (2003) Radiation dose is reduced with a single-pass whole-body multi-detector

row CT trauma protocol compared with a conventional segmented method: initial experience. *Radiology* **229**(3), 902–5.

Riddell AM, Khalili K (2006) Assessment of acute abdominal pain: utility of a second cross-sectional imaging examination. *Radiology* **238**, 570–7.

Schauer DA, Linton OW (2009) National Council on Radiation Protection and Measurements report shows substantial medical exposure increase. *Radiology* **253**(2), 1–4.

Shaneyfelt T, Center R (2009) Reassessment of clinical practice guidelines. *JAMA* **301**, 868–9.

Silva E, Silva G (2007) Eliminating unenhanced CT when evaluating abdominal neoplasms in children. *AJR Am J Roentgenol* **189**, 1211–14.

Sistrom CL, Dang PA, Weilburg JB *et al.* (2009) Effect of computerized order entry with integrated decision support on the growth of outpatient procedure volumes: seven-year time series analysis. *Radiology* **251**(1), 147–55.

Slovis TL, Frush DP (2007) Biological effects of diagnostic radiation on children. In *Caffey's Pediatric Diagnostic Imaging*, ed. TL Slovis (Philadelphia: Mosby, 2007) pp. 3–12.

Strauss KJ, Goske MJ, Frush DP, Butler PF, Morrison G (2009) Image Gently Vendor Summit: working together for better estimates of pediatric radiation dose from CT scans. *AJR Am J Roentgenol* **192**(5), 1169–75.

Studdert DM, Mello MM, Sage WM *et al.* (2005) Defensive medicine among high-risk specialist physicians in a volatile malpractice environment. *JAMA* **293**, 2609–17.

Thierry-Chef I, Simon S, Miller D (2006) Radiation dose and cancer risk among pediatric patients undergoing interventional neuroradiology procedures. *Pediatr Radiol* **36**(2), 159–62.

Thomas KE, Wang B (2008) Age-specific effective doses for pediatric MSCT examinations at a large children's hospital using DLP conversion coefficients: a simple estimation method. *Pediatr Radiol* **38**, 645–56.

Wagner L (2006) Minimizing radiation injury and neoplastic effects during pediatric fluoroscopy: what should we know? *Pediatr Radiol* **36**(2), 141–5.

General references for pediatric radioprotection

Frush DP, Huda W (2006) *Categorical Course in Diagnostic Radiology Physics: From Invisible to Visible—The Science and Practice of X-Ray Imaging and Radiation Dose Optimization* (Oak Brook, IL: Radiological Society of North America, 2006) pp. 7–241.

Strauss KJ, Kaste SC (2006) The ALARA (as low as reasonably achievable) concept in pediatric interventional and fluoroscopic imaging. *Pediatr Radiol* **36**(Suppl. 2), S107–239.

United Nations Scientific Committee on the Effects of Atomic Radiation Annex D: medical radiation exposures. In *Volume I: Sources of UNSCEAR 2000 Report to the General Assembly, with Scientific Annexes* (Vienna: UNSCEAR, 2000).

Willis CE, Slovis TL (2004) The ALARA concept in pediatric CR and DR. *Pediatr Radiol* **34**(Suppl. 3), S159–247.

Index

multiple hereditary exostoses 215, 217, 305–6

musculoskeletal system
ischemia 223–5
nontraumatic emergency 133–6

Mycobacterium avium intracellulare (MAI) 176

myelination 5, 6

myelon 15–16

myofibromatosis, infantile 212, 213

myositis ossificans 216

N

nail patella syndrome 315, 316

nasogastric tube (NGT) 364

nasojejunal tube (NJT) 364, 365–7

neck 8

necrosis, ischemic 220

necrotizing enterocolitis (NEC) 31, 32–3, 117

neonates 19–39
abdomen 31–9
ischemic brain injury 232–7
respiratory distress 19–30

nephroblastoma (Wilms tumor) 203–5

nephroblastomatosis 205, 206, 399

nephrocalcinosis 282, 284

neurenteric cyst 28

neuroblastoma 201, 202, 203

neurofibroma 212, 213

neurofibromatosis 1 (NF1) 191–2, 212, 213, 249

neutropenic colitis/typhlitis 338, 339

Niemann-Pick disease 260

Nit-Occlud coil (NOC) 378, 379

non-Hodgkin's lymphoma (NHL) 196, 199
HIV-related 175, 177
staging 198

nonseminomatous germ cell tumor (NSGCT) 200, 210

non-accidental trauma 93–5, 237–9, 244

nonossifying fibroma 214, 215, 217

Noonan syndrome 315–16

normal child 1

O

oculoauriculovertebral dysplasia (Goldenhar syndrome) 312, 313

oligodendroglioma 189, 190

Ollier's disease 215, 306–7

optic pathway glioma 191–2

orogastric tube (OGT) 360, 364

orthopedic device 380–9

ossification 14–15

ossifying fibroma 215

osteitis fibrosa cystica 276

osteochondroma 214, 215
multiple 215, 217, 305–6

osteodysplasty 300–1

osteogenesis imperfecta 301, 302, 303

osteoid osteoma 215, 217

osteolysis syndrome 316, 317

osteoma 215

osteomalacia 256

osteomyelitis 167–9
acute 166, 167
chronic 167
chronic recurrent multifocal 169
sickle cell disease 221, 223, 224
tuberculous 168
vertebral 167, 168

osteonecrosis (avascular necrosis of bone) 221, 223, 224–5
Cushing-related 268, 271
Gaucher disease 286
idiopathic 134

osteopetrosis 302–4

osteosarcoma 214, 215, 217, 218

ovaries 12
cyst 126–8
germ cell tumor 209, 210
masses 209
shielding 393–4
torsion 126–8, 209, 230–1

over ranging 1, 399

oxalosis 273

oxaluria 273, 274

P

pain, congenital insensitivity to 310

pancreas 11, 13
annular 34
transplant 346, 347
trauma 84–5, 94

paraduodenal hernia 115

paralytic ileus 104, 347

paranasal sinuses 2–3

paranasal sinusitis 341

parapneumonic effusion 150–1

parathyroid adenoma 276, 278

parathyroid glands 13

parathyroid hyperplasia 276, 279, 281

partial anomalous pulmonary venous return (PAPVR) 50–2, 53

Patau syndrome 318

patent ductus arteriosus (PDA) 46–9
closure device 378, 379
stenting 380

pelvic cyst 128

pelvic fracture 86, 87

pelvis 15

pelviureteric junction obstruction *see* ureteropelvic junction obstruction

perfusion imaging 250–1, 252

pericardial cyst 201

perinatal asphyxia 20–1, 24

peripheral arterial line (PAL) 369

peripherally inserted central venous catheter (PICC) 367–9

peritonitis, meconium 38

peritonsillar abscess 146–7

periventricular leukomalacia (PVL) 233–4

periventricular white matter injury of premature infants 232–4

persistent pulmonary hypertension of newborn (PPHN) 20–1

pes planus 385, 386

pharyngitis 146–7

pheochromocytoma 202

physeal fracture 89, 90
see also Salter fracture

physical abuse *see* non-accidental trauma

pin fixation (K-wires) 381, 382

pineal region masses 193–5

pineoblastoma 194, 195

pineocytoma 195

pituitary adenoma 267, 270, 271, 272

pituitary gland 13

plate fixation 383

pleomorphic xanthoastrocytoma (PXA) 189, 190

pleural recesses 8

pleuropulmonary blastoma 28, 30

pneumatocele 151

pneumatosis coli 231, 231

pneumatosis intestinalis (PI)
bone marrow transplant recipients 338, 339
bowel ischemia 230
neonates 32, 33
older children 159–60

Pneumocystis carinii pneumonia (PCP) 172, 173, 174

pneumomediastinum 101, 102, 103
neonatal 20, 24–5, 26
traumatic 82

pneumonia 149–52
bacterial 149–50
complications 150–1
HIV infection 174–5
neonatal 20, 24, 25, 149
transplant recipients 345, 346
viral 149

pneumopericardium 102, 103
neonatal 24–5, 27

pneumoperitoneum
bowel ischemia 230
neonatal 24–5, 33–4

pneumothorax 101–3
neonatal 20, 24–5
skinfolds mimicking 25, 27
tension 101, 103
traumatic 81, 82

Poland syndrome 316–17

poliomyelitis, enteroviral 146

portal hypertension 115, 118

portal vein 12, 13
gas 32, 33, 230

posterior urethral valve (PUV) 129, 130

post-transplantation lymphoproliferative disorder (PTLD) 348, 349

Potter's syndrome (renal agenesis) 22, 27

premature infants
brain development 3–5
ischemic brain injury 232–4, 235
surfactant deficiency disease 19–20, 22, 23

primitive neuroectodermal tumor (PNET) 186–9